Nutraceuticals

THE COMPLETE ENCYLOPEDIA

of Supplements, Herbs, Vitamins and Healing Foods

Nutraceuticals

THE COMPLETE ENCYLOPEDIA

of Supplements, Herbs, Vitamins, and Healing Foods

◉ ◉ ◉

ARTHUR J. ROBERTS, M.D., MARY E. O'BRIEN, M.D.,
AND GENELL SUBAK-SHARPE, M.S., EDITORS

A Perigee Book

A Perigee Book
Published by The Berkley Publishing Group
A division of Penguin Putnam Inc.
375 Hudson Street
New York, New York 10014

First edition: January 2001

Published simultaneously in Canada.

The Penguin Putnam Inc. World Wide Web site address is
http://www.penguinputnam.com

Library of Congress Cataloging-in-Publication Data

Roberts, Arthur J. (Arthur James)
    Nutraceuticals : the complete encyclopedia of supplements, herbs,
vitamins, and healing foods / Arthur J. Roberts, Mary E. O'Brien, and
Genell Subak-Sharpe.
        p.   cm.
    Includes index.
    ISBN 0-399-52632-3
    1. Dietary supplements.   2. Functional foods.   I. O'Brien, Mary E.
II. Subak-Sharpe, Genell J.   III. Title.
RM258.5 .R63   2001
613.2—dc21   00-062435

Printed in the United States of America
10 9 8 7 6 5 4 3 2 1

Contents

PART 1:

Nutraceuticals in Perspective

A NEW LOOK AT AN ANCIENT ART   3

PART 2:

Directory of Nutraceutical Remedies

COMMON DISORDERS   21

PART 3:
The Top 200 Nutraceuticals

VITAMINS 205

MINERALS 239

NUTRACEUTICAL SUPPLEMENTS 263

BOTANICAL MEDICINES   354

PART 4:

Nutraceuticals in Practice

NUTRACEUTICALS JUST FOR WOMEN   567

NUTRACEUTICALS JUST FOR MEN AND ATHLETES   609

ANTIAGING NUTRACEUTICALS   621

APPENDIX A: Resources and Guidelines on Buying and Using Nutraceuticals   635

Listings from the American Nutraceutical Association of brand-name
products used in clinical trials; how to read the labels and definitions of
terms; general rules to follow; what to expect.

APPENDIX B: Selected Bibliography   649

Acknowledgments

The creation of any book invariably involves the cooperation and efforts of many people, and *Nutraceuticals: The Complete Encyclopedia of Supplements, Herbs, Vitamins, and Healing Foods* is no exception. While it is impossible to cite the dozens of organizations and people who have supported this undertaking, there are those whose efforts have been especially invaluable. From the outset, the American Nutraceutical Association (ANA) has not only lent its imprimatur to the book, but the ANA's founder and CEO, Allen Montgomery, R.Ph., has devoted untold hours to helping the editors sort through mountains of research data and often-conflicting information to shape the book's content.

Our team of skilled and knowledgeable medical writers included Leslie Anders, M.S., R.D., Diana Benzaia, Dianne Lange, Susan A. Schwartz, Sarah E. Subak-Sharpe, M.D., Elizabeth Ward, R.D., and Densie Webb, Ph.D., R.D. We are grateful to Diana Benzaia and Susan Schwartz for the many hours they have spent researching hundreds of different nutraceutical topics. We are also grateful to Charles Loeber for sharing his considerable knowledge about nutraceuticals, especially botanical medicines.

Lois B. Morris has been invaluable in helping edit the manuscript, and Jeremy Katz, our editor at Penguin Putnam, further sharpened the manuscript and made invaluable additions. Our copyeditor, Sheila Moody, has done a stellar job in whipping the final manuscript into shape.

We are especially appreciative of the support of our literary agent, Barbara Lowenstein, whose unflagging enthusiasm and efforts made the book possible. Finally, we thank our respective family members for pitching in on the home front to give us the time and space needed to produce this book.

—The Editors

Editorial Advisory Board

IMPORTANT NOTICE
Nutraceuticals provide numerous benefits and play an important role in promoting personal health and well-being. The suggested dosages in this book are based on clinical experience and scientific research, but it should be noted that individual needs vary, and what may be a safe and

appropriate dosage for one person is not necessarily what's best for another. As with conventional pharmaceutical products, a health care provider experienced in the use of nutraceuticals is your best source of information on how best to incorporate these products into your personal health regimen. In any event, this book should not be considered a substitute for medical care from your doctor or other health care professional. Talk to your doctor before trying the remedies suggested on the following pages, especially if you have a chronic medical problem or are taking prescription or over-the-counter pharmaceutical products. Although most nutraceuticals are generally safe, some contain ingredients that interact with medications or other nutraceuticals.

Pregnant and nursing women should be especially diligent in checking with a doctor before taking any nutritional supplement or botanical medicine. While many may be safe during pregnancy or breastfeeding, most have not been specifically studied for their effects on a developing fetus or infant. Thus, the same precautions used when taking pharmaceutical products also applies to nutraceuticals. Caution is also needed in giving nutraceuticals to young children. As with pharmaceutical products, always check with your pediatrician or other health care provider before giving nutraceuticals to a baby or young child.

Finally, although the editors have made every effort to ensure that the information in this book is accurate and up-to-date, it should be stressed that new research is constantly revealing new information about nutraceuticals. Thus, the information in this book should not be substituted for, or used to alter, medical therapy without your doctor's advice. For a specific health problem, consult your physician for guidance.

Foreword

The American Nutraceutical Association (ANA) was established in February 1997, with a straightforward mission: to develop and provide educational materials and programs on nutraceuticals for health care professionals and consumers, with an emphasis on scientific validity and technology. Since our modest beginning at a meeting hosted by the Office of Continuing Education at the Medical University of South Carolina's College of Pharmacy, the ANA now has several thousand members scattered throughout the United States and in eight other countries.

Since its founding, one of the ANA's most important goals has been to empower consumers to make informed choices about preventive health care programs and products, and to guide health care professionals on using and recommending nutraceutical products to their patients. Toward this end, the ANA sponsors continuing education programs for health care professionals and publication of our peer-reviewed journal, *JANA*, and *The Grapevine*, our quarterly newsmagazine for consumers. We also provide expert speakers on nutraceuticals for health care professional organizations and consumer groups. But one of our most extensive efforts is represented in this official ANA guide to nutraceuticals.

Working with members of our ANA Medical Advisory Council, the editors—Drs. Mary E. O'Brien and Arthur J. Roberts and Genell Subak-Sharpe—a team of health care professionals, medical writers, and editors have compiled information on more than two hundred nutraceutical products and more than fifty common medical conditions that often benefit from their responsible use.

Although this book was created specifically to meet the informational needs of consumers, I am confident that health care professionals will find this reference book both informative and useful in their preventive health care programs. As a trained health care professional myself, I know that it is important to base decisions on good science. The majority of Americans, including a growing number of health care professionals, now include nutraceutical products in their wellness and preventive medicine programs.

An ever-growing body of scientific research documents the substantial benefits that can be obtained from nutraceuticals. The suggested dosages are based on findings from clinical studies and recommendations of consulting physicians and other health care professionals who use nutraceuticals in their practices. Although the material in this book has been carefully researched and is based on sound scientific data, it should be stressed that the information should not be a substitute for or used to alter conventional medical therapy without your doctor's advice. I encourage you to use nutraceutical products wisely by selecting quality products that have been produced under good manufacturing practices, and to look for those products that are supported by clinical studies, for when they are combined with good nutrition, exercise, and other components of a healthful lifestyle, nutraceutical products can help us obtain a longer, healthier, and more productive life.

I want to thank the many ANA members and advisers who have contributed to the development of this important project. The ANA is committed to providing you with continued guidance on these products that is based on good science and not marketing hype. The authors and review panel for this book have attempted to include all available updated information in this first ANA reference book. It is unrealistic, however, to assume that all clinicians, researchers, and other experts will always agree with the complete content. This book's editors and members of the ANA Medical and Pharmacy Advisory Councils realize that new information on nutraceuticals is surfacing daily and that new interpretations are forthcoming based on new research projects. Therefore, we encourage companies and clinicians to keep us informed about their research projects so that we can keep the consumer and health care professional community updated about the benefits of nutraceuticals that may have been omitted from this first edition of *Nutraceuticals*.

Allen Montgomery, R.Ph.
Pharmacist
Founder, CEO, and executive director
American Nutraceutical Association

PART 1

Nutraceuticals in Perspective

CHAPTER 1

A New Look at an Ancient Art

All of a sudden, health care consumers and medical practitioners alike are focusing on nutraceuticals—broadly defined as components of foods or dietary supplements that have a medicinal or therapeutic effect. In general, nutraceuticals are taken in amounts higher than what can be obtained from an ordinary diet. In common usage, the term *nutraceuticals* is being applied not only to a growing array of nutritional supplements, vitamins, and minerals, but also to a broad range of herbal or botanical medicines. In the following chapters, we will address specific medical conditions and the nutraceuticals that can help prevent or treat them. But first, here's an overview of nutraceuticals from prehistoric times to the dawning of this new millennium, and a discussion of how they fit into today's high-tech, science-based medicine.

History in a Nutshell

From the beginning of human history, healers of every culture in every corner of the world have recognized that plants, in addition to providing essential food, also have the power to heal or to poison. Through centuries of observation, trial, and sometimes fatal error, each culture has evolved a tradition of herbal, or botanical medicine. The earliest medical texts of India, China, Persia, Egypt, and Greece all contain healing formulas based on various plants. Some, such as Chinese healers, added animal parts, insects, and other ingredients to their formulas. In recent decades, archeologists have gleaned considerable insight into the importance of these medications by studying the contents of ancient tombs of royalty in Egypt and China. And there's mounting evidence that ordinary people also relied on healing plants. For example, the five-thousand-year-old mummified "ice man" who was discovered a few years ago in the Alps was carrying a bag of herbal medicines.

A brief look at the development of Western medicine shows the critical role of plant-based healing, or phytomedicine (*phyto* is the Greek term for "plant"). Hippocrates, called the "father of Western medicine," lived from about 460 to 400 B.C. and was one of the first to recognize the link between diet and health. While historians cannot separate fact from legend about Hippocrates, the enduring legacy of the Hippocratic school is clear. Its teachings laid the groundwork for future scientific medicine by rejecting superstition and the notion that disease was a punishment of the gods and could be cured by divine intervention and magic. Instead, Hippocrates taught that diet and lifestyle formed the basis of health and healing, and to treat a patient, the physician must understand the nature of the malady and prescribe the appropriate cures. To do otherwise might cause more harm than good. To this day, new doctors take the Hippocratic oath, which includes the admonition: "Above all, do no harm." Today, a growing number are also heeding his advice to "honor the healing power of nature."

One of the first European texts of herbal medicine, *De Materia Medica (The Materials of Medicine)*, was written in the first century A.D. by Pedanios Dioscorides, a Greek physician who served in the Roman legions. His travels with Nero's armies allowed him to study and adopt medicinal plants and their uses from the far reaches of the Roman empire—from North Africa and the eastern Mediterranean to northern Europe. Modern pharmacologists who have analyzed Dioscorides' phytoformulas agree that many include ingredients useful for treating pain, infection, digestive problems, and a number of diseases.

In the second century, Galen, another Greek physician who studied and traveled widely through the ancient Roman empire, is remembered for his considerable knowledge of anatomy and medicines. He codified herbal medicine into more than a dozen texts, and even though many other aspects of Greco-Roman medicine fell out of favor during the Middle Ages, doctors used Galen's texts until the so-called Scientific Revolution of the seventeenth and eighteenth centuries, which ushered in the age of discovery, scientific experiments, and increasing knowledge of chemistry.

In the early nineteenth century, chemists learned to identify and isolate the active ingredients from plants, beginning with isolating and extracting morphine from opium. For the first time, doctors could administer exact dosages of a specific phytochemical, thereby reducing the risk of over- or underdoses that often occur when using crude botanical medicines. For example, in 1785, a British doctor named William

Withering published his famous monograph, "Account of the Fox-glove," in which he confirmed that an old folk remedy of drinking tea brewed from foxglove, or digitalis, leaves was useful in treating certain heart disorders and swelling (edema). But he also recognized that simply brewing a tea from foxglove leaves could be lethal if it contained too much digitalis, the active ingredient in foxglove. (Interestingly, digitalis is still used to treat certain heart conditions, and patients must still be very careful not to exceed the effective dosage.)

The Emergence of Pharmaceuticals

Until the early part of the twentieth century, doctors and pharmacists were trained in botany and relied heavily on botanical medicines. Often, pharmacists and doctors would make medications themselves from various plant compounds. This began to change in the early 1900s, when pharmaceutical companies started to synthesize drugs from chemical compounds. Over the next few decades, drug formulas were standardized, tested, and patented. Today, we have an incredible array of thousands of different medications, and new ones are added monthly. Still, about half of the medications in our standard pharmacopoeia of pharmaceutical products trace their origins to plants, even though most of the ingredients used to make them are now being synthesized in the laboratory.

Of course, the promise of a pill to cure every ill has its understandable allure. There is no doubt that modern pharmaceutical products save countless lives from once deadly infections and diseases, ease pain and other symptoms, and make it possible for all of us to lead longer, healthier lives. But there is also a downside to our growing reliance on medications. The effectiveness of many drugs—especially antibiotics—wanes with use. Indeed, there is mounting evidence that all of us face a growing risk of contracting antibiotic-resistant "superbugs" due to the overuse and misuse of antibiotics.

Every medication, even simple aspirin, carries a risk of serious side effects. As we grow older and develop more ailments, we end up taking more and more medications, which often interact with each other to produce even more adverse side effects. A 1998 study published in *JAMA*, the *Journal of the American Medical Association*, estimated that adverse drug reactions account for a minimum of 76,000 to perhaps more than 100,000 hospital deaths in the United States each year. Depending upon which figure is correct, this means that adverse drug reactions suffered in hospitals are either the sixth or fourth leading cause of death among Americans. Undoubtedly, a large number of deaths from adverse drug reactions also occur outside hospitals. And each year, millions of Americans suffer severe medication-caused complications, such as internal bleeding, irregular heartbeats, permanent organ damage, and life-threatening allergic reactions.

Then there's the cost factor. Americans spend more than $80 billion a year for prescription drugs alone, and the figure rises constantly with the introduction of each better and more costly new medication. So while pharmaceutical products will certainly continue to play a central role in American medicine, it is understandable that many people are also looking for alternatives for at least some health problems.

The Pendulum Swings Back

Our increasing use of nutraceutical products is in keeping with a growing recognition among both consumers and health care professionals that alternative, or complementary, therapies can have an important place in our science-based medicine. In fact, integrative medicine—a blending of mainstream and alternative therapies—is now being practiced in many settings nationwide. Only a few years ago, however, most American doctors trained in the scientific method dismissed alternative medicine as unproved remedies whose successes were due mostly to the placebo effect. Naysayers still exist, but their cries of "unproven" and "quackery" are being gradually drowned out by the reasoned responses of a new breed of doctor and the demands of restive consumers.

To determine whether a drug or other treatment works, it is tested against a placebo, a dummy pill or treatment. In general, placebos work as well as proven remedies about 20 to 30 percent of the time. Until recently, many nutraceuticals and other natural remedies had not been subjected to rigorous scientific tests against placebos or proven therapies. Instead, alternative practitioners and consumers relied mostly on tradition, observations, and personal experience. While these are all valuable tools, doctors trained in science-based medicine are understandably reluctant to adopt them when it's easier and faster to reach for their prescription pads. But this attitude is changing rapidly for a number of reasons. For starters, there is a growing body of solid scientific evidence to validate the effectiveness of many alternative therapies. Much of the research so far has been conducted in Germany and other countries, but American researchers are also doing studies and are beginning to report their results in medical journals. In short, doctors can no longer dismiss a growing number of complementary therapies due to a lack of scientific validation that they work.

Patients themselves are pressing their doctors for information and guidance about using nutraceuticals and other complementary therapies. Even without a doctor's recommendation, millions of Americans are turning to these therapies on their own. According to a 1998 report by a group of Harvard researchers, at least 42 percent of all Americans had tried some form of alternative medicine in the previous year. They paid some 629 million visits to alternative medicine practitioners, more than the total visits to all primary care physicians. The report added that the total out-of-pocket cost for alternative therapies paid by American consumers was "conservatively estimated at $27 billion in 1997." This exceeded the uncovered costs of all hospitalizations, and was comparable to the out-of-pocket expenditures for all physician services.

With so many people trying myriad remedies on their own, doctors have noted an interesting phenomenon. Here's how a Minneapolis internist put it: "Patients that I had been treating for years with various ailments without much improvement suddenly started getting better. When I asked if they had been doing anything different I kept hearing similar stories: 'Well, Doctor, I read an article about taking this natural medicine for my arthritis (or back pain, or headaches, or asthma, or whatever), and it seems to be working.' I started following up these stories, and sure enough, I, too, was finding evidence that many of the remedies worked." This particular doctor has now opened a center of integrative medicine, which combines the best of mainstream and alternative practices. And he's not alone. Across the United States, a growing number of doctors are taking courses in complementary therapies, especially botanical (herbal) medicine, acupuncture, and homeopathy, so that they can offer patients a broader range of services.

So as not to be left behind, many leading pharmaceutical companies are jumping on the nutraceutical bandwagon, coming out with their own lines of products. They are also hiring ethnobotanists—professionals who study the botanical medicines of different ethnic groups—to search the rain forests and remote corners of the world for new drugs. Clearly, all this emphasis on nutraceuticals is more than just another fad.

The Search for Scientific Validation

As noted by Daniel B. Mowrey, Ph.D., in his book, *The Scientific Validation of Herbal Medicine*, from the beginning of modern scientific research during the Renaissance and until the early twentieth century, medicinal plants were studied extensively in both the United States and Europe. But the scientific interest in medical botany ground to a halt among most American scientists with the development of synthetic medications. Suddenly a vast array of heretofore lethal diseases could either be prevented by vaccines or cured by synthetic drugs. Most of these drugs were aimed at a specific disease or target organ, unlike many nutraceuticals and botanical medicines that are taken as panaceas for a variety of disorders or an entire body system or process. For example, ginseng is regarded as a panacea for the entire body—it is used to boost immunity, counter stress and fatigue, treat everything from asthma to digestive disorders, and enhance sexual performance, among other functions. SAM-e, whose 1999 introduction to the U.S. nutraceutical market was greeted with tremendous media coverage and a consumer rush on suppliers, is promoted as a treatment for both arthritis and mild depression. Raspberry leaf is a popular woman's tonic, taken for everything from premenstrual syndrome and cramps to fertility and pregnancy problems.

While some synthetic medications have multiple functions—aspirin, for example, lowers a fever, relieves pain and inflammation, and helps prevent blood clots—the more common goal is to use a single effective ingredient with a specific therapeutic target. Obviously, it is easier to conduct scientific studies using a single active substance, or a very controlled combination, than it is to work with a complex plant made up of thousands of chemicals and perhaps a dozen or more active ingredients.

In the United States, the profit motive very often dictates the focus of scientific research, especially in the area of medications. It costs many millions of dollars to take a drug through all of its mandated testing before gaining government approval to market it. Increasingly, these costs are borne by private industry rather than government funding and, understandably, companies want to recoup their research investments. Pharmaceutical companies cite this as the major reason for today's soaring drug prices.

Nutraceuticals are derived from natural products that cannot be patented. This greatly reduces any financial incentive for a pharmaceutical company or another manufacturer to invest millions of research dollars to validate the effectiveness of a product over which it has no market control, a major reason why nutraceutical research has lagged behind pharmaceutical studies. But, as noted earlier, Americans are now spending billions of dollars each year on nutraceutical products, prompting a growing number of the big pharmaceutical companies to move into this expanding market, and some are even funding studies to demonstrate the efficacy of certain products, such as glucosamine, a nutraceutical widely used to treat osteoarthritis.

Still, the bulk of nutraceutical research is being carried out abroad, led by Germany. In general, European doctors have been more receptive to nutraceuticals and other alternative therapies than American physicians. In Germany alone, more than six hundred different botanic medicines are available, and about 70 percent of German doctors prescribe specific products, most of which are covered by the national health insurance. In 1976, the German government decreed that herbal remedies were subjected to the same regulations as synthetic drugs and regulated compounds, such as morphine, that are derived from plants. An expert panel, known as Commission E, was appointed to evaluate the safety and efficacy of hundreds of herbal medicines. The commission, made up of physicians, toxicologists, pharmacists, pharmacologists, pharmaceutical representatives, and laypersons, is charged with checking the data on botanical medicines and preparing a detailed monograph on each. So far, more than three hundred monographs have been published; about two-thirds of them favorable. The American Botanical Council has translated the monographs into English and, in 1998, published them as *The Complete German Commission E Monographs*. There is also a new *Physicians' Desk Reference (PDR) for Herbal Medicine*.

The Question of Quality

Of course, a much different system prevails in the United States, where nutraceuticals are marketed as foods or food supplements, rather than drugs, and thus they are not subject to the same controls. In 1994,

Congress passed the Dietary Supplement and Health Education Act (DSHEA), which gives the Food and Drug Administration (FDA) the power to:

1. Stop any company from selling a dietary supplement that is toxic or unsanitary.
2. Stop the sale of a dietary supplement that has false or unsubstantiated claims.
3. Take action against dietary supplements that pose "a significant unreasonable risk of illness or injury."
4. Stop any company making a claim that a product cures or treats a disease.
5. Stop a new dietary ingredient from being marketed if FDA does not receive enough safety data in advance.
6. Require a dietary supplement to meet strict manufacturing requirements (Good Manufacturing Practices), including potency, cleanliness, and stability.

In addition, the Federal Trade Commission (FTC) has the power to:

1. Enforce laws outlawing "unfair or deceptive acts or practices" to ensure consumers get accurate information about dietary supplements so they can make informed decisions about these products.
2. Challenge and stop advertising that is not adequately substantiated.
3. Investigate complaints or questionable trade practices.
4. Following its own investigation, negotiate a consent order or proceed through an FTC adjudication resulting in a cease-and-desist order, which can be quite broad in scope.

Even so, nutraceuticals are not covered by the same stringent requirements that the FDA and other government agencies impose on the marketing of many pharmaceutical products. Thus, consumers can buy what are essentially medications without a prescription. In Europe, for example, consumers need a doctor's prescription in order to buy many of the products that are sold as over-the-counter nutritional supplements in the United States. And, despite DSHEA regulations, quality control can be lax. Consumers often have no way of knowing whether a particular product contains what its label purports. There have been numerous instances in which independent laboratories have analyzed an assortment of nutraceuticals only to find that a large percentage contained little or none of the intended active ingredient(s). In fact, quality sometimes varies from one pill to another within the same bottle. This is not a concern in Germany and other countries where nutraceutical products are manufactured according to standardized formulas and under the same quality control regulations as pharmaceuticals.

The good news is that quality control is one area in which competition is fostering improvement. Manufacturers who practice good quality control and produce standardized products win out in the end because consumers quickly learn what works and what doesn't. Organizations such as the American Nutraceutical Association are also pressuring manufacturers to practice good quality control and produce standardized products that consumers can trust. Still, it's a good idea to buy from established outlets, such as a pharmacy or health food store, and to look for products made by known and trusted manufacturers. (Also see Appendix A, "Resources and Guidelines on Buying and Using Nutraceuticals.")

Cautions and Precautions

There is another potential downside in the ready availability of certain nutraceuticals; namely, that it encourages self-diagnosis and self-treatment, often with potentially harmful substances. Many people mistakenly believe that "if it's natural it's safe." Of course, this is not true. While nutraceuticals and botanic medicines generally have a lower risk of adverse reactions and side effects than synthetic pharmaceuticals, it would be foolish to assume you can take them with impunity. Some interact with each other and with pharmaceutical products, alcohol, and certain foods. They can cause allergic or other adverse reactions in susceptible people. Some can be highly toxic when taken in excessive amounts or by people with certain medical problems, such as liver or kidney disorders. Some are dangerous if consumed during pregnancy or while breast-feeding. (See "The Top 200 Nutraceuticals," for more specific information on individual products.) As with pharmaceutical medications, it's a good idea to consult a knowledgeable health care professional before taking any nutraceutical product.

The Role of Personal Responsibility

As we enter this new millennium, we are developing a more holistic view of health and disease—one that echoes the ancient teachings of Hippocrates and many of his followers through the centuries. We are finally beginning to realize that good health is an individual responsibility. Poor health and diseases are not the punishments of the gods, but often the consequence of our faulty diets and unhealthy lifestyle habits, as well as heredity and other factors beyond our control. Still, it's our lifestyle that frequently works to lower immune resistance and make us vulnerable to a whole range of diseases and symptoms—headaches, fatigue, heart attacks, diabetes, stroke, cancer, and autoimmune disorders, to name but a few.

As Hippocrates taught, in order to achieve and maintain health, we need to look at the whole organism, rather than focus on a single organ or disease. While it's essential to assume responsibility for our own health maintenance, it's also necessary to establish a working partnership with our doctors and other health care professionals.

None of this means, however, that we should even consider turning back the clock and dispensing with medical specialists in favor of using only natural supplements and botanicals instead of synthetic pharmaceuticals. Such counterproductive actions would be akin to throwing out the baby with the bathwater. What is needed is a commonsense blending of the best of both worlds; in other words, the very essence of integrative traditional and science-based medicine and enlightened self-care. The goal of this book is to provide solid information about one of the most important aspects of sound preventive medicine; namely, the rational use of nutraceuticals. Use this book to talk to your doctor to arrive at what is the best approach for you and your loved ones.

Quick Reference Charts

The following two charts provide a ready-reference to the material presented in the following pages of NUTRACEUTICALS.

The first chart, "Ailment Guide," is organized by condition and gives a quick run-down of all the nutraceuticals that are connected with that ailment. **However, this is not a statement of endorsement or an assertion of effectiveness. This chart lists all nutraceuticals organized by ailment whether they work or not.** For value judgements and recommendations, see Part 2, "Directory of Nutraceutical Remedies" and Part 3 "The Top 200 Nutraceuticals."

The second chart, "Nutraceutical Guide," is organized by nutraceutical and lists most every condition that the nutraceutical has been claimed to treat. **Again, this is not an endorsement or an assertion of effectiveness. It is just a rundown of common uses and claims.** For guidance on each nutraceutical see its entry in Part 3 "The Top 200 Nutraceuticals" or an ailment listing in Part 2 "Directory of Nutraceutical Remedies."

AILMENT GUIDE

Acne Arnica, Tea Tree, Vitamin A, Burdock, Chaste Berry

Allergies Antihistamines, Decongestants, Vitamin C, Essential Fatty Acids, Flavonoids, Nettle, Licorice, Bee Pollen, Vitamin B_{12}, Bromelain, Cat's Claw, DMSO/MSM, Ginkgo Biloba, Grape Seed Extract, Pycnogenol

Alzheimer's Disease and Memory Loss Vitamin E, Vitamin B_{12}, L-Carnitine, Phosphotidyscribe, Gingko Biloba, Ashwagandha, Choline, Coenzyme Q_{10}, DHEA, Glutamine, Gotu Kola, Guarana, Lecithin, Melatonin, Rosemary

Anemia Iron, Folic Acid, Vitamin B_{12}, Vitamin B_2, Vitamin B_5, Vitamin B_6, Dandelion, Copper, Chlorophyll, Bee Pollen

Anxiety Benzodiazephrines, Antidepressants, Kava, St. John's Wort, Valerian, Chamomile, Cramp Bark, Devil's Claw, Eucalyptus, Ginseng, Lavender, Poppy

Arthritis Vitamin C, Vitamin E, Folic Acid, Vitamin D, Calcium, Glucosamine Sulfate, Chrondroitin Sulfate, GLA, SAMe, Omega-3 Fatty Acids, Capsaicin, Boswellia, Ginger, Vitamin B_5, Zinc, Bromelain, Bilberry, Black Carrot, Black Cohosh, Black Haw, Boneset, Borage, Burdock, Camphor, Cat's Claw, Devil's Claw, DMSO/MSM, Evening Primrose Oil, Feverfew, Flax, Grape Seed Extract, Guarana, Gugsul, Horseradish, Kelp, Kombuchu Mushrooms, Licorice, Nettle, Pycnogenol, Shark Cartilage, Spiralina, White Willow

Bronchitis Zinc, Echinacea, Goldenseal, Licorice, Slippery Elm, Vitamin A, Vitamin C, Magnesium, Bromelain, Chamomile, Goldenseal, Horseradish, Licorice, Marshmallow, Mushroom Extract, Mustard, Pycnogenol, Thyme

Cancer Calcium, Folic Acid, Selenium, Vitamin C, Vitamin E, Vitamin A, Vitamin D, Copper, Carotenoids, Isoflavones, Prebiotics and Probiotics, Pycnogenol and grape seed extract, Tea, IP-6, Astragalus, Garlic, Milk Thistle, Brewer's Yeast, Acidophilus, Chlorophyll, Vitamin B_{12}, Burdock, Boneset, Cat's Claw, Essential Fatty Acids, Flavonoids, Glutamine, Marijuana, Melatonin, Phytoestrogens, Poppy, Psyllium, Shark Cartilage, Soy Products, Spirulina

Carpal Tunnel Syndrome Vitamin B_6, Vitamin B_2, Bromelain, DMSO/MSM

Cataracts Vitamin C, Vitamin E, Vitamin B_2, Lipoic Acid, Beta Carotene, Lutein and Zeaxanthin, Bilberry, Selenium, Grape Seed Extract, Melatonin

Cholesterol Disorders and Atherosclerosis Statins, Bile-acting-binding Resins, Fibric Acids, Vitamin B_3, Vitamin B_5, Vitamin B_6, Vitamin B_{12} (Vitamin B-complex), Folic Acid, Vitamin E, Red Rice Yeast, Plant Sterol Esthers, Omega-3 Fatty Acids, Psyllium, Green Tea, Pycnogenol and Grape Seed Extract, Soy Protein, Gugulipid, Garlic, Magnesium, Acidophilus, Beta Glucan, Brewer's Yeast, Barley, Benecol, Butcher's Broom, Calendula, Carnitine, Chondroitin Sulfate, Coenzyme Q_{10}, Devil's Claw, DHEA, Fenugreek, Flavonoids, Flax, Ginger, Ginkgo Biloba, Glucomannan, L-Arginine, Lecithin, Melatonin, Mushroom Extracts, Oak, Oat Bran, Phytoestrogens, Wild Yam

Chronic Fatigue Syndrome Vitamin B-Complex, Magnesium, Calcium, Carnitine, Coenzyme Q$_{10}$, Astragalus, Licorice, Siberian Ginseng, Zinc, Vitamin C, 5-HTP, Ashwagandha, Brewer's Yeast, Choline, DMSO/MSM, Echinacea, Nettle, Pycnogenol

Circulatory Problems Vitamin C, Vitamin B$_3$, L-Arginine, Pycnogenol and Grape Seed Extract, Ginkgo Biloba, Butcher's Broom, Horse Chestnut, Bilberry, Coenzyme Q$_{10}$, Flavonoids, Gotu Kola, Kelp, Rosemary

Common Cold and Flu Vitamin C, Zinc, Vitamin A, Echinacea, Goldenseal, Garlic, Astragalus, Boneset, Camphor, Catnip, Chamomile, Fennel, Ginger, Horehound, Hyssop, Kava, Licorice, Marshmallow, Mint, Red Clover, Rose, Seneca Root, Slippery Elm, Thyme, White Willow

Constipation Laxatives, Stool Softeners, Lubricants, Kelp, Psyllium, Flax, Cascara Sagrada, Aloe, Senna, Brewer's Yeast, Basil, Cardamom, Cleavers, Dandelion, Dong Quai, Fenugreek, Goldenseal, Kelp, Marshmallow, Oat Bran, Rose, Slippery Elm

Depression Vitamin B-Complex, Phenylalanine, SAMe St. John's wort, Gingko Biloba, Carnitine, 5-HTP, Essential Fatty Acids, Ginger, Glutamine, Kombuchu Mushrooms, Lemon Balm, Rosemary, Sage

Dermatitis/Eczema Omega-3 Fatty Acids, Quercetin, Grape Seed Extract, Evening Primrose, Gingko, Licorice, Brewer's Yeast, Bee Pollen, Bilberry, Black Cohosh, Black Currant, Bloodroot, Borage, Burdock, Cleavers, Echinacea, Flavonoids, Goldenseal, Lavender, Marshmallow, Nettle, Oak, Red Clover, Slippery Elm, Spirulina, Tea Tree

Diabetes Vitamin A, Vitamin B Complex, Vitamin E, Magnesium, Chromium, GLA, Vitamin, Biotin, Alfalfa, Barley, Brewer's Yeast, DHEA, Fenugreek, Glucomannan, Goldenseal, Kombucha Mushrooms, Lipoic Acid, Marshmallow, Mushroom Extracts, Oat Bran, Pycnogenol

Diarrhea Acidophilus, Green Tea, Bilberry, Red Raspberry, Agrimony, Barley, Black Cohosh, Black Currant, Blackberry, Boswellia, Catnip, Cinnamon, Corriander, Dandelion, Goldenseal, Mullein, Oak, Poppy, Sage

Diverticular Disease Diet (Fiber and Fluid), Antibiotics, Acidophilus, Psyllium, Aloe Vera, Slippery Elm, Flax, Goldenseal, Wild Yam

Gallstones Vitamin C, Lecithin, Turmeric, Dandelion, Milk Thistle, Wild Yam

Gout NSAIDs, Corticosteroids, Colchicine, Uric Acid Inhibitors, Vitamin C, Omega-3 Fatty Acids, MSM, Bromelain, Billberry, Burdock, Horseradish, White Willow

Heart Disease Lifestyle, Blood Pressure Medicine, Surgery, Vitamin C, Folic Acid, Vitamin E, Flavonoids, Soy Products, Omega-3 Fatty Acids, Coenzyme Q$_{10}$, Oatbran, Grape Seed Extract, Hawthorn, Gugulipid, Vitamin B-Complex, Calcium, Magnesium, Copper, Selenium, Carnitine, Astragalus, Choline, DHEA, Fish Oil, Flavonoids, Garlic, Ginko, Green Tea, Hawthorn, L-Arginine, Lecithin, Melatonin, Poppy, Pycnogenol, Spirulina

Heartburn Anti-Acids, Histamine 2 Antagonists, Proton Pump Inhibitors, Surgery, Calcium carbonate, Licorice, Aloe Vera, Chamomile, Barberry, Alfalfa, Fennel, Slippery Elm, Turmeric

High Blood Pressure Diuretics, Beta-Blockers, Alpha-1 Blockers, Alpha-1 Beta-Blockers, Calcium Channel Blockers, ACE Inhibitors, Angiotension II Receptor Blockers, Calcium, Potassium, Vitamin C, Vitamin E, Essential Fatty Acids, Garlic, Barley, Black Haw, Coenzyme Q$_{10}$, Cramp Bark, Dandelion, DHEA, Dong Quai, Fish Oil, Garlic, Goldenseal, Hawthorn, Kombucha Mushrooms, L-Arginine, Mushroom Extracts, Valerian

Hypoglycemia Diet, Chromium, Magnesium, Brewer's Yeast

Inflammatory Bowel Disease Folic Acid, Zinc, Acidophilus, Omega-3 and -6 fatty acids, Psyllium, Aloe Vera, Licorice, Agrimony, Glutamine

Insomnia Calcium and Magnesium, 5-HTP, Melatonin, Valerian, Kava, Lavender, Catnip, Chamomile, Cleavers, Coriander, Dill, Ginseng, Lemon Balm, Mint, Mullein, Poppy, St. John's wort

Irritable Bowel Syndrome Psyllium, Acidophilus, Peppermint, Bilberry, Valerian

Kidney Disorders Calcium, Cranberry, Goldenrod, Parsley, Vitamin B$_6$, Phosphorus, Alfalfa, Dill, Ginko, Kelp, Mushroom Extracts, Nettle

Leg Cramps and Restless Legs Calcium and Magnesium, Vitamin E, Grape Seed Extract, Ginkgo Biloba, Garlic, Hawthorn

Liver Diseases Lifestyle, Vitamin A, Vitamin D, Vitamin K, Vitamin B-Complex, Coenzyme Q$_{10}$, Digestive Enzymes, Milk Thistle, Licorice, Cascarda Sagrada, Choline, Dandelion, Dong Quai, Glutamine, Horseradish, Lecithin, Mushroom Extracts, SAMe, Turmeric

Lupus Vitamin B$_6$, Folic Acid, Vitamin E, Vitamin A, Beta-carotene, GLA, DHEA, Vitamin B$_5$, Borage, Fish Oil, Flax, Kombucha Mushrooms

Macular Degeneration Vitamin C, Vitamin E, Vitamin B-Complex, Zinc, Lutein and Zeaxanthin, Flavonoids, Bilberry, Beta-carotene, Grape Seed Extract

Migraine Headaches Vitamin B$_2$, Magnesium, Omega-3 Fatty Acids, Feverfew, Ginkgo Biloba, Ginger, 5-HTP, Fish Oil, Kava, Phenylalanine

Mouth Sores Vitamin B-Complex, Vitamin C, Zinc, Chamomile, Goldenseal, Licorice, Myrrh, Barberry, Barley, Bilberry, Blackberry, Marshmallow, Red raspberry, Rose, Sage

Nausea Vitamin B$_6$, Ginger, Cinnamon, Peppermint, Goldenseal, Anise, Cascera Sagrada, Coriander, Fennel, Marijuana, Red Raspberry

Osteoporosis Calcium, Vitamin D, Magnesium, Soy Isoflavones, Fluoride, Vitamin K, Zinc, Copper, Manganese, Kelp, Flavonoids, Phytoestrogens, Red Clover

Psoriasis Vitamin A, Vitamin D, Zinc, Omega-3 Fatty Acids, Licorice, Capsaicin, Chamomile, Barberry, Burdock, Cleavers, Fish Oil, Gotu Kola, Kelp, Lavender, Nettle, Pycnogenol, Red Clover

Tooth Decay and Gum Diseases Calcium, Vitamin D, Vitamin C, Fluoride, Flavonoids, Coenzyme Q$_{10}$, Tea, Chamomile, Sage, Bloodroot, Phosphorus, Magnesium, Molyselenium, Cinnamon, Cloves, Licorice, Myrrh, White Willow

Ulcers Vitamin C, Iron, Acidophilus, Ciceria, Aloe Vera, Barberry, Beta Glucan, Calendula, Cat's Claw, Dong Quai, Fennugreek, Goldenseal, Horehound, Licorice, Mullein, Slippery Elm

Urinary Tract Infections Antibiotics, Vitamin C, Cranberry, Uva Ursi, Acidophilus, Alfalfa, Bilberry, Echinacea, Goldenseal, Licorice, Marshmallow, Rose

Varicose Veins Horse Chestnut, Butcher's Broom, Gotu Kola, Broom, Grape Seed Extract, Pycnogenol

Weight Problems Chromium, Carnitine, Psyllium, 5-HTP, Glucomannan, Gugulipid, Ephedra, Caffeine, Coenzyme Q$_{10}$, DHEA, Kelp, Lecithin, Oat Bran, Slippery Elm

Bladder Control Problems Wild Yam, Dong Quai, Kava

Breast Disorders (Benign) Vitamin E, Vitamin B-Complex, Iodine, Evening Primrose, Chaste Berry, Borage, Cleavers, Dong Quai, Fish Oil

AILMENT GUIDE

Endometriosis Vitamin B-Complex, Vitamin E, Iron, Magnesium, Flax Seed Oil, Wild Yam, Chaste Berry, Black Cohosh, Cramp Bark, Dandelion, Grape Seed Extract

Infertility Vitamin E, Selenium, Chaste Berry, Dong Quai, Red Raspberry

Menopause Vitamin E, Boron, DHEA, Soy Products, Black Cohosh, Chaste Berry, Dong Quai, Ginseng, Red Clover, Sage, Alfalfa, Fenugreek, Phytoestrogens, Wild Yam

Menstrual Problems Vitamin E, Calcium, Magnesium, Iron, Black Cohosh, Dong Quai, Uva Ursi, Shepherd's Purse, Vitamin K, Bee Pollen, Black Haw, Broom, Bugleweed, Caraway, Catnip, Chaste Berry, Cramp Bark, Devil's Claw, Fennel, Fenugreek, Ginger, Ginseng, Goldenseal, Grape Seed Extract, Guarana, Kava, Lemon Balm, Mint, Nettle, Poppy, Red Raspberry, Sage, Valerian, White Willow

Pregnancy NB: Check with your health care provider before taking any nutraceutical during pregnancy. General Supplements: Iron, Folatin, Vitamin B-Complex, Vitamin A, Vitamin C, Calcium, Phosphorous.

Morning Sickness: Peppermint, Ginger, Raspberry Leaf, Meadowsweet, Rosemary. Gestational Diabetes: Glucomannan. Post-Partum: Raspberry Leaf, Black Cohosh, Wild Yam, Black Haw. Lactation: Fennel, Sage

Pre-Menstrual Syndrome Vitamin B_6, Calcium, Black Cohosh, Chaste Berry, Evening Primrose, Vitamin E, Black Currant, Borage, Cramp Bark, Fennel, Ginseng, Licorice, Red Raspberry, Spirulina, Thyme, Uva Ursi, Wild Yam

Uterine Fibroids Vitamin B-Complex, Iron, Magnesium, Methionine, Choline, Inositol, L-Arginine, Chaste Berry

Vaginitis Acidophilus, Boric Acid, Iodine, Garlic, Tea Tree Oil, Echinacea, Goldenseal, Kava, Myrrh

Benign Prostate Enlargement Vitamin E, Selenium, Zinc, Saw Palmetto, Nettle, Pygeum, Soy Products, Lycopern, Bee Pollen, Alfalfa, Nettle

Sexual Dysfunction Vitamin C, Vitamin E, Vitamin B-Complex, Selenium, Zinc, Essential Fatty Acids, Ginkgo Biloba, Ginseng, Yohimbe, Fish Oil, Ginger

NUTRACEUTICAL GUIDE

VITAMINS

Vitamin A Vision, growth and development, immunity, cancer protection, metabolic and hormonal function; diabetes, bronchitis and asthma, acne.

Vitamin C Metabolism, connective tissue, immune function, bones and teeth, antioxidant; colds and flu, cancer, cardiovascular disease, diabetes, cataracts, asthma, wounds, arthritis, Parkinson's disease, gum disease, mouth ulcers, chronic fatigue syndrome, gallstones.

Vitamin D Bones and teeth, mineral absorption, immune function, cancer prevention; rickets, osteomalacia (adult rickets), tetany, osteoporosis, psoriasis, osteoarthritis.

Vitamin E Antioxidant, cancer protection, metabolism, anti-inflammatory; heart disease, diabetes, dementia and Alzheimer's disease, cataracts and macular degeneration, PMS and fibrocystic breast disease, leg pain and cramps.

Vitamin K Blood clotting, bone metabolism; surgery, osteoporosis, heavy menstruation.

Vitamin B-complex Maintain healthy nerves, muscles, skin, and liver; synthesis of adrenal hormones, cholesterol, and fatty acids; red blood cells and pernicious anemia prevention; reduce heart attack risk, spina bifida, carpal tunnel syndrome, stress.

Vitamin B_1 Metabolism, nerve and muscle function, mood and mental attitude; alcoholism, stress, mood disorders, congestive heart failure, high-carb diet, aging.

Vitamin B_2 Metabolism, antioxidant, hormone function, vision, immune-system function, blood manufacture, nerve function; cataracts, migraines, carpal tunnel syndrome, skin disorders, physical and emotional stress.

Vitamin B_3 Metabolism, brain and nerve function, appetite and digestion, circulation and blood pressure; lower blood cholesterol.

Vitamin B_5 Metabolism, immune function, nerve function, hormone function, red blood cell formation; lower blood cholesterol, arthritis, lupus.

Vitamin B_6 Metabolism, immune-system function, nerve function, blood cell manufacture, controlling homocysteine; carpal tunnel syndrome, mild depression, PMS, kidney stones, diabetes, tuberculosis.

Vitamin B_{12} Metabolism, nerve tissue maintenance, red blood cell manufacture; pernicious anemia, nerve and psychological disorders, sprue, fatigue, allergies, cancer protection in smokers, multiple sclerosis.

Biotin Metabolism; brittle nails, hair loss, diabetes.

Folacin Metabolism, growth and development, fetal development, red blood cell manufacture; megaloblastic anemia, sprue, heart disease.

MINERALS

Calcium Bones and teeth, muscle function, maintaining heartbeat, nerves, blood clotting, wounds, cell membrane permeability, synthesize hormones and enzymes for digestion, colon cancer protection; osteoporosis.

Phosphorus Bones and teeth, body cells, genetic material, lactation, muscle tissue, maintain body acid-base and fluid balances, metabolism; severe burns, kidney and digestive disease.

Magnesium Builds bones and teeth, metabolism, indigestion, prevent early birth, convulsions and rapid heartbeat; muscle and nerve function, calcium function, dental cavities, immunity and makes DNA, asthma, cardiac arrhythmias, high blood pressure, fibromyalgia, diabetes; atherosclerosis and heart disease, high blood pressure, insulin metabolism, migraine headaches.

Sodium Maintain body chemistry, nerve and muscle function, miscellaneous functions [absorption and metabolism of carbohydrates, component of sweat, tears, bile, digestive juices]; fluid loss through diarrhea, vomiting, excessive sweating; Addison's disease, low blood pressure.

NUTRACEUTICAL GUIDE

Chloride Maintain body acid-base and fluid balances, stomach, brain, and spinal cord function; red blood cell function, antibacterial and microorganism agent.

Potassium Nerve and cell function, heartbeat and blood pressure, metabolism, insulin secretion, protein synthesis, enzyme action.

Iron Red blood cell manufacture, transport O_2, metabolism; iron deficiency anemia, pregnancy, blood loss.

Zinc Healing wounds, immune-system function, reproduction, common cold and other infections, fibromyalgia, osteoporosis, rheumatoid arthritis, growth and development, maintain skin and bones, metabolism, taste and smell.

Iodine Thyroid maintenance and manufacture, metabolism regulation, growth and mental development, nerve and muscle function, reproduction, retardation and cretinism prevention.

Copper Metabolism, skin, nerves, wounds, skeleton formation, brain and spinal cord cells, blood vessels; anemia, hemoglobin manufacture, osteoporosis, high blood pressure, heart disease, and cancer prevention.

Manganese Metabolism, bones and connective tissues, antioxidant, insulin action, blood clotting; epilepsy, osteoporosis, tendon and joint disorders.

Molybdenum Metabolism, tooth enamel, dental cavity prevention, proper growth.

Fluoride Bone and tooth formation, dental cavity prevention; osteoporosis.

Selenium Antioxidant, detoxifier protects against cancer, heart disease, boosts immune function, prevents cataracts, fertility problems, protects newborns against SIDS.

Chromium Metabolism, protects genetic material, builds fatty acids and synthesizes cholesterol; weight loss, increase vitamin C absorption.

NUTRACEUTICAL SUPPLEMENTS

Acidophilus Digestion and ulcers, helps manufacture of vitamin K and other nutrients, cholesterol, immune system, yeast overgrowth, colon cancer; UTI, antibiotic-induced diarrhea, lactose intolerance, cholesterol; diverticular disease, inflammatory bowel disease.

Bee Pollen Immunity, athletic prowess and muscle strength, stamina; eczema and other skin problems, allergies, anemia, menstrual disorders and bleeding problems, enlarged prostate.

Benecol Lowers cholesterol; atherosclerosis.

Beta-Carotene/Carotenoids Certain cancers (prostate, colon, lung, cervical); immune system, cataracts, macular degeneration.

Beta Glucan Immune system, cholesterol, inflammatory and infectious skin disorders and ulcers, white blood cell production.

Brewer's Yeast Diabetes, fatigue, eczema, cancer, high blood cholesterol, constipation; hypoglycemia.

Bromelain Minor burns, sports injuries, bruises, sprains; digestive aid; arthritis, bronchitis; allergic reactions; carpal tunnel syndrome, gout.

Caffeine Mental alertness, athletic performance, energy booster, insomnia, painkiller enhancer, weight loss, diuretic.

Carnitine Fatty acid and blood cholesterol regulator, antioxidant booster, dementia and Alzheimer's disease, male fertility; athletic prowess, weight loss, chronic fatigue syndrome, heart-muscle disorders, depression, nerve disorders, AIDS.

Chlorophyll Antioxidant, deodorizer, wounds, infections, blood cleanser, anticancer agent, anemia.

Choline Cell membranes, metabolizes fats, nerves and muscles, heart function, memory, liver; athletic performance, fatigue.

Chondroitin Sulfate Cartilage, blood clots and fatty plaque build-up, osteoarthritis, pain reliever, arthritis.

Coenzyme Q$_{10}$ Cell energy production, vitamin E preserver, atherosclerosis, heart disease, high cholesterol, blood pressure, erratic heartbeat, angina, blood clots, Raynaud's disease, Parkinson's disease, cardiomyopathy, congestive heart failure, cardiovascular disease, Alzheimer's disease, fibromyalgia, chronic fatigue syndrome, dementia, AIDS, periodontal disease and tooth decay, weight loss; liver disease.

Creatine Muscle builder, athletic performance enhancer.

DHEA Libido and mood enhancer, heart attack and stroke, cholesterol, blood pressure, immune system, autoimmune disease (lupus), diabetes, aging disorders (Alzheimer's and Parkinson's diseases), weight control, menopause.

DMSO and MSM Antioxidant, muscle pain and inflammation of arthritis, interstitial cystitis, headaches, fibromyalgia, carpal tunnel syndrome, allergies, gout.

Essential Fatty Acids Brain development, hormone production, cell health, heart disease, cancer, diabetes, asthma, depression; arthritis, cholesterol disorders and atherosclerosis, dermatitis and eczema, diabetes, gout, heart disease, inflammatory bowel disease, lupus, migraine headaches, psoriasis, sexual dysfunction.

Fish Oils Anti-inflammatory, immune-system, heart disease, stroke, blood pressure, atherosclerosis, psoriasis, rheumatoid arthritis, lupus, inflammatory bowel disorders, fibrocystic breast disorders, breast and colon cancer, dermatitis and eczema, gout, migraine headaches, sexual dysfunction, psoriasis.

5-HTP Mood regulator, depression, sleep and eating disorders, migraine headaches, OCD, fibromyalgia, appetite suppressant, weight problems.

Flavonoids Antioxidant, cancer, heart disease, allergies, anti-inflammatory, viruses, anticoagulant, antibacterial, dilates blood vessels, anticarcinogenic, lowers cholesterol, osteoporosis, dermatitis and eczema.

Glucomannan Weight loss, cholesterol, glucose levels, diabetes, childhood obesity.

Glucosamine Sulfate Builds and repairs cartilage, tendons, and ligaments; osteoarthritis; arthritis.

Glutamine Metabolism, muscle tissue, blood plasma, energy booster, mental alertness, mood and memory booster, athletic supplement, inflammatory bowel disease, depression, prevents muscle loss, protects liver tissue; cancer, AIDS, chemotherapy.

Grape Seed Extract Antioxidant, cancer, aging, degenerative diseases, atherosclerosis, heart disease; heart attack and stroke, vascular disorders, cataracts and macular degeneration, anti-inflammatory, allergies, reduce blood clots; cholesterol disorders; dermatitis and eczema, heart disease, leg cramps and restless legs.

Green Tea Heart disease, cancer, atherosclerosis, heart disease, stroke, dental cavities; cholesterol disorders, diarrhea.

Kelp Calcium source, iodine source, inflammatory arthritis, psoriasis, circulatory and kidney disorders, constipation, indigestion, weight-loss aid, strong nails and hair.

Kombucha Mushrooms Infections, inflammatory arthritis, lupus, diabetes, high blood pressure, depression and emotional illness.

L-arginine Circulatory disease, coronary artery disease, atherosclerosis, high blood pressure, blood clots, heart attack and stroke, peripheral artery disease; circulatory problems.

Lecithin Heart disease, gallstones, obesity, Alzheimer's disease and memory loss, blood cholesterol, cirrhosis.

Lipoic Acid Antioxidant, blood sugar, cataracts, diabetes, diabetic neuropathy, AIDS, vegetarians, birth defects, exercise stress, AIDS, antiviral agent.

Melatonin Regulates body's circadian rhythms, jet lag and insomnia, immune-system function, antiaging supplement, antioxidant, cancer, heart disease and stroke, cataracts, degenerative disorders, Parkinson's and Alzheimer's diseases; breast cancer, atherosclerosis, SAD.

Mushroom Extracts Antibiotic, anti-inflammatory, asthma and bronchitis, cardiovascular disorders, cholesterol-lowering extracts, diabetes, high blood pressure, kidney function, liver disorders, stress, viral infections.

Oat Bran Lowers blood cholesterol, diabetes, constipation, weight control, lowers blood sugar, heart disease.

Phenylalanine Thyroid disorders, appetite suppressant, memory enhancer, painkiller; depression, alcoholism and addictions, libido, chronic back pain, migraine headache, menstrual pain, bipolar disorder.

Phosphatidylserine Normal cell function, regulates neurotransmitters and supports mental function (concentration, memory loss, dementia, Alzheimer's disease).

Phytoestrogens Menopause; breast, endometrial, and leukemia cancer prevention; lowers blood cholesterol.

Psyllium Constipation, hemorrhoids and fissures, lower blood cholesterol, boost immune system, colon cancer, gallstones, obesity, weight control, appetite regulator; cholesterol disorders and atherosclerosis, diverticular disease, inflammatory bowel disease, irritable bowel syndrome.

Pycnogenol Blood circulation, vision, flexibility, bruising, inflammation, skin tone and appearance, psoriasis, chronic fatigue syndrome, exercise endurance and injuries, heart disease, stroke, cancer, diabetic retinopathy, clotting problems, antiaging, sun damage, antioxidant, arthritis, hay fever and other allergies, bronchitis, asthma, ADHD, cholesterol disorders and atherosclerosis.

Red Rice Yeast Indigestion, diarrhea, abdominal pain, cardiovascular and cholesterol disorders, atherosclerosis.

SAM-e Depression, arthritis, osteoarthritis, liver function, cartilage.

Shark Cartilage Cancer, arthritis.

Soy Products Provides calcium, protein, lecithin, phytoestrogens. Cancer, menopause (hot flashes, osteoporosis), blood cholesterol reduction, antioxidant (atherosclerosis), benign prostate enlargement.

Spirulina Immune-system booster, heart disease, cancer, natural antibiotic, HIV, arthritis, PMS, eczema, colonic.

BOTANICAL MEDICINES

Agrimony Sore throat, diarrhea and intestinal disorders, inflammatory bowel disease and hemorrhoids, skin abrasions and ulcers, muscle aches, yeast infection.

Alfalfa Indigestion, heartburn, and loss of appetite; UTI and kidney, bladder, and prostate disorders; diuretic; diabetes; menopause; insect stings.

Aloe Vera Minor skin burns, scalds, sunburn; cuts and wounds; scarring; frostbite; skin irritations and inflammation; hemorrhoids; skin softener; stomach ulcers and intestinal problems, immune-system function.

Anise Nasal and lung congestion, cough suppressant; indigestion; gas and nausea; bad breath; food and liquor flavoring.

Ashwagandha Energy booster; endurance; immune-system function; regulate bodily functions; mental well-being; chronic fatigue syndrome; fibromyalgia; AIDS; Alzheimer's disease; infections.

Astragalus Immune-system function; colds and infections; heart attack; memory; diuretic; fibromyalgia, stress, chronic fatigue syndrome; skin abrasions

Barberry Sore throat and mouth ulcers; indigestion, ulcers, heartburn, intestinal inflammation; high blood pressure; coughs; skin disorders.

Barley Diarrhea and intestinal upset; blood sugar; blood cholesterol; sore throat and mouth ulcers.

Basil Appetite, digestion, and gas; stomach cramps and vomiting; constipation, diuretic; minor cuts, wounds, and insect bites; nasal congestion.

Bilberry Sore throats, mouth inflammation; night blindness, retinopathy, vision disorders; diarrhea; circulatory disorders; gastrointestinal, renal, and urinary tract problems; arthritis, gout, and dermatitis; cataracts, irritable bowel syndrome, macular degeneration.

Blackberry Wounds; hemorrhoids; diarrhea; sore throat and mouth sores and inflammation.

Black Cohosh PMS, dysmenorrhea, menopausal symptoms; diarrhea, lung congestion and cough suppressant; diuretic; arthritis; eczema and insect bites.

Black Currant Diarrhea, diuretic, arthritis pain and inflammation; PMS; sore throat; eczema and other inflammatory skin conditions.

Black Haw Menstrual cramps and uterine contractions after childbirth; miscarriage; high blood pressure; bronchial spasms and asthma; arthritis.

Bloodroot Oral bacteria, gum disease, gingivitis; skin disorders and infections; sore throat, coughs.

Boneset Fever, cold, flu; muscle aches; indigestion and appetite loss; diuretic and laxative; infections; cancer.

Borage Fibrocystic breast disease; neuropathy, eczema, rheumatoid arthritis, lupus; PMS.

Boswellia Musculoskelatal pain; ulcerative colitis; diarrhea and dysentery; lung disease; parasitic worms.

Broom Diuretic; cardiac arrhythmia; uterine contractions, heavy menstual bleeding; varicose veins.

Bugleweed Thyroid disease; breast enlargement; sedative; cough suppressant; nosebleeds and heavy menstrual bleeding.

Burdock Indigestion and appetite loss; diuretic and laxative; inflammatory skin conditions; gout, arthritis, rheumatism; antibiotic; cancer.

Butcher's Broom Hemorrhoids; varicose veins; atherosclerosis.

Calendula Skin abrasions; skin fungi; skin inflammation; stomach ulcers and intestinal inflammation; blood cholesterol; immune-system function.

Camphor Pain reliever; chapped lips; skin irritations; minor burns and skin wounds; colds and flu; insect repellant.

Caraway Menstruation, amenorrhea, menstrual cramps.

Cardamom Asthma; indigestion, flatulence, and constipation; spastic colon; bad breath.

Cascara Sagrada Nausea, intestinal cramps; laxative; digestive system tonic; liver and gallstone disorders.

Catnip Nerves, insomnia; coughs and colds; indigestion and diarrhea; menstrual and muscle cramps; minor cuts.

Cat's Claw Immune-system function; gastrointestinal symptoms; skin wounds; asthma; arthritis; bacterial, viral, and yeast infections.

Cayenne Arthritis, bursitis, fibromyalgia, diabetic neuropathy, shingles; skin rash, psoriasis; nerve pain syndromes; gastrointestinal distress.

Chamomile Skin abrasions [wounds, burns, scrapes, cuts]; skin rashes and inflammation; anxiety; insomnia; coughs, fevers, colds, bronchitis.

Chaste Berry Menstrual problems, PMS; ovulation; endometriosis; uterine fibroid tumors; menopausal symptoms; infertility; acne.

Chinese Cucumber Boils and abscesses; dryness; bronchial congestion; antibiotic, expectorant, laxative, and anti-inflammatory properties; HIV.

Cinnamon Upset stomach, gas, diarrhea; appetite stimulant, digestive aid; cuts and abrasions; tooth decay, gum disease; nausea.

Cleavers Diuretic; constipation; sunburn, blisters, psoriasis, eczema; fibrocystic breasts; insomnia.

Cloves Toothache, minor mouth irritation; sore throat; bad breath; indigestion; skin infections; insect repellant.

Comfrey Skin ulcers, bedsores, lesions; minor burn and wounds; bee stings, spider bites; skin infections; athlete's foot.

Coriander Appetite stimulant, indigestion, intestinal upset; nerves, insomnia; blood glucose; bad breath; joint and muscle pain; pancreatic function.

Cramp Bark Colic, muscle spasms, menstrual cramps, endometriosis; miscarriage; anxiety and nerves; PMS; palpitations; blood pressure.

Cranberry UTI; skin wounds; vitamin C deficiency.

Dandelion Wounds, warts, moles, pimples, calluses, sores, bee stings, blisters; diuretic; indigestion; constipation, diarrhea; liver disorders and gallstones; high blood pressure; breast-feeding; endometriosis; dental plaque.

Devil's Claw Arthritis; anxiety; diuretic; digestion and appetite stimulant; blood cholesterol; menstrual symptoms.

Dill Stomachache, intestinal gas and flatulence; bad breath; breast-feeding; colic; insomnia; kidney disorders.

Dong Quai Menstrual symptoms; sexual desire, fertility; liver disorders; inflammation; sciatica and rheumatism; stomachache, ulcers, and constipation; high blood pressure; fibrocystic breasts.

Echinacea Skin problems; cold and flu; recurrent infections [respiratory, ear, UTI, vaginal yeast]; immune-system function.

Elder Fever, nasal and bronchial congestion; diuretic; vomiting; skin inflammation, sprains, bruises; joint and muscle pain.

Eucalyptus Anxiety; minor skin infections, cuts, and abrasions; upper respiratory and nasal congestion; sore throat; bad breath.

Evening Primrose Skin itchiness, flaking, and eczema; PMS; rheumatoid arthritis.

Fennel Appetite stimulant, digestive, nausea, gas, flatulence; heartburn and indigestion; PMS and menstrual cramps; bad breath; colds; colic.

Fenugreek Digestive problems; bronchial congestion, coughs, sore throat; minor skin wounds and infections; blood cholesterol and triglycerides; diabetes; menstrual cramps, uterine contractions, menopausal symptoms.

Feverfew Migraine headache; arthritis and other inflammatory diseases; minor skin wounds, irritation, and inflammation; insect repellant.

Flax Skin irritation; constipation; intestinal diseases; high blood cholesterol; arthritis.

Garlic High blood pressure; blood cholesterol; blood clots, heart attack, stroke; cold symptoms; minor skin infections and wounds; coughs; ringworm; intestinal worms; fever; digestive disorders; swimmer's ear; athlete's foot; cancer; artherosclerosis; leg cramps and restless legs.

Ginger Nausea; digestive problems; colds and flu; menstrual irregularities; impotence; depression; arthritis pain; migraine headache; high blood cholesterol; dandruff, skin inflammation, minor burns; sore throat.

Ginkgo Memory; early Alzheimer's disease symptoms; mild depression; leg pains; erectile dysfunction; blood clots; inner ear disorders; allergies, asthma, inflammatory disorders; atherosclerosis; heart attack; ischemic stroke; shock; heart arrhythmia; hemorrhoids; leg ulcers; phlebitis, Raynaud's disease; anaphylaxis; kidney disease; graft rejection; circulatory problems, dermatitis and eczema; leg cramps and restless leg; migraine headaches.

Ginseng Physical stamina and mental alertness; stress; fatigue, insomnia, poor appetite, anxiety, restlessness; PMS, menstrual problems, menopause symptoms; chronic fatigue syndrome, menopause, sexual dysfunction.

Goldenseal Immune-system function; diverse infections; upper respiratory infections; minor eye infections; intestinal problems; sciatica, muscle and joint disorders; gynecological disorders; UTI; skin disorders; blood pressure; mouth canker sores; diabetes; bronchitis, nausea.

Gotu Kola Skin wounds, psoriasis, leprosy, surgical incision scarring; varicose veins, blood circulation; connective tissue; dementia and aging symptoms.

Guarana Mental alertness, drowsiness, memory; appetite suppressant; athletic performance enhancer; edema; painkiller, muscle ache; fever, malaria.

Guggul High blood cholesterol and triglycerides; obesity; arthritis; cardiovascular disease; atherosclerosis, heart disease.

Hawthorn Congestive heart failure; high blood pressure; edema; heart arrhythmia; leg cramps and restless legs.

Horehound Cold symptoms and congestion; coughing spasms; sore throat; appetite stimulant and digestive; GERD, peptic ulcers.

Horseradish Minor muscle aches and arthritis pain; sinus congestion; bronchitis and other upper respiratory disorders; appetite stimulant and digestive; gout, rheumatism, liver and gallbladder diseases.

Hyssop Coughs, bronchial congestion, cold and flu symptoms, sore throat; gas, stomachache; fever sweats; minor burns, bruises, and skin sores; insect repellant.

Kava Anxiety; insomnia; muscle tension; colds, migraine headaches, gonorrhea vaginitis, menstrual problems, nocturnal incontinence and other urinary problems, rheumatism.

Lavender Aromatherapeutic uses to calm nerves and upset stomach, relieve abdominal cramps and intestinal gas, promote digestion; tension headaches; mood elevator; sleep inducer; infection and healing of minor cuts, wounds, burns; eczema, psoriasis, skin inflammation, itching from insect stings and bites.

Lemon Balm Digestive problems; stress, anxiety, depression, insomnia; herpes cold sores, fever blisters, minor skin infections; itchy insect bites; muscle spasms, menstrual cramps; Grave's disease.

Licorice Eczema, minor skin infections; sore throat, mouth ulcers, gum disease, tooth decay; congestion, coughing, bronchitis, common cold symptoms; indigestion, heartburn, peptic ulcers, intestinal inflammation, urinary tract infections; PMS, chronic fatigue syndrome, fibromyalgia; arthritis; allergies, dermatitis, Inflammatory bowel disease, liver diseases, mouth sores, psoriasis, ulcers.

Marijuana Mild to moderate pain relief, inflammation; appetite stimulant; nausea from cancer therapy; glaucoma; muscle spasms; epileptic seizures; AIDS symptoms.

Marshmallow Minor skin irritations, eczema; mouth ulcers, sore throats, coughs, cold symptoms, bronchitis; intestinal disorders, UTI; diabetes [blood sugar]; constipation.

Milk Thistle Liver and gallbladder diseases; alcoholism; poison mushroom antidote.

Mint/Peppermint Digestive disorders; appetite stimulant; headaches, stress; nasal congestion from common cold, flu, sinusitis; muscle aches, hives, itchy insect bites; dry cough; bad breath; gingivitis, dry mouth; menstrual cramps; insomnia.

Mullein Minor skin abrasions, burns, insect bites; infection fighter; hemorrhoids; sore throats and throat irritations, coughs; diarrhea; ulcers; insomnia.

Mustard Chest congestion; muscle aches, inflammation, and joint pain; appetite stimulant; vomiting.

Myrrh Bad breath, canker sores, bed sores, skin ulcers, gingivitis, fever blisters; sore throat, intestinal inflammation; hemorrhoids; vaginitis; immune-system function; topical antiseptic; mouth sores.

Nettle Diuretic, kidney stones; benign prostate enlargement; skin wounds; bronchial congestion; allergies; inflammatory skin disorders; menstrual bleeding, postpartum hemorrhaging; muscle and joint pain; fatigue.

Oak Skin wounds; sore throat; hemorrhoids; diarrhea; blood cholesterol.

Poppy Pain [postoperative, broken bones, heart attack, cancer, menstrual]; anxiety; diarrhea; dry cough; muscle spasms; insomnia.

Red Clover Menopause; inflammatory skin disorders; cold and flu symptoms.

Red Raspberry Pregnancy; PMS, menstrual cramps; female fertility; intestinal upset [diarrhea, indigestion, nausea]; skin inflammation, fever blisters, hemorrhoids, mucous membranes]; mouth sores, sore throat.

Rose Common cold; UTI, diuretic; constipation; mouth ulcers, cold sores, sore throat.

Rosemary Intestinal disorders; blood circulation; skin wounds and bruises; insect repellant; joint and muscle pain; stress, depression, mental fatigue; male-pattern balding; memory loss.

Sage Mouth and throat inflammation, canker sores, gum disease, toothache; dry skin; insect bites; excess perspiration; fever; dry cough; digestive upset; menstrual discomfort; depression; joint and muscle pain; lactation; appetite stimulant.

St. John's Wort Depression; insomnia; anxiety; minor skin wounds and infections; HIV.

Saw Palmetto Benign prostate enlargement [BPH]; bladder irritation.

Seneca Root Expectorant; cold and flu symptoms; purgative.

Senna Constipation.

Slippery Elm Skin abrasions; eczema; cold and bronchitis symptoms; intestinal inflammation; constipation; weight loss; diverticular disease.

Tea Tree Minor skin infections; inflammatory skin conditions; skin irritations, bad breath, plaque, gingivitis, canker sores, herpes cold sores; fungal infections; sore throat; nasal and sinus congestion; muscle and joint pain and inflammation; hemorrhoids; dandruff, cradle cap.

Thyme Cold, flu, and bronchitis symptoms; indigestion; muscle aches, joint pain and inflammation; PMS; skin infection, minor wounds.

Turmeric Joint pain and inflammation; indigestion and heartburn; liver function; gallstones.

Uva Ursi UTI and cystitis; kidney and bladder stones; PMS; minor cuts and abrasions; muscle pain.

Valerian Insomnia; muscle spasm, menstrual cramps, irritable bowel syndrome; anxiety; ADHD, high blood pressure.

White Willow Cold and flu symptoms, joint inflammation [arthritis, bursitis, rheumatism]; common pain syndromes.

Wild Yam PMS, vaginal dryness after menopause; arthritis, muscle pain; high cholesterol; gallstones, diverticulosis, irritable bowel syndrome; bladder control problems, endometriosis.

Witch Hazel Hemorrhoids, minor skin burns and abrasions, muscle aches, bleeding and oozing from cuts and other skin conditions, insect bites, sore throat and intestinal inflammation.

PART 2

Directory of Nutraceutical Remedies

CHAPTER 2

Common Disorders

Practitioners of integrative medicine often prescribe nutraceuticals along with pharmaceutical products to treat everything from acne to vaginitis. But in most instances, there are no hard and fast rules: There are some disorders that should be treated only with conventional medications, and others where nutraceuticals may be more effective, safer, and less expensive. And in all instances, self-diagnosis and self-treatment should be approached with great caution or avoided entirely.

This chapter addresses more than forty of our most common disorders, with emphasis on those that are most likely to respond to nutraceuticals. For each, you will find descriptions of symptoms and diagnostic steps, an overview of conventional treatments, and listings of nutraceuticals arranged by vitamins and minerals, nutritional supplements, and botanical medicines. Within each of these categories, products are arranged according to their generally recognized importance. Each section also suggests strategies of relief. This material is based on the latest scientific research, and it has been carefully reviewed by conventional physicians and alternative practitioners. While every effort has been made to ensure that the information is accurate and relevant, it should not be used to alter or substitute for your doctor's prescribed therapy. Instead, it should be used as a basis of discussion with your health care provider. It may well be that he or she will recommend that you try some of the nutraceutical approaches described on the following pages; in other instances, your doctor may seek other opinions or point out why you should stick to your present regimen.

Remember, too, that nutraceutical products should be approached with the same caution as pharmaceutical medications by women who are pregnant or breast-feeding. In short, always check with your doctor before taking any high-dose vitamin or mineral product, other nutritional supplements, or botanical medicines. Similarly, nutraceuticals should not be given to children without first checking with your pediatrician or other health care provider.

ACNE

Acne is a virtually universal problem that, at one time or another, afflicts almost everyone. While an occasional whitehead, blackhead, or pimple is not medically serious, for some people, especially teenagers, acne can be unpleasant, embarrassing, and in severe cases, even disfiguring. Acne can strike at any age, but it most commonly starts during adolescence, between the ages of ten and thirteen, and it typically lasts anywhere from five to ten years and fades away on its own by the time a person reaches his or her twenties. But there are many exceptions—sometimes it lasts into adulthood, and some people experience their first bout of acne in middle age.

Acne, especially the more severe forms, tends to run in families. Young men are more likely to have severe, long-lasting acne, although young women are sometimes afflicted, too. Acne is closely related to shifting levels of androgens, the sex hormones that are most abundant in males, but which women also produce in small amounts. Androgen production rises sharply with the onset of puberty, which is when acne typically starts. Many women experience flare-ups of acne at specific times during the menstrual cycle, again a consequence of shifting hormonal levels.

Acne is basically a disease of the type of hair follicles that are especially abundant on the face and upper back—the favored sites of acne. Each follicle contains a tiny hair and a sebaceous gland, which produces an oily substance called sebum. The sebum travels along the hair follicle and exits to the skin's surface. In some people, androgens overstimulate the sensitive sebaceous glands, which then produce more sebum. The excess sebum picks up skin bacteria and dead skin cells, which also shed more rapidly during puberty. As the mixture travels up the hair follicle in an attempt to exit to the skin's surface, the follicle can easily become clogged, providing an ideal environment for bacteria, especially *Propiobacterium acnes,* or *P. acnes,* to multiply rapidly. The bacteria then irritate the follicle and the surrounding skin, resulting in either a blackhead (or an open comedo) or a whitehead (a closed comedo). If the comedo becomes inflamed, a pus-filled pimple (also called a papule or pustule) will form. In severe cases, large pus-filled cysts form—these can result in scarring.

Many things can aggravate or worsen acne. Many people note that

● ACNE MYTHS AND FACTS

According to the American Academy of Dermatology, these are some of the most common myths about acne:

Myth: Acne is caused by poor hygiene.
Fact: No amount of cleansing can wash away acne, which forms deep in the skin, and has little to do to with surface cleanliness.

Myth: Acne is caused by eating fatty foods or chocolate.
Fact: Acne is basically a hormonal disorder, and has little or nothing to do with diet. However, stress can lead to hormonal changes, and indirectly provoke an outbreak of acne. When under stress, many people crave chocolates or other foods, and then blame their eating indiscretion for the acne outbreak. In reality, the stress is the culprit for both the acne flare-up and the food craving.

Myth: Acne is just a cosmetic disease.
Fact: Acne can cause considerable emotional pain, especially during adolescence when young people are especially conscious of their appearance. The condition can be devastating for adults in the workplace as well.

Myth: You just have to let acne run its course.
Fact: Acne can almost always be controlled; if self-treatment doesn't work, a dermatologist should be consulted.

Myth: Sexual activity can worsen (or improve) acne.
Fact: Although sex hormones are responsible for acne, sexual activity has no effect on it.

acne often flares up during a period of undue stress, such as school exam week. This is probably due to stress-related hormonal changes. Cosmetic products, such as foundations, moisturizers, night creams, and blushes, can contribute to the clogging of pores. Environmental factors, such as grease floating in the air at a fast-food restaurant, can also contribute to clogged pores.

Diagnostic Steps

Acne can usually be diagnosed simply by observing the typical skin eruptions. Sometimes, however, rashes, allergies, and other skin conditions produce eruptions similar to acne. If in doubt, or if painful cysts develop, consult a dermatologist.

Conventional Treatments

According to the American Academy of Dermatology, Americans spend well over $100 million dollars a year for nonprescription acne treatments. This sum does not include special soaps and cleansers, which are rarely needed and may actually aggravate the condition.

■ NONPRESCRIPTION TREATMENTS

The two most commonly recommended ingredients found in over-the-counter acne preparations are benzoyl peroxide and salicylic acid; glycolic acid and sulfur may also be helpful. Examples of skin-care/acne systems that combine these four ingredients include Pro-Active and Serious Skin Care.

Benzoyl peroxide destroys the bacteria (*P. acnes*) thought to contribute to acne. It is available in creams, lotions, and gels and works best for mild acne. The affected area should be washed gently with a mild soap, rinsed thoroughly with lukewarm water, and patted dry before applying the benzoyl peroxide preparation. It can cause skin irritation, so it should be used sparingly for the first day or two. For dry or sensitive skin, start with a 5 percent solution and use only on affected areas. For oily skin, start with a 10 percent solution. If no redness or scaly, itching skin appears, it can usually be applied twice a day. It must be used daily, for an indefinite period of time, to control acne. If treatment is stopped too soon, the acne may return. Improvement is usually seen within two to four weeks; if not, consult a dermatologist.

Salicylic acid controls the abnormal shedding of skin cells and helps unclog pores that contribute to acne. It does not affect bacteria or sebum production. It is available in creams, lotions, and pads and works best for mild acne. Like benzoyl peroxide, it must be used long-term to keep acne under control.

◉ SYMPTOMS

▪ Eruptions of whiteheads, blackheads, or pimples. The face is usually the area most affected but acne also occurs on the neck, chest, back, shoulders, scalp, and upper arms and legs.

▪ Large, painful red or purple nodules. These are hallmarks of cystic acne, the most severe type, which goes deeply into the skin.

◉ STRATEGIES FOR RELIEF

The American Academy of Dermatology recommends the following self-help approaches:

▪ Do not pop, squeeze, or pick at acne. This can make it worse, by spreading infection. Blackheads and whiteheads should be removed only by an experienced health professional.

▪ Gently wash your face twice a day with a mild soap and pat dry. Vigorous washing and scrubbing can irritate your skin and make acne worse.

▪ Use nonoily cosmetics and toiletries.

▪ Avoid things that might aggravate acne, such as oily hair creams and skin moisturizers, airborne grease, irritating clothing, or hairstyles with long bangs.

▪ Give acne products enough time to do their job. See a dermatologist if over-the-counter preparations don't work, and realize that severe, disfiguring acne may require years of treatment.

▪ Some acne products, including antibiotics, can increase the skin's sensitivity to sunlight and ultraviolet light from tanning booths. Use protective clothing and sunscreens when outdoors and avoid tanning booths.

■ PRESCRIPTION MEDICATIONS

There are several prescription medications that a dermatologist might prescribe to treat acne, depending on the patient's age, gender, drug sensitivities, and severity of the condition.

Antibiotics are used either on the skin or taken as an oral medication; they work by destroying *P. acnes*. Erythromycin and tetracycline are the antibiotics most commonly prescribed to treat acne. Mild acne often can be controlled with a topical antibiotic cream, gel, pad, or lotion. Systemic antibiotics are usually reserved for the more severe types because they carry an increased risk of adverse side effects, and their use may contribute to the formation of antibiotic-resistant bacteria.

Vitamin A derivatives, collectively called retinoids, can be used topically or as oral drugs. Topical retinoid preparations, used to treat moderate to severe acne, help unclog pores and normalize the way skin grows and sheds. Oral retinoid drugs reduce sebum production, lessen the shedding of skin, and help control *P. acnes*. These drugs are powerful and can have serious side effects, so they are usually reserved for severe cases of acne. They can cause serious birth defects if taken just before or during pregnancy, so for women, doctors often prescribe oral contraceptives at the same time.

Oral contraceptives provide female hormones that help counteract the effects of acne-provoking male hormones. Obviously, they are an option only for women. Doctors generally don't recommend oral contraceptives solely to treat acne, but the presence of acne may be a factor in selecting this form of birth control. (The only oral contraceptive approved by the FDA for treatment of acne is Ortho Tri Cyclen.)

Nutraceuticals for Acne

There are few well-studied nutraceuticals for the treatment of acne. However, there are two that stand out as options to over-the-counter and prescription preparations for the treatment of mild to moderate acne.

■ BOTANICAL MEDICINES

Arnica (*Arnica montana L.*)

How it works. The dried flower heads have an established reputation as an effective treatment for acne, among other things. In the form of a tincture, they prevent and reduce inflammation of the skin as well as provide antibiotic properties.

Recommended dosages. The most commonly used dosage is a 1:10 tincture prepared with 70 percent ethanol. Ointments and creams with a maximum of 20 to 25 percent of the tincture or with a maximum of 15 percent arnica oil may also be used.

Possible problems. Arnica should be used only topically. Taken orally, it can be toxic to the heart. But even topical application, if used for a long period of time, especially on damaged or injured skin, can cause skin irritations that can become serious if not treated. The more concentrated the arnica solution or cream, the greater the risk of side effects.

Tea tree (*Melalueca alternifolia*)

How it works. The essential oil of this tree, a native of Australia, is a topical antiseptic agent and has been proven to have a wide variety of antimicrobial activities. It is said to have been used by the aborigines as a local antiseptic, and the early settlers in Australia used it for the treatment of cuts, abrasions, burns, insect bites, and athlete's foot.

Recommended dosages. One Australian study of 124 people with mild to moderate acne found a 5 percent tea tree oil gel to be almost as effective in treating the condition as a 5 percent benzoyl peroxide lotion and with fewer side effects.

Possible problems. Irritation of the skin can occasionally occur in sensitive people, though no other side effects have been observed.

ALLERGIES

Allergies are one of our most common afflictions, affecting more than 50 million Americans. Hay fever, or seasonal allergic rhinitis, is the most common, affecting some 25 million people. More than 17 million have asthma, which is often triggered by allergies. Millions of others develop hives, rashes, and allergic reactions when they are exposed to certain foods, chemicals, animal dander, and a variety of other allergy-provoking substances (allergens).

Although allergic responses vary greatly from one person to another, all stem from an overly sensitive immune system that mounts attacks against normally harmless substances (allergens). The immune system is a complex defense network that stands ready to protect the body from foreign substances such as bacteria, viruses, and cancer cells, which the body perceives as foreign. But an overly sensitive immune system views the likes of animal dander, pollen, dust mites, and other normally harmless substances as potential dangers that must be fought. Thus, when a person comes in contact with an allergen, the immune system goes into action to fight it off, resulting in a variety of symptoms.

Typically, allergy involves the gradual buildup in the body of immunoglobulin E(IgE), a type of protein known as an antibody. After a

⊙ **STRATEGIES FOR RELIEF**
- Try to identify your specific allergens and then avoid them as much as possible.
- Stay indoors when pollen counts are high.
- Use allergy-proof mattress and pillow covers; remove rugs and other dust catchers, especially from the bedroom.
- Try to keep stress under control. Although stress per se does not cause allergies, it can exacerbate reactions.
- If you are hypersensitive and in danger of anaphylaxis, wear a MedAlert bracelet and always carry a syringe of epinephrine (adrenaline) to use in case of an emergency.
- If you are allergic to molds, avoid mushrooms, blue cheese, and other mold-containing foods, which may provoke a reaction. Also, wipe down damp surfaces with chlorine or another mold-killing cleaner.

◉ DEALING WITH FOOD ALLERGIES

Food allergens are proteins in foods that can survive cooking and digestion to be absorbed by the bloodstream and travel to target organs. A reaction to food may begin with an itching or strange sensation in the mouth, or it may provoke a fit of sneezing after a meal. Hives, diarrhea, nausea, and indigestion are other possible symptoms; in some people, certain food allergies provoke asthma attacks.

The most common causes of food allergies are shellfish and fish; peanuts (a legume); tree nuts, including walnuts; and eggs. Children are most affected by peanut, egg, and milk allergies. However, the latter should not be confused with lactose intolerance, which entails an inability to digest milk sugar.

susceptible person's first close encounter with an allergen, IgE is produced. These antibodies attach to mast cells, which defend the body again and again as the allergen returns. Mast cells, which are concentrated in the nose, throat, lungs, skin, and intestinal tract, secrete a substance called histamine, and this is what produces the symptoms of an allergic reaction, which can range from annoying but minor to life-threatening attacks of asthma or anaphylaxis, a response that involves tissue swelling, vomiting, cramps, and a dramatic drop in blood pressure.

Symptoms

Symptoms vary from one person to another, and may include any or all of the following:

- Sneezing and nasal stuffiness, itching, and clear discharge.
- Itching of ears and/or roof of the mouth.
- Red, itchy, dry skin, typically on elbows, knees, and in skin folds.
- Red, itchy, watery eyes.
- Itchy welts on any body part.
- Wheezing, coughing, and difficulty breathing.
- Nausea, diarrhea, and other intestinal symptoms.
- Feelings of anxiety, especially when accompanied by difficulty breathing.

Diagnostic Steps

Allergies can show up at any age. Myriad substances cause allergies, including animals, cockroaches, or dust mites and their wastes; weeds, plants, grass and tree pollens; mold and mildew spores; stinging insects, including wasps and fire ants; common medications, especially aspirin, penicillin, and sulfa drugs; foods, most commonly eggs, peanuts and tree nuts, milk and milk products, and seafood; and chemicals present in dyes, cosmetics, and latex. Allergens may be difficult to pinpoint. That's why keeping a diary of symptoms and exposures can help identify specific allergens.

Doctors can often pinpoint what is causing an allergic reaction by asking questions and reviewing a diary of symptoms and exposures. To confirm a suspected allergen, however, allergy blood tests and skin scratch tests are usually needed.

Conventional Treatments

The best approach is simply to avoid the allergens. Of course, it is not always easy or even possible to stay away from the offending plants, dust, molds, animals, foods, and other allergens. Mild allergies, especially seasonal hay fever, usually can be controlled with antihistamines and decongestants. These medications are available in both nonprescription and prescription forms. Topical medications, such as corticosteroid creams and ointments, can help relieve itchy skin and rashes. Anaphylaxis, always a medical emergency, is treated with an injection of adrenaline and antihistamines.

Many allergy sufferers find relief with a course of allergy shots, known as allergen immunotherapy or desensitization. Tiny amounts of the offending allergens are injected at regular intervals—at first every week or two—until the body builds a tolerance to gradually increasing doses of the substance. The full course may take three to five years to administer, but after that, most patients do not react to normal exposure to the allergen. Studies have found that desensitization can also decrease the frequency and severity of allergic asthma. This approach, however, does not work for food allergies.

Nutraceuticals for Allergies

■ VITAMINS AND MINERALS

Vitamin C

How it works. Vitamin C is a powerful antioxidant that is also important in normal immune system function. It is the major antioxidant that protects cells in the respiratory system from free radicals; researchers theorize that it may also have an antihistamine effect.

Recommended dosages. The typical dosage calls for 200 to 500 mg a day, although hay fever sufferers may need higher doses during the allergy season.

Possible problems. Very high doses (1,000 mg or more) can cause diarrhea.

■ NUTRITIONAL SUPPLEMENTS

Essential Fatty Acids

How it works. These types of fats in the diet can reduce inflammatory and allergic reactions by reducing arachidonic acid, a substance needed to make prostaglandins; these are hormonelike body chemicals that are instrumental in producing inflammation. A diet high in omega-3 fatty acids, found in oily cold-water fish (salmon, tuna, mackeral, herring) or fish oil supplements and flaxseed or walnut oils, lowers levels of arachidonic acid.

Recommended dosages. Eating three or four servings of oily fish—salmon, trout, sardines, mackerel, among others—a week has been correlated with reduced allergic reactions. If supplements are taken, the usual dosages of fish oils range from 3 to 5 g a day. Take it in divided doses of 1 g at a time; taking too much at a time can cause belching and reflux. Flaxseed oil can be taken in capsule form, but a less expensive source is liquid oil, which can be used as a salad oil. The usual dosage ranges from 1 teaspoon to 1 tablespoon a day.

Possible problems. Omega-3 fatty acids have a blood-thinning effect, so they should be used cautiously by people who are taking low-dose aspirin or other anticoagulant drugs as well as high doses of vitamin E, garlic, and ginkgo biloba extract. Fish oil supplements can cause belching and acid reflux.

Flavonoids

How they Work. Flavonoids (or bioflavonoids as they are also known) are antioxidants found in many foods, especially brightly colored fruits and vegetables. Some, such as quercetin, which enhances the effects of vitamin C, are thought to be effective against hay fever. Precisely how they work is unknown, although some studies suggest they reduce inflammation and perhaps histamine production. Some flavonoids appear to facilitate absorption of vitamins C and E through all membranes.

Recommended dosages. Quercetin is found in black tea, apples, and onions, but is most concentrated in grapes. It is available in tablet or capsule form; the usual dosage calls for 300 to 400 mg two or three times a day.

Possible problems. There are no reports of adverse effects.

■ BOTANICAL MEDICINES

Nettle (*Urtica dioica*)

How it works. Nettle is high in quercetin, a flavonoid that reduces histamine production. Several studies have found that nettle can help reduce the nasal congestion, runny nose, watery eyes, and itching of hay fever.

Recommended dosages. The usual dosage calls for taking two or three 250-mg nettle capsules three times a day, prior to the start of the usual hay fever season. It may also be taken as a tea brewed from dried nettle leaves.

Possible problems. There have been some reports of diarrhea and indigestion caused by nettle, especially when it is taken in high doses. Some people are also allergic to nettle and should avoid it.

Licorice (*Glycyrrhiza glabra*)

How it works. Glycyrrhizin, the active ingredient in licorice root, helps counteract the symptoms of allergies and asthma by reducing inflammation. Other substances in licorice thin mucus; it is also a demulcent that coats and soothes respiratory passages and the intestines, thereby reducing irritation that may accompany an allergic reaction. It may also be applied to allergic rashes to ease itching and inflammation.

Recommended dosages. The usual daily dosage calls for 5 to 6 g, standardized to provide 22 percent glycyrrhizin, for up to a maximum of five or six weeks.

Possible problems. Glycyrrhizin can cause swelling, potassium loss, high blood pressure, headaches, heart failure, and even death when consumed in excess. Do not use licorice that contains glycyrrhizin if you have high blood pressure, edema, or liver, kidney, or heart disease. Also, do not take it if you are also are taking a thiazide diuretic to treat high blood pressure because glycyrrhizin increases the loss of potassium that occurs with these medications. Avoid taking licorice root for more than six weeks without medical advice. Deglycyrrizinated licorice, or DGL, does not contain glycyrrhizin and is safe to use to soothe irritated respiratory passages and digestive upsets.

ALZHEIMER'S DISEASE AND MEMORY LOSS

Although Alzheimer's disease gets the most attention, it is actually only one of several types of dementia that cause memory loss. In dementia, the brain's cognitive functions, such as reasoning, thinking, and judgment, progressively deteriorate. This decline can occur rapidly within months or slowly over years.

Alzheimer's disease affects some 4 million Americans. As the population ages, that number could climb to 8 to 10 million by the year 2020. Now known to be the chief cause of age-related dementia, until recently Alzheimer's was considered quite rare. Overall, an estimated 10 percent of the population over the age of sixty-five suffers from the disease. But the numbers are overwhelmingly weighted toward the over-eighty-five group, in which it affects an estimated 47 percent of the population.

It has long been known that Alzheimer's patients have abnormal protein deposits and clusters of dead tissue in their brains. The cause or causes remain unknown, although research is yielding clues on the molecular changes that occur in the brain as the disease unfolds. It is not completely clear whether Alzheimer's runs in families, with the exception of the early-onset form of the disease, which typically strikes several members of the same family beginning in middle age. However, at least one study found that if one identical twin develops Alzheimer's disease, the other's risk is as high as 50 percent, which strongly suggests a genetic predisposition. Alzheimer's occurs commonly in people with

◉ **SYMPTOMS**

The Alzheimer's Association has developed a list of warning signs suggestive of Alzheimer's disease. It is important to know that many of these symptoms may occur in a wide number of other illnesses or for other reasons. Also, age-related memory loss and forgetfulness are not in themselves abnormal. In Alzheimer's, the memory loss is more profound and serious, associated with problems communicating, learning, thinking, and reasoning, including:

- Memory loss that affects job skills.
- Difficulty performing familiar tasks.
- Problems with language, numbers, math, finances.
- Disorientation to time and place.
- Poor or decreased judgment.
- Problems with abstract thinking.
- Misplacing things.
- Changes in mood or behavior; increased irritability and depression.
- Changes in personality.
- Loss of initiative.
- Daytime sleepiness.
- Self neglect, decreased hygiene.

The Alzheimer's Association recommends nondrug approaches to managing behavioral problems as the first treatment option for Alzheimer's patients.

• *Family education and counseling* help family members learn what to expect and how to cope with the changes in behavior of a loved one. Help is available through local chapters of the Alzheimer's Association.

• *Controlling the environment,* by manipulating factors such as lighting, color, and noise, can have a major impact on the behavior of someone suffering from Alzheimer's disease. Low lighting may make some Alzheimer's patients feel uneasy. Loud noises can cause agitation and disorientation. Surrounding the patient with familiar personal belongings can have a calming and orienting effect.

• *Planned activities* may help alleviate depression and agitation, and prevent wandering off from home.

To keep the mind sharp and fight age-related memory loss:

• *Develop interests or hobbies* that stimulate both body and mind.

• *Limit the intake of alcoholic beverages.* They dull the senses, damage brain cells, and can increase the risk of bleeding into the brain.

• *Reduce stress.* It can rob the mind of its full potential and increase cortisol levels.

• *Eat a diet rich in fruits and vegetables,* which provide a vast array of antioxidant vitamins and phytochemicals.

• *Get treatment for depression.* Forgetfulness can be a symptom of depression.

• *Use memory triggers.* To-do lists, calendars, Post-it Notes, alarm clocks, and other common reminder tools can keep important information at hand and help relieve the stress that comes from forgetting things.

• *Exercise regularly.* Studies show that daily physical activity improves cognitive functioning.

• *Engage in problem-solving.* Traveling, gardening, playing cards, doing crossword puzzles, and learning anything new encourages the growth of new nerve (synaptic) connections in the brain.

Down's syndrome, and it also appears that having a close relative with Down's syndrome increases the risk.

Another common type of dementia is called multi-infarct dementia or vascular dementia. It is caused by a series of small strokes or changes in the brain's blood supply that cause brain tissue to die. The location in the brain where the small strokes occur determines the nature and seriousness of the symptoms. High blood pressure and diabetes are often to blame.

Dementia often accompanies other conditions as well. For example, up to 40 percent of people with Parkinson's disease will develop dementia as the disease progresses. Also, conditions such as heart disease, stroke, diabetes, and high blood pressure damage blood vessels in the brain, increasing the risk of dementia. Smoking can exacerbate all of these conditions.

Although it is not yet known how to prevent Alzheimer's, researchers have discovered that people who often use nonsteroidal anti-inflammatory drugs (NSAIDs), such as ibuprofen, may have as much as a 60 percent lower risk of developing Alzheimer's disease, compared to nonusers. It is thought that these drugs might reduce inflammation of brain tissue, which may play a pivotal role in the development of the disease. Women who take estrogen replacement therapy following menopause may have significantly lower rates of Alzheimer's disease.

Diagnostic Steps

No blood test, X ray, or brain imaging technique available can definitively diagnose Alzheimer's, although many are in development and appear promising. An absolute diagnosis can be made only by an autopsy of the brain after a person's death. A newly available urine test for a protein that is commonly elevated in people with the disease may prove helpful in identifying some people at high risk. In most cases, diagnosis generally depends on a person's medical history and the clinical judgment of an experienced physician.

Many other conditions can mimic some or many of Alzheimer's symptoms, such as depression, nutritional deficiencies, brain tumors, head injuries, thyroid problems, alcohol abuse, even use of some prescription medications. These must always be ruled out before a diagnosis of Alzheimer's disease can be made.

Conventional Treatments

There is no mainstream medical treatment available that has been proven to cure or stop the progression of Alzheimer's disease. However, there are two FDA-approved drugs—donepezil (Aricept) and tacrine (Cognex)—that may temporarily relieve symptoms in people with mild to moderate Alzheimer's.

Donepezil is taken once a day, at bedtime. It can promote improvement in cognitive function, overall ability to function, and behavior. It has few harmful side effects; although it can sometimes cause diarrhea, nausea, vomiting, insomnia, fatigue, and loss of appetite, these generally decline with continued use.

Tacrine is taken four times a day, and not everyone can tolerate it. The most common serious side effect is possible liver damage; other possible side effects include nausea, vomiting, diarrhea, abdominal pain, indigestion, and a skin rash.

For the associated psychiatric symptoms that often accompany Alzheimer's, such as agitation, aggression, paranoia, delusions, and depression, a variety of antipsychotics, antianxiety drugs, and antidepressants are often prescribed.

Many treatments, including a possible vaccine, are currently in development to prevent or slow the progression of Alzheimer's. In clinical trials are drugs such as galantamine, derived from daffodils. Trials using vitamin E (see p. 216) are proving very promising. Recently, researchers reported discovering an enzyme involved in the formation of the brain protein tangles characteristic of Alzheimer's. Ultimately, this and other basic-science discoveries could lead to development of drugs to prevent or treat the disease.

Nutraceuticals for Alzheimer's Disease and Memory Loss

■ VITAMINS AND MINERALS

Vitamin E

How it works. Vitamin E has antioxidant properties that may counteract destructive damage to brain cells from free radicals.

Recommended dosages. A major study, funded by the National Institute on Aging, is currently under way to test the effectiveness of 2,000 IU a day on mild cognitive impairment, believed to be a forerunner of dementia, including Alzheimer's disease. A 1997 study found this level of vitamin E slowed some aspects of cognitive decline in people with Alzheimer's.

Possible problems. Although the 2,000-IU dose was tolerated well in the 1997 study, it may be associated with increased risk of bleeding in some people, especially those taking anticoagulant medications.

Vitamin B$_{12}$

How it works. Vitamin B$_{12}$ is necessary for building and maintaining the protective shield (myelin) around nerve cells in the spinal cord and brain. Inadequate vitamin B$_{12}$, which is most common in people over sixty, causes neurological problems that can result in changes in behavior, loss of memory, and a diminished ability to think and process information properly. Studies have shown that B_{12} levels are low in some people with Alzheimer's.

Recommended dosages. For prevention or for mild memory problems, 6 mcg of B_{12} a day should be adequate for most people. Dosages from 100 to 1,000 mcg have been recommended, however. A high-potency B-vitamin-complex supplement will usually provide sufficient B_{12} along with folic acid and other B vitamins that are important to brain function.

Absorbing B_{12} through the stomach can be problematic for some people over sixty, who may require injections or a prescription for a nasal spray.

Potential problems. There are no reported adverse effects of taking large amounts of vitamin B_{12} either from food or supplements. However, as a precaution, a recommended safe limit has been set at 3,000 mcg a day.

■ NUTRITIONAL SUPPLEMENTS

L-Carnitine

How it works. Acetyl-L-carnitine, a derivative of carnitine, is similar in structure to the brain neurotransmitter acetylcholine, which is important for memory functions. Acetyl-L-carnitine protects brain cells from free radical damage that may contribute to memory loss. As well, the body is able to convert it to acetylcholine.

Recommended dosages. Several clinical trials suggest that doses of 1,500 to 3,000 mg of acetyl-L-carnitine a day may help slow the progression of Alzheimer's. One study found it to be most effective in younger Alzheimer's patients (sixty-one or younger).

Potential problems. No serious side effects have been seen in people taking these doses, although it may cause vomiting when taken on an empty stomach. However, it could cause overstimulation in people without Alzheimer's who take it for prevention.

Phosphatidylserine

How it works. Phosphatidylserine (PS) is a phospholipid, an essential component of cell membranes. PS is most concentrated in the brain, where it helps to keep brain cells fluid and to regulate neurotransmitters (brain chemicals that carry nerve messages). Research suggests it may improve concentration and memory in people suffering from age-related memory loss and dementia.

Recommended dosages. Studies suggest that 300 mg of PS a day, divided into three doses (100 mg three times a day) can offer modest improvement in cognitive function, especially in early stages of the disease. It may not be enough to improve day-to-day functioning, however. PS may be a greater aid to people suffering from normal age-related memory loss.

Potential problems. No side effects have been noted at this dosage.

Periwinkle Extract (Vinpocetine)

How it works. Vinpocetine has been shown to enhance memory and mental function, especially among older people who do not have Alzheimer's disease. Vinpocetine works in several ways: it protects brain cells against damage from normal metabolic changes; it increases cerebral blood flow and the brain's metabolism of energy and oxygen, and it speeds the brain's uptake of glucose, its major fuel. It appears to increase the production of neurotransmitters, brain chemicals such as serotonin, acetylcholine, and dopamine, which carry messages from one nerve cell to another.

Recommended dosages. The typical dosage calls for 15 mg a day, taken as 5 mg pills taken three times a day.

Potential problems. No major adverse effects have been found in more than 100 clinical studies worldwide involving more than 20,000 patients. However, some people who take high doses (more than 30 or 40 mg a day) have reported feeling hyperactive and overstimulated.

■ BOTANICAL MEDICINES

Ginkgo biloba extract

How it works. Flavonoids and ginkgolides in ginkgo leaves make capillaries less fragile, fight against free radical damage, and improve blood flow to the brain.

Recommended dosages. The recommended daily dosage for cerebral circulatory disturbances including early-stage dementia is 120 to 240 mg a day divided into two or three doses. It may take at least six to eight weeks of treatment, possibly as long as six months, for benefits to show. Two recent clinical studies have confirmed the effectiveness of ginkgo biloba extract in modestly improving cognitive function in Alzheimer's.

Possible problems. Side effects are not common, although they can include gastrointestinal disturbances, headaches, and allergic skin reactions. Some researchers have suggested that large doses may cause bleeding abnormalities in people already at risk for such problems. Persons taking NSAIDs, aspirin, and blood thinners, especially warfarin (Coumadin), should not take ginkgo biloba extract.

ANEMIA

The run-down, irritable, and exhausted feelings often associated with anemia result when the body's tissues do not get the oxygen they need from red blood cells. Anemic red blood cells may be deficient in number, poorly formed, or lack adequate hemoglobin, an iron-rich pigment that

- Fatigue that sleep won't cure.
- General weakness.
- Pale skin.
- Headaches.
- Always feeling cold.
- Chewing or craving ice.
- Brittle, spoon-shaped nails.
- Difficulty breathing upon exertion.
- Fainting spells.
- Irregular heartbeat.

carries oxygen to cells throughout the body. Although mild anemia may not be apparent or dangerous, severe anemia can be life-threatening.

There are numerous types and causes of anemia. Dietary deficiencies of iron and the B vitamins, especially folic acid and B_{12}, are at the root of most cases.

Iron-deficiency anemia reigns as the most common type of anemia, particularly among children, teens, and women in their childbearing years. An iron shortfall causes the body to form smaller red blood cells that are less efficient in delivering oxygen, which can be especially detrimental during periods of rapid growth and development. Blood loss is a common cause of iron-deficiency anemia, since nearly all of the body's iron is bound to red blood cells and recycled to help form new hemoglobin when old blood cells die. Blood loss during menstruation and childbirth puts women of childbearing age at high risk. Both men and women can lose significant amounts of blood from bleeding ulcers or tumors in the GI tract. Although adequate dietary iron can ordinarily offset iron losses, many people at high risk do not ingest sufficient iron or their bodies cannot absorb it.

Deficiencies of vitamin B_{12} and/or folic acid contribute to production of red blood cells that are oversized, fewer in number, and fragile. These two nutrients are required for healthy production of red blood cells in the bone marrow.

• *Vitamin B_{12} anemia,* also called *pernicious anemia,* is usually caused by poor absorption rather than inadequate consumption. Many people with B_{12} anemia lack a substance known as intrinsic factor, which is made in the stomach lining and is needed for proper B_{12} absorption. This type of anemia is most common among people over forty. In the elderly, pernicious anemia can cause confusion and other symptoms that may be mistaken for Alzheimer's disease. Diets low in vitamin B_{12} can also contribute to pernicious anemia, but usually only in strict vegetarians, since vitamin B_{12} is naturally present only in animal foods.

• *Megaloblastic anemia,* a condition induced by a poor supply of folic acid, can be the result of poor absorption, dietary deficiency, and an increased need for folic acid when demands are high, such as during pregnancy and breast-feeding.

Acute and chronic medical conditions also produce anemia. For example, hemolytic anemia results when the body destroys red blood cells faster than it can make them. Cancer, including leukemia, is one cause of hemolytic anemia, which can also be prompted by a malfunctioning spleen; autoimmune disorders, including lupus and rheumatoid arthritis; and kidney disease, among others.

Genetic Disorders, such as sickle-cell disease and thalassemia, can also cause severe forms of anemia. These two conditions are characterized by abnormal hemoglobin production.

Diagnostic Steps

A variety of blood tests will confirm anemia, depending on its cause. These ordinarily begin with a complete blood count and a blood smear, which will show the size and shape of the blood cells. Tests for iron deficiency include blood levels of ferritin and total iron binding capacity, and transferrin saturation. A complete medical workup may be necessary to detect the underlying cause of iron deficiency. Testing for blood levels of folic acid and vitamin B_{12} will determine whether deficiencies in these nutrients are present.

Conventional Treatments

When anemia results from nutritional deficiency, supplements are the primary treatment. For B_{12} or other deficiencies resulting from poor absorption, however, the vitamin must often be given by injection. Iron-deficiency anemia resulting from menstruation may be mitigated by increasing iron in the diet. Other possible sources of chronic blood loss must be pinpointed and treated, to preserve iron stores. And, of course, any underlying illness or condition that is associated with the anemia must be treated. In cases of severe anemia, blood transfusions may be needed to quickly restore the blood's hemoglobin. Periodic injections of erythropoietin, a hormone that stimulates red blood cell production, may also be used to treat severe anemia.

Current medications may need adjustment, since some, including aspirin, may interfere with vitamin or mineral absorption or cause chronic bleeding. Alcoholics are at special risk for folic acid deficiency, so alcohol moderation or counseling may be advised. Even excessive coffee and tea—more than two or three cups a day—can reduce iron absorption and contribute to anemia.

Nutraceuticals for Anemia

■ VITAMINS AND MINERALS

Iron

How it works. Iron is imbedded in hemoglobin, the portion of the red blood cell that binds with oxygen in the lungs and transports it to every cell. In food, iron comes in two forms: heme and nonheme. Heme iron is the primary type found in animal foods such as seafood, meat, and poultry. It is absorbed by the body at three times the rate of non-heme iron, the dominant form in foods of plant origin, including dried apricots, raisins, green leafy vegetables, breads, grains, and cereals.

Recommended dosages. Ordinarily, women in their childbearing years need 15 mg of iron daily; 30 mg when pregnant to reduce iron deficiency risk. After age fifty, a woman's iron needs drop to 10 mg a day, which is the same amount adult men require throughout life. Higher doses, which should be determined by a doctor or clinical dietitian, are needed to treat iron-deficiency anemia. Do not take iron supplements with coffee or tea, which contain tannins that decrease the body's iron uptake. Instead, swallow iron pills with orange, grapefruit, or vitamin C–fortified juice, as vitamin C–rich foods and beverages boost iron absorption. To that end, pair vitamin C–rich foods such as tomatoes, oranges, grapefruits, strawberries, kiwi, and green pepper with enriched breads, cereals, and grains to boost the availability of nonheme iron from these foods.

Possible problems. Supplemental iron irritates the stomach. Taking pills with food often prevents or reduces indigestion. Consuming a high-fiber diet helps alleviate supplemental iron's constipating qualities, but too much bran interferes with iron absorption.

Folic acid

How it works. Folic acid helps make hemoglobin and DNA, the cells' blueprint for replicating themselves. Folic acid is the synthetic form of its naturally occurring cousin, folacin or folate. The body is much better at absorbing folic acid, making it the form of choice to correct anemia. By law, folic acid must be added to enriched breads, pastas, grains, and cereals, and it is the form found in vitamin supplements. Folate is plentiful in legumes, dark green leafy vegetables, and orange juice.

Recommended dosages. Adults need 400 mcg of folic acid a day in addition to a folacin-rich diet. Pregnancy boosts folic acid requirements to 600 mcg daily; while lactating women need 500 mcg. Higher doses may be needed to treat megaloblastic anemia, however; these should be determined by a doctor or clinical dietitian.

Possible problems. Long-term use of high-dose folic acid supplements can mask a vitamin B_{12} deficiency, which can cause permanent nerve damage. In general, excess intake of one B vitamin may interfere with the absorption of others, so supplements should be balanced. In one study of excess folic acid, more than 15 mg a day for a month was associated with sleep problems, mental changes, and stomach upset. The National Academy of Sciences Food and Nutrition Board has established a daily tolerable upper intake level of 1,000 mcg. (See Folacin, p. 237.)

Vitamin B_{12}

How it works. Vitamin B_{12} works closely with folic acid to ensure healthy blood cells; a shortfall decreases cell production and compromises their quality. Vitamin B_{12} is unique to animal foods. However, it is a common ingredient in fortified cereals, soy milks, and other fortified nondairy milks. Check the labels. Up to 30 percent of older people don't fully absorb the vitamin B_{12} found naturally in foods, but can absorb the synthetic version of the vitamin. Thus, people over age fifty should get their vitamin B_{12} largely from fortified foods or supplements, which contain forms that are easy to absorb.

Recommended dosages. Adults need 2 mcg of vitamin B_{12} daily. However, oral supplementation may not work to prevent vitamin B_{12} deficiency or correct anemia in those who lack the intrinsic factor necessary for absorption. To treat pernicious anemia, doctors typically give daily injections of 1,000 mcg, for three days, then weekly for three weeks, then monthly until the anemia abates. Alternative forms include a nasal B_{12} spray or sublingual tablets, which are placed under the tongue. These forms are absorbed directly into the bloodstream, and do not require intrinsic factor.

Possible problems. Excess vitamin B_{12} from food or supplements produces no known side effects.

■ BOTANICAL MEDICINES

Herbalists recommend a number of herbal tonics to help build healthy blood and prevent or treat anemia. Most of these botanicals are rich in iron or the B vitamins needed to build and maintain red blood cells; if you have been diagnosed as having anemia, check with your doctor before taking any nutraceutical product to avoid possible interactions or adverse effects.

Dandelion (*Taraxacum officinale*)

How it works. Dandelion root extract and tea have long been used to prevent or treat anemia as well as liver disease and numerous other disorders. Dandelion is a good source of iron as well as vitamin C, which promote iron absorption.

Recommended dosages. Herbalists typically recommend 1 teaspoon of dandelion tincture diluted in a cup of water to be taken morning and night. To bolster dietary intake of iron and numerous other greens, serve lightly cooked dandelion greens as a vegetable dish.

Possible problems. Dandelion greens are generally safe and cause few if any problems. However, they can act as a diuretic and lower potassium levels, and should not be used by patients taking blood pressure or cardiac medications. The root extract, which increases the flow of bile and gastric juices, should be used with caution—if at all—by people who suffer from gallstones, gastritis, and peptic ulcers.

◉ STRATEGIES FOR RELIEF
Because the causes of anemia are so varied, self-medicating is never a good idea. If changing to a more healthy, balanced diet does not relieve symptoms, consult a health professional. Left unchecked, inadequate nutrition or other medical problems causing anemia can be life-threatening.

ANXIETY

Anxiety disorders are our most common psychiatric illnesses, affecting more than 15 million Americans at any given time. Now and then, we all experience feelings of nervousness, dread, or apprehension—hallmarks of anxiety. Most of the time, these feelings are a perfectly normal response to stress. When faced with what the brain perceives as a potential danger, the body is programmed to react by preparing to either fight or flee—the heart beats faster, muscles tense, blood pressure rises, and adrenaline and other stress hormones flood the body. Anxiety becomes a disorder when the feelings get out of hand and interfere with normal life.

Anxiety disorders take different forms; some of the more common include:

- *Generalized anxiety disorder (GAD),* a chronic free-floating feeling of dread and apprehension with no identifiable cause.
- *Panic attacks,* in which the feelings of dread seem to strike "out of the blue" and are far more intense than in GAD.
- *Phobias,* which are persistent and irrational fears of an object, activity, or situation, such as intense fears of spiders, flying, or leaving home.
- *Obsessive-compulsive disorder (OCD),* in which a person becomes preoccupied, or obsessed, with a specific thought or behavior, such as obsessive hand washing or constantly checking a stove to make sure it's turned off. Phobias are often a component of OCD.

Many researchers believe that anxiety disorders have organic rather than psychological origins, but the precise cause is unknown. Because anxiety disorders tend to run in families, there may well be a genetic component. Other possible culprits include an imbalance in brain chemicals; a tendency to overbreathe (hyperventilation), which results in abnormal carbon dioxide in the blood; and a buildup of lactic acid, a body chemical that is normally produced during vigorous exercise.

Diagnostic Steps

Some anxiety disorders, such as phobias and OCD, are easily diagnosed based on their symptoms. Others, such as generalized anxiety and panic attacks, may not be so obvious because the physical symptoms often mimic heart attacks, intestinal disorders, and other illnesses. In such cases, a thorough physical examination and tests are needed to rule out heart disease and other serious disorders.

Conventional Treatments

Anxiety disorders are usually treated with a combination of psychotherapy and medication; common choices include benzodiazepine drugs, such as alprazolam (Xanax), or antidepressants, such as fluoxetine (Prozac) or sertraline (Zoloft). These drugs should be taken only under the supervision of a physician, especially in the beginning; some people experience bizarre reactions, including suicidal urges. Psychotherapy may take the form of one-on-one counseling, behavior modification, and group therapy. Alternative therapies, such as hypnosis, guided imagery or visualization, and music, drama, or art therapies, may also be tried.

Nutraceuticals for Anxiety

■ BOTANICAL MEDICINES

Many herbal medicines have a calming effect, and are age-old folk remedies for anxiety. These are some of the most effective.

Kava (*Piper methysticum*)

How it works. German studies indicate that the plant's kavalactones work to mildly depress action of the brain's limbic system, which controls emotions. In effect, it calms jittery nerves in much the same manner as pharmaceutical antianxiety drugs, but without causing dependency and withdrawal symptoms when kava is stopped. Kava has been used in the South Pacific for centuries to promote feelings of well-being and relaxation.

Recommended dosages. Look for a kava extract standardized to provide at least 30 percent kavalactone. A typical dosage calls for 300 mg of kava extract three times a day.

Possible problems. Kava should not be used with alcohol or other drugs that depress the central nervous system. Because it can cause sleepiness, it should not be taken before driving or operating dangerous machinery. It is also contraindicated in people suffering from clinical depression, and should not be used during pregnancy or breast-feeding. Some cases of paradoxical hypertension linked to kava use have been reported; blood pressure returns to normal when the kava is stopped. A kava abuse syndrome has been identified and results in confusion, memory loss, conjunctivitis, yellow nails, scaly skin, and seizures.

St. John's wort (*Hypericum perforatum*)

How it works. A number of European studies, as well as some in the United States, show that St. John's wort is an effective treatment for mild depression. Because free-floating anxiety is often a component of depression, it's commonly assumed that St. John's wort can also combat these on-edge feelings. Researchers do not know precisely how St. John's wort works, but researchers theorize that extracts of the flowering tops act as selective serotonin reuptake inhibitors (SSRIs), similar to the action of Prozac and other SSRI antidepressants. Hypericin is considered the active ingredient, but other compounds such as hyperforin in the plant probably also contribute to its action.

Recommended dosages. Look for pills, capsules, or extract that is standardized for 0.3 percent hypericin or a whole-plant extract. The

- Engage in regular exercise, such as brisk walking, jogging, tai chi, cycling, swimming, or other aerobic activities. Exercise has a calming effect and also causes the brain to increase its output of chemicals that have a calming effect.
- Cut back on or eliminate alcohol and caffeine (coffee, colas, tea) from the diet.
- Take time out each day for ten to fifteen minutes of deep breathing, meditation, visualization, or another relaxation exercise.
- Consider learning yoga and meditation, time-honored methods of quelling anxiety.
- Look at the stressors in your life and assess how well you are coping with them.

typical adult dosage calls for 300 mg of the standardized extract to be taken three times a day. St. John's wort causes stomach upset in some people, so it's a good idea to take it just before eating. Some people experience improvement in only a few days, but plan to allow four to six weeks to begin to notice results.

Possible problems. In theory, St. John's wort may make the skin more sensitive to sunlight or ultraviolet lamps, although this phenomenon has not been reported among any of the participants in numerous medical studies. Still, it's a good idea to always apply a sunblock with an SPF (sun protection factor) of at least 15 before going outdoors because, with or without St. John's wort, the sun damages the skin and increases the risk of skin cancer. Some experts caution that St. John's wort may interact with foods high in tyramine, such as aged cheeses, red wine, and yeast. Again, this is a theoretical risk that has never been observed in humans.

St. John's wort should not be taken with antidepressant drugs like Prozac or Zoloft, or drugs such as lithium, demerol, or dextromethorphan because they may magnify their effects. It should not be used during pregnancy or breast-feeding.

Valerian (*Valeriana officinalis*)

How it works. Valerian is an ancient remedy for anxiety and insomnia, but researchers do not know how it works. One prevailing theory holds that it binds to certain receptors in the brain to exert its calming and sedating effects.

Recommended dosages. Look for extracts containing 0.8 percent valerenic acids. The standard dosage is 150 to 300 mg, although up to 500 mg is considered safe. It is generally taken before bedtime to quell restlessness and promote sleep.

Possible problems. Valerian should not be consumed with alcohol or other drugs that depress the central nervous system. As with kava, it should not be taken before driving or operating machinery. Both kava and valerian should be avoided for one week before undergoing anesthesia.

ARTHRITIS

Arthritis, which literally means inflammation of the joint, is an umbrella term commonly used to cover nearly one hundred different disorders that affect the joints and bones. Rheumatic disease is a more accurate term for these disorders, however, since not all involve inflammation.

According to the Arthritis Foundation, some 40 million Americans suffer from one or more types of arthritis. Women are affected more than men, accounting for 23.5 million sufferers. The two most common types—osteoarthritis and rheumatoid arthritis—are discussed here; gout is covered on page 115 and lupus on page 157.

Osteoarthritis, also called degenerative joint disease, affects about 16 million Americans, most of them over the age of forty-five. It affects only joints and their surrounding tissue, and it may or may not be accompanied by inflammation. Traditionally, physicians have considered it a "wear-and-tear" disease and a normal part of aging. Recent research, however, dispels this notion, indicating that it is actually a disorder that impairs normal cartilage regeneration, but what causes the destructive process remains unknown. Any sport or occupation that involves chronic trauma or repetitive motions can cause premature osteoarthritis. For example, ballerinas may suffer arthritis in their ankles, football players in their knees. Assembly line workers who perform repetitive movements show far more degeneration in their dominant hands.

Rheumatoid arthritis (RA), which affects about 1.2 million Americans, is an autoimmune disease, in which the immune system attacks healthy tissue. The result is painful inflammation, starting in the joints and often extending to other tissues throughout the body. What starts the destructive process remains unknown but likely involves a genetic predisposition triggered by one or more environmental agents, such as a virus. Although RA lasts for life, it is a disease that tends to come and go, with periodic remissions, when symptoms abate, interspersed between flares, when symptoms worsen. Severe rheumatoid arthritis can be crippling, and its damage may extend to the lungs, skin, blood vessels, muscles, heart, and eyes.

Diagnostic Steps

Because there are so many different types of rheumatic disease, it's important not to self-diagnose. Chronic aches and pains are not a normal part of growing older, so always consult a health professional. Diagnosis is based on a complete physical examination, description of your symptoms, blood tests, and X rays.

Conventional Treatments

Together with lifestyle modifications, such as losing excess weight and regular exercise, mainstream treatments involve several types of drugs. Most provide relief of symptoms rather than cure of the underlying illness. Several new types of drugs and many that are in development, however, also directly attack the disease process underlying inflammatory types of arthritis. Vaccines that may help curtail the autoimmune response are currently in development.

◉ SYMPTOMS

Osteoarthritis
- Mild aching to severe pain and loss of mobility, especially in the evening, due to joint stiffness.
- Usually afflicts weight-bearing joints, such as the hips, knees, and spine, as well as the finger joints.

Rheumatoid arthritis
- Swelling, stiffness, tenderness, redness and pain in several or many joints throughout the body. Usually most severe in the morning.
- Pain is usually symmetrical; that is, the same joint—the wrist or knee, for example—is affected on both sides of the body.
- Fever.
- Weight loss.
- Fatigue.
- Joint deformity.
- General malaise, especially during a flare-up of symptoms.

● STRATEGIES FOR RELIEF

▪ *Exercise.* Numerous studies have shown that exercise can be critically important in improving the quality of life in people with arthritis. Exercise maintains flexibility, improves mobility, and combats the debilitating fatigue that is associated with the disease itself, the accompanying pain, and deconditioning that follows excessive rest. Most people report that once they achieve an exercise routine, they find that activity energizes them. Many people start with a walking program, beginning at just ten minutes a day and slowly increasing. Working with weights can strengthen muscles that support the joints and ease the stress on them, lessening the chronic pain. A physical therapist can help you plan a safe regimen.

▪ *Eat a healthful diet.* Some research suggests that diets low in fat, especially animal fat, can help reduce the inflammation that causes pain. A study of people with rheumatoid arthritis showed that those who most closely followed the Dr. Ornish Healthy Heart diet had the least pain, swelling, and disability. So reduce your intake of meat, poultry, and dairy, increase your intake of fish, and eat lots of fresh fruits and vegetables and whole grains.

▪ *Lose weight.* A healthy diet and regular exercise can also promote weight loss. Extra weight puts an extra burden on your hips, knees, ankles, and feet. Gradual weight loss from better eating and more activity results in lower joint stress and less pain.

▪ *Take a hot bath or shower* first thing in the morning to ease joint stiffness and help you get moving.

▪ *Sleep and rest.* To reduce fatigue, get at least eight hours of sleep at night and balance your day with one or more half-hour rest breaks between periods of activity.

▪ *Reduce stress.* Stress triggers flare-ups. Learn relaxation techniques to practice during your rest breaks. Support groups, sponsored by the Arthritis Foundation, may help.

• *Nonsteroidal anti-inflammatory drugs (NSAIDs),* which include aspirin, ibuprofen, and other nonprescription painkillers as well as more potent prescription formulations. These drugs can increase the risk of stomach upset, ulcers, and potentially catastrophic bleeding. Rarely, these drugs cause damage to kidneys and liver, especially in older adults. (Note: Although acetaminophen does not quell inflammation, it may relieve osteoarthritis that is not causing inflammation.)

• *COX-2 inhibitors.* These, the newest types of NSAIDs, are supposed to cause fewer side effects, and early studies suggest that gastrointestinal side effects are indeed less of a problem than with conventional NSAIDs. The full side-effect profile of these drugs is not likely to emerge until they've been in use for some time, however. Potential risks to kidneys and liver remain, particularly among the elderly. Celebrex and Vioxx are two drugs in this category, and more are on their way.

• *Joint-fluid injections.* Used to treat osteoarthritis of the knees, Synvisc and Hyalgan are synthetic versions of hyaluronic acid, a normal part of joint fluid. The fluid is injected directly into the knee joint once a week for three to five weeks; they seem to improve the viscosity and elasticity of joint fluid, the way oil keeps car engines lubricated and running smoothly. The result can be freedom from pain for six months or more.

• *Corticosteroids,* such as prednisone, prednisolone, methylprednisolone, and dexamethasone, reduce inflammation and suppress the immune system. They can produce dramatic results in treating acute arthritis. However, because long-term use increases the risk of diabetes, osteoporosis, cataracts, and other problems, these are used at the lowest possible dose for the shortest period of time. For people with rheumatoid or other inflammatory types of arthritis, a corticosteroid injection directly into the joint can help, especially when only one or two joints are involved.

• *DMARDs* (disease modifying antirheumatic drugs) are increasingly the drugs of choice for rheumatoid or other inflammatory types of arthritis. They appear to slow the disease and bring it into remission. Drugs in this category include gold compounds, hydroxychloroquine, penicillamine, and sulfasalazine. DMARDs require periodic testing to monitor possibly serious side effects. These drugs usually take months to produce beneficial effects, and their effectiveness often diminishes over the long term.

• *Immunosuppressants,* in the DMARDs category, are given to those with the most severe rheumatoid arthritis; drugs in this category include methotrexate, azathioprine, and cyclophosphamide. Frequent monitoring for potentially severe side effects, including dangerous infections, is required. These drugs, too, may lose their effectiveness over time.

• *Biologicals*—the newest approach to treating severe rheumatoid arthritis—work by targeting specific parts of the immune system. For example, Enbrel targets tumor necrosis factor (TNF), a protein that attaches itself to cells that cause inflammation in joints and that is produced in excess in rheumatoid arthritis. Arava is another drug in this category, and others are being developed.

• *Surgery* can be useful to clean out a joint damaged by arthritis debris. In the worst cases, a severely affected joint can be replaced surgically. With the painful joint substituted with a metal and plastic prosthesis, most people can return to a normal, active life.

Nutraceuticals for Arthritis

■ VITAMINS AND MINERALS

Several studies have shown that people with various types of arthritis, especially rheumatoid arthritis, have underlying vitamin and/or mineral deficiencies. It is not known whether these deficiencies stem from poor nutrition or from how nutrients are absorbed or metabolized. A daily multivitamin supplement with minerals is commonly recommended. Specific vitamin and mineral supplements that may be helpful include the following.

Vitamin C

How it works. Vitamin C is one of the antioxidant vitamins that can neutralize free redicals, which can damage or destroy cells. It also helps synthesize collagen, the gluelike substance in cartilage. Data from the large, ongoing Framingham study found that vitamin C intake was associated with reduced risk of osteoarthritis progression as well as reduced risk of developing osteroarthritis-related knee pain.

Recommended dosages. As little as 100 mg of vitamin C a day made the difference in the Framingham study, but some practitioners recommend 500 to 1,000 mg a day.

Possible problems. Large doses (over 1,000 mg) can cause gastrointestinal problems, including cramps and diarrhea, and increase the risk of kidney stones in susceptible people.

Vitamin E

How it works. Vitamin E, another important antioxidant, also protects against cell damage from free radicals. Studies have shown that people with some forms of inflammatory arthritis, including lupus, may have abnormally low levels of vitamin E.

Recommended dosages. A German study of people with rheumatoid arthritis showed that 1,500 IU of vitamin E daily yielded improvements in pain, grip strength, and morning stiffness equal to that of standard doses of diclofenac (a powerful NSAID drug) without the stomach upset of NSAIDs.

Possible problems. High doses have sometimes been associated with risk of bleeding, especially in those taking anticoagulant medications. In general, 1,500 IU of natural (d-alpha) vitamin E is the maximum safe dose, and many doctors advise against taking more than 1,000 IU a day.

Folic acid

How it works. Folic acid supplements are essential for people taking the drug methotrexate, often prescribed for rheumatoid arthritis. Methotrexate reduces levels of this important B vitamin in the body. Folic acid supplements also help reduce methotrexate side effects, such as nausea and diarrhea.

Recommended dosages. Dosing will vary depending on your methotrexate dosage and schedule.

Possible problems. Prolonged, excessive folic acid can mask pernicious anemia. It can also cause sleep problems, mental changes, and stomach upset. (See Folacin, p. 237.)

Vitamin D

How it works. Another study based on the Framingham population found that the risk of osteoarthritis progression was three times higher in people with low vitamin D intake. Vitamin D is necessary for the body to absorb and use calcium, and anyone taking calcium supplements (see below) will need to supplement with vitamin D.

Recommended dosages. Doctors recommend 200 to 400 IU twice a day with calcium.

Possible problems. Prolonged intake of dosages greater than 1,000 IU a day can lead to vitamin D toxicity; symptoms include headaches, weight loss, kidney stones, and possibly, in rare cases, blindness, deafness, and death. Anyone suffering from sarcoidosis or hyperparathyroidism should not supplement with vitamin D.

Calcium

How it works. If you are taking corticosteroid drugs such as prednisone for your arthritis, you need calcium supplements to help prevent bone loss.

Recommended dosages. Depending on your diet and risk factors for such diseases as osteoporosis (p. 175), your doctor may recommend 500 mg taken two or three times a day. Virtually all women need 1,200 to 1,500 mg daily.

Possible problems. Calcium should not be taken if you have hyperparathyroidism, sarcoidosis, or calcium-based kidney stones.

■ NUTRITIONAL SUPPLEMENTS

Glucosamine sulfate

How it works. Glucosamine is a form of a natural body chemical that plays a critical role in building cartilage, the spongy material that cushions bone ends. Glucosamine seems to help repair the cartilage damage caused by osteoarthritis. Over the past two decades more than a half dozen controlled clinical studies have demonstrated its ability to relieve the pain of osteoarthritis. In addition, a number of well-controlled studies have found that it works best when given along with chondroitin sulfate (see below).

Recommended dosages. The starting dosage is usually 500 mg three times daily. Symptom relief begins in two to four weeks. The dosage can often be reduced to twice a day after a few months. Improvement progresses with continued use, but benefits last only about a month after stopping.

Possible problems. Most people have no problems taking glucosamine. A small minority experience stomach upset, which can usually be remedied by taking it with meals. People with diabetes should use glucosamine with caution, since it can increase blood glucose levels.

Chondroitin sulfate

How it works. Chondroitin sulfate is another building block of cartilage and may work best when taken with glucosamine sulfate.

Recommended dosages. The starting dose is usually 400 mg three times daily. Many health food stores carry capsules that combine this dose with 500 mg of glucosamine, but caution is needed in selecting these products as laboratory analyses have found that many do not contain therapeutic amounts of one or both ingredients. (See Appendix A, "Resources and Guidelines on Buying and Using Nutraceuticals.") After a few months, twice-daily dosages may be sufficient.

Possible problems. Capsules may be too large for some people to swallow. If so, open the capsule and mix the contents with food or juice.

GLA (gamma-linolenic acid)

How it works. Several studies have shown benefits from use of supplements of gamma-linolenic acid (GLA), a fatty acid found in seed oils such as evening primrose oil and borage oil. Because abnormal fatty acid levels have been shown in various types of inflammatory arthritis, researchers have tested the benefits of supplements in people with rheumatoid arthritis and lupus, with good results. The body converts GLA to one form of prostaglandin, a hormonelike substance that acts as an anti-inflammatory.

Recommended dosages. If you want to try it, you must take high doses and be prepared to give it plenty of time to work. Studies showing benefits, which appear within four to eight weeks, have used from 525 mg to 2,000 mg of GLA daily. Some suggest taking at least 1,300 mg daily.

Possible problems. None are known. (See Essential Fatty Acids, p. 295)

SAM-e

How it works. S-adenosyl-methionine, commonly called SAM-e, is a substance produced in the body from protein. It is involved in a host of body processes, including the transmission of mood-boosting chemicals in the brain and promotion of healthy cartilage in joints.

Recommended dosages. Generally, dosages of 200 mg two or three times a day have been used.

Potential problems. SAM-e has been used in Germany and other European countries as a prescription drug for years, but it has only recently been made available in the United States. So far, no problems have been reported; in fact, in contrast to NSAIDs, SAM-e may protect the stomach instead of pose hazards.

Omega-3 fatty acids

How they work. Found in cold-water fish, such as tuna, salmon, mackerel, herring, and anchovies, and in flaxseed, omega-3 fatty acids have anti-inflammatory properties. As with GLA, above, studies have shown some benefit in rheumatoid arthritis.

Recommended dosages. Again, you need high doses taken over a period of time for benefits. Some studies suggest as high as 2.5g daily.

Possible problems. May increase bleeding problems in people taking anticlotting drugs. Some people find even modest doses may cause an upset stomach, including belching and indigestion. (See Essential Fatty Acids, p. 295.)

■ BOTANICAL MEDICINES

Capsaicin

How it works. Capsaicin is the substance in cayenne peppers that gives these hot chilies their "bite." When diluted and applied to the skin, it alleviates arthritis pain in at least two ways: it acts as a counterirritant that distracts from the underlying joint pain, and it also interferes with the action of substance P, a nerve chemical (neurotransmitter) that transmits pain messages to the brain.

Recommended dosages. Look for products that contain at least 0.025 percent capsaicin. Gently apply the cream directly to painful areas three or four times a day. Be sure skin surface is dry.

Potential problems. Be very careful not to let capsaicin come in contact with the eyes, delicate mucous membranes, or damaged or broken skin; such contact can result in tissue burning. Temporary stinging or burning of the skin is normal, but stop using the cream if it causes excessive or prolonged burning or a rash. (See Cayenne, p. 411.)

Boswellia (*Boswellia serrata*)

How it works. The gummy resin of this tree is high in boswellic acids, which have anti-inflammatory actions similar to NSAIDs, but without the stomach irritation and bleeding problems commonly caused by these drugs. Boswellic acids have long been used in Ayurvedic medicine to treat arthritis, bursitis, and other inflammatory disorders.

Recommended dosages. Practitioners typically recommend taking 150 mg of boswellic acid three times a day. Boswellia extracts are usually standardized to contain 37.5 to 65 percent of the active ingredient. Thus, it would take 400 mg of an extract standardized to contain 37.5 percent to provide 150 mg of boswellic acids. Improvement should be seen in a few weeks, and a typical course of treatment lasts twelve weeks.

Potential problems. Boswellia is generally safe; possible side effects include a skin rash, diarrhea, and nausea.

Ginger (*Zingiber officinale*)

How it works. Ginger can have a powerful anti-inflammatory impact on the body and has long been recommended, especially in Chinese medicine, for many types of arthritis.

Recommended dosages. An average dose is 1 to 2 g of powdered ginger a day, but some people report successful treatment of inflammatory conditions with higher doses taken over several months.

Potential problems. High doses may cause a burning sensation in the stomach; to minimize this, take ginger with food.

BRONCHITIS

Bronchitis is a common respiratory disorder in which one or more of the lung's airways (bronchi) become inflamed. Acute infectious bronchitis—the most common type—may be caused by bacteria, chlamydia or other bacterialike organisms, or viruses, often the same ones responsible for colds, flu, and other upper respiratory infections. In fact, bronchitis often starts as a cold or bout of flu. It may also be due to irritants, such as tobacco smoke, dust, air pollution, and noxious fumes. Asthma or allergies can also lead to bronchitis.

Bronchitis generally occurs in winter, and most healthy people recover fully in a week or two, although the cough sometimes lingers for several weeks. It usually is not a serious health threat except when it occurs in the frail elderly and persons with heart disease or a chronic lung disorder, such as emphysema. In these people, bronchitis can fur-

⊙ SYMPTOMS

- Initially, a runny nose, sore throat, chills, achy muscles, possible fever, and other symptoms of a cold or flu.
- An irritating cough that is dry (nonproductive) at first, but after a day or so, produces lots of thick phlegm, or sputum.
- Possible greenish or thick yellow sputum, an indication of a secondary bacterial infection.
- Possible high fever (101° to 102°F) that can last for three to five days, or longer if pneumonia develops.
- Burning chest pain, which worsens when coughing.
- Wheezing and shortness of breath, especially after coughing.

ther obstruct the flow of air in and out of the lungs, and also develop into pneumonia.

Bronchitis also poses a serious threat if it becomes chronic, defined as symptoms lasting three months or longer and occurring two years in a row. Smokers are especially vulnerable to chronic bronchitis, which is classified as a form of chronic obstructive pulmonary disease (COPD). It is often accompanied by emphysema, another form of COPD in which the tiny air sacs (alveoli) lose their elasticity and become filled with stale air.

Diagnostic Steps

In general, you should see a doctor for any productive cough that lasts longer than seven to ten days. Go sooner if you have a history of heart disease or asthma or other COPD; a high fever (over 102°F) that lasts more than two days; or sputum that becomes a thick, greenish yellow and has an unpleasant odor. A doctor can usually diagnose simple bronchitis on the basis of the cough and other typical symptoms. A chest X ray may be ordered to rule out pneumonia. A sputum culture can identify a bacterial infection.

Conventional Treatments

Doctors typically recommend aspirin (for adults only) or acetaminophen to relieve muscle aches and lower a fever. (Remember, abstain from alcohol when taking acetaminophen; combining the two can cause serious liver problems.) During the acute, feverish phase, you should increase your intake of fluids—water, broth, juices, weak tea, and other nonalcoholic drinks—to at least twelve glasses a day. This helps loosen phlegm and prevent dehydration due to the fever.

Antibiotics are prescribed to treat a bacterial infection. Prophylactic antibiotics are sometimes prescribed for patients with a history of chronic bronchitis, as well as those who have COPD or heart disease, to prevent a secondary bacterial infection. This practice is becoming increasingly controversial because, while it may prevent an infection, it can also foster development of superinfective strains of bacteria that are antibiotic-resistant and difficult to treat.

Cough suppressants are not recommended for any productive cough because coughing helps clear the airways of mucus. However, an over-the-counter expectorant—a medication that thins phlegm and makes it easier to cough up—may help. For obstructed breathing, a doctor may prescribe a bronchodilator, a medication that relaxes and widens the airways.

Nutraceuticals for Bronchitis

There are many home remedies and herbal products that help ease the inflammation of bronchitis and loosen phlegm. Some of the more common are discussed below.

▪ VITAMINS AND MINERALS

Zinc

How it works. Zinc is thought to boost the immune system and thereby shorten the duration of a cold and help prevent bronchitis.

Recommended dosages. Look for lozenges containing 15 to 20 mg of zinc gluconate, and take one every two to three hours during waking hours. A double-blind study, reported in 1996 in the *Annals of Internal Medicine* and involving one hundred persons suffering from cold symptoms, found that this approach cut in half the number of days the colds lasted.

Possible problems. Some people using zinc lozenges develop mouth sores and an upset stomach. High doses of zinc (more than 300 mg a day) actually reduce rather than boost immune function. Long-term use of excessive zinc can inhibit absorption of copper; to compensate, take 2 mg of copper a day. Zinc may also inhibit iron, magnesium, and calcium absorption. Using up to ten 15- to 20-mg lozenges for a few days to shorten the course of a cold and help prevent bronchitis is unlikely to be harmful, but consult a doctor or qualified nutritionist before exceeding the zinc RDA of 12 to 15 mg for any length of time.

▪ BOTANICAL MEDICINES

Echinacea (*E. purpurea; E. angustifolia, E. pallida*)

How it works. Echinacea stimulates the immune system, and numerous studies indicate that it is effective in shortening the course of a cold, flu, or other respiratory infection. Taken at the first sign of a cold or flu, it can help prevent bronchitis from developing. It may also help shorten the course of infectious bronchitis.

Recommended dosages. Dosages vary according to the form and potency of the echinacea product. For bronchitis, herbalists typically recommend preparations made with echinacea tincture (30 to 60 drops taken three times a day) or a daily dose of 6 to 9 ml of pressed juice (in a 2.5:1 concentration).

Possible problems. Because echinacea stimulates the immune system, it should not be used by people with autoimmune diseases, such as lupus, or progressive disorders, such as multiple sclerosis, TB, or AIDS, unless prescribed by a physician. It can also provoke a rare reaction in people allergic to plants in the Asteraceae family, which includes chamomile, yarrow, tansy, and goldenrod.

◉ STRATEGIES FOR RELIEF

▪ Don't smoke, and avoid secondhand smoke and other irritants. If you have chronic bronchitis, it is imperative that you quit smoking for good. Otherwise, you risk developing progressive emphysema.

▪ Stay in bed, or at least rest quietly, getting as much rest as possible, especially if you have a fever.

▪ Use a humidifier, especially in your bedroom, to keep air moist. To ease a bad coughing spell, take a steamy shower or sit in a steamy bathroom for a few minutes.

▪ To help clear the airway, practice postural drainage two or three times a day. Start by applying a heating pad or warm compress to the chest for fifteen or twenty minutes. Then lie on your stomach with the upper part of your body hanging over the edge of the bed and supporting yourself with your forearms on the floor. Simply being in this position for five to ten minutes helps drain mucus from the airways. If possible, have someone tap your back, starting just above the waist and moving systematically toward the shoulders. The tapping helps loosen phlegm.

Goldenseal (*Hydrastis canadensis*)

How it works. Goldenseal is rich in berberine and hyprastine, alkaloids that are reported to have an antibiotic effect, especially against chlamydia, a common cause of infectious bronchitis. It also soothes irritated and inflamed mucous membranes, such as those lining the throat and respiratory tract.

Recommended dosages. Look for an extract that contains 8 to 10 percent berberine and hyprastine. The typical dosage is 2 to 4 ml of extract three times a day. It can be added to warm water to make a tea to soothe the sore throat that often accompanies bronchitis. Powdered goldenseal root or rhizome supplements are available in pill or capsule form; the daily dosage is 4 to 6 g. Pills or powdered capsules can be dissolved in warm water to make a tea. The most effective of these preparations are dried extracts.

Possible problems. The alkaloids in goldenseal can cause stomach upset. It should not be taken for more than two to three weeks.

Licorice (*Glycyrrhiza glabra*)

How it works. Among other things, licorice root contains glycyrrhizin, which gives licorice its sweet flavor. It is thought to have antiviral properties, which may shorten the course of virus-caused bronchitis. Licorice is also a soothing demulcent that coats the irritated linings of the throat and respiratory tract, thereby easing a sore throat and quieting a hacking cough.

Recommended dosages. Look for extracts that contain glycyrrhizin, rather than the DGL (deglycyrrhizinated licorice) form. A soothing tea is made by boiling a half ounce of licorice root in a pint of water for ten to fifteen minutes; let cool, and drink two to three cups a day. Licorice root is also available in capsule form; the daily dosage is 5 to 6 g, with a total glycyrrhizin content of about 200 mg.

Possible problems. Licorice containing glycyrrhizin should not be taken by anyone with edema or liver, kidney, or heart disease, or used during pregnancy. Do not use it if you take thiazide diuretics, drugs often used to treat high blood pressure, because it increases the body's loss of potassium. It should be used with extreme care, if at all, by anyone with high blood pressure or edema—conditions that are worsened by as little as 1 g of glycyrrhizin (about 10 g of licorice root) a day.

Slippery elm (*Ulmus rubra*)

How it works. Tea made from slippery elm is a demulcent that coats and soothes irritated mucous membranes. The inner bark of the slippery elm tree is rich in soothing mucilage, which relieves a sore throat and helps calm a hacking cough.

Recommended dosages. For bronchitis and coughs, slippery elm can be taken as a lozenge or consumed as a tea. To make a tea, use 1 to 2 g of bark per cup of water. Boil for ten minutes, and then cool before drinking. Herbalists generally recommend three or four cups of tea a day. It is often combined with other botanicals because its mucilage prolongs their contact with the membranes.

Possible problems. No adverse effects have been reported.

CANCER

Cancer is the second-leading cause of death in the United States—led only by heart disease—killing an estimated 1,500 people a day. The risk of a person developing cancer in his or her lifetime is one in two for men and one in three for women. Although it is often discussed as if it were one disease, cancer is actually a collection of more than one hundred different diseases. The National Institutes of Health has estimated that yearly national costs for all types of cancer exceed $107 billion. In recent years, death rates from several types of cancer have begun to decline.

Cancer occurs when something causes cells to rapidly develop and divide without control or order. If the rapid growth and division of cells continue unchecked, a mass of tissue called a malignant tumor forms. (Tumors can also be benign, or noncancerous, meaning they do not spread to other parts of the body and can usually be removed.) Cancer cells can invade and damage nearby tissues and organs, or travel to other parts of the body and grow there. If the spread is not stopped or brought under control, it can kill. Cancers of the lung, colon, breast, and prostate are the most common in the United States, but cancer can occur in any organ in the body as well as in the blood, connective tissues, and lymph system. Though the exact cause of most cancers isn't known, it may be triggered by exposure to chemicals, radiation, viruses, hormones, immune conditions, inherited factors, and genetic mutations. Such factors may act together or in sequence to either initiate or promote cancer, and it may take ten years or more for developing cancer to be detected.

Although some causes of cancer cannot be avoided, cancers caused by cigarette smoking and heavy use of alcohol can be prevented completely. The American Cancer Society has estimated that in 1999, for example, about 173,000 cancer deaths were caused by tobacco use and 20,000 were related to excessive use of alcohol. Evidence suggests, too, that a healthy diet can be protective, reducing the chances of developing the disease. Screening tests that have been developed for the most common types of cancers are the best forms of what experts call "secondary prevention"—catching the disease early in its course while it is still curable (see Strategies for Relief, p. 54)

◉ SYMPTOMS

Often cancer presents no symptoms until the disease is advanced. Depending on the type and stage of a cancer, symptoms vary considerably. Pain is not necessarily a symptom of cancer in its early or even late stages. Common warning signs include:

- Changes in bowel or bladder habits.
- A sore that doesn't heal.
- Unusual bleeding or discharge.
- Thickening or lump in the breast or any other part of the body.
- Indigestion or difficulty swallowing.
- Obvious change in a wart or mole.
- Nagging cough or hoarseness.

Nutraceuticals to Counter Effects of Cancer Therapy

It's a well-known fact that patients undergoing cancer treatment suffer from severe fatigue and a variety of other adverse side effects, including nausea and vomiting. Recent studies, including one at Harbor-UCLA Medical Center in Torrance, California, indicate that patients given a regimen of high-dose vitamins, minerals, and other nutrients suffered fewer adverse effects than patients taking a placebo.

The supplement used in these studies is called Propax with NT Factor. It provides large amounts of all the major vitamins and minerals plus a variety of nutraceuticals—boron, coenzyme Q_{10}, creatine, grape seed extract, green tea extract, DHA and phosphoglycolipids, among others. The added NT Factor is a proprietary food tablet that contains nutrients derived from plants and other sources. In one study, a double-blind crossover study involving thirty-five cancer patients, those taking the supplement experienced significant improvement in energy levels and decreased episodes of nausea, diarrhea, mouth sores, skin changes, and other common side effects. When switched to the placebo group, most of the patients reported increased fatigue and a worsening of side effects. The researchers concluded that "this nutritional approach as a support for chemotherapy is promising and deserving of further study."

Diagnostic Steps

The best way to detect abnormal conditions that suggest cancer include regular checkups, self-examinations (for breast, skin, mouth, and testicular cancers), and screening tests for common cancers. For someone with symptoms suggestive of cancer, a doctor will do a physical exam, get a medical history, and most likely order one or more diagnostic tests and examinations. To locate the tumor and determine its impact, any of the following procedures may be used:

• *Imaging.* Including conventional X rays, computed tomography (CT scan), radionuclide scanning, ultrasonography, magnetic resonance imaging (MRI), these are increasingly high-tech procedures that in different ways provide an inside view of various areas of the body and pinpoint abnormal tissues.

• *Endoscopy,* often combined with imaging procedures, allows the doctor to get a direct look at certain areas of the body, such as the throat or the colon, by inserting a thin, lighted tube.

• *Blood and urine tests.* Damage to some organs can show up in elevated or reduced levels of substances normally found in the blood and urine. Increasingly, doctors have begun testing for biochemical "tumor markers" in the blood that suggest the presence of specific types of cancer. One of the most common such tests, for example, is the prostate-specific antigen (PSA). A dramatic rise in PSA levels indicates possible prostate cancer.

• *Biopsy.* All the diagnostic procedures mentioned above give a better picture of the size, location, and impact of a tumor, but only a biopsy can confirm that it is cancer. In a biopsy, the doctor removes a small piece of tissue from the tumor for examination under a microscope. If it is cancer, a pathologist will likely be able to tell what kind of cancer it is and whether it is likely to grow fast or slow.

Staging of a cancer is the next important phase of the diagnostic process. Based on the results of these tests (such as a biopsy of lymph nodes to see if a cancer has spread), a cancer will be designated as stage I, II, III, or IV. The higher the stage, the more likely the tumor is large and has spread, and the more aggressive the treatment will probably be. Cancer that is present only in the layer of cells where it originally developed and has not spread to other areas of that organ or to other parts of the body is cancer in situ. If cancer cells have spread beyond the original layer of tissue, then the cancer is considered invasive.

Conventional Treatments

There are several options for the treatment of cancer. They can be administered individually or in combination, depending on the type and stage of the cancer and a person's age and overall health. A person diagnosed with cancer is often treated by a team of specialists, which may include an oncologist (a doctor specializing in the treatment of cancer), a surgeon, and a radiation oncologist (a doctor specializing in the use of radiation to treat cancer). Some cancer patients may opt to take part in a clinical trial, a research study using new treatments or combinations of treatments. Treatments for cancer may include any of the following:

• *Surgery* removes the tumor and the tissues surrounding it. Nearby lymph nodes may be removed as well. In many cancers that are detected early, surgery can provide a complete cure.

• *Radiation therapy* employs high-energy rays to damage cancer cells and stop them from growing and dividing. Radiation may come from a machine or from an implant placed directly into or near the tumor, or both. For internal radiation therapy, a brief hospital stay is required. The implant may be temporary or permanent. Because the level of radiation is highest during the hospital stay, patients may not be able to have visitors or may have visitors for only a short time. The amount of radiation goes down to a safe level before the patient leaves the hospital. Once the implant is removed, there is no radioactivity in the body.

• *Chemotherapy* uses a variety of very potent drugs, sometimes alone, sometimes in combination, to kill cancer cells. Most chemotherapy is injected into a vein (IV), but some types are taken by mouth. Patients who require several doses of IV chemotherapy may have a catheter (a thin, flexible tube) implanted in a large vein in the chest. The other end is outside the body or attached to a small device just under the skin. The drugs are then administered through the catheter. The drugs travel through the bloodstream to most parts of the body. Chemotherapy is

⊚ **INFORMED DECISIONS**
If the diagnosis is cancer, the National Cancer Institute recommends patients ask their doctors these questions:

- What is my diagnosis?
- What is the stage of the disease?
- What are my treatment choices? Which do you recommend for me? Why?
- What are the chances that the treatment will be successful?
- Would a clinical trial be appropriate for me?
- What are the risks and possible side effects of each treatment?
- How long will treatment last?
- Will I have to change my normal activities?
- What is the treatment likely to cost?

Focus on prevention—it's the only sure "cure" for cancer. Prevention techniques may also help avoid a recurrence or progression of the disease once it has been diagnosed. Primary prevention includes avoidance of substances or situations that are linked to cancer (see suggestions below). Secondary prevention includes getting frequent checkups, performing self-exams, and following all guidelines for screening to detect cancers that can be eliminated early but may be killers if found late.

It's been estimated that about one-third of all cancers are related to diet. Nutrition is critical in prevention of cancer and in battling the disease.

▪ Avoid barbecued meats, cured meats, and saturated fats. Charring and curing meats produces carcinogenic compounds. A diet high in saturated fat has been linked to colon, breast, prostate, pancreatic, and endometrial cancers.

▪ Eat a healthful diet that includes at least five servings of fruits and vegetables each day and three servings of whole-grain foods, such as whole-grain cereal, breads, and pastas. A diet rich in plant foods provides a collection of nonnutritive substances called phytochemicals that may help prevent cancer. Research has shown that people who eat lots of fruits and vegetables, for example, have about one-half the risk of cancer of those who don't.

▪ Healthy diet is particularly important while undergoing cancer treatments, which frequently interfere with absorption of nutrients. Eating may be difficult, however, especially if you have no appetite or if you are suffering from side effects such as mouth sores, changes in taste, and nausea. Consult your doctor about taking supplements, work with a dietitian, and consider a nutritionally oriented health practitioner in addition to your standard treatment (but with full knowledge of your oncologist). To cope with nausea and vomiting related to chemotherapy, your doctor may prescribe antinausea drugs. Marijuana works for many people to prevent this common side effect of chemotherapy. However, although some states have passed medical marijuana initiatives, it remains illegal by federal law. Marinol, a prescription drug containing the major active ingredient in marijuana, is believed by many people to be less effective, in part because it must be swallowed and because it takes a much longer time to work.

▪ The amino acid N-acetyl cysteine (NAC), a purported hangover cure, has been shown

generally given in cycles. A treatment period is followed by a recovery period, then another treatment period, and so on. Chemotherapy is usually administered on an outpatient basis at a hospital, doctor's office, or at home.

• *Hormone therapy* is effective for cancers that depend on hormones to grow, such as breast and prostate cancers. Drugs are prescribed that stop hormone production or change the way hormones work. Like chemotherapy, hormone therapy travels throughout the body, affecting all the body's cells.

• *Biological therapy* is a form of treatment that uses the body's natural ability to fight infection and disease or to protect the body from some of the side effects of treatment. It is also called immunotherapy.

• *Bone marrow transplant,* once used only for cancers of the blood (leukemia) and lymphatic systems, is now an option for a number of cancers, although frequently on an experimental basis. High doses of chemotherapy destroy the patient's bone marrow. Then a small amount of bone marrow is removed via a large needle from a donor and its blood-making cells are injected into the patient, where they eventually find their way to the marrow and begin to replenish its ability to form new blood cells. Bone marrow transplant is a direct treatment for blood cancers. For other types of cancers, it enables doctors to treat patients with extremely high levels of chemotherapy, whose effects on blood production in the bone marrow would ordinarily be deadly.

• *Gene therapy* is available in clinical research trials. Healthy genes are delivered via viruses into human cells, where they replace defective, cancer-causing genes.

Most conventional cancer treatments have serious and painful side effects that may lower the quality of life and cause other health problems during treatment. Doctors treat these side effects and conditions as well.

Nutraceuticals for Cancer

Many of the following nutraceuticals can be taken by anyone for cancer prevention. Some are effective in people with active cancer either as possible cancer fighters, as methods to promote health while undergoing aggressive treatment, or as relief for the side effects of treatment. However, if you are currently undergoing treatment for cancer, never take supplements of any kind for any reason without your doctor's knowledge. Some nutraceuticals may interact or interfere with treatments, or contribute to side effects.

Calcium

How it works. Calcium supplementation may help prevent precancerous cells in the colon from developing further, in part by altering the composition of bile acids and slowing the division and growth of cells.

Recommended dosages. Several studies have found a reduced risk of colon and rectal cancer, and risk factors associated with colon and rectal cancer, in people taking between 1,200 and 2,000 mg of supplemental calcium a day. Experts recommend between 1,200 and 1,500 mg a day for all adults. Calcium citrate is the form most readily absorbed.

Possible problems. No problems have been associated with taking calcium supplements of up to 2,000 mg a day. However, some calcium supplements (principally those derived from oyster shell, dolomite, and bonemeal) have been found to be contaminated with lead.

Folic Acid

How it works. Folacin or folate, a B vitamin, may influence changes that lead to cancer in some tissues. Generally, studies show that the risk of colon cancer goes down as folate intake goes up. It has also been suggested that low folate may be related to cervical dysplasia, a forerunner of cancer of the cervix. And two recent studies have suggested that low folate may significantly increase the risk for breast cancer.

Recommended dosages. In the case of this B vitamin, natural is not better. Folacin found naturally in food is absorbed by the body only about half as well as folic acid, the form of folate found in fortified foods and supplements. The recommended dosage of folic acid is 400 mcg, although some practitioners recommend higher doses to treat specific problems.

Possible problems. If there is a deficiency of vitamin B_{12}, folic acid supplements may mask the symptoms of the deficiency and lead to permanent neurological damage. Seniors and vegetarians are most at risk for B_{12} deficiencies. (See Folacin, p. 237.)

Selenium

How it works. It isn't known exactly how selenium might fight cancer, but there are several theories. Selenium is an essential component of an antioxidant enzyme in the body. It also works with vitamin E to provide antioxidant activity. It may also help in the body's attempts to kill off cancer cells, a process known as apoptosis. And it may play a role in boosting the immune system.

Recommended dosages. The Recommended Dietary Allowance is 70 mcg a day for men and 55 mcg a day for women. However, one study of 1,400 people taking a daily dose of 200 mcg found them to

in one study to prevent nausea and vomiting induced by chemotherapy for lung cancer.

■ For mild cases of nausea, try ginger tea. (Also see Nausea, p. 172.)

Other preventive strategies include these precautions:

■ Don't smoke. Tobacco causes cancer and it is the most preventable cause of death in the United States. Smoking tobacco, using smokeless tobacco, and being regularly exposed to secondhand tobacco smoke are responsible for about one-third of all cancer deaths in the country each year.

■ Use alcohol only in moderation, if at all. Drinking large amounts of alcohol increases the risk of cancer of the mouth, throat, esophagus, and larynx through direct contact. People who smoke and drink are at especially high risk. Drinking has also been linked to breast, liver, and colon cancers.

■ Exercise regularly. Research shows that people who are active are healthier overall and have a lower risk of several kinds of cancer, including cancer of the breast and colon, two of the most common types. Even limited exercise also proves helpful in coping with chemotherapy and recovery of well-being following treatment.

■ Lose excess weight. Obesity is a risk factor for several cancers, including breast cancer, both because of its association with intake of dietary fat and because fat cells contain estrogen.

■ Stay out of the sun, especially during the hours of eleven A.M. to three P.M., when the sun's rays are strongest. Ultraviolet radiation from the sun causes skin damage that can lead to skin cancer. Repeated exposure to UV rays increases the risk of skin cancer, especially if you have fair skin or freckle easily.

■ Manage stress. Stress definitely affects health status. Although there is no proven link between stress and the development of cancer, research does show that stress affects recovery and even survival once you have the disease.

■ Try alternative and complementary therapies—but don't give up conventional treatments for something unproven. Don't rush into treatments that promise instant "cures"; evaluate claims rationally—if it sounds too good to be true it probably is. Always keep your doctors informed of what you're doing.

● STRATEGIES FOR RELIEF (cont.)

■ Finally, play an active role in your treatment, rather than letting your doctor or family members make decisions for you. Find out about treatments and their side effects and what you can do to relieve discomfort and improve your physical and emotional well-being. Read books; join support groups; attend hospital or American Cancer Society education groups; go to cancer sites online for information, support, and suggestions. Involve your family members, too. Cancer affects the whole family and everyone needs to learn how to cope.

have much lower rates of prostate, colon, and lung cancer than those who took placebos.

Possible problems. A daily dose of 200 mcg of selenium is safe, but it can be toxic at levels of 800 mcg. Symptoms of selenium toxicity include fatigue, nausea, nerve damage, and nail and hair loss.

Vitamin C

How it works. Studies from several countries have found a connection between diets rich in vitamin C and reduced risk of cancer, including cancer of the gastrointestinal tract (mouth, pharynx, esophagus, stomach, and pancreas), lung, and cervix. The strongest evidence is for prevention of stomach cancer. High doses of vitamin C inhibit the growth of *H. pylori,* the bacterium that causes most ulcers and may cause some stomach cancer. The vitamin also blocks the formation of some carcinogens and it fights free radicals that may cause cellular damage that can lead to cancer.

Recommended dosages. The Recommended Dietary Allowance is 70 to 90 mg a day (100 mg a day for smokers). However, several experts recommend an intake of 200 to 500 mg a day for saturation of the body's tissues and optimum benefit. It appears that doses above 500 mg a day offer no additional benefit and may be dangerous for cancer patients.

Possible problems. Recent research suggests that taking high doses of vitamin C can make cancer cells resistant to chemotherapy and radiation treatment, so do not take supplements if you are undergoing cancer treatment. Daily doses of 1,000 mg or more a day can cause diarrhea. People with kidney stones or kidney disease should also avoid high doses. Finally, large doses may also interfere with the action of anticoagulant medications such as Coumadin.

Vitamin E

How it works. Vitamin E is thought to protect cells against free radical damage by acting as an antioxidant, boosting the immune system, and regulating critical enzyme systems that control the growth of cancer cells.

Recommended dosages. The current Recommended Dietary Allowance is 15 IU for men and 12 IU for women. However, in a recent study, more than twenty-nine thousand men taking 50 IU a day for five to eight years were about 40 percent less likely to die of prostate cancer than those who took no vitamin E. Dosages up to 1,500 IU of natural vitamin E are considered safe.

Possible problems. Vitamin E has a blood-thinning effect, so large doses should not be taken with other blood-thinning medications or supplements.

Carotenoids

How they work. Carotenoids—which are responsible for the red, orange, and yellow pigments in fruits and vegetables—act as antioxidants, protecting cells and compounds in the body from free-radical damage. Carotenoids also are thought to enhance the immune system and prevent the changes that occur in some cells leading to cancer. The evidence for a cancer-preventive effect is strongest for lung cancer and prostate cancer. Over five hundred carotenoids have been identified in plants, but only a handful are used by the human body. The major ones are beta-carotene, alpha-carotene, lutein, zeaxanthin, cryptoxanthin, and lycopene. Lycopene has been found to have the greatest antioxidant activity; cooked tomatoes are an especially rich source of lycopene.

Recommended dosages. There is no currently recommended intake for carotenoids. But some researchers have suggested that an intake of about 6 mg a day of beta-carotene should be recommended for optimal health. A daily diet that includes broccoli, carrots, tomato juice, watermelon, and pink grapefruit can provide more than 11 mg of beta-carotene and more than 20 mg of other carotenoids. Supplements, even natural ones, do not contain all of the components found in foods. The best approach is to get as many carotenoids from foods and make up any deficits with natural supplements.

Possible problems. The only common side effect from a high intake of carotenoids (30 mg or more per day) from either supplements or food is yellowing of the skin. More seriously, two studies actually found an increased risk of lung cancer among current and previous smokers taking synthetic beta-carotene supplements. However, in another study of more than twenty-two thousand male physicians, there were no major side effects associated with taking an average of 25 mg of beta-carotene a day.

Isoflavones

How they work. Isoflavones are phytochemicals that are found in abundance in soy foods. In Asia, where people have been eating soy foods for almost five thousand years, there is a lower rate of cancer than in the United States. Researchers believe regular consumption of soy foods among some Asian populations may be the reason. Chemically, isoflavones are remarkably similar to the body's own estrogen, though they are only about one-thousandth as potent. Isoflavones displace some of the more potent estrogen in cells, preventing it from triggering precancerous changes in the breast and uterus, for example. Isoflavones may also trick the body into thinking that there's plenty of estrogen on hand, reducing estrogen production. On the other hand, if estrogen levels in the body are low, isflavones can actually provide estrogenlike benefits for the heart and bone.

Recommended dosages. Most experts believe that getting about 30 to 50 mg of isoflavones a day may be enough to provide benefit and possibly reduce the risk of hormone-sensitive cancers like cancer of the breast, prostate, and uterus. In Japan, where the incidence of these cancers is low, the typical diet contains 25 to 50 mg of isoflavones daily.

Possible problems. Although no problems have been seen with people taking isoflavone supplements or eating lots of soy foods, some experts have expressed concern that the estrogenlike effects of isoflavones could potentially cause problems in people with undiagnosed hormone-dependent cancer, particularly in postmenopausal women. These concerns have not been proven, but many experts suggest getting isoflavones naturally from soy products (including soy protein) rather than from supplements. One gram of uncooked soybeans contains approximately 1 mg of isoflavones. (See Soy Products, p. 349.)

Prebiotics and probiotics

How they work. The intestinal tract is home to hundreds of different kinds of good and bad bacteria. Harmful bacteria, such as staphylococci, can cause diarrhea and infection. Beneficial bacteria, such as lactobacilli (acidophilus and bifidus), inhibit the growth of bad bacteria, enhance immune function, and possibly help prevent colon cancer. If the number of good bacteria decrease, the bad bacteria can flourish and cause problems ranging from diarrhea to possibly colon cancer. Prebiotics and probiotics can help shift the balance of bacteria in the intestinal tract in the right direction.

Prebiotics are nondigestible food ingredients, such as fructooligosaccharides (FOS for short), a type of carbohydrate, which are a favorite food for the beneficial bacteria and promote their growth and activity. They are present in fruits, vegetables, and grains. FOS are also found in capsule or powder form. A lot of animal research has shown that regular consumption of FOS has wide-ranging health benefits.

Probiotics are products or supplements that contain live, active beneficial bacterial cultures. The most common probiotics are yogurt and fermented milk products. Acidophilus may help control diarrhea that is a common side effect of radiation treatment.

Recommended dosages. The typical dose for prebiotics, such as FOS, is about 1 teaspoon a day of powder. FOS are widely used in Japan, where they are added to more than five hundred food products. Although no recommended dose has ever been established for probiotics, such as yogurt and fermented milk, it is known that consumption must be on a regular basis to maintain the population of good bacteria in the intestinal tract and have a beneficial effect. Probiotic and prebiotic supplements are sold separately and together.

Possible problems. No serious side effects have been reported with the regular consumption of pre- or probiotics. However, they can cause gas and bloating in those not accustomed to taking them. (See Acidophilus, p. 263.)

Pycnogenol and grape seed extract

How they work. Pycnogenol is the trademarked name for an extract from the bark of a French maritime pine tree. It is quite similar to grape seed extract. Both contain a powerful combination of naturally occurring phytochemicals, mainly flavonoids, that may help prevent free-radical damage that can lead to disease. Though the research is promising, it is far from conclusive. One recent review of studies using pycnogenol (in cell cultures, animals, and humans) suggests that the pine bark extract has the potential to inhibit the spread of cancer cells and reduce the cancer-causing ultraviolet damage to skin cells. Also known as proanthocyanidim, pycnogenol and grape seed extract appear to protect the structural integrity of small blood vessels, or capillaries.

Recommended dosages. The typical dose of pycnogenol is 50 to 100 mg a day, although it has not been proved that this dose will lower the risk of cancer. Grape seed extract is recommended at 200 mg a day for people with cancer, 100 mg for prevention.

Possible problems. These substances appear to be safe, even in large doses. Although no allergic reactions have been documented, some herbal experts caution that people who are allergic to pine products should exercise caution before taking pycnogenol.

Tea

How it works. Laboratory research has shown that the polyphenols found in both green and black teas have cancer-fighting capabilities. And dozens of animal studies indicate that the compounds, including catechins in green and black tea, and theaflavins and thearubigins in black tea, may help protect against cancers of the breast, lung, mouth, and pancreas. Tea has greater antioxidant power than some fruits and vegetables. It may help delay cancer by preventing damage to DNA.

Recommended dosages. It isn't known how much tea is needed to help prevent cancer, but some researchers have suggested that as much as ten cups a day, or the equivalent in a tea supplement, may be required to make a difference.

Possible problems. The polyphenols in tea can interfere with the absorption of iron. Tea contains caffeine, about 40 mg per 6-ounce cup (a cup of drip coffee contains about 100 mg). However, adverse effects are rarely seen in people who regularly drink several cups of tea a day. (See Green Tea, p. 312.)

IP-6 (*inositol hexaphosphate*)

How it works. This substance appears to work by improving immunity and boosting the cancer-fighting activity of the body's own tumor-fighting killer cells. IP-6 is extracted from rice bran. Cereal grains, legumes, cantaloupe, and oranges are especially rich sources. Though animal and laboratory studies show that IP-6 reduces the frequency of tumors or beneficially alters levels of chemicals in the blood that suggest the presence of cancer, there's no human research that shows IP-6 has the ability to fight cancer cells.

Recommended dosages. The manufacturer of IP-6 recommends four capsules a day, equivalent to 1,600 mg of IP-6. But there is no research to back up this dosage for the prevention or treatment of cancer in humans.

Possible problems. People who are taking blood thinners or who are undergoing chemotherapy should not take IP-6.

■ BOTANICAL MEDICINES

Astragalus (*A. membranaceus*)

How it works. In China, the root of this plant is used to enhance effectiveness of cancer treatments and at the same time to reduce their toxic side effects. Animal research has shown it to be a potent immune-system stimulant. In Chinese medicine, it is often dispensed in combination with other herbal medicines.

Recommended dosages. Dosages range from 1 to 4 g of dried root three or four times a day.

Possible problems. Used for centuries throughout Asia, astragalus appears to be safe. It may act as a blood thinner, so avoid it if you are taking Coumadin. It may interact adversely with some medicines to control blood pressure as well as with some anesthesia agents, so stop taking it before undergoing surgery.

Garlic (*Allium sativum*)

How it works. Studies in the laboratory show that garlic slows the growth of malignant cells and disarms carcinogens (cancer-causing chemicals). It also contains powerful antioxidant compounds that may help fight free-radical damage. Garlic is also rich in phytochemicals that block the formation of nitrosamines, themselves powerful carcinogens. Studies in China have found that people who regularly consume garlic have a reduced risk of several kinds of cancer, including cancer of the stomach and esophagus. A recent French study found that women who ate the most garlic had a lower risk for breast cancer, compared to those who ate little. One recent study in the United States of more than forty thousand women determined that those who consumed the most garlic had the lowest risk of colon cancer.

Recommended dosages. There is no recommended dosage of garlic to prevent cancer. Most studies have simply compared what people eat and found that those who consume the most garlic have less risk of cancer than those who eat the least. In the Chinese study, those who ate about seven cloves a day (20 g) received the greatest benefits. To get the beneficial effects, eat it raw or slightly cooked, or take supplements.

Possible problems. Eating moderate amounts of garlic, as someone would use in cooking, poses no health risk for healthy people. However, because garlic has a blood-thinning property, there is a potential interaction with prescription anticoagulants and some over-the-counter painkillers such as aspirin. Consumption of five or more cloves of garlic a day can cause heartburn, gas, and gastrointestinal upset. In large doses, garlic can also lower blood sugar.

Milk Thistle (*Silybum marianum*)

How it works. Silymarin is the active ingredient of milk thistle, which protects liver cells from toxins and provokes the production of proteins to aid in liver-cell regeneration. It fights inflammation and seems to improve liver function in people with a variety of liver diseases. In cancer patients taking chemotherapy, milk thistle may help protect them from liver damage.

Recommended dosages. Although there is no established dosage for use along with chemotherapy, the recommended dose for liver diseases is 450 mg daily of a supplement standardized to 70 percent silymarin. Take it alone or in a so-called liver complex or lipotropic (fat-metabolizing) supplement, which may also contain dandelion, and B vitamins choline, inositol, and methionine.

Possible problems. When used properly, there are no known side effects.

CARPAL TUNNEL SYNDROME

Carpal tunnel syndrome is usually a repetitive strain injury. It is the fastest-growing occupational illness in the United States, affecting more than 250,000 workers a year. Anyone who performs forceful, repetitive tasks with their hands is at risk. Data processors, secretaries, cashiers, assembly-line workers, meat packers, writers, and piano players are especially vulnerable.

Two-thirds of the victims of carpal tunnel syndrome are women. Although this gender difference may reflect the type of jobs women tend to hold, experts believe that the hormonal changes experienced by women also increase their risk. Indeed, carpal tunnel syndrome occurs most often in women who are pregnant, menopausal, or taking oral contraceptives. Arthritis, diabetes, thyroid problems, or other diseases

◉ SYMPTOMS

Early or mild cases of carpal tunnel syndrome may cause only a few symptoms on an intermittent basis. Symptoms can become persistent and severe if the condition is not treated. In some cases, symptoms may worsen at night, awakening you from sleep, or first thing in the morning.

- Discomfort ranging from a dull aching to severe pain in the fingers, hand, wrist, and/or elbow.
- Shooting pain in the wrist and arm.
- Decreased hand strength, especially thumb weakness and an inability to grasp properly.
- Numbness in the hand, resulting in weakness or clumsiness.
- Tingling in all but the little finger.
- Dry and pale hand skin.
- Swollen fingers.

that cause joint or hand swelling or inflammation also may predispose someone to carpal tunnel syndrome.

The carpals are small bones in the wrist. They form a tunnel together with a ligament that runs from the forearm through the wrist. The median nerve, which controls sensation in the fingers and movement in some of the muscles in the hand (especially the thumb), passes through this tunnel. Repeated hand or wrist movement can put stress on the ligament or surrounding muscles and tendons, causing them to swell. Those swollen structures then press on the median nerve. Such pressure can cause pain or numbness, and may impair movement in the hand and fingers. If untreated, carpal tunnel syndrome can lead to severe muscle weakness, pain, and hand and finger disability. As disabling as carpal tunnel syndrome can be, it is often preventable if you know how to position your hands properly during repetitive tasks and how to recognize and treat early signs of trouble. See your doctor if you have hand or wrist symptoms that persist for more than a few weeks and are not alleviated by rest and a normal dose of pain reliever.

Diagnostic Steps

Referral to an orthopedist is often necessary for diagnosis, which is based on a complete history and examination. The doctor will want to know what types of movement cause symptoms and when they are most likely to occur, as well as what eases them. For example, ice packs are likely to ease carpal tunnel discomfort. If hot applications relieve pain, your symptoms are most likely not caused by carpal tunnel syndrome but rather by another condition producing similar symptoms. X rays and other tests may be necessary to rule out other potential causes of the symptoms. Electrodiagnostic tests for nerve conduction may be helpful in determining who would most benefit from surgery.

Conventional Treatments

If you have any underlying disease that may contribute to carpal tunnel syndrome, such as diabetes or arthritis, treatment for those conditions may alleviate carpal tunnel symptoms. Other treatments are designed to reduce inflammation and stress in the carpal tunnel.

Anti-inflammatory drugs are the first approach. Aspirin or other over-the-counter or prescription nonsteroidal anti-inflammatory drugs (NSAIDs), such as ibuprofen, can help relieve both the pain and the underlying inflammation and swelling that is causing it. In some cases, your doctor may inject steroid drugs, such as prednisone, directly into the wrist to reduce the inflammation. Such injections should be given by a rheumatologist, orthopedist, hand specialist, or other physician who is experienced in the procedure. Sometimes a short course of oral steroid drugs may be prescribed.

Diuretics, such as trichlormethiazide, help reduce fluid in the body and, therefore, may reduce pressure within the carpal tunnel.

Physical or occupational therapy can serve as a treatment and help prevent progression of the problem. The therapist may prescribe a wrist splint, which keeps the wrist straight or slightly extended, to be worn when at rest or at work for proper hand-positioning at work. A therapist can also teach you exercises to strengthen your wrists and techniques to reduce stress on them in your daily activities. Physical therapy also may include exercises to improve your overall balance and posture.

Surgery to relieve pressure on the nerve may be necessary if conservative treatments are ineffective, or if you develop weakness in your thumb at any time. By one of several techniques, the surgeon cuts the carpal tunnel ligament, which covers the median nerve, to relieve the pressure on that nerve. This is usually a simple operation that can be done on an outpatient basis. Whether and when to have surgery is controversial because there is no test that can determine whether symptoms will resolve or become worse in most people. In general, surgery is recommended if symptoms persist for four to six months and if muscles begin to atrophy in the base of the palm. Surgery does not cure all patients and, because it permanently cuts the carpal ligament, some wrist strength may be lost.

Nutraceuticals for Carpal Tunnel Syndrome

■ VITAMINS AND MINERALS

Vitamin B_6

How it works. Some studies have found that deficiencies of vitamin B_6 are associated with carpal tunnel syndrome, and that high levels of B_6 are associated with fewer symptoms. Multiple studies have shown B_6 supplementation to be helpful in many cases, although it may take as long as three months to produce a benefit.

Recommended dosages. Some doctors believe that B_6 supplements of 100 to 200 mg per day, taken in divided doses, should be the initial treatment of choice for carpal tunnel syndrome.

Possible problems. Pregnant or breast-feeding women should not take more than 100 mg of vitamin B_6. Megadoses of B_6 (1 to 5 g daily for months) can damage nerves. But doses of up to 200 mg a day have been successfully prescribed by many doctors for years to help ease carpal tunnel syndrome without side effects. One study found that even 500 mg a day was safe.

◉ STRATEGIES FOR RELIEF

▪ Never ignore wrist pain. Immediately stop any activities that trigger hand or wrist symptoms. If you cannot stop the activity, try to change the way you do it so that your wrist is not stressed.

▪ Try to alternate tasks so that you don't spend more than one to two hours at a time doing one that involves your hands.

▪ Avoid repetitive hand motions that involve a bent wrist. Try to keep the wrist straight and relaxed when you write, type, draw, drive, use tools, play musical instruments, or do needlework.

▪ Take frequent breaks (five minutes each hour) from repetitive hand motions. During your breaks, stretch your fingers and thumb and rotate your wrists in slow circles. Several brief respites do your wrists more good than a single long break.

▪ If you work at a computer, set up your keyboard so it is flat rather than slanted down at the front. While typing, your wrists should be straight, your forearms parallel to the floor, and your elbows bent at right angles. Use a wrist-support pad to help maintain a straight alignment of your wrist. However, do not place your wrists on the pad while you work; rather, let them hover about a half inch above it. Another option is a movable forearm rest that attaches to your chair to help keep your wrists straight and in place. Ergonomic keyboards may be helpful as well.

▪ Workplace specialists can come to your work site to analyze the conditions that may be causing your problems and recommend remedies.

▪ For acute pain relief, apply ice or a cold pack to the palm side of the wrist for five to ten minutes to help reduce swelling in the area. A bag of frozen peas is an effective ice pack because it can flex over the joint.

▪ Avoid over-the-counter splints; an improper fit may worsen your problems.

▪ Be aware of dietary factors that can interfere with vitamin B_6 absorption in the body. For example, avoid a high protein intake and tartrazine (FDC & yellow dye #5).

▪ Acupuncture has helped some people relieve carpal tunnel pain.

How it works. The effectiveness of B$_6$ may be boosted by taking it along with other B vitamins, especially B$_2$ (also called riboflavin) which converts B$_6$ to its more active form.

Recommended dosages. The Recommended Daily Allowance of B vitamins are usually present in a standard one-a-day multivitamin. Some practitioners recommended 20 mg of riboflavin daily.

Possible problems. No adverse effects occur when taken at the recommended dosages.

▪ NUTRITIONAL SUPPLEMENTS

Bromelain

How it works. Bromelain, an enzyme found in pineapple, has well-documented anti-inflammatory benefits. After surgery, for example, it can reduce bruising, swelling, and healing time. It may be used as a conservative treatment for carpal tunnel syndrome.

Recommended dosages. Different tablets contain different amounts of the active ingredient—the MCU (milk-clotting units) or GDU (gelatin-digesting units). Practitioners recommend 250 to 750 mg tablets twice daily between meals. If you are having surgery, start its use three days before the procedure and continue it for at least three weeks afterward. Some authorities recommend taking it along with 400 mg of turmeric (p. 540), an herb in the ginger family, with each dosage.

Possible problems. No adverse effects have been reported.

CATARACTS

More than half of all Americans over age sixty-five, and three-fourths of those over seventy-five, have cataracts. In fact, treatment for cataracts constitutes one of the largest expenditures in the Medicare budget. Although a simple surgical procedure can remove them, cataracts remain the leading cause of blindness throughout the world.

Cataracts occur in the lens of the eye. A healthy lens is transparent, allowing light to pass through it and focus on the retina, which then sends visual signals to the brain. The lens consists mostly of water and protein. Over time, the protein tends to clump together, creating an opaque area—a cataract—and clouding the lens. Gradually, the cataract grows larger and makes it much more difficult to see clearly. Cataracts can develop in one or both eyes, although not necessarily at the same time or at the same rate.

There are four types of cataracts:

◉ SYMPTOMS
The most common symptoms include:

- Cloudy or blurred vision. Sometimes close vision is more affected than distance vision, and vice versa, or the cataract may reduce both kinds of vision.
- Problems with light, such as headlights that seem too bright at night, glare from lamps or the sun, or a halo or haze around lights.
- Colors that seem faded.
- Double or multiple vision (this symptom goes away as the cataract grows).
- Frequent changes in eyeglasses or contact lens prescriptions.

- *Age-related.* This is by far the most common type. Although most people will develop cataracts, they are not inevitable.
- *Congenital.* Some babies are born with cataracts or develop them in childhood, often in both eyes. They may not affect vision, but if they do, they can be removed to improve vision. Cataracts in babies and young children are generally due to metabolic diseases or an infection—especially rubella, or German measles—during pregnancy.
- *Secondary.* Cataracts are a common complication of diabetes as well as other eye diseases. They are also linked to excessive alcohol consumption and long-term use of prescription corticosteroid drugs.
- *Traumatic.* Damage to the lens from accidents or even eye surgery can result, immediately or eventually, in cataracts.

Diagnostic Steps

An eye examination will easily reveal cataracts.

Conventional Treatments

Aside from surgery, no medical treatment has been proven to prevent, delay, or reverse the development of cataracts in adults. For an early-stage cataract, a change in eyeglass prescription, magnifying lenses, or stronger lighting may improve vision. Surgery to remove cataracts—performed when they have begun to interfere with daily activities—is one of the most common operations performed in the United States. More than 90 percent of people who have the surgery are able to see better, although vision may never return to what it was before the cataract began to develop.

Surgery, which takes less than an hour, is usually done on an outpatient basis, under local anesthesia. The newest and most common procedure uses ultrasound—high-frequency sound waves—to break up the cataract. The lens is removed and replaced with an artificial one specifically corrected for your vision, although most people will still need to wear glasses or contact lenses, which are fitted after recovery from the surgery. It's normal to feel itching, sticky eyelids and discomfort for a while following surgery. Recovery time is minimal, although it takes about six weeks for the eye to heal completely.

Nutraceuticals for Cataracts

■ VITAMINS AND MINERALS

Studies have found that some vitamins appear to protect against cataracts, although none totally prevent them.

Vitamin C

How it works. A Tufts University study of women between fifty-six and seventy-one who had taken vitamin C supplements (400 to 800 mg per day) for at least a decade found they had a substantially lower incidence of cataracts. Researchers theorize that the apparent protective effect of vitamin C is due to its antioxidant properties, which protect cells against the damage of unstable molecules (free radicals) formed when the body burns oxygen. Vitamin C is sixty times more concentrated in the lens of the eye than in blood. These levels normally drop with age, and people with cataracts tend to have lower blood levels of vitamin C than those without cataracts. It's also known that vitamin C boosts vitamin E's antioxidant activity, which may be an indirect cataract connection. Although the logical conclusion may seem that getting enough vitamin C would protect the eye and delay cataract development, a direct connection has yet to be demonstrated.

Recommended dosages. The Recommended Dietary Allowance for adults is 75 to 90 mg a day. Although supplements of 1,000 mg or more are sometimes recommended, several experts now advise that an intake of 200 to 500 mg a day is sufficient to saturate the body's tissues and provide optimum benefit.

Possible problems. Daily doses of 1,000 mg or more a day can cause diarrhea and stomach upset. People with kidney stones or kidney disease should avoid such high doses of vitamin C. Large doses may also interfere with the action of anticoagulant medications such as Coumadin.

Vitamin E

How it works. Like vitamin C, vitamin E shows promise in preventing cataracts through its ability to act as an antioxidant and prevent free radical damage to the eye.

Recommended dosages. The current Recommended Dietary Allowance is 15 IU for men and 12 IU for women. However, a four-year study of more than seven hundred people, funded by the National Eye Institute, found that those who regularly took 400 IU of vitamin E cut their risk of developing cataracts in half. Other studies have confirmed that persons who have high blood levels of vitamin E have a reduced incidence of cataracts.

Possible problems. Vitamin E has a blood-thinning effect, so large doses should not be taken with other blood-thinning medications or supplements.

■ NUTRITIONAL SUPPLEMENTS

Lipoic acid

How it works. Lipoic acid, also called alpha-lipoic acid, is a vitaminlike substance that aids in metabolism and is also a powerful antioxidant. Animal studies indicate that it may prevent cataracts; other studies have found that it improves insulin metabolism and blood-sugar control in diabetes and protects against diabetes-related nerve damage. Because cataracts are a common complication of diabetes, it seems logical that alpha-lipoic acid may be a beneficial adjunctive treatment in this disease.

Recommended dosages. Supplements of 50 to 150 mg a day are considered sufficient to protect against cataracts. However, higher doses of 100 to 200 mg, taken three times a day, are recommended for persons with diabetes.

Possible problems. No serious adverse effects have been reported, although some people may experience mild stomach upsets.

Lutein and zeaxanthin

How they work. Lutein and zeaxanthin are carotenoids, which act as antioxidants and may protect the eye from damage from free radicals. They are particularly concentrated in the retina, where they help filter out the most damaging portion of the ultraviolet rays from the sun. People with cataracts tend to have low levels of both lutein and zeaxanthin in their retinas and low dietary intakes of these carotenoids.

Recommended dosages. Although there are no recommended intake levels for lutein or zeaxanthin, people whose diets contain a lot of fruits and vegetables rich in the carotenoids tend to have a lower risk of cataracts than those who eat little. Natural food sources include dark green leafy vegetables, corn, broccoli, green peas, papaya, oranges, carrots, and zucchini. As supplements, mixed carotenoids (including beta-carotene, lycopene, cryptozanthin, and alpha-carotene) in dosages to provide 15,000 IU of vitamin A activity are most often recommended.

Possible problems. There have been no reports of side effects from consuming foods rich in lutein or zeaxanthin or from taking supplements. (See Beta-carotene/Carotenoids, p. 270)

■ BOTANICAL MEDICINES

Bilberry (*Vaccinium myrtillus*)

How it works. This relative of the blueberry contains anthocyanosides, flavonoid compounds that act as antioxidants and may help to protect the lens from cataracts. One study found that bilberry effectively slowed or prevented cataracts when taken along with vitamin E.

Recommended dosages. Look for standardized extracts containing 25 percent anthocyanosides. There is no recommended intake level, although doses of 80 to 160 mg and higher, taken two or three times a day, are often suggested. Bilberry tea can be made from fresh or dried berries steeped in hot water and strained.

Possible problems. Bilberry appears to be quite safe. However, it may interfere with iron absorption.

◙ SYMPTOMS

Abnormal cholesterol levels cause no noticeable symptoms in most people until atherosclerosis is advanced. Then, severely diminished blood flow may cause:

- Angina or chest pain.
- Leg pain (intermittent claudication) when walking.
- Formation of xanthomas, clumps of fatty tissue under the skin, especially on the eyelids.

◙ FAMILIAL HYPERCHOLESTEROLEMIA: INHERITED DANGER

About one in five hundred Americans inherits a metabolic defect that results in an inability to clear LDL cholesterol from the bloodstream, resulting in extremely high LDL levels and a higher-than-average risk of heart disease. Those with a very severe form of the disorder often develop heart disease—and even heart attacks—in childhood. This form of high cholesterol is marked by telltale pinkish-yellow deposits (xanthomas) under the skin, especially on the eyelids or in the tendons of the lower leg. They can also occur in the eye on the cornea.

In addition to dietary changes, treatment for familial hypercholesterolemia usually requires cholesterol-lowering drugs to reduce the risk of premature heart disease.

◙ LIPID LEVELS: WHAT THEY MEAN

Total cholesterol
Less than 200 mg/dl = Desirable blood cholesterol
200 to 239 mg/dl = Borderline-high blood cholesterol
240 mg/dl and over = High blood cholesterol

HDL cholesterol
Less than 35 mg/dl = Low HDL cholesterol (higher levels are desirable)

LDL cholesterol
Less than 100 mg/dl = Desirable for people with heart disease
Less than 130 mg/dl = Desirable for people with no heart disease
130 to 159 mg/dl = Borderline-high risk
160 mg/dl or more = High risk

Triglycerides
Recent research suggests that levels over 100 mg/dl may increase risk for some people. Generally, however:

CHOLESTEROL DISORDERS AND ATHEROSCLEROSIS

Cholesterol, a lipid (fatlike substance) that is produced in the liver and absorbed from food, is a necessary building material for all of the body's cells and for some hormones. At elevated levels, however, cholesterol and other lipids, including triglycerides, may constitute disorders in themselves and increase the risk for heart disease and stroke. High cholesterol conditions are referred to as hypercholesterolemia. Excess levels of lipids in general is termed hyperlipidemia. All lipids circulate in the blood attached to proteins. The fat-protein complexes are called lipoproteins. They include: high-density lipoprotein (HDL), low-density lipoprotein (LDL), and very low density lipoprotein (VLDL).

HDL is known as the "good" lipoprotein because it tends to transport cholesterol away from arterial walls and back to the liver. LDL is known as "bad" because it tends to carry serum cholesterol from the liver to the arteries, where it is deposited on arterial walls. When LDL cholesterol in the blood is elevated, and the HDL cholesterol is low, the risk of atherosclerosis—fat-clogged arteries—increases. Coronary heart disease caused by atherosclerosis is the single leading cause of death in both men and women in the United States.

Often referred to as hardening of the arteries, atherosclerosis is derived from the Greek words *athero,* meaning paste, and *sclerosis,* meaning hardening. It is a narrowing of the arteries from a buildup of fatty deposits called plaque. The process, which can begin in childhood, usually shows no symptoms until it is quite advanced, in middle or old age. Heart attack and stroke are frequent, often fatal results of blocked arteries that completely restrict blood flow and thus cut off oxygen supply to the brain and heart. Sometimes this blockage is caused by blood clots—thromboses—that form on the surface of the arterial plaque.

It isn't known for sure what starts this chain of events that leads to clogged arteries. But some experts think it starts when the inner layer of an artery, the endothelium, is damaged by high blood levels of cholesterol (especially LDLs) and triglycerides, high blood pressure, or cigarette smoking.

According to the American Heart Association, an estimated 98.1 million American adults have elevated cholesterol levels, putting them at risk for atherosclerosis. Other risk factors for both atherosclerosis and high cholesterol are family history (see box, Familial Hypercholesterolemia), obesity, diabetes, diet, inactivity, and smoking. Additional atherosclerosis risk factors include high blood pressure (which can also be a consequence of the disorder), high cholesterol, and high triglycerides; risk is also greater for men and for anyone with a stressful lifestyle.

High cholesterol is also linked to kidney disease, hypothyroidism, and alcoholism, and it may increase the risk for hearing loss, impotence, and gallstones. Certain medications also may increase cholesterol levels, including progesterone, isotretinoin, corticosteroids, and thiazide diuretics. Most experts think, however, that the most common form of hypercholesterolemia is linked, at least in part, to eating foods containing cholesterol and fat, especially animal (saturated) fat.

Diagnostic Steps

Checking blood levels of cholesterol and triglycerides is the first and simplest screening test to determine risk for atherosclerosis. Although at-home cholesterol testing kits are available, results are not necessarily reliable, and they only indicate total cholesterol levels, not the amounts of LDL and HDL, which are more informative. In general, a desirable lipid profile is defined as a total serum cholesterol level of under 200 mg/dl, with an LDL level under 130 mg/dl and an HDL over 50 mg/dl. If HDL levels are particularly high, and LDL levels correspondingly low, a higher total serum cholesterol level may be acceptable. In such cases, it is the ratio that is important. Triglyceride levels above 250 mg/dl are considered abnormal.

In a physical examination, the doctor finds evidence of poor circulation using a stethoscope and feeling for weakened pulses in various parts of the body. If atheroslerosis is suspected, other tests may include an exercise stress test, an ultrasound examination of the heart, and possibly angiography, a more invasive examination in which the coronary arteries are x-rayed after injection of a dye to make them visible on film.

Conventional Treatments

As yet there is no cure for atherosclerosis. The principal goal of treatment is to prevent further narrowing of the arteries and damage to vital organs. Diet and exercise are the main focus, as described in Strategies for Relief (p. 69). Medication is prescribed when cholesterol levels are very high or when moderately elevated levels do not respond to lifestyle changes. The addition of medications does not mean that a careful diet should be abandoned; it remains the cornerstone of cholesterol-lowering therapy.

Commonly prescribed cholesterol-lowering drugs include:

• *Statins,* which inhibit an enzyme essential in the body's manufacture of cholesterol, are now the most widely prescribed class of cholesterol-lowering drugs. They include lovastatin (Mevacor), pravastatin (Pravachol), simvastatin (Zocor), atorvastatin (Lipitor), fluvastatin (Lescol), and cerivastatin (Baycol). Depending on the dose and your individual response, these drugs may reduce LDL cholesterol by

◉ LIPID LEVELS: WHAT THEY MEAN (cont.)

Less than 200 mg/dl = Normal triglycerides
200 to 400 mg/dl = Borderline-high triglycerides
400 to 1,000 mg/dl = High triglycerides
Greater than 1,000 mg/dl = Very high triglycerides

◉ STRATEGIES FOR RELIEF

A heart-healthy lifestyle can often prevent or cure cholesterol disorders. It may even be able to halt or reverse atherosclerosis.

Diet

The American Heart Association recommends two levels of dietary control. In both, no more than 30 percent of your total calories should come from fat. In the Step I diet:

- Of the maximum 30 percent of calories from fat: limit saturated fat to 8–10 percent, polyunsaturated fat to 10 percent, and monounsaturated fat to 15 percent.
- Eat no more than 300 mg per day of cholesterol.
- At least 55 percent of calories come from carbohydrates.
- Protein should account for 15 percent or less of calories.

If this diet doesn't lower blood cholesterol, try the Step II diet, which further restricts saturated fat to 7 percent and cholesterol to 200 mg.

Some experts recommend a much stricter diet for controlling cholesterol. Dr. Dean Ornish of the Preventive Medicine Research Institute in California has conducted several studies to see if a program of extreme lifestyle changes, such as a vegetarian diet with less than 10 percent of calories from fat, stress management, psychological counseling and support, and regular moderate exercise, could make a difference. His research has found that such a program significantly lowers cholesterol, and can stop and in some cases reverse the progression of atherosclerosis and reduce the risk of heart attack. But the program is not for everyone. It is a strict, life-altering program that may not be palatable over the long haul. And some experts worry that the extremely low-fat, high-carbohydrate diet may cause a dangerous rise in triglyceride levels. Care must also be taken to avoid deficiencies of essential fatty acids which are crucial for normal nerve function.

Other recommendations for reducing cholesterol include:

- Eating plenty of soluble fiber. Oat bran, oatmeal, beans, peas, rice bran, barley, citrus fruits, strawberries, and apples are good sources of soluble fiber.
- Reducing your intake of meat, whole milk and cheese, butter, and eggs. This is the most important step you can take, since saturated fats stimulate the liver to produce LDL.
- Avoiding trans fatty acids, which act like saturated fats but are even worse. They raise LDL and also lower HDL. They are found in most margarines, vegetable shortening, deep-fried foods, and the partially hydrogenated vegetable oils used in almost all commercial snack items, such as crackers, cookies, chips, and cake.
- Eating more fish, poultry, and mono-unsaturated vegetable oils such as olive oil.
- Increasing your intake of soy, from tempeh, tofu, soy milk, soybeans, or other sources.

Other lifestyle changes

- Even if you can't get down to your ideal weight, losing ten or fifteen pounds can improve your health and lower your cholesterol levels.
- Exercise regularly to strengthen your heart muscle, help maintain ideal weight, prevent or control high blood pressure and diabetes, and improve the balance of good vs. bad cholesterol in your blood. In particular, exercise can play a major role in raising HDL levels.
- If you smoke, quit. Smoking increases total cholesterol and decreases HDL cholesterol. The risk of heart disease may be as much as three hundred times greater for the heavy cigarette smoker. Within a few years after giving up the habit, the ex-smoker appears to have no greater risk than the nonsmoker.
- Learn to relax. Stress, anger, and hostility have been shown to increase the risk of heart disease. Exercise, prayer, meditation, guided imagery, visualization, and a host of relaxation techniques can enhance the effectiveness of diet and medication.

up to 60 percent. They can also lower triglyceride levels and raise HDL levels. The most common adverse side effects are gastrointestinal upset, muscle aches, and liver damage. If one of the statins causes serious problems, another can often be tried.

• *Bile-acid-binding resins,* which include colestipol (Colestid) and cholestyramine (Questran, LoCholest, and Prevalito), work by binding with bile acids and interrupting the liver's cholesterol-making activities. They are now used mostly as adjuncts for persons taking statins who need further lowering of their cholesterol levels. The most common adverse side effects are feelings of fullness, gas, and constipation, which can be minimized by lowering the dose and increasing fiber intake.

• *Fibric acids,* also called fibrates, increase the liver's oxidation of fatty acids, which ultimately results in a lowering of LDL and triglycerides. They include clofibrate (Atromed-S), gemfibrozil (Lopid), and fenofibrate (Tricor). The most common side effect is upset stomach. Some men also may experience erectile dysfunction (impotence); these drugs may increase the risk of gallstones as well.

Nutraceuticals for Cholesterol Disorders and Atherosclerosis

Because nutrition is the cornerstone of therapy for abnormal cholesterol levels and atherosclerosis, the proven effectiveness of some dietary supplements is not surprising.

■ VITAMINS AND MINERALS

Nicotinic acid (niacin, vitamin B_3)

How it works. Large doses of this B vitamin, usually in the form of nicotinic acid, are often prescribed as a conventional treatment not only to lower LDLs and triglycerides but also to raise HDL levels. It works by mobilizing fatty acids from tissues around the body, thereby reducing the liver's production of triglycerides and lowering LDL levels. It also increases HDL more effectively than any other drug, by up to 30 percent.

Recommended dosages. To effectively lower LDL cholesterol and triglycerides and raise HDL cholesterol, nicotinic acid must be taken in very high amounts, usually 1,000 to 2,000 mg two or three times a day.

Possible problems. High doses of nicotinic acid can cause the skin to feel warm and flush, especially on the face and neck, and very high doses (e.g., 3,000 mg a day) can cause serious flushing and itchiness. Taking a standard aspirin a half hour beforehand, or taking a time-release form of nicotinic acid, may reduce the flushing. Nicotinic acid can also trigger a headache and in large doses can cause dizziness, diarrhea, itching, and irregular heartbeat; it may also cause liver problems and increase the risk of type 2 (adult-onset) diabetes. Persons taking high-dose nicotinic acid should see their physician regularly for blood tests to monitor for liver damage, diabetes, and other adverse effects. Also, never take any form of niacin when you are taking cholesterol-lowering drugs. (See Vitamin B_3, p. 226.)

Folic acid, vitamin B_{12}, and vitamin B_6

How they work. Several studies have shown that low intakes of these B vitamins are associated with increased blood levels of homocysteine and an increased risk of atherosclerosis and coronary heart disease.

Recommended dosages. Supplements that provide more than the RDAs for these nutrients may be needed to lower high homocysteine levels. Many doctors recommend 800 mcg of folic acid; 1,000 mcg of vitamin B_{12}, and 50 mg of vitamin B_6.

Possible problems. Because folic acid can mask the symptoms of pernicious anemia, some experts are concerned that taking folic acid supplements could cause anemia to go undetected and result in permanent neurological damage. Getting enough vitamin B_{12} eliminates that risk. More than 15 mg a day of folic acid taken for a month has been associated with sleep problems, mental changes, and stomach upset. People over sixty may have trouble absorbing B_{12} and may require injections or a nasal spray, which are available by prescription. Vitamin B_6 can cause reversible nerve damage at high dosages (as little as 500 mg a day for some people, as much as 2,000 mg for others). (For more information on folic acid, see Folacin, p. 237.)

Vitamin E

How it works. The antioxidant action of vitamin E is believed important in preventing damage to LDLs. (Recent research suggests that damaged, or oxidized, LDLs are an important first step in the development of atherosclerosis.) Several studies have found that people taking vitamin E supplements have a reduced risk of heart attacks and death from coronary artery disease. Some studies, however, have failed to show any benefit.

Recommended dosages. An intake of 200 to 400 IU a day may reduce the risk of atherosclerosis, and some doctors recommend up to 1,000 IU for patients with coronary heart disease. These high levels of vitamin E intake can be obtained only through supplements, which should be the natural, or d-alpha, form to assure maximum absorption.

Possible problems. Vitamin E appears to be safe in doses up to 1,500 IU. However, it does have an anticoagulant effect and should not be combined with other nutraceuticals that reduce clotting such as ginkgo biloba extract, or other anticoagulant medications, such as Coumadin or aspirin.

■ NUTRITIONAL SUPPLEMENTS

Red rice yeast

How it works. Red rice yeast, or Chinese red yeast, is sold under the brand name Cholestin. It is prepared from a strain of red yeast fermented on rice. It contains a compound that seems to act identically to the statin class of cholesterol-lowering drugs. This supplement lowered total cholesterol by an average of 16 percent and LDL by 12 percent, plus raised HDL by nearly 15 percent, in eight weeks, according to Tufts University researchers.

Recommended dosages. The studies were done with two capsules of 600 mg of Cholestin.

Possible problems. The most common side effect is gastrointestinal upset. It can be minimized by taking Cholestin with meals. However, do not take Cholestin if you have any liver problems, because it sometimes causes liver damage. For the same reason, don't have more than two alcoholic drinks daily if you use this supplement. Long-term safety has not been tested. The manufacturer recommends its use only for healthy men and women with borderline-high cholesterol levels; anyone with levels over 240 should check with their doctor. Do not take it if you are taking any of the statin drugs or if you are pregnant.

Plant sterol esters

How they work. Benecol and Take Control are two new brands of margarines, salad dressings, and, in the case of Benecol, candy bars that can help control cholesterol. All contain plant sterol esters that inhibit the absorption of LDL cholesterol from the intestines and, therefore, promote its excretion. The sterol esters in Benecol come from pine trees, while those in Take Control come from soybeans. The appropriate dose can lower LDL levels by about 10 to 15 percent in less than a month.

Recommended dosages. The doses of the margarinelike spread used in clinical trials were about 2 tablespoons per day, although the packages recommend 1 to 2 tablespoons per day.

Possible problems. So far, no adverse effects have been seen. A product similar to the spreads has been used safely in Finland for five years. Though it is believed safe for everyone, pregnant women should first discuss it with their doctors, as should anyone currently taking medications. An 8-g serving of Benecol spread (it comes in prepackaged servings) provides 45 calories and 5 g of fat. Adding these products to your diet without eliminating other fats will boost total fat and calories. (See Benecol, p. 268.)

Omega-3 fatty acids

How they work. The principal fatty acids found in fish (especially in cold-water fish), omega-3 fatty acids such as EPA and DHA inhibit inflammation, have anticlotting actions, and lower triglyceride levels, all of which reduce the risk of developing atherosclerosis. Plant sources of omega-3s include flaxseed, rapeseed, and evening primrose oils as well as walnuts.

Recommended dosages. Studies suggest that a daily dose of 1 to 3 of omega-3 fatty acids may lower triglycerides and provide cardiovascular benefits. A 3½-ounce serving of salmon provides 1.8 grams of omega-3s. One study of two thousand men found that those eating about 8½ ounces of fish a week had half the risk of dying from a heart attack compared to men who ate little or none.

Possible problems. Because omega-3s have an anticlotting effect, there could be an interaction with medications having a similar action. Large doses of fish oil can cause a fishy body odor or a fishy aftertaste. (See Essential Fatty Acids, p. 295.)

Psyllium and other soluble fibers

How they work. Soluble fibers help prevent the absorption of fats as they move through the gastrointestinal system, thus reducing the available fat used by the liver to make cholesterol. Studies have found that after six weeks of regular use, 10 g a day of ground psyllium lowered LDL cholesterol by up to 20 percent. While psyllium husks are most commonly used in soluble-fiber preparations, oat bran, flaxseed, guar gum, pectin, and other fruit and vegetable fibers have the same result. Ground psyllium husks are the active ingredient in Metamucil and other commercial products used to help prevent constipation and lower cholesterol levels. The natural husks, without sugar and other additives, are available in health food stores.

Recommended dosages. Follow label directions, which depend on the potency of the product. In general, your goal is to get 7 to 10 g of soluble fiber a day through a combination of diet and supplements. For example, 1 tablespoon of ground flaxseeds contains 3 g of soluble fiber. Psyllium and other soluble fibers, along with insoluble fibers, are often added to commercial breakfast cereals; check the labels. Be sure to drink at least eight to ten glasses of water or other fluids a day.

Possible problems. Some people report bloating and gas with these products. Starting with a low dose and gradually increasing allows the body to gradually get accustomed to the increased fiber.

Green tea

How it works. Green (unfermented) tea contains several compounds that may interfere with the process that leads to atherosclerosis. Much of the research into green tea's medicinal properties has focused on its phytochemicals, called polyphenols. They appear to lower cholesterol, improve metabolism of lipids, and act as antioxidants. The amount of polyphenols in black and green tea are about the same; only the types of compounds differ. A recent study at Harvard found that black tea is also effective, suggesting that the fermented forms of polyphenols are themselves medicinally potent.

Recommended dosages. How much green tea it takes to prevent or treat atherosclerosis isn't known. Some sources recommend drinking several cups daily or taking 240 to 320 mg of green tea in capsule or pill form. The Harvard study found that people who drank only one cup of black tea a day had half the risk of heart attack compared to those who drank no tea at all. Decaffeinated tea may contain fewer polyphenols than regular tea.

Possible problems. The compounds in tea can bind with iron from food or supplements, making it less available to the body. Heavy tea drinkers may have a problem getting enough of this mineral, especially if tea is consumed with meals.

Pycnogenol and grape seed extract

How they work. Pycnogenol is the registered trademark for an extract from the French Maritime pine tree bark. According to some studies, Pycnogenol and grape seed extract, which is closely related, have more antioxidant power than vitamins C and E and can help relax blood vessels and prevent damage to LDLs. No long-term clinical trials have been done to see if these substances actually prevent atherosclerosis or reduce the risk of coronary artery disease, however.

Recommended dosages. The recommended dosages of either product range from 50 to 100 mg a day.

Possible problems. There have been no reported side effects from taking Pycnogenol or grape seed extract.

Soy protein

How it works. The isoflavones found in soy, daidzein and genistein, have estrogenlike effects that may help reduce the risk of atherosclerosis. Genistein is also an antioxidant, which may play a role in preventing the oxidation of LDLs. Soy protein increases bile acid secretion, helping to lower blood cholesterol levels.

Recommended dosages. An analysis of thirty-eight soy studies found that soy protein intakes of about 47 g a day lowered total cholesterol by about 9 percent and LDLs by about 13 percent. The Food and Drug Administration has determined that only 25 g of soy protein a day, as part of a diet low in saturated fat and cholesterol, may lower cholesterol and help reduce the risk of heart disease.

Possible problems. Asian populations have consumed soy as a regular part of their diets for thousands of years, with no safety problems. (See Soy Products, p. 349.)

■ BOTANICAL MEDICINES

Gugulipid (*Commiphora mukul*)

How it works. Gugulipid is a standardized extract of a resin from the mukul myrrh tree of India. Its effects are similar to those of lipid-lowering drugs because it increases the liver's metabolism of LDL cholesterol. One clinical study of people with high cholesterol found that along with a heart-healthy diet, gugulipid lowered LDLs and triglycerides about 12 percent compared with diet only.

Recommended dosages. Dosage is based on the guggulsterone content. Clinical trials have demonstrated benefits with capsules standardized to contain 25 mg of guggulsterone per 500-mg tablet, taken three times a day.

Possible problems. No side effects have been reported when purified preparations are used. Crude guggul may cause rashes, diarrhea, and other gastrointestinal problems. (See Guggul, p. 476.)

Garlic (*Allium sativum*)

How it works. Studies have shown that garlic has blood-thinning properties, making clots less likely to form in the arteries. Some, but not all, studies suggest that the herb can help lower cholesterol. Its benefits are linked to its sulfur compounds, alliin in particular. When raw garlic is crushed, cut, or chewed, it is converted to allicin, which produces its characteristic odor as well as its medicinal effects.

Recommended dosages. The daily dose suggested for lowering cholesterol blood levels is 4 g a day (about one average-size clove) of fresh garlic. Cooking garlic substantially reduces allicin levels. Dozens of garlic supplements are available, but they vary greatly in their garlic content and allicin yield. One German study found that of eighteen garlic preparations, only five produced an allicin yield equal to 4 g of fresh garlic. Garlic preparations in oil contain little or no allicin. Dried garlic products are best if enteric-coated, allowing them to break down in the intestines rather than the stomach. Look for a product with an allicin yield of 5,000 mcg, the equivalent of one clove of fresh garlic. Doses of 600 to 900 mg a day of standardized powdered supplements have been shown in some studies to lower total cholesterol by 12 percent.

Possible problems. Eating moderate amounts of garlic poses no health risk for healthy people. However, because garlic has a blood-thinning property, there is a potential interaction with prescription anticoagulants such as Coumadin and some over-the-counter painkillers such as aspirin. Consumption of five or more cloves of garlic a day, or equivalent amounts of supplements, can cause heartburn, gas, and gastrointestinal upset. Enteric-coated supplements may help prevent these side effects. In large doses, garlic can also lower blood sugar.

CHRONIC FATIGUE SYNDROME

Although chronic fatigue syndrome (CFS) has probably been around a long time, it wasn't until the mid-1980s that it hit the headlines. Nicknamed the "yuppie flu," it was often written off as burnout or depression. Many people with CFS looked so healthy that they were told their symp-

Symptoms may develop within a few hours or days and last from months to several years. The Centers for Disease Control defines CFS as the presence of profound fatigue for at least six months that does not improve with bed rest; physical or mental activity may worsen the condition, often necessitating substantially lower activity levels than prior to the onset of illness. Four or more of the following symptoms must also be present:

- Substantial impairment in short-term memory or concentration.
- Sore throat.
- Tender lymph nodes in the neck and/or armpits.
- Muscle pain.
- Pain in many joints without swelling or redness.
- Headache of a type, pattern, or severity not experienced before.
- Sleep that is not refreshing.
- Feelings of exhaustion and illness that last twenty-four hours or more following exertion.

In addition, some people may have one or more of the following symptoms, which are not considered part of the official definition of CFS:

- Unusual nervous system symptoms, such as increased sensitivity of eyes to light, confusion, "fuzzy" or "foggy" thinking, or dizziness.
- Abdominal pain, bloating, nausea, or diarrhea.
- Alcohol intolerance.
- Chest pain.
- Chronic cough.
- Dry eyes or mouth.
- Earaches.
- Irregular heartbeat.
- Morning stiffness.
- Psychiatric symptoms, such as irritability, anxiety, depression, or panic attacks.
- Shortness of breath.
- Skin sensations, such as tingling.
- Sleep disturbances, such as insomnia, excessive sleep, or night sweats.
- Weight loss.

toms were "all in their heads." But time has shown that it's a real, if mysterious, illness.

Chronic fatigue syndrome is a debilitating and complex disorder characterized by prolonged and severe tiredness that is not relieved by rest and is not directly caused by any current physical or psychological disorder. In academic research circles, it is called chronic fatigue and immune dysfunction syndrome; in Britain, it is called myalgic encephalomyelitis. The prevalence remains unknown, but it has been estimated that anywhere from 100,000 to 2 million Americans currently have the condition. It most commonly arises between the ages of thirty and fifty, and women seem to be affected three to seven times as often as men.

The cause of CFS remains unknown. Some researchers suspect it may be caused by a virus, but early theories that it might be caused by Epstein-Barr virus or a herpes virus have not been proved. Allergies may play a role, because about 65 percent of those afflicted have a history of allergies. Multiple abnormalities of immune system function have been found in these patients, but they don't occur among everyone who has CFS and they are not specific to people with the illness. Other disease mechanisms under investigation include abnormalities in endocrine function, neurotransmitter imbalances, blood pressure abnormalities, and inflammation of the nervous system. Other factors, such as age, health history, stress, genetics, and environmental factors may play a role.

Diagnostic Steps

There are no specific tests to confirm the diagnosis of CFS. However, because many illnesses have incapacitating fatigue as a symptom, a variety of tests are usually performed to exclude them: infections; immune or autoimmune disorders, such as lupus; tumors; muscle or nerve diseases, such as multiple sclerosis; endocrine diseases, such as hypothyroidism; psychiatric disorders; drug dependence; or heart, kidney, or liver diseases. Further, the doctor may look for a pattern of findings on certain tests. While they are not specific enough to diagnose CFS, they are seen frequently in people who are eventually diagnosed with the disorder. These include: higher levels of specific white blood cells; swelling in the brain or destruction of part of the nerve cells shown by a brain MRI; and active forms of herpes virus-6 in lymphocyte cell cultures.

Conventional Treatments

There is currently no therapy that has been proven to be effective in curing CFS. Instead, the symptoms are treated. Most people do get better, although that may take one to five years. CFS is usually worse at its onset and then tends to wax and wane until it finally disappears.

Antidepressants are the conventional drugs that have been used most successfully. As many as 80 percent of patients experience benefits. By modifying biochemistry in the central nervous system, they can reduce pain and enhance energy as well as treat depression, if present. Often several types need to be tried before finding relief.

Immunologic drugs have been studied but results have been inconclusive. These include immunoglobulins, amphigen, interferons, isprinosine, and corticosteroids. Some researchers are studying the use of medications that prevent low blood pressure.

Nutraceuticals for Chronic Fatigue Syndrome

■ VITAMINS AND MINERALS

Vitamin B-complex

How they work. The B-complex vitamins help support the adrenal glands, which are among the major organs in the body connected with stress. These vitamins are also instrumental in metabolism and energy production, which can make them valuable for people with CFS.

Recommended dosages. Take a supplement containing the entire B-complex. You can get these vitamins in most multivitamin/mineral supplements. Make sure you are getting at least 50 mg each of thiamin, pantothenic acid, and vitamin B_6, and 50 mcg of vitamin B_{12}. You may need an additional B-complex supplement when you're under stress.

Possible problems. No side effects are associated with these dosages.

Magnesium

How it works. Magnesium is essential for proper muscle function and energy-producing activities in cells. Levels have been reported to be low in CFS sufferers, and supplements have been reported to improve symptoms in some people.

Recommended dosages. Start with 500 mg daily, divided into two dosages. Take it with calcium (see below).

Possible problems. Taking too much magnesium often leads to diarrhea. Occasionally, this can happen at doses as low as 350 to 500 mg per day. Reducing the dose usually eliminates the problem. If you have heart or kidney problems, check with your doctor before taking magnesium supplements.

◉ STRATEGIES FOR RELIEF

• Practice moderation in your daily activities. Because symptoms of CFS can vary so dramatically from person to person—and even from day to day—some people find the "morning test walk" useful. To assess what kind of day you're going to have, take a short walk each morning. Plan your day's activities according to how you react to the exertion.

• Exercise is important to prevent physical deconditioning, which can worsen fatigue. Many people report feeling better after undertaking a regular, moderate exercise regimen. However, start slowly and build your strength and endurance gradually. But don't overdo, especially early on. At the beginning, just getting out of bed and walking around your room for a few minutes may be all you can handle. Many doctors recommend a program leading to thirty minutes of aerobic activity, such as walking, at least five times a week.

• Practice energy conservation. For example, use a luggage carrier or cart with wheels to carry heavy books or groceries. Sit down whenever possible, on the job and at home. Keep a tall stool in the kitchen so that you can prepare meals or do the dishes sitting down. Get a shower stool so that you can sit when you bathe. You may benefit from discussing alternatives with an occupational therapist.

• Plan for downtime when it's likely to be needed. If you have to attend an important but energy-draining function, keep the day before the event, and the day after, free for rest.

• Watch your sugar intake. Some research suggests that people with CFS are deficient in an enzyme needed to metabolize sugar. When you're going to have sugar, always do so after a meal, rather than on an empty stomach. That slows down the absorption of the sugar, making it easier for your body to handle.

• Reduce your fat intake. Fatty foods are difficult to digest and can cause a general sluggish feeling. Further, there's some evidence that too much fat in the diet can have an adverse effect on immunity.

• Eat a balanced diet with a variety of foods that is high in fiber and complex carbohydrates, with lots of fruits, vegetables, beans, and whole grains.

• Get tested for food and other allergies.

• Beware of caffeine. When you're tired all of the time, it's tempting to depend on caffeine to make you more alert. But it's also important to avoid or cut back on foods that may cause a loss of minerals, as caffeine can do.

- If you suffer from low blood pressure, include some salty foods in your diet to help maintain a normal pressure.
- Stay socially active to avoid isolation, which can contribute to depression.
- Ask for help when you need it. Don't hide your problems from family members and friends.
- Find a support group, through your local hospital or online. Talking with others who also have chronic health problems can be very valuable in keeping your spirits up.
- Try to avoid highly stressful situations. You may also benefit from relaxation training and behavioral therapy to help you improve your coping mechanisms for dealing with stress.
- If you have memory problems, use memory aids. For example, make lists and write notes to yourself, and post them prominently. Organize your home, labeling drawers and storing necessities in visible places.

Calcium

How it works. Taking more magnesium intake increases the body's need for calcium, a mineral that is essential to maintain healthy bones, support proper muscle function, and carry out other bodily functions.

Recommended dosages. Practitioners usually recommend taking them in a 2:1 ratio—1,000 mg of calcium if you're taking 500 mg of magnesium. (Calcium citrate is the form most easily absorbed.)

Possible problems. Calcium, whether from the diet or supplements, is absorbed best by the body when it is taken several times a day in amounts of 500 mg or less, but taking it all at once is better than not taking it at all.

■ NUTRITIONAL SUPPLEMENTS

Carnitine

How it works. Carnitine (acetyl-L-carnitine) is required for energy production in cells, and some CFS sufferers have been found to have a carnitine deficiency.

Recommended dosages. Taking 1g of carnitine three times daily led to improvement in CFS symptoms among participants in a recent study.

Possible problems. Carnitine appears to be safe and has not been consistently linked with any toxicity symptoms. But it may cause vomiting when taken on an empty stomach.

Coenzyme Q_{10}

How it works. This natural substance is involved in energy-production at the cellular level. It is an antioxidant with a chemical makeup similar to that of vitamins E and K. It reacts with another enzyme to help cells convert protein, fat, and carbohydrates into energy. Although people with CFS have not been shown to be deficient in coenzyme Q_{10}, they may have functional shortages of the enzyme it reacts with.

Recommended dosages. Try 100 to 200 mg daily, taken in divided doses under the tongue. Since coenzyme Q_{10} is fat-soluble, it should be taken with a little bit of fat or oil (although some supplements come in an oil base).

Possible problems. Give this nutrient at least a two-month trial before expecting results.

■ BOTANICAL MEDICINES

Astragalus (A. membranaceus)

How it works. Astragalus is derived from the root of a plant grown mostly in northern China that has been aged between four and seven years. Although few well-controlled scientific studies using human subjects can confirm its precise effects, basic science and animal studies suggest that astragalus bolsters the immune system by increasing production and action of a type of white blood cell.

Recommended dosages. Boil astragalus root for a few minutes, and then make a tea from the fluid. In powdered form, 200- to 500-mg capsules or tablets taken two or three times a day are commonly prescribed. Alternatively, 3 to 5 ml (¾ to 1 teaspoon) of astragalus tincture daily is often recommended.

Possible problems. There are no known side effects to astragalus, but there is also a dearth of reliable scientific information about this botanical.

Licorice (*Glycyrrhiza glabra*)

How it works. Many people with CFS experience a drop in blood pressure when standing, which can result in light-headedness or even fainting. Licorice that contains glycyrrhizin (as opposed to deglycyrrizinated, or DGL-type, licorice) can occasionally cause an elevation of blood pressure if used in high enough amounts.

Recommended dosages. A case study has reported that taking 2.5 g of licorice each day helped one patient who did not respond to any other therapy.

Possible problems. Long-term intake of products more than 5 or 6 weeks containing more than 1 g of glycyrrhizin per day can cause serious side effects, including a dangerous rise in blood pressure. Such a regimen should only be undertaken with help from a properly trained health care professional, given its complexity and potential dangers.

Siberian Ginseng (*Eleutherococcus senticosus*)

How it works. This popular herbal medicine is used as a general tonic in China to increase energy and vigor, in Russia to help withstand stress, and in Germany to counteract fatigue. Experiments in humans have shown that it boosts some immune system components.

Recommended dosages. Some practitioners recommend 100 to 300 mg once or twice a day. As a tincture in an alcohol extract, one expert suggests taking ½ to 6 ml one to three times a day. Take it for only a month, then resume after a break of at least two weeks.

Possible problems. Rarely, temporary drowsiness has been reported immediately after taking it. Otherwise, the herb appears to be safe at this dosage. Anyone with high blood pressure, heart disease, thyroid disorders, or migraine headaches should avoid taking ginseng products. (See Ginseng, p. 466.)

Intermittent claudication

- Cramping, aching, painful, and/or tired sensations in the leg, calf, foot, buttock, hip, or thigh occurring during physical activity and when the leg is elevated.
- Intensifying pain when walking, especially when climbing stairs or going up-hill.
- Pain relief at rest, early in the disease.
- Cold, numb foot with dry, peeling skin.

Chronic venous insufficiency

- Swelling of the legs.
- Dull aching, heavy feeling or cramping.
- Discoloration of the ankles.
- Ulcers in the skin of the legs.
- Chest pain and difficulty breathing, if a blood clot breaks loose and lodges in the lungs, which is a medical emergency.

Raynaud's disease/phenomenon

- Skin that becomes extremely pale and turns reddish blue when exposed to cold.
- Numbness, tingling, and pain.

Circulatory problems, which are generally known as vascular disorders, occur when insufficient blood supply is available to the brain, the heart, the leg muscles or other parts of the body. Blood circulates throughout the body by way of an intricate system of arteries and veins. Arteries are responsible for distributing oxygen-rich blood from the heart to all parts of the body, while veins collect and return oxygen-depleted blood to the heart. When the flow is blocked or arteries and veins do not dilate properly, the parts of the body served by those vessels can no longer get enough blood to function properly.

Circulatory problems are often caused by arteries that have narrowed from atherosclerosis. But they can also result from a clot that blocks blood flow through an artery or vein, or from damaged valves. When the blocked arteries are in the heart, the resulting pain is called angina, which is often a warning sign of heart attack risk (see Heart Disease, p. 118). Specific circulatory disorders include:

• *Intermittent claudication.* Blocked arteries in the pelvis, thighs, or calves lead to this characteristic pattern of leg pain and weakness. Most at risk are men of any age, women past menopause, anyone over sixty, smokers, and people with diabetes or high blood pressure. Other risk factors include excess weight and sedentary lifestyle. The pain of intermittent claudication is likely to indicate the presence of diseased arteries in the heart or brain as well. It is progressive and will not go away unless treated.

• *Chronic venous insufficiency.* The valves of veins channel the flow of blood in one direction only, toward the heart. But when these valves are damaged or blocked, blood leaks and pools. In the absence of normal blood flow, painful skin ulcers may develop. Problems in the legs are most common, since the deep leg veins and calf muscles must pump blood back to the heart when a person is standing. People who are bedridden or even those who sit for long periods may also be vulnerable, because their calf muscles aren't doing the necessary work of compressing the veins and sending the blood back to the heart. For a discussion of varicose veins, a type of venous disorder, see page 194.

• *Raynaud's disease and Raynaud's phenomenon.* Raynaud's disease and Raynaud's phenomenon cause the same condition, which occurs when tiny arteries just below the skin overreact to cold. Although the normal reaction of the body to cold is to slow blood flow and preserve body heat, in people with Raynaud's symptoms, the blood vessels constrict too much and begin to spasm, causing the skin to turn pale and take on a red-blue tint. In Raynaud's phenomenon, symptoms are secondary to some other disease; Raynaud's disease is the term used when no precipitating cause can be found. The condition affects mostly women between the ages of fifteen and fifty. It frequently occurs in conjunction with heart disease, migraine, scleroderma, lupus, rheumatoid arthritis, pulmonary hypertension, or medications prescribed for these conditions. Raynaud's can also be aggravated by stress, by the use of vibrating tools such as chain saws or power drills, and even by playing the piano or typing. In most cases, it is simply an uncomfortable nuisance, but in some extreme cases, the condition can become chronic, leading to death of tissue from a lack of oxygen.

Diagnostic Steps

If intermittent claudication or venous insufficiency is suspected, a doctor is likely to check the blood flow in the legs. For intermittent claudication, first the pulses in the feet will be checked. Then the blood pressure in the arm is compared to that in the ankle. If the pressure in the ankle is much less than that in the arm, it's a sign that the arteries in the legs are narrowed and not enough blood is getting to the legs and feet. To better identify which artery or vein is blocked, an ultrasound scan may be performed. Special imaging studies (X rays of the blood vessels using radioactive contrast material) will be ordered if blood flow to the heart or lungs is affected.

Raynaud's disease/phenomenon is usually diagnosed by description of the symptoms. Sometimes arterial blood flow tests will be performed before and after exposure to cold.

Conventional Treatments

If circulatory problems are caused by atherosclerosis, diet and lifestyle changes are important to slow the progression and perhaps even reverse the buildup of plaque on artery walls. (See Cholesterol Disorders and Atherosclerosis, p. 68.) Numerous medications are available for increasing circulation. For intermittent claudication in particular, Pentoxifylline (Trental) is prescribed to improve blood flow through the blood vessels in the arms and legs. The medication often takes two to three months before any improvement can be seen; side effects may include nausea, loss of appetite, constipation, headaches, dizziness, or blurred vision.

The primary treatment for chronic venous insufficiency and leg ulcers is the use of compression bandaging and hosiery, which improve circulation. Medical treatment is not required unless there are complicating factors, such as a blood clot or severe bleeding. About 15 percent of people with poor circulation will require surgery to increase blood flow, using procedures such as balloon angioplasty, arterial bypass, or replacement of blocked blood vessels.

◉ STRATEGIES FOR RELIEF

- Exercise regularly. Walking or cycling are especially good activities that can help improve circulation.
- Maintain a healthy weight. Extra weight places stress on the legs and makes activity difficult.
- Don't sit cross-legged; this position reduces the circulation in the legs.
- Don't smoke. It affects blood circulation throughout the body.
- Make sure that high blood pressure and diabetes are kept under control. Both diseases increase the risk of circulatory disorders.
- Keep blood cholesterol levels within desirable ranges. Cholesterol contributes to the buildup of plaque on artery walls, which reduces blood flow.
- For Raynaud's, taking evening primrose oil is sometimes recommended. There have also been reports that rubbing evening primrose oil directly into fingertips may help ease symptoms.
- Avoid taking cold pills that contain decongestants, which constrict blood vessels and can worsen circulatory problems.
- If you suffer from Raynaud's symptoms, discuss the advisability of taking birth control pills. Some studies suggest that these medications, especially those high in estrogen, may worsen the condition. Similarly, taking postmenopausal estrogen replacement may also worsen symptoms.

Nutraceuticals for Circulatory Problems

■ VITAMINS AND MINERALS

Vitamin C

How it works. Vitamin C prevents the destruction of nitric oxide, a powerful relaxer of blood vessels, making it more available to the body. The vitamin is known to strengthen capillaries and prevent bruising.

Recommended dosages. The Recommended Dietary Allowance is 75 to 90 mg a day (100 mg a day for smokers). However, several experts recommend an intake of 200 mg a day for saturation of the body's tissues and optimum benefit. It appears that doses above 500 mg a day offer no additional advantage.

Possible problems. Daily doses of 1,000 mg or more a day can cause diarrhea. People with kidney stones or kidney disease should avoid such high doses of vitamin C. Large doses may also interfere with the action of anticoagulant medications such as Coumadin.

Nicotinic acid (niacin, vitamin B$_3$)

How it works. Niacin is an umbrella term for various forms of vitamin B$_3$, which promotes increased circulation by relaxing blood vessels.

Recommended dosages. The preferred form for Raynaud's phenomenon, intermittent claudication, and other circulatory disorders is time-release nicotinic acid or inositol hexaniacinate, a form in which nicotinic acid is bound to inositol, another member of the B-complex family. Take 500 mg three times a day.

Possible problems. High doses of nicotinic acid can cause intense flushing of the skin, itching, nausea, and liver damage. Taking it as inositol hexaniacinate reduces these risks, but check with your doctor if you are taking it. Large doses of inositol hexaniacinate can thin the blood, which is a problem if you are taking medicines such as Coumadin. (See Vitamin B$_3$, p. 226.)

■ NUTRITIONAL SUPPLEMENTS

L-Arginine

How it works. The body uses this amino acid to produce nitric oxide, a powerful relaxer of blood vessels, which helps keep arteries relaxed and blood flowing freely. Nitric oxide also keeps platelets and white blood cells from sticking to artery walls, reducing the risk that atherosclerosis will develop. Finally, nitric oxide improves blood flow to the legs.

Recommended dosages. In addition to L-arginine obtained through dietary proteins, 3 to 6 g a day of supplementary L-arginine is recommended by some practitioners.

Possible problems. Research to date has found supplemental L-arginine to be safe for people with heart disease or diseases of the blood vessels. However, L-arginine has not been tested on people with other medical conditions. It can cause mild diarrhea and trigger a herpes outbreak in those infected with the virus. There's even a possibility it could increase blood flow to undiagnosed tumors.

Pycnogenol and grape seed extract

How they work. In the United States, Pycnogenol is a registered trademark for a French pine tree extract. Grape seed extract is similar in antioxidant compounds. Each can help relax blood vessels and prevent the oxidation of LDLs, which leads to atherosclerosis and reduction of blood flow. These two botanical medicines also appear to help the body utilize vitamins C and E. No long-term clinical trials have been done to see if Pycnogenol or grape seed extract actually prevents atherosclerosis or improves circulatory problems, however.

Recommended dosages. Dosages range from 50 to 200 mg a day.

Possible problems. There have been no reported side effects from taking either Pycnogenol or grape seed extract.

■ BOTANICAL MEDICINES

Ginkgo (G. biloba)

How it works. Flavonoids and ginkgolides in ginkgo leaves make capillaries less fragile, fight free-radical damage, and improve peripheral blood flow, which may make them useful for Raynaud's and other circulatory problems.

Recommended dosages. The recommended daily dosage of standardized gingko biloba extract (GBE) for cerebral circulatory disturbances is 120 to 240 mg a day divided into two or three doses. It may take six to eight weeks for effects to become apparent.

Possible problems. Although side effects are not common, they can include gastrointestinal disturbances, headaches, and allergic skin reactions. Large doses may cause bleeding abnormalities in people already at risk for such problems, such as those taking low-dose aspirin, NSAIDs or other blood thinners, such as warfarin (Coumadin).

Butcher's broom (Ruscus aculeatus L.)

How it works. The roots of this shrub are believed to increase the strength of blood vessel walls and to have an anti-inflammatory effect.

Recommended dosages. Extracts standardized to contain 9 to 11 percent of ruscogenin at a dosage of 100 to 150 mg three times a day are recommended.

Possible problems. Though it is generally considered safe, it can cause a rise in blood pressure and stomach upset.

Horse chestnut (Aesculus hippocastanum)

How it works. Seeds from the horse chestnut tree contain a compound called aescin, which has the ability to reduce the activity of certain enzymes that destroy the elastic tissue of the veins and damage blood-vessel valves. Horse chestnut has also been shown to reduce swelling and improve the overall tone of the veins and improve return blood flow to the heart.

Recommended dosages. Start with a dose that contains the equivalent of 90 to 150 mg of aescin. If circulatory problems begin to improve, reduce the dosage to 35 to 70 mg a day.

Possible problems. Side effects are not common, although gastrointestinal upset can occur. Do not take higher than recommended doses for extended periods. Never eat the horse chestnut seeds that fall from trees—they're poisonous and require processing before they can be ingested.

COMMON COLD AND FLU

◉ SYMPTOMS

Cold

- Usually comes on slowly, beginning with a sore, scratchy throat.
- Increasing nasal discharge and congestion; difficulty breathing through the nose, swelling of mucous membranes in sinuses.
- Sore throat and cough.
- Possible headache.
- Fever, when present, is low.

Flu

- Begins suddenly, with headache, chills, dry cough, and exhaustion.
- Fever as high as 104°F begins to decline on second or third day.
- Nasal congestion and sore throat follow.
- Fatigue, which may linger for weeks.

◉ WHEN TO CONSULT A DOCTOR

Some telltale signs medical attention is necessary include:

- Chest pain upon breathing.
- Trouble swallowing or breathing.
- Inner ear pain.
- Significantly swollen glands in the neck.
- Severe facial pain in the sinus area.
- A fever over 100°F lasting more than seventy-two hours.
- Severe headache.
- A cough that produces green, yellow, or bloody phlegm.

Colds and flu share a number of symptoms—congestion, aches and pains, malaise, and, sometimes, fever—that can make them hard to distinguish one from the other. In addition, both are highly contagious respiratory infections caused by viruses. Colds and flu are spread from person to person by coughing or sneezing, or by touching surfaces containing the virus, such as people's hands, and then touching your own eyes, nose, or mouth. Commonsense precautions, such as washing your hands and promptly disposing of used tissues, as well as bolstering the immune system, are the keys to prevention.

Colds strike on average four times a year, no matter what the season. According to the National Institute of Allergy and Infectious Diseases, children can have up to twelve colds in as many months. Women tend to catch more colds than men, and the risk of all upper respiratory infections is high among smokers, in part because smoking dries the nasal and sinus passages.

Although colds are usually a short-lived and minor illness, there are exceptions. For example, colds can lead to secondary ear and sinus infections, and they can pose special threats to people with asthma, emphysema, and other chronic lung disorders.

The flu season generally lasts from December to March, with up to half the population contracting the virus during that time. While a cold is annoying, the flu, or influenza, can be very serious, even life-threatening among the very young, the elderly, and persons whose resistance is lowered by a chronic disease such as diabetes, heart disease, or AIDS. While most people recover from flu in under two weeks, fatigue and weakness may linger, and people in high-risk groups may be sicker for longer periods or suffer from complications such as pneumonia. Flu shots help fend off viruses that cause flu, but because flu viruses undergo almost constant mutations, a new vaccine is needed each year.

Diagnostic Steps

Diagnosis is usually based on the symptoms. Generally, it is not necessary to consult a doctor unless you have other health problems or if the symptoms are very severe or fail to abate in a few days.

Conventional Treatments

Although new antiviral medications are coming on the market, the conventional way to recover remains to rest, drink large amounts of fluids, and take aspirin, ibuprofen, or acetaminophen for fever and body aches. However, children and teenagers with flu symptoms should not take any product containing aspirin, since they could develop a rare but sometimes fatal disease called Reye's syndrome.

Because colds and flu are caused by viruses, antibiotics are of little or no value unless the cold or flu gives rise to a bacterial infection, such as sinus and inner ear infection. In such cases, antibiotic treatment may be appropriate.

For the flu, the best conventional offense is defense: a flu vaccination shot given prior to the flu season. Flu shots are effective in preventing the disease in 70 to 90 percent of healthy adults. For people who cannot take the vaccine (because of allergies to eggs or current illnesses such as pneumonia), or those at high risk who have not had the shots, prescription antiviral medications may help. Amantidine and rimantadine can shorten type A strains of the flu if they are administered within the first few days of illness. Newer drugs—zanamivir (Relenza), administered through an inhaler; and oseltamivir (Tamiflu)—appear to inhibit both type A and type B flu viruses; treatment must begin within the first two days that symptoms appear. Relenza is not recommended for anyone with asthma or breathing problems, or for children. For flu prevention in children, an apparently effective vaccine in the form of a nasal spray (FluMist) may soon be on the market.

Otherwise, for both colds and flu, over-the-counter decongestants and cough suppressants may ease symptoms, but they should be used with caution, if at all, by persons with high blood pressure, glaucoma, diabetes, heart disease, and a number of other disorders. Depending upon the medication, side effects may include drowsiness, dizziness, or insomnia. If these products are used, look for formulations designed to combat only your most troublesome symptoms. For example, a nonprescription antihistamine works against a runny nose and watery eyes; aspirin or acetaminophen ease achiness.

◉ STRATEGIES FOR RELIEF

- *Avoid transmitting germs.* Many of the viruses that cause colds and flu can survive up to three hours outside the body, even on inanimate objects, and on skin. Simple hand-washing goes a long way to prevent respiratory illness. Avoid touching your nose and eyes; it's easy for germs to enter your body at these points.

- *Drink fluids.* To prevent and to speed recovery from colds and flu, sip on at least 64 ounces of nonalcoholic, caffeine-free fluids each day. You know you've got enough fluid on board when your urine is nearly clear in color. For prevention, staying well hydrated is especially important if you fly often or work or live in a dry environment; dry air promotes minute cracks in the membranes of your nasal passages, allowing germs to gain entry into your system. When you are ill, warm fluids help loosen phlegm. In fact, chicken soup contains a substance that helps temporarily relieve congestion by thinning out mucus.

- *Try hot peppers (chilies) and slippery elm for symptom relief.* Chilies contain capsaicin, which can loosen nasal and sinus congestion. To soothe sore throat symptoms, try slippery elm tablets, tea, or tincture. Be aware of its laxative effect, though.

Nutraceuticals for Common Cold and Flu

■ VITAMINS AND MINERALS

Vitamin C

How it works. Decades of scientific research have failed to prove that high doses of vitamin C can prevent the common cold or flu. Even so, millions of Americans persist in taking large amounts of the vitamin in the firm belief that it helps. There is some evidence that vitamin C, taken early in the course of a cold, may shorten its duration and perhaps lessen the symptoms. Some researchers theorize that high-dose vitamin C has some antihistamine properties, which may help to relieve a runny nose and watery eyes.

Recommended dosages. Suggested dosages range from 500 to 2,000 mg three times daily during the active illness period.

Possible problems. Too much vitamin C in pill form may cause bloating and diarrhea. Start with a low dose of 200 mg three times a day, and gradually work up to a total of 1,000 mg a day. Reduce the dosage if diarrhea and other intestinal problems develop.

Zinc

How it works. Zinc is part of more than two hundred enzymes that drive the bodily functions supporting good health and a strong immune system. Studies suggest that zinc consumption slacks off with age, even though keeping the immune system strong is essential as one grows older. Taking zinc gluconate lozenges several times a day during the first few days of symptoms may reduce the duration of a cold, although studies are equivocal.

Recommended dosages. About 15 mg of zinc per day, through diet or supplements, is generally sufficient to prevent zinc deficiency. Although dosages to treat colds or flu have not been established, many experts recommend taking 10 to 25 mg of zinc gluconate, in lozenge form, every two or three hours during the first few days of a cold. In general, you should not take more than 150 mg a day, and these large amounts should not be taken for more than a week or so.

Possible problems. Too much zinc is detrimental to immune-system functioning, so don't take high doses on an ongoing basis. Experts note that taking more than 100 mg a day for more than a few weeks may lower resistance to infections. Lozenges and high-dose supplements may cause mouth sores and intestinal discomfort. High doses may interfere with absorption of copper, so look for supplements that contain that mineral.

Vitamin A

How it works. Among its myriad functions, vitamin A boosts the immune system; some researchers theorize that it may have a direct effect on the viruses that cause colds and flu. Vitamin A is available in foods and supplements as retinol, the preformed version, or as beta-carotene, which the body converts to vitamin A on an as-needed basis.

Recommended dosages. Some vitamin A proponents recommend taking 50,000 to 150,000 IU of vitamin A per day for a minimum of three, and a maximum of five, days when trying to rid yourself of a virus. This approach, however, has not been subjected to controlled clinical studies.

Possible problems. Vitamin A is fat-soluble, and as such, excess amounts are stored primarily in the liver tissue. A buildup of retinol can cause severe liver damage; it can also cause severe birth defects when taken before or during early pregnancy. When taking high doses of vitamin A, even short-term, select products that are mostly beta-carotene, which is nontoxic even in large doses. (It may, however, temporarily turn the skin a yellowish orange.)

■ BOTANICAL MEDICINES

Echinacea (*E. purpurea, E. angustifolia, E. pallida*)

How it works. Commonly called purple or prairie coneflowers, several species of echinacea may help protect against colds, flu, and other viral infections by bolstering the immune system. When taken at the first hint of a cold or flu, echinacea has been shown to shorten the duration and severity of infection. In one study, people who ordinarily suffered colds almost monthly reduced their bouts by 35 percent and also almost doubled the time between colds. In another double-blind study of one hundred people with upper respiratory infections, taking echinacea when symptoms first appeared shortened the duration of the colds by about three days.

Recommended dosages. A typical dosage calls for 800 to 1,000 mg a day, taken in 200-mg dosages during the course of the day. It can be taken in capsule, tablet, lozenge, or liquid form. It should not be taken for more than eight weeks at a time because it tends to lose its effectiveness with prolonged use.

Possible problems. Echinacea is a potential allergen for people sensitive to ragweed. More importantly, experts say to avoid it if you have an autoimmune disease, including multiple sclerosis; lupus and other collagen disorders; or rheumatoid arthritis. Echinacea may worsen such disorders by stimulating the immune system to step up its attack on healthy tissue. Prolonged use (more than eight weeks at a time) may actually lower immune resistance. Those with TB or HIV should avoid echinacea until more is known about its effects on immune function.

Goldenseal (*Hydrastis canadensis*)

How it works. Native Americans have long used the dried root of this plant to soothe inflamed mucous membranes and as a general tonic to prevent colds, flu, and other infections. Goldenseal is high in berberine and hydrastine, alkaloids that are thought to bolster the immune system. Herbalists often prescribe it in combination with echinacea to increase the effectiveness of both herbs, although there is little scientific proof of this.

Recommended dosages. A typical dosage calls for taking 125 mg of goldenseal, along with 200 mg of echinacea, four or five times a day beginning at the first sign of a cold and continuing for five days or until symptoms abate.

Possible problems. Some people taking very high doses develop digestive disorders, such as diarrhea and constipation. It may also irritate the mucous membranes.

Garlic (*Allium sativum*)

How it works. Animal studies suggest garlic protects against viruses by increasing antibody production. Its healing properties are ascribed to one of its sulfur compounds, alliin, which converts to allicin when it is crushed or chewed.

Recommended dosages. Raw or barely cooked garlic is most beneficial, since cooking and processing decreases allicin potency. In lieu of the recommended one to ten raw garlic cloves a day, try enteric-coated supplements containing allicin. About 5,000 mcg of allicin are equivalent to one clove of fresh, raw garlic.

Possible problems. Garlic can affect platelet function. If you take anticoagulants like Coumadin or daily aspirin, or if you have surgery planned within one or two weeks, adding garlic to the mix may cause internal bleeding. Check with your doctor before using raw or supplemental garlic in large amounts. People with diabetes must consider that large garlic doses can reduce blood glucose levels, which can enhance the effects of the medication you take to control diabetes. Heartburn and intestinal tract distress are also common side effects of eating raw garlic or taking certain supplements.

Astragalus (*A. membranaceus*)

How it works. Astragalus is derived from the root of a plant grown mostly in northern China that has been aged between four and seven years. Although few well-controlled scientific studies using human subjects can confirm its precise effects, basic science and animal studies suggest that astragalus bolsters the immune system by stimulating production of a type of white blood cell. Astragalus may not be as beneficial for actually combating colds and flu as it is for preventing them.

Recommended dosages. Boil astragalus root for a few minutes, and then make a tea from the fluid. In powdered form, 200- to 500-mg capsules or tablets taken two or three times a day are commonly prescribed. Alternatively, 3 to 5 ml (¾ to 1 teaspoon) of astragalus tincture daily is often recommended.

Possible problems. There are no known side effects to astragalus, but there is also a dearth of reliable scientific information about this botanical.

CONSTIPATION

According to the National Institutes of Health, constipation is the most common digestive problem in the United States, resulting in about 2 million doctor visits each year and prompting Americans to spend $725 million a year on laxatives. Almost everyone experiences constipation at some time in their lives, with about 4.5 million people reporting they are constipated most or all of the time.

Constipation is generally defined as bowel movements that are small, dry, and difficult to pass. Although frequency is not necessarily a factor, most people who are constipated report having fewer than three bowel movements a week. As food moves through the colon, the colon absorbs water while forming waste products, or stool. Muscle contractions in the colon push the stool toward the rectum. By the time stool reaches the rectum, it is semisolid because most of the water has been absorbed. The hard, dry stools of constipation occur when the colon absorbs too much water, usually because the colon's contractions are too slow or sluggish.

Among the most common causes of constipation are:

• *Diet.* The most common cause of constipation is a diet low in fiber, the parts of fruits, vegetables, and grains that the body can't digest. Experts recommend a daily intake of 20 to 35 g of fiber. Yet the average intake falls somewhere between 5 and 20 g a day. People who eat a high-fiber diet are less likely to become constipated. Soluble fiber found in fruits, vegetables, oats, and psyllium dissolves easily in water and takes on a soft, gel-like texture in the intestines. Insoluble fiber, found in whole-grain foods, passes virtually unchanged through the intestines. Both kinds of fiber help prevent the formation of hard, dry stools.

• *Inadequate liquids.* Fiber absorbs large amounts of fluids, adding bulk to the stool and making it softer and easier to pass. Experts recommend a daily intake of at least eight 8-ounce glasses of fluid a day. However, caffeine-containing beverages like coffee and soft drinks may have a dehydrating effect.

• *Inactivity.* Though it isn't known exactly why, a lack of exercise can lead to constipation. It is a common complication following an accident

◉ SYMPTOMS
- Infrequent, painful, and difficult-to-pass stools.
- Abdominal bloating and discomfort.

◉ STRATEGIES FOR RELIEF
- Eating a diet rich in high-fiber foods is important for both preventing and treating constipation. The goal should be to get 20 to 35 g of fiber a day from such high-fiber foods as whole-grain breads, cereals, rice, corn, peas, Brussels sprouts, broccoli, cauliflower, apples, strawberries, prunes, dates, kiwifruit, raspberries, and bananas. Some bran cereals are very high in fiber; compare nutritional information on the boxes.
- Exercise daily; even just walking around the block may help stimulate bowel movements.
- Try dried dandelion root tea, made from about 1 teaspoon per cup of hot water.
- If you are taking antacids containing aluminum, change to types containing magnesium, which has a slight laxative effect.
- When traveling or having a busy day, plan to take bathroom breaks at the time you usually have a bowel movement, and head there when you get the urge. When traveling across time zones, it may take time for your body clock to get back on its usual schedule. Bring psyllium, bran, or flaxseed products with you to get things going more quickly.

or an illness, when someone is confined to bed. Getting some exercise every day can help keep sluggish bowels moving.

• *Medications.* Pain medications (especially narcotics), antacids that contain aluminum, antispasmodics, antidepressants, iron supplements, diuretics, and anticonvulsants are among the many medications that can slow passage of bowel movements.

• *Irritable bowel syndrome.* The condition can cause colon spasms that affect bowel movements. Constipation often alternates with diarrhea.

• *Changes in routine.* Traveling, stress, and overwork can often lead to constipation as the normal diet and daily routines are disrupted.

• *Life change.* Constipation is common during pregnancy as a result of hormonal changes and pressure from the expanding uterus pressing on the intestine. Aging can affect bowel regularity because of a loss of muscle tone and a decrease in intestinal activity.

• *Overuse of laxatives.* With chronic use, laxatives can damage nerve cells in the colon and interfere with its natural ability to contract. They should be limited to single uses and be taken only as a last resort.

• *Delaying bowel movements.* Ignoring the urge to go to the toilet because of a hectic schedule or discomfort using facilities in unfamiliar surroundings can eventually lessen the urge to go and lead to constipation.

• *Diseases.* Among the conditions and diseases that can cause constipation are neurological disorders such as multiple sclerosis, Parkinson's disease, stroke, and spinal cord injuries. Metabolic and endocrine conditions such as diabetes and an underactive or overactive thyroid can also cause constipation, as can systemic disorders such as lupus and scleroderma.

• *Problems with the colon and rectum.* Intestinal obstruction, scar tissue, diverticulosis, tumors, or cancer can compress, squeeze, or narrow the intestine and rectum, causing constipation.

• *Problems with intestinal muscles.* Though rare, there are people who are chronically constipated and do not respond to standard treatment. Such a case is referred to as chronic idiopathic constipation. It may be caused by problems with hormonal control or with nerves and muscles in the colon, rectum, or anus. It occurs in both children and adults, but is most common in women.

Diagnostic Steps

Extensive testing is usually not needed; a decision of whether to recommend tests depends upon the duration and severity of the constipation, your age, whether there is blood in stools, changes in bowel habits, or recent unexplained weight loss. If a digital rectal exam detects tenderness, obstruction, or blood, tests such as a barium enema followed by X rays or sigmoidoscopy or colonoscopy—tests in which a viewing tube is used to inspect the inside of the colon—may be performed to detect the cause or to rule out cancer.

Conventional Treatments

If a change in diet and activity have not brought relief, some doctors recommend laxatives or enemas for a limited period of time. There are a wide variety of laxatives available in liquid, tablet, gum, powder, and granule form:

• *Bulk-forming agents.* These are generally considered the safest among the over-the-counter laxatives, but they can interfere with the absorption of some medications. Two of the most common ingredients are psyllium and methylcellulose, which absorb water in the intestine and make stools softer.

• *Stimulants.* These over-the-counter products contain cascara, senna, or bisacodyl, which trigger rhythmic contractions in the intestines. This type of laxative is most associated with overuse, dependency, and abuse. The ingredient phenolphthalein, which used to be commonly used in laxatives, was found to increase the risk of cancer in animals and was removed from the market. Many over-the-counter products that used to contain phenolphthalein now contain bisacodyl or senna.

• *Stool softeners.* These enhance the penetration of water into the stool, making it softer and easier to pass. These are often recommended for people who shouldn't strain during a bowel movement, such as women after childbirth, people who have had surgery, and some cardiac patients.

• *Lubricants.* Mineral oil is the most commonly used lubricant. It greases the stool, allowing it to move more easily through the intestinal tract.

• *Osmotic laxatives.* These draw water into the bowel to soften stool. Lactulose is a commonly prescribed osmotic laxative.

Nutraceuticals for Constipation

■ NUTRITIONAL SUPPLEMENTS

Kelp

How it works. There are several varieties of kelp and all contain a compound called algin or sodium alginate, which forms a thick gel in water and is responsible for its laxative effect.

Recommended dosages. Though no dose has been established as safe and effective for the treatment of constipation, several kelp products suggest a dose of about 500 to 1,200 mg a day. It is typically available in tablets and capsules.

Possible problems. Be sure to drink eight to ten glasses of water a day. Kelp is high in iodine. Regular consumption of large amounts could result in iodine overdose and thyroid dysfunction.

Psyllium

How it works. The psyllium seed is filled with a thick gel that is not digested in the intestinal tract, so it acts as a bulk-producing laxative. When it comes in contact with water, it swells and provides bulk and lubrication.

Recommended dosages. The usual dose is 1 to 2 heaping teaspoonfuls each day stirred into a glass of water, juice, or milk. The mixture must be consumed quickly before it has time to gel and become thick. (Psyllium is the main ingredient in Metamucil and similar laxatives.)

Possibly problems. Psyllium can trigger allergic reactions in a small number of people, such as hospital workers, who are exposed regularly to psyllium powder. A full glass of water or juice should be consumed with psyllium to prevent the formation of blockages in the esophagus or intestines. For it to work properly, additional fluid—eight to ten glasses—should be taken during the course of the day.

■ BOTANICAL MEDICINES

Flax (*Linum usitatissimum*)

How it works. Flaxseed, like psyllium, swells in liquid and becomes a bulk laxative. It requires several glasses of water throughout the day to prevent blockage.

Recommended dosages. Take 1 to 2 tablespoons of whole or crushed flaxseed in 5 to 8 ounces of water two or three times a day. Drink several glasses of water during the course of the day to prevent blockage.

Possible problems. Flaxseed is generally considered safe when used over a short or long term.

Cascara sagrada (*Rhamnus purshiana*)

How it works. Like aloe, cascara also contains anthraquinone glycosides, chemicals that powerfully stimulate the colon and increase water absorption.

Recommended dosages. The dose is based on the anthraquinone content of the plant, which is typically at least 8 percent. Recommended daily doses range from 100 to 500 mg of the aged bark. It should not be used for more than a few days at a time. Drink plenty of water throughout the day.

Possible problems. It should not be used during pregnancy or breast-feeding or by children under the age of twelve. Chronic use or abuse can cause a severe loss of potassium and make some medications such as cardiac glycosides more potent. The total dose of anthraquinones should not exceed 20 to 30 mg.

Aloe vera (*A. vera, A. barbadensis*)

How it works. Aloe latex (but not aloe gel), usually in dried form, is a very powerful laxative. It contains compounds called anthraquinone glycosides, which act directly on the intestinal lining to stimulate contractions and increase water absorption, putting aloe in the category of a stimulant laxative. It can cause loose, watery stools.

Recommended dosages. The dose is based on the anthraquinone content of the plant, which is typically between 20 and 40 percent. Recommended daily doses range from 50 to 200 mg of dried aloe latex, taken at bedtime. Use it only for a few days, and drink several glasses of water throughout the day.

Possible problems. It can increase menstrual bleeding and during pregnancy may increase the risk of miscarriage. Like any stimulant laxative, it can create dependence if used over a long period of time.

Senna (*Cassia senna*)

How it works. Senna contains compounds called dianthrone glycosides, which have a cathartic action. It is considered a stimulant-type laxative, but it has a stronger laxative action than cascara.

Recommended dosages. Though it is available as a tea, it is difficult to get a standardized dose this way and it has an extremely unpleasant taste unless it is masked by other flavors. Of the over-the-counter preparations that contain senna, most contain standardized amounts of the herb's active ingredients and package directions for dosing should be followed. Drink a lot of water throughout the day.

Possible problems. Like cascara, it can cause problems if used chronically or abused. And it should not be used by pregnant or breast-feeding women, or children under the age of two. Senna can cause abdominal discomfort even at low dosages.

DEPRESSION

Depression is one of our most common health problems, and one that can cause both emotional and physical symptoms. It is estimated that each year some 15 million Americans suffer a bout of clinical depression, but most of these never seek the professional help they need. About 25 percent of the population will suffer at least one episode of clinical depression during their life; women are affected about twice as often as men.

Clinical depression should not be confused with the "blue" moods that everyone experiences now and then, often for very good reasons, such as the loss of a job or loved one. In contrast, clinical depression often starts seemingly without reason, is more intense, lasts longer, and significantly interferes with day-to-day activities. Without treatment, depression can lead to a downward spiral of ever-worsening symptoms.

The causes of depression are not entirely clear. Many studies suggest that genetic and biochemical factors play a role in its development, but the precise mechanisms are largely unknown. Some people may be more prone to depression because of their environment and personal needs, but it's likely that a combination of factors are involved. In addition to genetics, these may include body chemistry, certain medications, and a triggering sad event, such as a serious illness, a death in the family, or another loss.

Diagnostic Steps

The first step should be a visit to a primary-care physician for a thorough checkup to rule out a possible underlying illness. Just knowledge that one is in sound physical health can improve mood. If depression is suspected, the primary-care doctor may suggest seeing a psychiatrist or another mental-health professional, who will ask numerous questions or use a standardized questionnaire to assess mood. Diagnosis is based on a rating of symptoms and general mood. The diagnostic process also involves identifying whether the person is suffering from a variation of clinical depression, which may include any of the following:

- *Dysthymia,* a chronic state of mild depression that often lasts for years and is characterized by many of the symptoms of clinical depression, but are not as severe. It is the most common form of depression.
- *Seasonal affective disorder,* or SAD, which occurs during the winter months and is linked to a lack of exposure to sun.
- *Atypical depression,* which is marked by excessive sleepiness and food cravings, especially for carbohydrates.
- *Bipolar disorder,* or *manic-depression,* in which periods of deep depression alternate with periods of euphoria, or mania.

Conventional Treatments

Treatments vary according to the type of depression. SAD, for example, is often cured by exposure to special full-spectrum lights for a few hours each day. Most other types of depression, however, are treated with a combination of psychotherapy and antidepressant medications. Although antidepressant drugs have revolutionized the treatment of this disorder, some also have a number of unwanted side effects, most commonly drowsiness, sexual dysfunction, and dry mouth, among others. The major classes of prescription drugs for depression include:

◉ SYMPTOMS

The presence of four or more of the following for more than two weeks indicates possible clinical depression:

- Appetite changes, with weight gain or weight loss not attributable to dieting.
- Changes in sleeping habits—either getting more or less sleep or awakening much earlier than usual.
- Lack of interest and pleasure in activities formerly enjoyed.
- Chronic feelings of fatigue and lack of energy.
- Feelings of worthlessness.
- Feelings of hopelessness.
- Inappropriate feelings of guilt.
- Inability to concentrate or indecisiveness.
- Overwhelming feelings of sadness or grief.
- Unexplained physical symptoms, such as headaches or stomachaches.
- Preoccupation with or recurring thoughts of death and suicide, always a sure sign that immediate professional help is needed.

- Selective serotonin reuptake inhibitors (SSRIs), such as fluoxetine (Prozac), sertraline (Zoloft), paroxetine (Paxil), and citalopram (Celexa).
- Tricyclic antidepressants, such as amitriptyline (Elavil), desipramine (Norpramin), imipramine (Tofranil), and nortriptyline (Pamelor).
- Monoamine oxidase (MAO) inhibitors, such as phenelzine (Nardil) and tranylcypromine (Parnate).
- Sedating antidepressants may be prescribed for those with severe sleep problems. They include trazodone (Desyrel), nefazodone (Serzone), and mirtazapine (Remeron).
- Miscellaneous other drugs used to treat depression include: bupropion (Wellbutrin), which does not affect sexual function; and venlaxafine (Effexor).

While antidepressant drugs can help a person overcome depression, the best long-term results are obtained when the drug therapy is combined with some form of psychotherapy, which may range from short-term therapy to help the patient sort out his or her problems to group therapy, in which people with similar problems give each other understanding and support.

Nutraceuticals for Depression

While many nutraceuticals can help ease the anxiety that often occurs with depression (see p. 37), experts generally agree that it is better to focus on products that attack the depression directly. The following are commonly recommended for mild depression and to prevent a recurrence of symptoms during and after recovery. (Note: The more severe forms of depression usually require stronger pharmaceutical products.)

■ VITAMINS AND MINERALS

Vitamin B-complex

How they work. The B vitamins are important for energy metabolism and proper nerve functions. Their precise role in mood is unknown, but studies show that people who suffer from clinical depression often have low levels of one or more of the B vitamins.

Recommended dosages. Most multiple vitamins provide the Recommended Dietary Allowances of the B-complex vitamins, but higher doses are needed during times of unusual emotional stress. Look for a B-50 (or B-100) formula. These provide 50 (or 100) mcg of vitamin B_{12} and biotin, 400 (or 800) mcg of folic acid, and 50 (or 100) mg of the other B vitamins.

Possible problems. B vitamins taken in these dosages are safe; very high doses of vitamin B_6 can cause nerve damage, and high doses of

It's important to recognize that depression is a clinical disease, and not a personal failing or something you can "tough" out. Seeking professional help is without doubt the most important step in overcoming the disease. Self-care strategies include:

- Depression often responds to structure. Get busy doing things you previously enjoyed. Develop a schedule that eliminates long empty stretches of time with nothing to do.
- Find a family member or trusted friend with whom you can share your feelings. Don't let yourself become isolated from family and friends. Attend activities with others even if you don't feel like talking.
- Engage in regular physical exercise, which prompts the body to increase its production of endorphins, mood-elevating brain chemicals.
- Watch your diet. Eat plenty of foods rich in B vitamins, such as beans and dark green vegetables like spinach and broccoli. B vitamins help maintain high levels of neurotransmitters, the chemicals that promote healthy brain and nerve function.
- Avoid alcohol, which not only interacts with medications and supplements to treat depression, but which also has a depressing effect of its own.
- Learn about depression and about yourself. Pick up self-help books and tapes that can help you better understand your emotions and overcome problem areas in your life.

folic acid can mask a deficiency of vitamin B_{12}, a relatively common problem among older people who do not fully absorb this vitamin.

■ NUTRITIONAL SUPPLEMENTS

Phenylalanine

How it works. Phenylalanine is an amino acid that is abundant in the human diet. Phenylalanine is a precursor of tryptophan, which helps make serotonin. Some studies have found that phenylalanine supplements are useful in treating mild depression, especially when they are given with St. John's wort (see below). There are three forms of phenylalanine: D, L, and DL, a mixture of the other two that is commonly referred to as DLPA. This is the type most used in the United States.

Recommended dosages. The typical daily dosage calls for 150 to 400 mg of DLPA, divided into two or three doses.

Possible problems. DLPA must be avoided by people with phenylketonuria (PKU), a rare metabolic disorder. Otherwise, it is generally safe; possible side effects include headaches and a mild rise in blood pressure. It should not be taken during pregnancy or breast-feeding, and its safety for people with liver or kidney disease has not been established.

SAM-e

How it works. SAM-e, which stand for S-adenosylmethionine, is a molecule found in all living cells that is essential for a number of body processes. European studies show that SAM-e can be faster and more effective in overcoming depression than many standard antidepressant drugs. It is thought to work against depression by enhancing the action of mood-elevating brain chemicals, such as serotonin and dopamine.

Recommended dosages. Most experts recommend starting with 400 mg a day, taken in two dosages, and if this doesn't help within a few weeks, gradually working up to a maximum of 400 mg taken four times a day, for a total of 1,600 mg. It is most effective when taken on an empty stomach; for example, an hour or so before a meal.

Possible problems. Stomach upset is the most common problem. This can be minimized by taking it as an enteric-coated pill that does not dissolve until it reaches the small intestine.

■ BOTANICAL MEDICINES

St. John's wort (*Hypericum perforatum*)

How it works. Numerous studies attest to this herb's ability to relieve mild depression. The active incredient is hypericin, which some studies suggest may have an effect on seratonin levels. Researchers are uncertain, however, whether this explains why St. John's wort works against depression. Still, many European studies have found that it is even more effective than some prescription antidepressants, and it has an added advantage of having only a minimal risk of side effects.

Recommended dosages. The standard dosage calls for 300 mg of St. John's wort to be taken three times a day. Look for products that are standardized to provide 0.3 percent hypericin. Allow six weeks for results to be noticed.

Possible problems. Although problems in humans have not been reported, animal studies suggest that people who are fair-skinned or photosensitive should avoid exposure to bright sunlight when using St. John's wort. Some people complain of stomach irritation from St. John's wort; this can be minimized by taking it with meals. St. John's wort should never be combined with prescription antidepressants, demerol, lithium, or dextromethorphan (an ingredient in some cough syrups). A dangerous condition known as serotonin syndrome can result.

Ginkgo (G. biloba)

How it works. It is not known how ginkgo works, although a number of studies have shown that it increases peripheral circulation as well as blood flow to the brain. Animal studies suggest that the herb produces a lowering of stress hormone activity, which may explain its effectiveness in treating some symptoms of mild depression. A Swiss study found that the herb helped depressed people improve their sleep patterns and cognitive function. After only five weeks of treatment, the number of awakenings was significantly reduced, and short- and slow-wave sleep increased. When tested, the study participants also showed substantial improvement in cognitive and psychomotor functions. Other studies suggest ginkgo is most effective in treating depression in older people, specifically, patients over age fifty. Ginkgo has also been shown to be an antioxidant and reduces plate aggregation, or "stickiness," which can cause blood clots.

Recommended dosages. The dosage most often recommended for mild depression is 40 to 80 mg of ginkgo, standardized to contain 24 percent glycosides, three times a day. It can be taken as a capsule, a tablet, or liquid extract. It can be made into a tea by dissolving a capsule in a cup of warm water.

Possible problems. A study involving more than 9,700 patients found that the most common side effects were mild stomach upset (in 0.2 percent of patients); even smaller numbers reported dizziness and headaches. A word of warning, however: Because ginkgo thins the blood, it should not be taken by people with bleeding problems or those who are on other blood-thinning medications such as warfarin (Coumadin) or low-dose aspirin therapy. Allergic skin reactions can also occur, but are rare.

⊙ SYMPTOMS

Depending on the severity of dermatitis, one or more of the following symptoms may appear:

- Reddened skin areas (termed erythema).
- Itching (pruritis), usually worse at night.
- Blisters that may burst and ooze, leading to crusts and scabs.
- Thickening of the skin.
- Peeling.
- Change in skin color.

⊙ OTHER TYPES OF DERMATITIS AND THEIR TREATMENT

Seborrheic dermatitis, in its most common, mild form, causes dandruff. The skin develops dry or greasy scales, which come off in flakes and may itch. In more severe cases, symptoms extend to the eyebrows, in and behind the ears, in the skin folds that extend from the nose to the lips, in the underarms, and in other body folds. A variant in infants is called cradle cap. Dandruff is treated with frequent shampooing with preparations containing zinc pyrithione, selenium sulfide, sulfur, salicylic acid, or tar. Severe seborrheic dermatitis may require daily applications of a corticosteroid lotion or cream.

Nummular dermatitis causes coin-shaped plaques almost anywhere on the body. It is most common in middle-aged people who have dry skin. It is occurs more frequently in winter, although at any time of year attacks may be triggered by stress, a dry environment, or other skin diseases. Treatment may involve oral antibiotics; topical, injected, or oral steroids; ultraviolet radiation; and oral psoralen.

Chronic dermatitis of the hands and feet includes, among other manifestations, "dishpan hands." Although worsened by frequent immersion in water, it may be due to such diverse causes as allergy, irritants, viral or fungal infections, psoriasis, or contact dermatitis. Treatment depends on the cause.

Stasis dermatitis afflicts primarily the ankles and lower legs and is associated with varicose veins in middle-aged and older people. Although it may initially appear as mildly annoying red patches, if untreated it can lead to increasing swelling, secondary infection, and ulceration. The condition often responds well to support stockings and cool wet compresses, topical steroids, or zinc preparations.

Lichen simplex chronicus emerges from a vicious cycle of itching and scratching, leading to increased itching and scratching and

DERMATITIS/ECZEMA

Dermatitis is an umbrella term used to describe skin inflammation, which typically causes an itchy, red rash. It may occur occasionally or last for years. Eczema is another name for dermatitis, although some doctors use that term only to define a serious, chronic form called atopic dermatitis.

Irritant contact dermatitis is the most common type. It is the body's response to direct contact with any substance that irritates the skin or provokes allergic reaction. Irritant contact dermatitis is especially common among restaurant workers, hairdressers, and others whose skin is often exposed to detergents, dyes, acetone, acids, alkalis, and other irritating chemicals. This type can be quite unpredictable, flaring up suddenly even after years of using the offending substances.

Allergic contact dermatitis can occur dramatically within hours of exposure to plants such as poison ivy or poison oak. But it can also develop after repeated exposure to everyday materials that have caused no problems in the past. Common offenders include nickel (in jewelry), rubber, latex, cosmetics, leather, materials used in clothing manufacture, and even medications in skin creams. Until the offending substance can be identified and contact eliminated from daily activities, treatment may be required for relief of symptoms.

Atopic dermatitis (eczema) often runs in families and is more common in those with a personal or family history of allergic disorders such as hay fever and asthma. It may begin in infancy, with patches of an itchy rash on the face and scalp. The rash may worsen after immunizations and during teething, but it disappears in almost half of all children between the ages of two and four. Alternatively, infantile eczema may continue beyond or even appear for the first time in early childhood. At this age, the areas most severely afflicted are the creases in the elbows and behind the knees, where skin may become brownish-gray, dry, scaly, and thickened. Again, the problem may disappear only to arise again in adolescence or adulthood, with similar symptoms that may also occur on the face, neck, and upper chest. Although most people are finally free of eczema by the age of thirty, some must put up with it throughout life.

Diagnostic Steps

Dermatitis usually can be diagnosed simply by examining the rash and a description of what contact provokes or alleviates it. Sometimes, however, a dermatologist or an allergist may be consulted for tests, such as a skin biopsy. Allergy tests also may be performed to identify the substances that cause or contribute to the dermatitis.

Conventional Treatments

In general, therapy for dermatitis is designed to suppress the inflammation that causes the symptoms and to reduce or eliminate the underlying factors that triggered it. It is important to alleviate the itching, because scratching worsens the rash and leads to the itch-scratch-itch cycle. For forms of dermatitis that are associated with dry skin, treatment also involves enhancing skin moisture. For types associated with stress, efforts should be made to ease anxiety. Treatment also varies depending on the areas affected and the degree of itching. Avoid over-the-counter medications unless recommended by your doctor; some contain benzocaine or lanolin, which can make some dermatitis problems worse. The following medications may be prescribed:

• *Corticosteroids.* These drugs suppress inflammation. They may be prescribed as topical creams or ointments of varying strengths, injected directly into severe lesions, or taken as pills for chronic dermatitis problems. Long-term use of corticosteroids, however, can cause serious side effects, even when used only topically. So work with your doctor to slowly reduce your dose to the minimum amount effective, and carefully follow guidelines for stopping within a specific time.

• *Antihistamines.* Numerous over-the-counter and prescription varieties are available for allergies. These drugs help reduce itching.

• *Tranquilizers.* Various drugs in this category ease anxiety that may be triggering or worsening dermatitis symptoms. They can also help you to sleep without scratching.

• *Tar compounds, petrolatum, and simple vegetable cooking oils.* Any of these may be prescribed to help moisturize the skin, especially between applications of corticosteroids.

• *Phototherapy.* This treatment employs ultraviolet light to help heal atopic dermatitis. Sometimes the drug psoralen (PUVA) is taken beforehand to enhance light sensitivity. Since some skin problems are aggravated by ultraviolet light (including sunlight), phototherapy should never be self-prescribed.

• *Antibiotics.* If scratching has caused bacterial infection, you may need antibiotics, such as penicillin, cephalosporin, or tetracyline.

Nutraceuticals for Dermatitis/Eczema

Although some of the nutraceuticals below may help for temporary symptomatic relief, most treatment plans focus on chronic conditions. The best evidence supports the use of essential fatty acids to reduce inflammation and one or more flavonoids to reduce histamine release.

◨ OTHER TYPES OF DERMATITIS AND
    THEIR TREATMENT (cont.)

worsening irritation. It usually begins between the ages of twenty and fifty, more often in women than men. The cycle can usually be broken with topical steroids, with the rash areas covered by tape or a bandage to prevent scratching. Oral antihistamines also may be prescribed.

◉ STRATEGIES FOR RELIEF

If you or your doctor can identify any substances or situations that tend to trigger outbreaks, try to avoid them. Keeping a daily diary of activities—what you eat, how you feel, what you wear, how you wash, and what chemical substances you come into contact with—may enable you to identify such triggers. Prevention is the best approach to dermatitis. The following strategies also may help prevent triggering or worsening dermatitis:

• Develop a regular skin care routine, following your practitioner's guidelines and including cleansing, moisturizing, and medication. Skipping even one day of therapy can allow your dermatitis to flare out of control, leading to weeks of discomfort until you get it under control again.

• People with dermatitis often have skin that is easily irritated by soap, detergents, and rough clothing, especially wool and certain synthetics, all of which should be avoided. If you must use detergent, use a mild one and make sure clothing is well rinsed. Further, avoid washing or drying your clothes with fabric softeners, which also may irritate the skin.

• To avoid drying the rash areas with soap, use soap substitutes that do not remove skin oils. Wash with lukewarm, not hot, water. Apply prescribed moisturizers and medications to the skin immediately after your bath or shower—within three minutes, advise some doctors. When rashes clear, continue to remember to keep your skin well moisturized daily.

• Hot, cold, and very humid weather often aggravates dermatitis, so try to protect yourself from weather extremes. Keep temperatures in your home as constant as possible.

• Avoid working around dust, industrial chemicals, fumes, sprays, and solvents—all of which tend to aggravate eczema.

• Try to avoid exposure to colds and flu. Upper respiratory infections can lower your body's resistance and aggravate your skin rash. Avoid contact with people who have cold sores or other forms of herpes, because the viruses that cause them can provoke very serious eruptions of eczema.

• If your skin comes in contact with any known irritant, wash it immediately.

• Learn stress-reduction techniques, such as progressive relaxation and meditation, to help reduce your anxiety.

• Keep your fingernails short to decrease skin damage if you absentmindedly scratch the rash. In children, it may be necessary to cover the area with bandages to prevent scratching. Consider sleeping with while cotton gloves on to prevent scratching.

• If you have other allergies—such as hay fever or asthma—follow your doctor's advice for keeping them under control. Flare-ups of either can contribute to worsening of eczema.

• Unless you are allergic to fish, increase your intake of fatty fish, such as mackerel, herring, tuna, and salmon, to help balance your essential fatty acids and reduce inflammation.

• Unless you are allergic to ragweed, try chamomile cream or lotion, which some people find very soothing.

■ NUTRITIONAL SUPPLEMENTS

Omega-3 fatty acids

How they work. Contained in fish oils and flaxseed, these work on the same principle as evening primrose oil, by changing the character of inflammatory prostaglandins in the body. Indeed, in some studies even greater benefit was found with fish and flaxseed oils.

Recommended dosages. Practitioners recommend 1 tablespoon of flaxseed oil daily, or extracts of the fish oils containing 540 mg EPA and 350 mg DHA daily. These oils should be taken with food.

Possible problems. Again, allow several weeks for them to have an impact on prostaglandin metabolism. (See Essential Fatty Acids, p. 295.)

Quercetin

How it works. Quercetin is a flavonoid (or bioflavonoid) that helps inhibit the body's release of histamine. Thus, it can act in a manner similar to antihistamine drugs prescribed by doctors.

Recommended dosages. Practitioners recommend 400 mg taken twenty minutes before meals.

Possible problems. None are known. (See Flavonoids, p. 302)

Grape seed extract

How it works. This is also a flavonoid that can have an antihistaminic effect.

Recommended dosages. Look for products standardized to 95 percent procyanidolic oligomers content and take 50 to 200 mg three times a day.

Possible problems. None have been reported.

■ BOTANICAL MEDICINES

Evening primrose (*Oenethera biennis*)

How it works. Prostaglandins are hormonelike substances in the body that contribute to inflammation in many disorders, including dermatitis. The body uses essential fatty acids as building blocks to make prostaglandins. Changing the balance of fatty acids in your body can create a less inflammatory environment. That's why many practitioners recommend supplements of evening primrose oil for the benefits of its active ingredient, gamma-linolenic acid (GLA), which also can be found in borage seed oil.

Recommended dosages. Several double-blind studies have shown improvement in eczema symptoms with dosages of at least 3,000 mg of evening primrose oil daily. Check the label to make sure you are getting at least 270 mg of GLA in your dosage, which may require multiple capsules.

Possible problems. Because you are trying to change the way your body makes prostaglandins, improvement will not occur overnight. Be prepared to wait several weeks for benefit.

Ginkgo (*G. biloba*)

How it works. Ginkgo contains terpene molecules that may block key chemical mediators in eczema. Studies have shown that ginkgo biloba extract standardized to contain 24 percent ginkgo flavone glycosides and 6 percent terpene lactones demonstrated clinically significant antiallergy effects.

Recommended dosages. Practitioners recommend 80 to 120 mg of the extract divided into two to three doses.

Possible problems. Some people have mild stomach upset when using ginkgo. Rarely, allergic skin reactions occur—so stop using it immediately if your dermatitis worsens. Ginkgo should not be used by people who take blood-thinning medications.

Licorice (*Glycyrrhiza glabra*)

How it works. Licorice may have both internal and external beneficial effects for dermatitis. When you take it orally, it has anti-inflammatory and antiallergic benefits. When applied topically, it acts similarly to hydrocortisone creams in the treatment of several different types of dermatitis.

Recommended dosages. Orally, licorice can be taken three times a day either as 1 to 2 g of the powdered root, 2 to 4 ml of the fluid extract, or 250 to 500 mg of the powdered extract. Topically, glycerrhetinic acid can be used in a gel formula and applied as needed to ease symptoms.

Possible problems. Ingested licorice can raise blood pressure when it is taken at the above recommended dosages for a prolonged period, typically five or six weeks. It should not be taken orally by people who have high blood pressure, liver or kidney disorders, or are pregnant. It also should not be taken with diuretics or oral corticosteroids.

DIABETES

Diabetes is a group of serious diseases in which the body does not properly convert sugar, starches, and other foods into the energy needed for life. When excess blood sugar (glucose) builds up in the blood, it damages structures throughout the body. Diabetes results from defects in the body's ability to produce or properly use insulin, a hormone that

Symptoms of type 1 diabetes usually develop suddenly and provoke a crisis demanding immediate care. In contrast, type 2 diabetes develops slowly, over many years. Many people who don't have regular checkups, including a blood sugar test, often don't discover they have the disease until one of its complications develops, such as a heart attack, stroke, or eye or kidney problems. When symptoms occur, they include:

- Excessive thirst and urination.
- Unexplained loss of weight.
- Itching.
- Changes in vision.
- Slow healing of cuts and bruises.
- Excessive hunger.
- Frequent or lingering skin infections.
- Tiring easily.
- Numbness, tingling, or pain in the hands or feet.
- Recurring vaginal infections.
- Abnormal drowsiness or weakness.
- Extreme hunger.
- Delivery of a large infant weighing nine pounds or more, an indication of gestational diabetes.

allows blood sugar to enter the cells of the body and be used for energy. Insulin is produced by the pancreas, an organ just below the stomach.

Some 16 million Americans have diabetes. About half of them—8 million—are "hidden diabetics," people who have the disease but don't know it because they have not had a simple blood test. Too many don't discover they have diabetes until they are hit with one of its complications—such as a heart attack, stroke, or kidney failure. The cause of diabetes remains unknown; however, it is assumed to have a genetic component because it often runs in families. In addition, some environmental agent, such as a virus for type 1 or obesity for type 2, seems to trigger the inherited predisposition.

Type 1 diabetes is also known as *juvenile-onset* or *insulin-dependent diabetes*. It usually starts in children or young adults who are slim. Type 1 is an autoimmune disease in which the insulin-producing cells in the pancreas are destroyed. Fewer than a million Americans have type 1.

Type 2 diabetes is also known as *adult-onset* or *non-insulin-dependent diabetes,* despite the fact that many do require daily insulin injections. It usually occurs in those over forty and overweight. While it was once thought that those with type 2 diabetes did not make sufficient insulin, it is now clear that most have normal or above normal supplies. But their bodies fail to use it properly due to insulin resistance, also known as reduced insulin sensitivity. Type 2 is the most common type of diabetes.

Gestational diabetes occurs only during pregnancy and usually disappears thereafter, but tends to lead to type 2 in later years. All pregnant women should have a test for diabetes. If they develop gestational diabetes, they need special care to help assure a healthy baby.

What can be done about diabetes? Most people with diabetes can lead normal lives by carefully balancing their diet, exercising and—if necessary—using medication.

Diagnostic Steps

Doctors often diagnose diabetes based on a simple blood test to check for blood sugar levels. In some cases, they prescribe a more complicated test called the OGTT—oral glucose tolerance test. It involves taking repeated blood samples over several hours, before and after drinking a special amount of liquid glucose.

Conventional Treatments

Research has shown that people who keep their blood sugar levels as close to normal as possible with good control can dramatically reduce their risk of serious diabetes complications.

The two mainstays of diabetes treatment are a careful diet to control sugar intake, balanced with adequate exercise to use energy. In addition, people who have type 1 diabetes require daily insulin injections to survive. Treatment of gestational diabetes depends on blood sugar levels; in some cases, insulin injections are needed. Many people who have type 2 can be treated by diet and exercise alone, especially if they lose weight. Others may need oral medication to help their insulin function more effectively; some of these drugs increase the body's production of insulin while others help you to use your insulin more effectively. Others may need insulin injections.

Nutraceuticals for Diabetes

■ VITAMINS AND MINERALS

Vitamin A

How it works. Diabetes may drive up or change the body's needs for vitamin A. Diabetes involves problems with islet function in the pancreas and glucose synthesis by the liver. Women with diabetes have a greater risk of miscarriages and malformed offspring—and vitamin A plays a role in all these processes.

Recommended dosages. The Recommended Dietary Allowance of 5,000 IU is present in most multivitamins.

Possible problems. Because vitamin A is stored in the body, rather than excreted, toxic levels can build up in the body. So don't supplement beyond the RDA without your doctor's advice.

Vitamin B-complex

How they work. High levels of the amino acid homocysteine, a protein precursor, increase the risk of heart attacks in the general population. So reducing the levels are likely to offer bonus benefits for people with diabetes, who are at greater risk of heart disease. Further, high homocysteine levels are related to the abnormal secretion of urinary protein, an early indicator of potentially serious kidney problems. Three B vitamins work synergistically to control homocysteine levels. Folic acid converts it to methionine, which is used to make new proteins for use by the body, thus lowering the fasting homocysteine. B_{12} helps folate do its job. B_6 helps the body get rid of extra homocysteine after a meal by promoting its excretion in the urine.

Recommended dosages. Recent research suggests the RDAs for the various B vitamins are not enough for people with high homocysteine levels. In people with early heart disease, moderately large doses of the B vitamins have been used, such as 1,000 mcg of folic acid, 25 mg of B_6, and 25 mcg of B_{12} daily.

Possible problems. Taking extra folic acid can mask anemia due to B_{12} deficiency. It corrects the anemia but can allow accompanying neurological damage to progress. It's rare, but the simple solution is to always take extra B_{12} when you supplement with folic acid. Because B vitamins are water-soluble, excess is excreted through the urine and there are virtually no toxicity problems.

Vitamin E

How it works. When vitamin E levels are low, the risk of developing type 2 diabetes rises dramatically. Supplements can improve sugar metabolism and reduce the risk and severity of several diabetic complications. Researchers theorize that the same oxidative stress that contributes to heart disease—free radicals damaging cells—may also play a role in blood flow in the eye and kidney. They have found improvements in blood flow abnormalities in the eye and in kidney function among people with type 1 diabetes.

Recommended dosages. Studies have used supplements of up to 1,500 IU daily, which is the maximum safe dosage when taking the natural (d-alpha) form.

Possible problems. People who have blood-clotting problems or who are taking blood-thinning medication should discuss vitamin E dosing with their doctors.

Magnesium

How it works. Many people with type 2 diabetes have low levels of magnesium, which may contribute to insulin resistance. Low levels also may worsen in people with poorly controlled diabetes because magnesium is excreted in the urine. Further, because insulin is involved in moving magnesium into cells, the process may not work as well in people with diabetes. Other complications of diabetes may affect dietary intake and/or absorption of the mineral.

Recommended dosages. Normally, you don't need to supplement beyond the RDA of 280 to 350 mg daily. But ask your doctor about a blood test for magnesium deficiency and discuss further supplementation depending on the results.

Possible problems. Doses above 600 mg can cause diarrhea. Reduce the risk by dividing the amount into two or three doses to be taken throughout the day. High doses should not be taken by persons with kidney disease.

Chromium

How it works. Chromium is a mineral essential for carbohydrate and fat metabolism, but normal intake may be suboptimal in the typical American diet. Some research has indicated that chromium supplements can help control blood glucose levels.

Recommended dosages. Four months of high doses—500 mg of chromium picolinate twice daily—helped many people with type 2 diabetes completely normalize their blood glucose levels. Some doctors have used chromium supplements to help keep women with mild insulin-resistant (type 2) diabetes off insulin.

Possible problems. Chromium is one of the safest nutrients, although prolonged high doses may reduce iron and zinc absorption.

■ NUTRITIONAL SUPPLEMENTS

GLA (gamma-linolenic acid)

How it works. Diabetic neuropathy is a nerve disorder that affects the majority of diabetic patients, although under 40 percent have significant symptoms—ranging from uncomfortable tingling in the fingers and toes to severe pain. Studies have shown that supplements of evening primrose oil can improve symptoms in mild cases. The key ingredient is gamma-linolenic acid (GLA) a fatty substance needed by nerves.

Recommended dosages. In one study, multiple capsules of evening primrose oil—containing a total of 480 mg daily—markedly improved symptoms.

Potential problems. You may have to take a dozen capsules daily to get this much GLA. It's also available in other seed oils, such as borage. (See Essential Fatty Acids, p. 295.)

DIARRHEA

Diarrhea is characterized by the frequent passage of loose, watery stools. Typically, the sufferer is hit with a sudden and very urgent need to go to the bathroom. Diarrhea occurs at all ages but it is especially common in babies and young children. Healthy people can usually weather a bout of diarrhea without ill effects, but it can be debilitating and very uncomfortable while it lasts. Prolonged or severe diarrhea can result in dehydration and a potentially life-threatening upset in body chemistry, especially in babies and the elderly, and is a major cause of death worldwide.

Diarrhea is usually a symptom of some other underlying condition, rather than a disease in and of itself. Typically, it is self-limiting, with a rapid (acute) onset and a return to normal bowel function in twenty-four to forty-eight hours. This type of diarrhea is most often due to the effects of a bacterium, such as *E. coli* or salmonella, or a so-called stomach virus. But there are many other causes of diarrhea, including stress, a reaction to certain foods, allergies, and intestinal disorders, such as irritable bowel syndrome (IBS) (see p. 143). In general, a doctor should be consulted if acute diarrhea lasts more than a day in a child under twelve months or two days in an older child or adult. Of course, a doctor

◎ **SYMPTOMS**
- The passage of more than three abnormally loose and watery stools a day.
- Possible abdominal pain or cramps, fever, and other symptoms depending upon cause.

should be called earlier if there are other symptoms, such as a high fever, vomiting, or blood in the stool.

Some people, especially young children, have chronic diarrhea, defined as the passage of several loose bowel movements a day. Often, tests cannot find a cause of this type of diarrhea. It should be noted that bowel function varies greatly from one person to another, and some people have several bowel movements a day while others may go for two or three days without one. Both may be variations of normal if there are no other symptoms. Doctors generally are not concerned if a young child with chronic diarrhea is growing normally and has no other symptoms. In an older child or adult, a change in diet or another lifestyle change, such as stress management, may be in order.

Diagnostic Steps

Doctors start by asking about the nature of the diarrhea and any other symptoms. For example, diarrhea alternating with constipation and periods of normal bowel function points to stress or irritable bowel syndrome as possible causes. Blood in the stool may indicate an intestinal infection, colon polyps, cancer, or an inflammatory bowel disease. Tests may include a stool analysis, a stool-based digestive analysis, blood studies, imaging studies (e.g., barium-enhanced X rays, MRI, or a CT scan), and colonoscopy (examination of the colon with a fiberoptic viewing instrument).

Conventional Treatments

There are a number of antidiarrhea medications, both prescription and over-the-counter, that can stop an attack. One of the most common is paregoric, a tincture containing opiates that is sold as a controlled prescription drug. Some antidiarrhea preparations work by slowing intestinal motility; others increase intestinal absorption of fluids, thereby making the stool firmer. However, doctors often advise letting a bout of acute diarrhea run its course, as the diarrhea may be the body's way of ridding itself of the effects of an infectious organism.

Nutraceuticals for Diarrhea

■ NUTRITIONAL SUPPLEMENTS

Acidophilus

How it works. Acidophilus is one of the many friendly bacteria that live in the human intestinal tract and vagina, where it helps maintain

◉ STRATEGIES FOR RELIEF

■ Avoid solid foods, milk, wheat products, fruit juices, coffee, and alcoholic beverages until the diarrhea subsides.

■ To avoid dehydration, take frequent sips of fluids. Good choices include plain water, flat (defizzed) ginger ale or cola, green tea, rice or potato water (the fluid drained from boiled rice or potatoes), and chicken broth or other clear salty soups.

■ When you resume solid foods, try starting with binding foods, such as bananas, rice, applesauce, toast, soda crackers, and skinless chicken or turkey white meat. Avoid fatty foods, raw fruit or vegetables, fruit juices, and milk until the bowels are normal for at least two days.

■ If stress is responsible for periodic flare-ups of diarrhea, strive to adopt more effective coping techniques. Set aside time for regular exercise and take one or two breaks during the course of the day to sit quietly and practice deep breathing or progressive relaxation exercises.

a normal balance of microorganisms. Diarrhea may develop when this balance of organisms is upset, which often happens when a person takes antibiotics. Although experts debate the usefulness of acidophilus supplements, some studies do show that they can relieve diarrhea, especially when combined with *Lactobacillus bifidum,* presumably by restoring the normal balance of intestinal organisms.

Recommended dosages. Some doctors and alternative practitioners recommend eating one or two cups of plain yogurt containing live acidophilus cultures a day to prevent diarrhea when taking antibiotics. Acidophilus is also available in capsules that combine *Lactobacillus acidophilus* and *Lactobacillus bulgaris,* since a combination of *L. acidophilus* and *L. bifidum* is probably more effective than acidophilus alone. A typical preventive dosage calls for taking one or two capsules a day. Make sure that they are enteric-coated, which means they do not dissolve until reaching the small intestine; this prevents exposing the bacteria to the strong stomach acids that can kill them. Also, time the acidophilus dosages so they are not taken within two or three hours of an antibiotic.

Possible problems. No problems have been reported from taking acidophilus supplements or eating yogurt containing the live cultures.

Green tea

How it works. Green tea has a much higher tannin content than black tea, a form in which the green tea leaves are fermented. Thus, green tea is thought to help normalize bowel function in much the same manner as dried bilberries. Green tea also contains theophylline, a muscle relaxant. Thus, some experts theorize that green tea helps calm diarrhea by reducing intestinal motility. Others, however, counter that the amount of theophylline in tea is too small to have a marked effect on the intestines. Finally, green tea helps normalize the levels of the colon's natural bacteria, another mechanism that helps counter diarrhea.

Recommended dosages. Studies have found that drinking six to eight cups of strong green tea (made with 1 g of tea leaves per liter of water) significantly reduced diarrhea. To release as much of the tannin as possible, the tea should be steeped for at least fifteen minutes. This will make it taste quite bitter. Drinking the tea cold makes it more palatable; steeping it with a sliver of fresh ginger root gives the tea a refreshing flavor. The ginger also helps settle an upset stomach (see Nausea, p. 172), which is an added benefit if the diarrhea is accompanied by nausea and vomiting.

Green tea can be obtained in capsules (standardized for 50 percent polyphenols). While green tea capsules confer many of the health benefits as the brewed tea, the latter is probably more effective against diarrhea because the drink often delivers more tannin than the pills. For those who cannot tolerate the bitter taste of strong green tea, black tea, while not as effective, is a possible alternative. Although tea has a mild diuretic effect, sipping it throughout the day helps prevent dehydration by replacing the fluids lost during acute diarrhea.

Possible problems. Tea, both green and black, is one of our safest drinks. Billions of people worldwide consume tea every day without adverse effects. Indeed, its consumption is second only to water among all beverages. People who are very sensitive to caffeine may find that drinking large amounts of tea makes them nervous and jittery. Still, the caffeine content is much lower than that of coffee and colas.

■ BOTANICAL MEDICINES

Bilberry (*Vaccinium myrtillus*)

How it works. Dried bilberries (a relative of blueberries) are rich in tannins, such as catechins and anthocyanins, and flavonoids. Researchers are uncertain as to the precise mechanism by which bilberry counters diarrhea. One theory holds that the astringent action of the tannins causes proteins to be deposited on the epithelial surface of the mucous membranes lining the intestinal tract. These proteins form a protective coating against irritants, and also help restore normal bowel motility. The pectin (a soluble fiber) in bilberries helps firm the stool.

Recommended dosages. Europeans have long recommended taking 20 to 60 g (1 to 2 teaspoons) of dried bilberries a day during a bout of diarrhea. The bilberries are soaked in water and then chewed, a little at a time, five or six times a day. A more practical dosage is to take bilberry capsules or a tea brewed from bilberry extract, standardized for 25 percent anthocyanins. A standard dosage for diarrhea calls for 240 to 480 mg a day in capsule form or 1 to 2 ml of the tincture twice a day.

Possible problems. Fresh bilberries can cause or worsen diarrhea, a problem not encountered when the fruit is dried.

Red Raspberry (*Rubus idaeus, R. strigosus*)

How it works. Raspberry leaves are yet another rich source of tannins, so it is reasonable to assume that it works in much the same way as dried bilberries, green tea, and other high-tannin remedies. Tea made from raspberry leaves is also an ancient remedy for menstrual disorders, morning sickness, and to "tone" the uterus during pregnancy.

Recommended dosages. Raspberry tea is made by pouring a cup of boiling water over 1 to 2 teaspoons of dried raspberry leaves and letting it steep for ten to fifteen minutes. A typical regimen to treat diarrhea calls for five or six cups of the tea per day.

Possible problems. No problems have been reported from drinking raspberry tea in the recommended dosages.

DIVERTICULAR DISEASE

Diverticulosis is characterized by the formation of many small sacs along weakened segments of the colon, or large intestine. Many people have diverticulosis without knowing it. If, however, one or more of the sacs becomes inflamed, a condition called diverticulitis may develop, causing pain, fever, and other symptoms.

Diverticulosis is increasingly prevalent with age; an estimated 50 percent of all Americans aged sixty to eighty have diverticulosis. The direct cause is a progressive pressure increase within the intestine, causing small sacs to form at weakened segments. Chronic constipation increases intestinal pressure and the risk of diverticulosis.

While the condition can exist for years without causing symptoms, one or more of the sacs can unpredictably become impacted, resulting in inflammation and infection—a condition called diverticulitis. Sometimes a pouch ruptures, allowing the intestinal contents to spill out. This can cause peritonitis, a life-threatening infection of the tissue lining the abdominal cavity.

Diagnostic Steps

The diagnostic process starts with taking a detailed medical history and conducting a thorough physical examination. Depending upon the circumstances, a doctor may order a computed tomography (CT) scan, magnetic resonance imaging (MRI), or X-ray studies of the intestines using barium, a chalky substance that is either drunk or infused into the colon as an enema to coat the intestine and make the sacs visible on X rays. Keeping a careful diary of symptoms prior to seeing the doctor can aid in making an accurate diagnosis.

Conventional Treatments

Diet is the cornerstone of treating diverticular disease. Fiber and fluid top the therapeutic list, although how you use them varies according to the state of the disease. For example, when diverticulitis develops, a doctor will usually order rest, antibiotics, and a low-fiber (low-residue) diet to give the colon a chance to heal. In a small number of cases, surgery is necessary to repair a sac that has perforated.

Otherwise, a high-fiber diet that emphasizes whole-grain breads and cereals, fruits, and vegetables is prescribed. Fiber helps the digestive system maintain the tone and strength it needs to avoid the weak spots

◉ SYMPTOMS

Diverticulosis is often symptom-free. When the signs appear, they may jnclude:

- Episodes of abdominal tenderness, bloating, and excessive gas.
- Changes in normal bowel habits, often marked by constipation alternating with diarrhea.

Diverticulitis is marked by:

- Persistent and increasing abdominal pain and tenderness.
- Bloating.
- Diarrhea.
- Fever.
- Nausea and vomiting.
- Blood in the stool.

◉ STRATEGIES FOR RELIEF

- Try to minimize stress. Although stress does not cause diverticulosis, it can provoke a flare-up of symptoms.
- Engage in regular exercise. This not only improves muscle tone throughout the body but it also relieves stress and enhances a sense of well-being.
- Follow your doctor's dietary recommendations. Some people find that foods with seeds and kernels—for example, whole-kernel corn, sesame and poppy seeds, raspberries, strawberries, and figs—worsen diverticulosis when the tiny, hard particles get trapped in the diverticular sacs. Such foods should be avoided during a flare-up of diverticulitis or if they provoke symptoms; otherwise, most people can eat them without encountering problems.
- Drink ample fluids—at least eight to ten 8-ounce glasses of juice, water, herbal teas, among others—a day. Fluid is especially important if you are taking psyllium or other high-fiber supplements. Without enough fluids, a fiber-rich diet can result in an intestinal blockage.

FIBER CONTENT OF COMMON FOODS

Food	Fiber (in grams)
All-Bran or other bran cereal, 1 ounce	4
Apple, medium, with skin, 1	3
Banana, medium, 1	2
Brown rice, cooked, 1 cup	4
Chickpeas, cooked, 1/2 cup	6
Figs, dried, 2	4
Lentils, cooked, 1/2 cup	4
Pear, medium, 1	4
Peas, cooked, 1/2 cup	2
Potato, medium, baked, with skin, 1	4
Prunes, dried, 3	4
Strawberries, sliced, 1 cup	4

where troubling sacs form. Fiber also produces soft, bulky stools that move easily through the colon without the need for strong muscle contractions or straining. Thus, larger, easier-to-pass stools reduce colonic pressure, while maintaining the tone of the intestine. In turn, sac formation is kept to a minimum, and so is straining during a bowel movement. Most adults should consume between 25 and 30 g of dietary fiber daily to avoid diverticulosis; people with diverticulosis should do the same to prevent flare-ups. (See the accompanying table for a selection of high-fiber foods.)

Nutraceuticals for Diverticular Disease

■ NUTRITIONAL SUPPLEMENTS

Acidophilus

How it works. Acidophilus is a strain of lactobacilli, bacteria that normally live in the intestinal tract where they help maintain a healthy balance of microorganisms and carry out other important functions, including the manufacture of some of the B vitamins. It also reduces intestinal inflammation due to diverticulitis and inflammatory bowel disease.

Recommended dosages. Dosages range from one to two capsules, containing at least 1 billion live acidophilus organisms, two or three times a day.

Possible problems. Acidophilus is generally safe, although very high doses can sometimes cause diarrhea.

Psyllium

How it works. Psyllium is the dried husk of psyllium seeds, also known as plantago seeds. The husks, high in soluble fibers, absorb large amounts of fluids to form bulky, soft stools that move easily through the colon. Psyllium is the ingredient in Metamucil and certain other laxatives; it can also be purchased in bulk in health food stores and is an ingredient in some high-fiber cereals.

Recommended dosages. The typical dose calls for 1 to 3 rounded teaspoons of psyllium, or about 7.5 to 10 g. Stir the powdered psyllium into a full glass of water, juice, or other fluid, and drink quickly before it thickens.

Possible problems. Just as too little fiber can cause problems, so too can too much. Excessive psyllium and other dietary fiber can cause cramps, bloating, and diarrhea. Also, be sure to drink at least eight to ten 8-ounce glasses of fluid daily when taking psyllium. Without adequate fluid, psyllium can cause an intestinal obstruction.

■ BOTANICAL MEDICINES

Aloe vera (*A. vera, A. barbadensis*)

How it works. Aloe vera gel extract promotes healing of inflamed intestines; it also has mild antibacterial properties that help prevent the sacs from becoming infected.

Recommended dosages. The typical regimen calls for one-third to one-half cup of aloe vera gel extract twice a day, or an equivalent amount of aloe capsules or softgel. Look for products that contain 98 percent aloe vera gel extract and are free of aloin or aloe-emodin. Also, do not take products containing the bitter aloe latex, a powerful laxative that can worsen diverticulosis symptoms.

Possible problems. Be sure to use only aloe vera gel extract for internal use. Aloe vera *juice* causes cramps and diarrhea. Aloe should not be taken during pregnancy.

Slippery elm (*Ulmus rubra*)

How it works. Slippery elm is rich in mucilages that coat and soothe inflamed mucous membranes that line the intestinal tract. It is also a mild laxative.

Recommended dosages. One-half cup of powdered elm bark can be sprinkled on oatmeal and other cereals. It can also be brewed into a tea; use 1 to 2 teaspoons of powdered bark per cup, and drink three or four cups a day.

Possible problems. Excessive slippery elm may cause diarrhea; start with a low dosage and gradually increase the amount up to one-half to three-fourths of a cup of powdered bark a day.

GALLSTONES

Gallstones are clumps of solid material, mostly cholesterol, that form in the gallbladder, a small, pear-shaped organ that sits under the liver on the right side of the abdomen. The gallbladder stores and releases bile, which is produced by the liver, into the small intestine to aid digestion. Bile contains numerous compounds, including bile salts that break down dietary fats; it travels from the gallbladder via tubes called bile ducts. Bile also serves as a vehicle for carrying cholesterol out of the body.

Gallstones form when the bile becomes supersaturated with cholesterol and the bile salts can no longer dissolve it. Cholesterol then begins to crystallize into rocklike particles. This supersaturation may be caused by an inherited tendency to develop an imbalance of substances in the bile or by the gallbladder's inability to contract enough to empty its bile on a regular basis.

About one in ten people develops gallstones, though many are unaware of them, since about 80 percent of gallstones are without symptoms (these are called silent gallstones) and don't require treatment. Though gallstones are generally not a medical problem, there can sometimes be serious, even life-threatening complications. In some cases, gallstones escape from the gallbladder and enter the ducts connecting it to the liver, pancreas, and small intestine. These blockages provoke severe pain and may even be fatal.

A diet low in fiber and high in fat is believed to contribute to the development of gallstones. They are also likely to occur in the presence of other digestive diseases. Other major risk factors for developing gallstones include:

- *Gender.* Women are twice as likely as men to develop gallstones. Estrogen, a female hormone, causes the liver to remove more cholesterol from the blood, which becomes concentrated in the gallbladder.
- *Pregnancy.* Estrogen levels are high during pregnancy, increasing risk even more.
- *Overweight.* While it's not exactly clear why being overweight increases risk, experts believe that the liver produces too much cholesterol, which leads to supersaturation of bile. Several studies have shown that women who are obese have at least double the risk of developing gallstones as do those of normal weight.
- *Dieting.* Although being overweight is a great risk, people who lose weight rapidly are also at an increased risk for developing gallstones. Dieting and weight loss may cause an increase in cholesterol and a decrease in bile salts.
- *Skipping meals.* Going for long periods without eating, and skipping

⊚ SYMPTOMS

Gallstones are usually asymptomatic. When severe symptoms develop, they may indicate medical emergencies. Symptoms can include:

- Intense, escalating, and long-lasting attacks of pain in the upper abdomen that may spread to the right shoulder blade or back. Pain occurs after meals and can last several hours.
- Nausea and vomiting.
- Gas, heartburn, cramps, and bloating.

Signs and symptoms that suggest potentially serious complications of gallstones include:

- Tea- or coffee-colored urine.
- Fever and chills.
- Yellowing of skin and eyes, which indicates jaundice.

meals (which is common among dieters), may decrease gallbladder contractions, making it more likely that gallstones will form.

- *Inactivity.* New research shows that women who exercise the most are about 30 percent less likely to require gallstone surgery than women who are the least active.
- *Age.* The chances of developing gallstones increase with age.
- *Ethnic background.* Native Americans have a higher incidence of gallstones than whites, and whites have a higher incidence than African Americans.
- *Family history.* People whose family members have gallstones are at increased risk of developing stones themselves.

Diagnostic Steps

An ultrasound examination of the gallbladder and bile ducts is the most common diagnostic technique. Cholecystography, an X ray taken after swallowing a contrast material, may also be done.

Conventional Treatments

Gallstones that cause no symptoms are left alone. If gallstones are causing symptoms, the gallbladder is typically removed in a procedure called a cholecystectomy. More than half a million cholecystectomies are done each year in the United States, and two-thirds of them are performed on women. Most cholecystectomies are now performed using a laparoscope, which requires only a few small incisions for the insertion of a thin tube and surgical instruments. There is little pain, minimal scarring, and a short recovery time. The body's ability to digest food carries on without the gallbladder, although a period of adjustment during which stools may be loose is not unusual. Persons who are unable to undergo gallbladder surgery may take drugs to dissolve the gallstones. However, this usually takes months or even years, and the stones recur when the drugs are stopped.

Nutraceuticals for Gallstones

■ VITAMINS AND MINERALS

Vitamin C

How it works. A few animal and human studies suggest that eating a diet rich in vitamin C or taking vitamin C supplements makes it less

◉ STRATEGIES FOR RELIEF

▪ Exercise regularly. Recent research shows that women who exercise regularly have a significantly lower risk of developing gallstones than do inactive women. The more activity, the better, but experts recommend at least two to three hours of exercise, such as brisk walking, a week.

▪ Maintain a healthy weight. Because obesity is a proven risk factor for developing gallstones, maintaining a healthy weight is important for reducing risk.

▪ Lose weight slowly. Rapid weight loss can trigger the development of gallstones. Losing weight slowly may reduce the risk associated with weight loss.

▪ Eat lots of fruits and vegetables and limit fats and meat. A large Harvard study a few years ago found that women who had the highest intake of fruits and vegetables were the least likely to have gallstone symptoms. The healthful combination of phytochemicals and fiber may be the reason behind the reduced risk. Eating fatty foods and meats often triggers gallbladder attacks once you've had them.

▪ Drink moderate amounts of coffee and other caffeinated beverages. Some studies suggest that caffeine triggers gallbladder contractions, providing fewer opportunities for gallstones to form. A Harvard study found that men who drank one to three cups a day of caffeinated coffee were 40 percent less likely to have symptoms of gallstones than those who didn't drink caffeinated coffee. If you already have gallstones, though, drinking caffeinated coffee can actually bring on gallbladder pain.

likely that gallstones will form. Researchers theorize that vitamin C reduces the risk of gallstones by lowering levels of bile cholesterol.

Recommended dosages. No dose has been set for the prevention or treatment of gallstones. However, one study in which vitamin C reduced the risk of developing gallstones used 2 g (2,000 mg) a day.

Possible problems. Vitamin C at these high dosages can cause diarrhea; if it develops, lower the dosage to 500 mg a day. Large doses may also interfere with the action of anticoagulant medications such as Coumadin. In addition, people with kidney stones or kidney disease should avoid such high doses of vitamin C.

■ NUTRITIONAL SUPPLEMENTS

Lecithin

How it works. Low levels of lecithin, an important component of bile, have been associated with gallstones. Some studies have found that lecithin can reduce the pain of a gallbladder attack and possibly help dissolve the stones. Lecithin is a fatty substance manufactured in the body. Food sources include soybeans, whole grains, egg yolks, and peanuts, and it is frequently added to processed foods to hold fat and water together. Lecithin consists of compounds called phosphatidylcholines and is the primary source of the B vitamin choline.

Recommended dosages. Usual dosages are 1,200 mg twice a day, in capsule form, although larger dosages are often suggested. Alternatively, 1 teaspoon to 1 tablespoon of granular lecithin can be eaten with food.

Possible problems. More than 20 g of lecithin may caused digestive problems and sweating.

Lipotropic combination

How it works. Lipotropic means "fat metabolizing." The typical combination is made up of milk thistle, dandelion, and members of the B-complex family, such as choline and inositol (IP-6). The combination is said to promote bile flow; in addition, some of the ingredients, such as milk thistle, reduce the risk of gallstones by altering the composition of the bile. Choline and inositol are instrumental in fat and cholesterol metabolism.

Recommended dosages. The usual dosage calls for 1 or 2 pills a day, with at least 250 mg of milk thistle.

Possible problems. This combination is safe when taken in the recommended dosage.

Taurine

How it works. This amino acid is thought to improve bile flow and may help dissolve small cholesterol gallstones.

Recommended dosages. The typical regimen calls for taking 1,000 mg of L-taurine twice a day for up to three months.

Possible problems. No side effects have been reported from taking L-taurine in the recommended dosages.

■ BOTANICAL MEDICINES

Turmeric (*Curcuma longa*)

How it works. This herb may help prevent gallstones by stimulating contractions of the gallbladder and stimulating bile flow.

Recommended dosages. A daily dose of 2 g has been set by the German Commission E to treat gallbladder disease. Traditional Chinese medicine typically recommends larger doses of 3 to 9 g a day.

Possible problems. While turmeric may be effective in preventing gallstones, it's not recommended for people who already have gallstones or who have blockages of the bile ducts, since it can aggravate the condition and cause pain.

GOUT

Sudden, excruciating pain marks gout, a genetic form of arthritis that initially targets the feet—particularly the big toe—but may also strike the knees, wrists, ankles, and elbows. Men are far more likely to suffer from gout, which generally develops in middle age. Excess body weight and high blood pressure increase the risk for gout in both sexes. Women become vulnerable to gout mostly after menopause.

Gout is triggered by an accumulation in the blood of uric acid, a by-product of cell turnover and protein digestion. Uric acid is also formed from eating foods high in purines, nitrogen-containing amino acids that are especially abundant in organ meats, anchovies, dried beans and other legumes, and wine and beer.

Under normal circumstances, uric acid is washed away in the urine. As excess uric acid floods the bloodstream, it seeps out and settles in the fluid surrounding joints, forming crystals that cause inflammation and pain. The uric acid builds up either because it is overproduced or because the kidneys fail to clear it.

Gout often runs in families, probably resulting from an inherited metabolic disorder. Leukemia and some cancer treatments can also cause it. Kidney disease is often present in people with gout, among whom

◉ SYMPTOMS
Gout tends to come and go; a typical attack is marked by:

- Extreme sensitivity in the affected joints to the slightest touch, with excruciating pain that can last from five to ten days.
- Warmth and redness over the joint.
- Increasingly frequent attacks of pain and swelling.
- Lumpy deposits of calcified uric acid appearing around affected joints and on ears.

STRATEGIES FOR RELIEF

- Avoid or limit foods rich in purines, which include anything that is high in protein, including meats, poultry, and legumes (beans). Organ meats are especially to be avoided; these include liver, kidneys, sweetbreads, and brains. High-purine fish include: sardines, fish roe, anchovies, herring, and mackerel. Chocolate, asparagus, cauliflower, mushrooms, and spinach may also be problematic. Work with a registered dietitian to come up with a gout-control diet you can live with.

- Avoid alcohol. Even a moderate amount of alcohol increases uric acid production. Limit intake to one drink a day, and abstain from alcohol during an acute attack.

- Increase fluids. Fluids, including water, milk, and juice, reduce the likelihood of kidney stones from high uric acid levels by diluting the urine while promoting your body's excretion of problematic uric acid. Gout management dictates a minimum of eight glasses (64 ounces) of fluids daily, but you may need more during a gout attack. Look for nearly clear urine as a sign of adequate hydration.

- Lose excess weight. Uric acid levels rise in overweight people, so your doctor may suggest a weight loss diet to achieve, and maintain, a healthy weight. Avoid severe calorie cutbacks, though, since rapid weight loss results in diminished uric acid excretion from the body.

- Try cherries and berries. Cherries have long been a folk remedy for gout, and a small study many years ago found that they lower uric acid levels. A half pound or more of fresh or canned cherries every day or a half cup to a cup of cherry juice a day have been recommended. Cherry fruit extract can serve the same purpose. Strawberries and blueberries may have similar benefits.

- Drink nettle tea. Nettle, which is rich in vitamin C, is a mild diuretic. To make nettle tea, steep 2 to 3 teaspoons of nettle leaves in a cup of drinking water. Two or three cups of the tea a day may help reduce uric acid.

kidney stones are very common. People with high blood pressure, and those who take diuretics, are also at increased risk of gout.

Diagnostic Steps

To make a definitive diagnosis, doctors often order blood tests. Your physician may remove fluid from inflamed joints to examine under a microscope for uric acid crystals.

Conventional Treatments

Pain relief is the first step in conventional treatments, generally starting with nonsteroidal anti-inflammatory drugs (NSAIDs), such as naproxen or ibuprofen, to reduce inflammation. Corticosteroids may also be used and can sometimes be effective when injected directly into the painful joint. Colchicine is a prescription drug that has long been used to treat gout pain. Once pain is controlled, drugs to prompt elimination of uric acid are prescribed as maintenance medications to prevent further bouts of gout. These include such drugs as probenecid and sulfinpyrazone. Allopurinol, which inhibits uric acid production, may be helpful for some people, although it can cause stomach disturbances and liver damage.

Nutraceuticals for Gout

■ VITAMINS AND MINERALS

Vitamin C

How it works. Vitamin C may help to eliminate uric acid, as one small study suggested.

Suggested dosages. Some experts recommend starting with a 250-mg dosage and gradually increasing it to 500 to 1,000 mg a day.

Possible problems. Initially high doses of vitamin C may provoke kidney stones in people with gout. High doses may also cause diarrhea; they may also interact with Coumadin and other anticlotting drugs.

■ NUTRITIONAL SUPPLEMENTS

Omega-3 fatty acids

How they work. Found primarily in cold water fatty fish, omega-3 fatty acids may inhibit inflammation. Many studies suggest that omega-3 fats can reduce the joint tenderness and morning stiffness suffered by people with rheumatoid arthritis; gout victims may also benefit. If you're not a fish lover, don't despair. Walnuts, flaxseed oil, soybeans, and evening primrose oil supply a fatty acid (gamma-linolenic acid, or GLA) that the body converts to beneficial omega-3 fats, although in limited quantities.

Recommended dosages. Try to dine on modest portions of allowed types of fish (see Strategies for Relief, p. 116) two to three meals a week. Or add 1 tablespoon of flaxseed daily to food. Evening primrose oil is generally recommended at dosages of 1,000 mg taken three times a day. Avoid fish oil supplements because they may be derived from types of fish that are high in purines.

Possible problems. Many fatty fish that are the richest sources of omega-3 fatty acids, including mackerel, anchovies, sardines, herring, and shellfish, are off-limits to people with gout, since they harbor high levels of purines. Nevertheless, it pays to eat nearly any allowable fish, including haddock and sea bass, since seafood has more omega-3 fats than poultry or meat. To avoid stomach upset from some types of oil supplements, take them with food. (See Essential Fatty Acids, p. 295.)

MSM (*methylsulfonylmethane*)

How it works. Veterinarians count on MSM (methylsulfonylmethane) to reduce muscle pain and inflammation in horses, and it may help deaden the pain of gout. MSM is found in dark green leafy vegetables, nutritional supplements, creams, and lotions. To date, however, there are very few well-controlled human studies that prove MSM's efficacy, mechanism of action, or safety.

Recommended dosages. You can purchase MSM as a capsule or gel, or in a powder form that's mixed with fluid. Some experts claim that up to 2 g a day of MSM on a long-term basis is safe.

Possible problems. Eating more dark green vegetables for their MSM content probably poses little, if any, risk. Supplements may result in rashes, diarrhea, and stomach upset; dividing up your daily dose may help limit side effects. MSM doesn't work as quickly as prescription medications to soothe joints. It may take weeks of supplements before inflammation abates, therefore MSM is not an appropriate therapy for gout. (See DMSO and MSM, p. 293.)

Bromelain

How it works. Bromelain, an enzyme found in pineapples, is a natural anti-inflammatory that may ease symptoms during a gout flare-up.

Recommended dosages. The typical dosage calls for 500 mg every three hours during an acute attack. After symptoms subside, reduce the dosage to two 500-mg pills a day to help prevent future attacks. Adding quercetin, a flavonoid, to the regimen helps control uric acid; bromelain aids in its absorption.

Possible problems. There have been some reports of nausea, diarrhea, skin rashes, and heavy menstrual periods among a few people taking very high doses of bromelain.

HEART DISEASE

Heart disease is most prevalent in developed countries, leading many experts to believe it's a condition largely of lifestyle. Despite a dramatic drop in cardiovascular mortality in the last thirty years, heart attacks remain the leading cause of death in the United States, claiming about five hundred thousand lives a year. Most of these heart attacks are due to atherosclerosis, a clogging of the coronary arteries with fatty plaque. Numerous studies have found that atherosclerosis starts early in life, and is affected by many factors, most notably diet, exercise, smoking, and other lifestyle factors. Aging and genetics, or family history, are also important, but studies also show that lifestyle changes can reduce risk even for people who have a strong family history of heart disease.

Diagnostic Steps

Doctors have at their disposal a multitude of tests for heart disease, ranging from simply listening to the heart sounds through a stethoscope, measuring blood pressure, ordering blood studies, doing an electrocardiogram (ECG), and taking a chest X ray, to extensive or invasive procedures, which may include:

- *A Holter monitor,* in which a person wears a portable ECG recorder for twenty-four hours or longer.
- *An exercise stress test,* in which an ECG is taken during increasingly intense exercise.
- *Imaging studies,* such as computed tomography (CT) scan, magnetic resonance imaging (MRI), magnetic resonance angiography, and echocardiography.
- *Cardiac catheterization and coronary angiography,* in which a catheter is threaded through a blood vessel until it reaches the heart, followed by taking dye-enhanced X rays of the coronary blood vessels and other heart structures.

Conventional Treatments

Heart disease often can be managed with a combination of diet, exercise, and other healthy lifestyle habits. Medication may be prescribed to lower blood pressure and alleviate symptoms, such as chest pain (angina). More advanced cases often require procedures such as heart bypass surgery or coronary balloon angioplasty to increase blood flow through the coronary arteries.

◉ SYMPTOMS

Heart disease can reach an advanced stage without causing obvious symptoms; when symptoms develop, they may include:

- Chest pain, especially during exercise or a time of emotional stress, after a heavy meal, or when going out in the cold or wind, that usually abates with rest.
- Shortness of breath.
- Leg pains when walking or climbing stairs.
- An irregular heartbeat.

Call 911 immediately if you or someone you are with experiences the following symptoms of a possible heart attack:

- Chest pain that persists for more than a few minutes and does not ease with rest. It may be most intense in the upper chest and radiate to the shoulder or arm (usually the left one), jaw, back, and stomach.
- Profuse sweating.
- Shortness of breath.
- Nausea or vomiting.
- Dizziness and possible loss of consciousness.
- Rapid or irregular pulse.
- Anxiety and a feeling of impending doom.

Nutraceuticals for Heart Disease

▪ VITAMINS AND MINERALS

Vitamin C

How it works. Vitamin C appears to reduce heart attack risk in several ways. It is an antioxidant that protects against cellular damage caused by free radicals, unstable substances that are a by-product of oxygen metabolism. It helps preserve the strength and elasticity of blood vessels. Some studies suggest that supplemental vitamin C may raise blood levels of the beneficial HDL (high-density lipoprotein) cholesterol, which carries fatty material away from the blood vessel walls. It may also lower the risk of abnormal blood clotting. A recent study also reported that vitamin C can lower high blood pressure, a major risk factor of heart attacks and strokes.

Recommended dosages. The Recommended Dietary Allowance is 75 mg a day for women and 90 mg for men. However, supplements of 200 to 500 or more mg a day are recommended to benefit the heart.

Possible problems. Large doses—1,000 mg or more—of supplemental vitamin C may promote formation of kidney stones in susceptible people, including those with a personal or family history of kidney stones. They also should be avoided by people with a genetic tendency to store too much iron, a condition called hemochromatosis. Excessive vitamin C can also cause intestinal upset and diarrhea, and may interact with anticoagulant medications.

Folic acid

How it works. Folic acid is the synthetic form of folacin or folate, a B vitamin found naturally in legumes, dark green leafy vegetables, orange juice, strawberries, and other foods. With the assistance of vitamins B_6 and B_{12}, folic acid helps control blood levels of homocysteine, an amino acid that promotes atherosclerosis and heart disease. A study involving one thousand adults aged sixty-seven to ninety-six showed that the higher the blood homocysteine, the greater the congestion or blockage of neck arteries.

Recommended dosages. All adults need at least 400 mcg of folic acid a day. Many cardiologists recommend increasing intake to 800 mcg a day, especially if a person has elevated homocysteine. It should be taken along with 1,000 mcg of vitamin B_{12} and 50 mg of vitamin B_6 to prevent an imbalance of B vitamins.

Possible problems. High doses of supplemental folic acid can mask the signs of vitamin B_{12} deficiency, a relatively common problem among older people. When left untreated, a deficiency of vitamin B_{12} causes anemia and possible nerve damage. (See Folacin, p. 237.)

◉ STRATEGIES FOR RELIEF

Lifestyle changes can often alleviate angina and other symptoms of heart disease. Changes recommended by the American Heart Association include these:

▪ Adopt a low-fat diet that provides at least five to nine servings of fruits and vegetables a day, along with starchy, high-fiber foods.

▪ Consider switching to margarine and salad dressings that contain Benecol, a substance that lowers blood cholesterol levels. Other heart-healthy fats include olive, canola, flaxseed, grape seed, and walnut oils.

▪ If you smoke, make every effort to stop; smoking is the leading cause of premature death from heart disease and cancer.

▪ If you have high blood pressure and/or diabetes, work with your doctor to keep them under control—both disorders greatly increase the risk of a heart attack and stroke.

▪ Learn ways to keep stress in check. Set aside quiet time for relaxation each day.

▪ Exercise for at least thirty minutes most days of the week. Walking, cycling, swimming, and tennis are good choices.

Vitamin E

How it works. Vitamin E is an antioxidant that helps prevent the oxidation of LDL cholesterol, a critical step in the development of fatty plaque, the material that clogs coronary arteries and other blood vessels. It reduces inflammation, which is thought to be a factor in heart disease. It also reduces clot formation, which may protect against heart attack and strokes.

Recommended dosages. Experts generally recommend 400 to 800 IU of vitamin E a day. Natural (d-alpha or RRR-alpha) vitamin E is more adsorbable than the synthetic dl-vitamin E.

Potential problems. Vitamin E may affect platelet function, which could result in excessive bleeding in some people. Vitamin E supplements should not be taken with blood-thinning medications, such as low-dose aspirin or Coumadin, or herbal products, such as ginkgo biloba or ginger.

■ NUTRITIONAL SUPPLEMENTS

Flavonoids

How they work. Also known as bio flavonoids, these are the pigments that give many fruits and vegetables their bright colors. Researchers have identified more than four thousand bioflavonoids, which include quercetin, polyphenols, genistein, and carotenoids. They are powerful antioxidants, which help prevent the harmful effects of free radicals, including the damage to the artery walls that fosters atherosclerosis.

Recommended dosages. Consuming at least five and preferably more servings of brightly colored fruits and vegetables every day should provide ample flavonoids. However, some experts recommend that people with heart disease also take supplements high in certain flavonoids; for example, carotenoids sufficient to supply 25,000 IU of vitamin A activity. Tea, soy, and red wine are also rich sources of flavonoids.

Possible problems. There are no known adverse effects of flavonoids.

Soy products

How it works. The protein in soy foods, such as tofu, tempeh, and soy milk, protects cardiovascular health in a number of ways. Pooling the data of thirty-eight well-controlled studies on soy, researchers found that 25 g of soy protein daily lowered heart disease risk. Soy reduces blood levels of the harmful LDL cholesterol and raises levels of the beneficial HDL cholesterol. Soy is also high in isoflavones, which are chemically similar to estrogen, the female sex hormone that is thought to protect against heart disease.

Recommended dosages. Studies indicate that 25 g of soy protein a day can help prevent heart disease, especially if it is incorporated into a diet low in saturated fat. That's about the amount found in three cups of soy milk, or a half cup of roasted soybeans, or an ounce of soy protein isolate; or 10 ounces of tofu.

Possible problems. People allergic to soy should avoid it. Remember, too, that soy products contain calories, so if weight control is a concern, substitute them for an equivalent number of calories from meat or other protein foods.

Omega-3 fatty acids

How they work. Omega-3 fatty acids, found primarily in cold water fatty fish, prevent blood cells from sticking together to choke off arteries that supply heart muscle with blood. Wheat germ, walnuts, flaxseed oil, and soybeans also supply a fatty acid that the body converts to one of the beneficial omega-3s.

Recommended dosages. Studies have shown that people who consume two or three servings of salmon, sardines, bluefish, and other cold-water fatty fish a week have a reduced incidence of heart disease. Alternatively, you can take three 1,000-mg capsules of fish oil a day.

Possible problems. Omega-3 fatty acids, when taken in high-dose supplements of fish oils, reduce platelet aggregation and can result in serious bleeding problems among people who are taking other blood thinners, such as aspirin, high-dose vitamin E, and ginkgo biloba extract. They may also pose a risk to people with a genetic tendency to bleed easily. High-dose fatty acid supplements can also cause diarrhea. (See Essential Fatty Acids, p. 295.)

Coenzyme Q_{10}

How it works. Coenzyme Q_{10}, often referred to as CoQ_{10}, is a natural substance found in all living creatures, who synthesize it in their cells. It plays an essential role in energy metabolism, producing ATP at the cellular level; it also helps maintain healthy muscles, including the heart. Studies have found that it is especially beneficial for patients with congestive heart failure, a disorder in which the weakened heart muscle is unable to pump enough blood to meet the body's needs.

Recommended dosages. Dosages of 50 to 100 mg twice a day are typically recommended for persons with heart disease.

Possible problems. CoQ_{10} is generally safe, although there have been reports of stomach upset, diarrhea, and nausea in a few people taking very high doses.

Oat bran

How it works. Oat bran is a soluble fiber that helps control levels of blood cholesterol, thereby reducing the risk of atherosclerosis. Soluble fiber is also found in beans, peas, and other legumes; rice bran and barley; and the pectin in apples and some other fruits.

Recommended dosages. Daily dosages of 25 to 100 g of oat bran have been shown to reduce total cholesterol by 6 to 12 percent and the harmful LDL cholesterol by 16 percent. Alternatively, the recommended amounts of soluble fiber can be obtained by consuming a cup and a half of cooked oatmeal or one-third cup of cooked beans. (See also Psyllium, p. 338.)

Possible problems. Abruptly increasing fiber intake can result in bloating, gas, and other intestinal problems. Start with a small amount and gradually increase intake until you reach the desired amount. Also, be sure to drink at least eight glasses of water, juice, or other nonalcoholic fluids a day; otherwise, there is a risk of intestinal blockage.

Grape seed extract

How it works. Grape seed extract is rich in proanthocyanidins, bioflavonoids that are potent antioxidants. These substances increase the effectiveness of vitamins C and E; they also help strengthen blood vessels and retard clotting by reducing platelet clumping.

Recommended dosages. The typical dosage calls for 100 to 200 mg a day of extract standardized to provide 92 to 95 percent proanthocyanidins. Pycnogenol, an extract made from the bark of the French maritime pine tree, is another source of proanthocyanidins, and can be taken as an alternative to grape seed extract.

Possible problems. No adverse effects have been reported.

■ BOTANICAL MEDICINES

Hawthorn (*Crateagus oxyacantha*)

How it works. Hawthorn extract appears to be an all-round heart tonic. Herbalists have used it for centuries to treat chest pain, irregular heartbeat, and congestive heart failure. It increases blood flow and lowers blood pressure by widening (dilating) blood vessels; it achieves this effect by blocking the action of ACE, the angiotensin-converting enzyme (pharmaceutical ACE inhibitors are a mainstay of heart medications). It strengthens the heart muscle by blocking other enzymes. It also helps block the buildup of fatty plaque in the arteries.

Recommended dosages. The typical dosage for heart patients ranges from 300 to 450 mg a day in pill form or liquid extract. Lower dosages of 100 to 150 mg a day are recommended as a preventive measure for persons with a high risk of heart disease.

Possible problems. Hawthorn appears to be quite safe and it does not seem to interact with pharmaceutical heart medications. However, to be on the safe side, check with your doctor before taking it—or any other nutraceutical product.

Gugulipid (*Commiphora mukul*)

How it works. Gugulipid, which is derived from the sap of a thorny shrub native to India, contains substances (for example, lignans, diterpenoids, and plant sterols) that have been shown to reduce blood cholesterol. While more research is needed to solidify gugulipid's role in heart disease prevention, one promising study involving sixty-one subjects with high cholesterol found that those receiving gugulipid while on a heart-healthy diet for about six months lowered their LDL cholesterol levels by 12 percent.

Recommended dosages. Study recipients received 50 mg a day of gugulipid for twenty-four weeks.

Possible problems. Some people experience mild nausea, headache, hiccups, or, rarely, skin rash. More importantly, gugulipid could decrease the efficacy of prescription drugs used to treat heart disease; these include Inderal and Cardizem. (See Guggul, p. 476.)

HEARTBURN

Heartburn—often called acid indigestion, acid reflux, or gastrointestinal reflux—is a burning feeling or pain in the chest that usually occurs or worsens after eating. Nearly 40 percent of Americans experience heartburn at least once a month, and about 50 percent of pregnant women report experiencing heartburn during the later stages of pregnancy. An estimated 25 million people suffer daily heartburn pain. Though the symptoms can be mistaken for a heart attack, heartburn actually has nothing to do with the heart.

While eating, food normally travels from the mouth down the esophagus—a ten-inch-long muscular tube—to the stomach. At the opening to the stomach, food passes through a special one-way valve called the lower esophageal sphincter (LES). The LES may, for a variety of reasons, become weak, allowing acid to back up from the stomach. This so-called reflux causes painful heartburn and indigestion.

Heartburn is generally worse after meals, especially when lying down or bending over. Smoking, caffeine, and alcohol can increase the acidity of the stomach, aggravating heartburn further. In otherwise healthy people, poor eating habits can trigger heartburn. Overeating, especially high-fat meals, or overindulging in alcohol can bring on the symptoms, as can consuming coffee (both regular and decaffeinated), citrus juices, spicy tomato products, peppermint, or chocolate. A lack of saliva and slow emptying of the stomach can worsen heartburn. A hernia of the esophageal hiatus—the opening in the diaphragm near the juncture of the stomach and esophagus—can allow the top of the stomach to push upward, causing a backflow of stomach acid and contributing to heartburn.

Other factors may increase the pressure in the stomach or relax the muscle tone of the LES, such as normal aging, coughing, frequent vomiting, and lifting heavy objects. Drugs that relax the smooth muscles (for example, theophylline and the oral bronchodilators used to treat

◉ SYMPTOMS

Heartburn and GERD represent two ends of the same spectrum. Common symptoms of heartburn include:

- Burning pain in the chest that starts in the upper abdomen and radiates into the neck.
- Burning that lasts one to four hours after eating.
- Discomfort immediately after drinking citrus juice.
- Frequent belching.

Heartburn that recurs at least twice a week may be GERD. Symptoms may include:

- Painful burning sensation in the upper chest (heartburn) and/or frequent indigestion.
- Coughing and/or choking while lying down.
- Increased salivation.
- Regurgitation.
- Difficulty sleeping after eating.
- Asthmalike symptoms and recurring or chronic bronchitis.
- Persistent hoarseness.

◉ IS IT HEARTBURN? OR A HEART ATTACK?

Heartburn is often mistaken for a heart attack. But there are some important differences in symptoms. A heart attack usually does not cause a burning sensation. Instead, the pain is more intense and likely to be centered in the upper chest, traveling perhaps to the arm (usually the left one), the face or jaw, or perhaps the back. The pain is often severe and accompanied by difficulty breathing, dizziness, nausea, and possible loss of consciousness.

Even so, any unexplained sudden pain in the chest or arm warrants a trip to the doctor or emergency room. More than half of all heart attack deaths occur before the victim reaches the hospital, very often because of a delay in seeking medical help.

◉ STRATEGIES FOR RELIEF

- Check the possible side effects of any medications you may be taking. Some may irritate the lining of the stomach or esophagus.
- If you smoke, make every effort to quit; nicotine can promote the backflow of stomach acid by relaxing the LES.
- Limit your intake of fried and fatty foods and avoid peppermint, chocolate, alcohol, coffee, citrus fruit and juices, and tomato products.
- Don't lie down or go to bed right after a meal. Wait two to four hours.
- Raise the head of your bed six inches using blocks.
- Eat small, frequent meals.
- Drink fluids between meals, rather than with meals.
- Chew gum to stimulate saliva, which helps neutralize stomach acid.
- Don't wear tight belts or clothes that bind around the abdomen.
- Try teas brewed from lemon balm, ginger, or slippery elm, which contain ingredients that soothe inflamed GI tissue.
- If indigestion is contributing to your heartburn, consider taking digestive enzymes.

asthma, calcium-channel-blockers to treat hypertension, and Valium) may also contribute to heartburn.

Although occasional heartburn is harmless, recurrent bouts can lead to inflammation, scarring, bleeding, esophageal ulcers, precancerous changes in the esophagus, and even breathing problems if the nearby lung tissue becomes inflamed. When heartburn is severe enough to cause these problems, it is known as gastroesophageal reflux disease, or GERD. In such severe cases, the burning sensation is often accompanied by a sour-tasting fluid in the throat and difficulty swallowing.

Diagnostic Steps

GERD, a hiatal hernia, ulcer, or other diseases that can cause recurring heartburn are often diagnosed with the following tests:

- *An upper GI series*—X rays taken after swallowing a substance, usually barium, that coats the esophagus and stomach and makes them more visible on X-ray film.
- *An ultrasound examination*—high-frequency sound waves used to map internal structures.
- *Endoscopy*—a long, thin, lighted tube is used that allows a doctor to inspect the inside of the esophagus, stomach, and upper part of the small intestine. Samples of tissue and stomach fluids may be collected during the examination.
- *Esophageal manometry*—a measurement of the muscle tone and functioning of the LES. A thin tube is passed from the nose to the stomach, and muscle action is measured as the patient swallows water.
- *Monitoring of pH*—a thin probe is inserted in the esophagus for up to twenty-four hours to record how much acid washes back from the stomach.

Conventional Treatments

For occasional heartburn, antacids, such as Tums and Rolaids, offer rapid relief. Though they neutralize stomach acid, when used chronically they can cause either constipation (if they contain aluminum) or diarrhea (if they contain magnesium). Other treatments include:

- Histamine$_2$ antagonists, such as Pepcid or Zantac. These medications, which reduce production of stomach acid, don't work as fast as antacids but they can provide more long-lasting relief. These are available in both over-the-counter and prescription strengths.
- Proton pump inhibitors, including such brands as Prevacid and Prilosec, may help strengthen the LES and prevent the backflow of stomach acid.
- Antireflux surgery, which strengthens the lower esophageal sphinc-

ter, may be an option for those who don't get relief from medication.

Nutraceuticals for Heartburn

■ VITAMINS AND MINERALS

Calcium carbonate

How it works. This form of calcium is the main ingredient in many popular antacids, including Tums. It helps neutralize stomach acid to make it less irritating.

Recommended dosages. The usual dosage is 300 to 500 mg of calcium carbonate, taken after meals.

Possible problems. Large amounts of calcium carbonate—e.g., dosages of 1,000 mg a day—cause constipation in some people. (See Calcium, p. 241.)

■ BOTANICAL MEDICINES

Licorice (*Glycyrrhiza glabra*)

How it works. The DGL (deglycyrrhizated) form of licorice helps alleviate heartburn by decreasing the levels of stomach acids. In this form of licorice, the glycyrrihizin, which raises blood pressure, has been removed, making it safer than the whole root.

Recommended dosages. The usual dosage calls for one to two wafers of DGL three to five times a day after eating.

Possible problems. This form of licorice is probably safe. Do not confuse it with glycyrrihizin-containing licorice, however, which at large dosages taken for five or six weeks can cause hypertension, edema, loss of potassium, and muscle weakness. (See Licorice, p. 491).

Aloe Vera (*A. vera, A. barbadensis*)

How it works. When taken internally, aloe vera gel extract is thought to inhibit stomach acid secretion; it also has anti-inflammatory properties that can soothe an inflamed esophagus.

Recommended dosages. Aloe vera can be taken in liquid or capsule form. The typical dosage is one-third to one-half cup of liquid gel extract or two capsules taken after meals.

Possible problems. If you decide to try aloe vera for internal use, make sure that you use the purified gel extract or capsules made from that, and not the bitter aloe latex or juice, which is a powerful laxative.

Chamomile (*Matricaria chamomilla, M. recutita, Chamomilla recutita*)

How it works. Chamomile has anti-inflammatory and antispasmodic properties.

Recommended dosages. There is no standardized dosage. Most commonly prepared as a tea, it is best ingested several times a day. It may need to be taken for several weeks before improvement is noted.

Possible problems. Although rare, allergic reaction is possible in anyone who reacts to ragweed.

Barberry (*Berberis vulgaris*)

How it works. Barberry has been used by folk healers throughout the world for a wide range of ailments, including heartburn, although its medicinal effects have yet to be scientifically proved.

Recommended dosages. For internal use, it is available as root, bark, extract, tincture, or powder. Follow label instructions. For tea, steep 1 teaspoon of the bark for about fifteen minutes, and drink two or three cups a day. Do not take this much tea for more than two weeks.

Possible problems. Barberry should not be used by pregnant or nursing women. No side effects from taking low doses of barberry supplements have been reported. Add honey to mask the bitter taste.

HIGH BLOOD PRESSURE

Blood pressure—the force of the blood pushing against the walls of arteries as it is pumped through the body—is controlled by the arterioles, the body's smallest arteries. When flow through these tiny vessels is impaired, more pressure is required to force blood through the larger vessels. Blood pressure varies greatly during the course of a day. It is typically highest in the early morning, and lowest during the first few hours of sleep. A blood pressure reading is stated in two numbers, such as 120/80. The higher number is the *systolic pressure,* which occurs when the heart contracts and forces a few ounces of blood into circulation. The lower number is the *diastolic pressure,* which occurs when the heart rests momentarily between beats.

About 60 million Americans have high blood pressure, but many are unaware that they have this potentially fatal disease. Long-term high blood pressure, or hypertension as it is known medically, damages the blood vessels and greatly increases the risk of a heart attack, stroke, kidney disease, and blindness. It is often called a silent killer because it usually produces no symptoms until it has caused severe damage, such as a stroke.

Anyone can develop high blood pressure, but the risk is especially

◉ SYMPTOMS

High blood pressure rarely has symptoms or warning signs. When symptoms do occur, they may include:

- Unexplained headaches.
- Frequent unexplained nosebleeds.
- Eye hemorrhages and vision problems.

RATING BLOOD PRESSURE READINGS
(for adults 18 and older)

Category	Blood Pressure Level (mmHg)	
	Systolic	*Diastolic*
Normal	<130	<85
High normal	130–139	85–89
High blood pressure		
Stage 1	140–159	90–99
Stage 2	160–179	100–109
Stage 3	>180	>110

high among people with a family history of the disease and people who have diabetes and/or are overweight. The disease is more common and more severe among African Americans than whites.

In 80 percent or more of cases, there is no apparent cause of the high blood pressure; this is known as primary or essential hypertension. Secondary hypertension is most often due to a kidney disorder, a hormonal disorder, certain drugs, and pregnancy. Treating the underlying cause often cures secondary hypertension, but there is no cure for the more common primary hypertension. However, it can almost always be managed through diet, lifestyle changes, and—if needed—antihypertensive medications.

Diagnostic Steps

Diagnosing high blood pressure is simple, quick, and painless. Using an instrument called a sphygmomanometer, a blood pressure cuff is wrapped around the upper arm and inflated to stop the blood flow in the artery for a few seconds. A valve is opened and air is then released from the cuff. The sounds of blood rushing through an artery are heard through a stethoscope, and pressure readings are taken as the heart contracts and again when it rests for a fraction of a second. A blood pressure reading of less than 140/90 is considered normal, although the American Heart Association recommends 120/80 as an optimal reading.

The blood vessels in the retina are the only ones that can be directly viewed. By examining the changes in retinal blood vessels with a magnifying instrument with a bright light (an ophthalmoscope), the doctor can estimate the damage to organs elsewhere in the body.

Conventional Treatment

If high pressure can't be moderated by diet and lifestyle changes (see Strategies for Relief, below), it is conventionally treated with prescription drugs called antihypertensives. There are seven major classes of drugs commonly used to treat high blood pressure, each with its own benefits and potential side effects. Because people respond differently to

◉ STRATEGIES FOR RELIEF

Lifestyle change is always the first focus for relief. Even when taking antihypertensive medications, it's very important to institute the following changes:

- Adopt a low-fat diet that emphasizes fruits, vegetables, and starchy foods (see The DASH Diet below).
- Cut back on salt. The American Heart Association recommends limiting sodium to no more than 2,400 mg (the amount in about 1 teaspoon of table salt) a day as a preventive measure. For people with high blood pressure, lower intakes of sodium may be prescribed.
- Engage in at least twenty to thirty minutes of moderate to vigorous aerobic exercise at least three or four times a week.
- If you smoke, make every effort to stop.
- Lose excess weight; trimming down even five or ten pounds can result in lowered blood pressure.
- Abstain from alcohol or drink only in moderation.
- Incorporate stress-relieving practices (e.g., meditation, tai chi, guided imagery) into your daily routine.

◉ THE DASH DIET

A recent landmark study investigated the effects on blood pressure of a diet high in fruits, vegetables, whole grains, and low-fat dairy products, and low in fats and meat products. Called DASH (Dietary Approaches to Stop Hypertension), the study found that people with high blood pressure who followed the diet experienced a significant lowering of their blood pressure readings.

The Daily DASH Diet

4 to 5 servings of vegetables
4 to 5 servings of fruits
7 to 8 servings of whole-grain foods
2 to 3 servings of nonfat and low-fat dairy products
2 servings or less of fish, poultry, or lean meat (or 4 to 5 servings a week of nuts, seeds, and beans)

these drugs, and because the choice may be determined by the presence of other diseases, treatment is always tailored to the individual patient. If one medication doesn't work or is difficult to tolerate, another drug will be tried.

• *Diuretics* rid the body of excess fluids and sodium and are considered one of the first-line drugs for people who have no complicating health factors.

• *Beta-blockers,* also a first-line therapy, reduce the heart rate as well as lower the output of blood from the heart. However, African Americans typically respond less well to these drugs than do Caucasians. And people over the age of sixty-five may not tolerate the drugs as well as younger people.

• *Alpha 1 blockers* trigger dilation of blood vessels, which increases blood flow. They appear to be safe and well tolerated.

• *Alpha 1 beta-blockers* are combination drugs that provide some of the advantages of both beta-blockers and alpha 1 blockers. They are not used as much as some other antihypertensives, in part because of their high cost.

• *Calcium channel blockers* decrease the force of the heart's contractions, dilate blood vessels, and increase blood flow. There are several types of calcium channel blockers; they vary in the way they work and in their side effects. Long-acting types appear to be safer than the short-acting variety.

• *ACE inhibitors* work via the kidneys to decrease sodium and water retention; they also decrease potassium excretion and widen (dilate) blood vessels.

• *Angiotensin II receptor blockers* are the newest class of antihypertensive drugs and they act similarly to ACE inhibitors but with fewer side effects.

Nutraceuticals for High Blood Pressure

■ VITAMINS AND MINERALS

Calcium

How it works. Calcium helps the kidneys regulate sodium and water balance in the body. The kidneys help control blood pressure and are themselves damaged by it.

Recommended dosages. Many practitioners recommend 1,000 to 1,500 mg a day.

Possible problems. More than 2,000 mg a day may cause problems for people who are prone to constipation.

Potassium

How it works. This mineral helps maintain fluid balance and reduces calcium loss.

Recommended dosages. There is no Recommended Dietary Allowance for potassium, but 2,000 to 3,000 mg a day is generally regarded as safe and adequate. Studies indicate that a diet that provides at least 2,500 mg of potassium a day reduces the risk of developing primary hypertension. Extra potassium, in amounts averaging 2,300 mg a day from a combination of high-potassium foods and supplements, has been shown to lower systolic pressure by 4.4 points and diastolic pressure by 2.5 points. However, do not take more than 500 mg of supplemental potassium a day; instead, increase potassium intake by making sure you eat at least eight or nine servings of fruits and vegetables a day.

Possible problems. Too much potassium can actually trigger a heart attack. Supplements should not be taken by persons with kidney disease or who are also taking antihypertensive medications unless a doctor specifically prescribes them.

Vitamin C

How it works. Vitamin C lowers high blood pressure by helping to relax constricted blood vessels.

Recommended dosages. Recent studies suggest that 250 to 500 mg a day should be sufficient, although dosages up to 1,000 to 2,000 mg a day are sometimes recommended.

Possible problems. Large doses of 1,000 mg a day or more can increase the formation of kidney stones in susceptible people. It can also trigger diarrhea and interfere with the results of certain blood tests. People who have a genetic tendency to conserve iron—a condition called hemochromatosis—also should avoid taking extra vitamin C because it promotes iron absorption.

Vitamin E

How it works. Vitamin E slows the progression of atherosclerosis, which increases the risk of developing high blood pressure.

Recommended dosages. For most people, 100 to 400 IU of natural vitamin E a day is sufficient, although dosages up to 1,000 IU may be prescribed.

Possible problems. It has blood-thinning effects and should not be combined with other blood-thinning nutraceuticals or prescription medications without the advice of a physician. Otherwise, no serious side effects have been reported, even when taken in large doses up to 1,500 IU of natural (d-alpha) vitamin E, the maximum safe amount.

Essential fatty acids

How they work. Omega-3 and other fatty acids—found in fatty cold-water fish and flaxseed, evening primrose, rapeseed, and borage oils—reduce damage to blood vessel walls and prevent blood platelets from sticking together and clogging arteries.

Recommended dosages. Take 1 tablespoon of flaxseed oil or 2 to 5 g of fish oil daily. Eating fish at least twice a week may be sufficient.

Possible problems. Because fatty acids are mild blood thinners, supplements should not be combined with other blood-thinning nutraceuticals such as garlic and vitamin E or with prescription blood thinners like Coumadin.

■ BOTANICAL MEDICINES

Garlic (*Allium sativum*)

How it works. The principal healing ingredient in garlic is believed to be allicin, a sulfur compound that is released when a bulb is crushed or chewed. Studies have shown that garlic can reduce blood pressure, but it is not known exactly how it works.

Recommended dosages. Eat at least one clove of raw or very slightly cooked garlic a day. (Cooking destroys the allicin. Instead, add crushed raw garlic to salads, pasta sauce, and other dishes just before serving.) In supplement form, to get the equivalent of one garlic clove, take at least 4,000 mg a day standardized to an allicin yield of at least 5,000 mcg.

Possible problems. Raw garlic gives the breath and skin an unpleasant odor. Allergic skin reactions may occur, as may nausea, light-headedness, heartburn, nausea, and diarrhea. Excessive amounts (one report cited 2 g of garlic a day) can cause bleeding problems. Garlic can affect liver enzymes, which in turn might affect the body's ability to metabolize some prescription drugs properly.

Hawthorn (*Crateagus laevigata*)

How it works. Hawthorn is rich in flavonoids. It is thought to work by widening (dilating) arteries, thereby lowering blood pressure by improving blood flow.

Recommended dosages. Studies indicate that a daily dose of 500 to 900 mg of hawthorn extract may produce a moderate lowering of blood pressure in about six weeks. It may also be consumed as a tea prepared by infusing 1 teaspoon of leaves and flowers in a cup of water; three to four cups a day are needed to produce results.

Possible problems. Although it may have a sedative effect, hawthorn appears to be a safe heart tonic that herbalists use to treat high blood pressure and many other heart disorders. However, some authorities caution not to take it for more than six weeks and not to take it along with other blood pressure or heart medications without first consulting a doctor knowledgeable in the use of nutraceuticals.

HYPOGLYCEMIA

Glucose, also called blood sugar, is the body's main fuel. Hypoglycemia refers to abnormally low blood sugar. Although hypoglycemia used to be a fairly common diagnosis, today that is a matter of great dispute. According to the American Diabetes Association, true hypoglycemia is a condition that mostly affects people with diabetes, a metabolic disease that is marked by wide swings in blood sugar. For them, hyperglycemia (abnormally high blood sugar levels) is the more common problem. However, diabetics may suffer serious drops in glucose when their levels of the hormone insulin fluctuate with the amount of available carbohydrates—the major source of blood sugar.

Less common, but also well recognized among health professionals, is low blood sugar affecting people who have had stomach surgery; those with rare tumors or conditions of the pituitary, adrenal, liver, or kidneys; and those who consume too much alcohol without eating. In rare instances, hypoglycemia can also be triggered by large doses of aspirin or use of sulfa drugs, which are often prescribed to treat urinary tract infections. It can also sometimes occur in early pregnancy, after prolonged fasting, and following long periods of strenuous exercise.

More controversial is the contention that low blood sugar affects a broader group of genetically susceptible people and can be triggered by eating too much sugar, stress, or a diet that is lacking in certain vitamins and minerals. For most people, however, blood sugar levels are maintained within a narrow range that is controlled by a complex interaction involving several organs and hormones. The pancreas secretes insulin and glucagon, hormones that have opposite effects on blood sugar. After you eat, blood sugar levels rise, which prompts the pancreas to immediately release insulin. This hormone lowers blood sugar by prompting body cells to take it up. In contrast, when blood sugar levels drop too low, the pancreas releases glucagon, which prompts the liver to release stored glucose back into the blood. Other hormones, especially epinephrine (adrenaline), which is secreted by the adrenal glands especially during times of stress as part of the fight-or-flight hormone response, also affect glucose levels.

Reactive hypoglycemia is sometimes diagnosed when low blood sugar occurs two to five hours after eating foods high in sugar and all other possible causes of low blood sugar have been ruled out. Studies have shown, however, that many people who experience symptoms of hypo-

⦿ SYMPTOMS
Normal blood sugar levels range between 60 and 120 mg per 100 ml of blood. If levels fall below 40 to 50 mg, symptoms include:

- Shakiness, dizziness, and irregular heartbeat.
- Mental confusion and anxiety.
- Profuse sweating and pallor.
- Unexplained headache.
- Poor coordination and tingling sensations around the mouth.

In addition, more severe hypoglycemia may cause:

- Increasing mental confusion.
- Weakness.
- Loss of consciousness and coma.

- Instead of three large meals a day, eat five or six small ones—one every two to three hours. Make sure that each meal provides a balance of protein and a small amount of fat, which are metabolized more slowly than carbohydrates.
- Build your diet around high-fiber complex carbohydrates (e.g., whole-grain products) and minimize your intake of all forms of sugar, including so-called natural or brown sugar, honey, maple syrup, and other syrups and sugars. Check food labels for ingredients ending in -ose, a suffix for sugar.
- Avoid eating high-sugar foods by themselves. Eating them with other foods will lessen their effect on blood sugar.
- Limit caffeine and alcohol, especially on an empty stomach, which can cause or aggravate symptoms.
- Reduce stress by meditation, relaxation, or reading.
- Exercise regularly. It improves insulin sensitivity and relieves stress.
- Licorice root, ginseng, or astragalus may be helpful for hypoglycemia that is aggravated by stress, although these herbs have not been scientifically studied for this purpose and no standard dose has been set.

glycemia after eating sugar-rich foods have normal levels of blood sugar. Some researchers have suggested that these people may be unusually sensitive to the body's normal release of epinephrine (adrenaline) after a meal, resulting in hypoglycemia symptoms even in the presence of normal blood sugar levels. In addition, unusual stress and anxiety can cause symptoms similar to hypoglycemia even when blood sugar levels are normal.

Diagnostic Steps

Some practitioners make a diagnosis of hypoglycemia based strictly on clinical symptoms. An oral glucose tolerance test used to be the standard diagnostic test. Experts now say it often gives too many false positives (a diagnosis of hypoglycemia where none exists) and can actually trigger hypoglycemic symptoms in people with no actual disorder. According to some experts, the best method to check for low blood sugar is a do-it-yourself blood glucose kit (available at most pharmacies), used as soon as symptoms appear. If low blood sugar levels repeatedly coincide with symptoms that disappear within five to fifteen minutes after eating, then you know you have hypoglycemia. Other experts, however, believe that problems occur more from a rise in insulin than a drop in blood sugar. If this is suspected, laboratory tests may be ordered to measure insulin production. In such cases, other tests may be done to rule out diseases that produce the low blood sugar.

Conventional Treatments

Consuming any type of sugar (candy, fruit juice, sugar water, or milk) will provide immediate relief of symptoms within minutes. Diabetics frequently keep glucose tablets with them for emergencies. Doctors often advise eating fast-acting sugars along with or followed by bread or crackers or other grains, which provide carbohydrates that will last for a more sustained period. Long-term treatment involves dietary changes (see Strategies for Relief).

Nutraceuticals for Hypoglycemia

■ VITAMINS AND MINERALS

Chromium

How it works. Chromium is an important nutrient for the production of insulin and as such is critical for the regulation of blood sugar. Research suggests that supplementation with chromium can help normalize blood sugar levels.

Recommended dosages. One study of people diagnosed with hypoglycemia found that supplementing with 200 mcg of chromium a day can help regulate blood sugar levels.

Possible problems. Chromium is generally considered safe in amounts up to 300 mcg a day. Animal studies suggest that larger doses may cause genetic damage, but this hasn't been confirmed in humans. People with diabetes should consult a doctor before taking chromium because it may interact with insulin and other drugs that treat the disease. Supplements may also interfere with iron and zinc absorption.

Magnesium

How it works. This mineral may keep blood sugar levels from falling too low in people with hypoglycemia.

Recommended dosages. A daily dosage of 340 mg of magnesium has been found beneficial in controlling blood sugar.

Possible problems. High doses of magnesium can trigger diarrhea in some people. People suffering from kidney disease should not take magnesium supplements.

■ NUTRITIONAL SUPPLEMENTS

Brewer's yeast

How it works. Brewer's yeast is a rich source of chromium and several B vitamins that are important for the regulation of blood sugar.

Recommended dosages. Experts suggest taking 1 to 2 tablespoons a day.

Possible problems. Brewer's yeast can cause gas, bloating, and diarrhea, so start off with a small amount (about ⅛ to ¼ teaspoon a day) and build up slowly to the recommended dosage. Some people may also experience allergic reactions. (Brewer's yeast is unrelated to *Candida albicans*, the organism that causes yeast infections.)

INFLAMMATORY BOWEL DISEASE

Inflammatory bowel disease (IBD) is an umbrella term that refers to chronic disorders that involve inflammation of the intestines. The two most common forms of IBD are ulcerative colitis and Crohn's disease. They produce similar symptoms, but ulcerative colitis is usually confined to the large intestine, or colon, while Crohn's disease usually affects the small intestine, but may arise anywhere in the intestinal tract, from the mouth to the anus. In ulcerative colitis, the inflammation causes sores, called ulcers or erosions, only in the inner lining, or mucosa, of the colon or rectum. In Crohn's disease, which is more severe, the inflammation extends into the deeper layers of the intestinal wall and the ulcers can cause permanent scarring of the intestines, narrowing or totally obstructing the channel.

An estimated 1 to 2 million Americans suffer from inflammatory bowel disease, with about equal numbers afflicted with the two types. IBD is most often diagnosed in young people between the ages of fifteen and forty, with a lesser peak occurring between ages fifty and eighty. The cause is unknown, but genetics is thought to play a role because IBD often runs in families. Up to 25 percent of people with IBD have family members with the disease. Furthermore, Jewish people of European descent have a five times greater risk than the general population. IBD seems to be more common among urban than rural populations and occurs more frequently in developed than in less developed nations, suggesting that environmental conditions, such as diet, also are involved. Some researchers believe that the disease develops in people who have a genetic susceptibility that enables an environmental agent, such as a virus or bacterium, to trigger an abnormal immune response. However, some studies have suggested that dietary factors may play a role, including high intakes of fat (particularly animal fat) and high sugar intake (from nonfruit sources).

In most IBD patients, symptoms tend to come and go, with intermittent attacks lasting for a few days to several weeks alternating with symptom-free intervals. Some, however, have continuous symptoms, and many of these people develop serious complications. For example, a complication called toxic megacolon involves inflammation in the deeper layers of the colon, causing it to enlarge, become paralyzed and, in the worst cases, rupture, requiring immediate surgery. Fistulas, channels that can develop between the loops of the small and large intestines and interfere with absorption of nutrients, are a common complication of Crohn's disease. Fistulas also can form pockets of infection or abscesses, which may become life-threatening without treatment. Both disorders also can lead to intestinal blockage due to scar tissue, and both increase the risk of colon cancer. People with Crohn's disease may also develop complications outside the intestinal tract; these include inflammation in the joints, skin, eyes, liver, and kidneys. While emotional and neurologic complications are also seen in Crohn's disease, it is not clear whether they are a part of the disease process or the result of coping with the symptoms of the disease and its treatment.

Diagnostic Steps

Diagnosis can be difficult and usually requires blood tests, laboratory examination of the stool, special X rays, and colonoscopy, an examina-

◉ SYMPTOMS

Both types of IBD
- Severe bouts of bloody diarrhea, alternating with constipation.
- Abdominal pain and cramps.
- Fever.
- Loss of appetite and weight.

Crohn's disease
- Hemorrhoids and anal abscesses.
- Joint pain and inflammation, similar to that of arthritis.
- Skin or eye inflammation.
- Delayed growth and sexual maturation in children.

tion in which a viewing tube is inserted into the colon. During colonoscopy, samples of tissue from the colon lining may be taken to help confirm the diagnosis.

Conventional Treatments

Drugs cannot cure inflammatory bowel disease, but they are effective in reducing symptoms and decreasing the inflammation that causes symptoms in the majority of patients. Surgical removal of the colon is the only cure for ulcerative colitis. Crohn's disease cannot be cured even with surgery. Medications that may be used to alleviate symptoms include these:

• *Acetaminophen* is most commonly recommended for mild pain. Aspirin and other nonsteroidal anti-inflammatory drugs (NSAIDs), such as ibuprofen, should be avoided. While NSAIDs are often used against other inflammatory disorders, they can irritate the gastrointestinal system and worsen the underlying condition.

• *Anticholinergic drugs* which relieve muscle spasms, abdominal cramps, and diarrhea, and also may indirectly relieve pain. These include diphenoxylate, loperamide, opium tincture, and codeine.

• *Hydrophilic mucilloids* are substances that increase the firmness and bulk of stools and may help prevent anal irritation and constipation. They include psyllium preparations (such as Metamucil) and methylcellulose.

• *Mesalamine compounds* inhibit substances in the immune system that cause inflammation. One type, sulfasalazine, has long been a mainstay of IBD therapy, treating acute attacks and maintaining remission. However, it is not effective in the small intestine and does not prevent recurrences. Furthermore, none of the mesalamine compounds can be taken by people allergic to aspirin or sulfa drugs. Side effects depend on which of the mesalamine compounds are used. Withdrawal of sulfasalazine when the disease is still active can trigger a severe relapse. Newer mesalamine formulations, including some given rectally rather than orally, may provide benefits with fewer problems.

• *Corticosteroids* are powerful anti-inflammatory drugs and include prednisone, prednisolone, hydrocortisone, and methylprednisolone. Steroids can produce rapid symptom relief. However, their long-term use is limited by their serious side effects, which include lowered immunity, high blood pressure, osteoporosis, diabetes, cataracts, muscle wasting, and weight gain, among others. Some of these side effects can be lessened by administering the drugs by rectal suppositories or enema infusions. Newer steroids, such as budesonide, beclomethasone, and tixocortol, may affect only local areas in the intestine, without circulating throughout the body. If they prove to be effective, such drugs may improve the outlook for many IBD patients.

• *Antibiotics* such as ciprofloxacin and metronidazole, may be useful

◉ STRATEGIES FOR RELIEF

▪ Diet may play a significant role in the development of IBD and its treatment. It would be wise to keep a food diary, noting what you eat each day and what symptoms you develop to see if any correlations exist, and then eliminating the offending food from your diet. Such elimination diets may be able to bring Crohn's disease into remission and reduce or eliminate medication. Foods most often blamed for aggravating existing symptoms are milk and milk products, spicy foods, fats, sugars, and grains. When symptoms erupt, physicians recommend a bland, low-fiber diet, avoiding raw fruits and vegetables, which can cause mechanical trauma to the intestinal lining.

▪ Ongoing diarrhea can cause dehydration. So drink plenty of fluids throughout the day.

▪ Surgery for IBD may increase your absorption of oxalate, a substance that reacts with calcium to form kidney stones. After surgery, avoid foods high in oxalates, including spinach, rhubarb, beets, coffee, tea, diet sodas, and chocolate.

▪ Liquid diets that are fully absorbed in the small intestine and provide complete nutrition are sometimes helpful in improving symptoms, reducing relapses, and improving nutrition in Crohn's disease patients. Your doctor can prescribe special "elemental diet" formulas, although they have an unpleasant metallic taste. Some doctors recommend adding flavored toppings or instant coffee and drinking the liquid cold to improve its taste. Over-the-counter liquid diets, such as Ensure and Sustacal, may also be beneficial, but their effectiveness has not been documented by research.

▪ If you have very severe Crohn's disease and find it difficult to tolerate any food, ask your doctor about total parenteral nutrition (TPN), or hyperalimentation, which is the intravenous administration of nutrients through a catheter.

▪ These are stressful diseases that may be worsened by stress. Get plenty of rest and practice relaxation techniques, such as meditation, daily.

for people with Crohn's disease whose condition is accompanied by bacterial infection and abscesses. (Antibiotic therapy does not seem to offer many benefits for patients with ulcerative colitis.)

• *Immune suppressants* are used for very active inflammatory bowel disease that does not respond to standard treatments. The two most commonly used immunosuppressants for IBD are azathioprine and mercaptopurine. Others include cyclosporine and methotrexate. The use of these drugs may enable control of the disease with a lower dose of steroid. In some studies, immunosuppressants have been effective in maintaining IBD remissions for several years. However, immunosuppressants also can yield serious side effects, especially increased risk of infection.

• *Biological therapies* are the newest approach to IBD treatment. These are genetically engineered drugs designed to interfere in the abnormal immune process. The first to be FDA approved is infliximab, which uses a monoclonal antibody attack substance called TNF, a major player in the inflammatory process. It is given intravenously and is only recommended for those with moderate to severe Crohn's disease that has not responded to other treatments.

Nutraceuticals for Inflammatory Bowel Disease

■ VITAMINS AND MINERALS

IBD and surgical procedures to treat it can inhibit absorption of vitamins, fats, calcium, and magnesium, leading to a need for supplementation. At the very least, a daily multivitamin with minerals should be taken. Depending on the severity of the disease and the medications being taken, other supplements may be needed. Children with IBD often need special diets and supplements to prevent malnutrition and to grow and develop normally. It's a good idea for anyone with IBD, regardless of age, to consult a clinical dietitian to devise a diet and supplements to meet individual needs. Vitamins and minerals that are usually needed are discussed below.

Folic acid

How it works. Because they often must restrict intake of fresh fruits and vegetables, folacin deficiency is very common among IBD patients. Absorption and utilization may be impaired not only by the disease but also by medications such as sulfasalazine. Supplements are important because folate deficiency itself promotes malabsorption and diarrhea.

Recommended dosages. At least 400 mcg of folic acid should be taken daily. If lab testing still shows a deficiency, up to 2 to 5 mg daily can be taken safely.

Possible problems. Taking extra folic acid can mask a certain type of anemia due to B_{12} deficiency. The simple solution is to always take extra B_{12} when supplementing with folate. Some doctors recommend 200 to 1,000 mcg daily. But those with Crohn's disease may need monthly injections instead, because B_{12} is absorbed in the part of the intestine most commonly damaged by the disease and surgically removed. (See Folacin, p. 237 and Vitamin B_{12} p. 233.)

Zinc

How it works. Due to low dietary intake, poor absorption, and excess fecal losses, zinc deficiency occurs in about 45 percent of IBD patients. Some IBD complications may be a direct result of such a deficiency, including poor healing of fissures and fistulas, skin lesions, delayed sexual development, growth retardation, retinal dysfunction, and appetite loss.

Recommended dosages. The usual dosage calls for 30 mg of zinc picolinate taken daily.

Possible problems. Avoid zinc sulfate, which may not be absorbed and utilized properly. Zinc hinders the absorption of copper; to compensate, add 2 mg of copper to the daily regimen.

■ NUTRITIONAL SUPPLEMENTS

Acidophilus

How it works. Acidophilus helps restore the normal balance of beneficial bacteria in the colon, especially when taking antibiotics. It also helps prevent diarrhea, a common symptom of IBD and a possible complication of antibiotic therapy.

Recommended dosages. Take one or two capsules containing at least 1 billion live organisms three or four times a day until symptoms subside.

Possible problems. Very large doses can provoke diarrhea; otherwise, acidophilus is quite safe.

Omega-3 and -6 fatty acids

How they work. Hormones called prostaglandins play a pivotal role in inflammation. Animal fats and some polyunsaturated vegetable oils favor the body's synthesis of prostaglandins that stimulate inflammation. In contrast, some essential fatty acids—specifically the omega-3s and omega-6s—tend to promote inhibitory prostaglandins. One study found that large doses of fish oil, which is rich in omega-3 fatty acids, improved Crohn's disease. In another, a coated preparation of fish oil was found to prevent relapse for at least a year in 60 percent of patients. Omega-3 fatty acids may also be useful for ulcerative colitis. The gamma-linolenic acid in omega-6 seed oils, such as evening primrose and black currant oils, also favor inhibitory prostaglandins.

Recommended dosages. At least eight to ten capsules of fish oils or an equivalent amount of GLA, taken over the course of the day, are needed to produce anti-inflammatory benefits. Another option is 1 tablespoon of flaxseed oil daily. It may take six to twelve weeks before results are apparent.

Possible problems. Large doses of some fish oil capsules produce fishy breath and such side effects as flatulence, heartburn, belching, and diarrhea. Look for coated capsules or focus on seed oils. (See Essential Fatty Acids, p. 295.)

Psyllium

How it works. Ground psyllium seeds and husks absorb water in the intestine, thus helping to treat diarrhea. Nonetheless, because it adds bulk to the stool, it helps reduce constipation. Further, the mucilage in psyllium is soothing to the intestines, which may help reduce cramps.

Recommended dosages. Dissolve 1 tablespoon of ground psyllium in an 8-ounce glass of water or juice each morning. Stir and drink quickly. If some psyllium is left in the bottom of the glass, add another 4 ounces of water to drink it. Drink another eight to ten glasses of water during the course of the day; psyllium absorbs large amounts of water and can cause intestinal obstruction without adequate fluids.

Possible problems. If any adverse allergic symptoms occur after the first use, forgo this remedy.

■ BOTANICAL MEDICINES

Aloe vera (*A. vera, A. barbadensis*)

How it works. Aloe vera juice is soothing and may help heal intestinal inflammation.

Recommended dosages. Drink one-half cup of juice between meals during a flare-up of symptoms. Alternatively, aloe vera pills can be taken; follow the product's dosage recommendations.

Possible problems. Be careful not to consume the aloe vera latex, the thick yellow extract from the inner leaf; this is highly laxative and should be avoided.

Licorice (*Glycyrrhiza glabra*)

How it works. Licorice root has soothing and healing properties that help counter intestinal inflammation.

Recommended dosages. The usual dosage calls for chewing two wafers (usually 380 mg) of deglycyrrhizinated licorice (DGL) licorice after each meal during a flare-up of symptoms.

Possible problems. Plain licorice can raise blood pressure, and its long-term use should be avoided. DGL does not pose this risk. (See Licorice, p. 493.)

INSOMNIA

About half of all Americans have significant sleep problems at some time in their lives, and at least 10 percent have chronic insomnia, generally defined as a persistent difficulty in falling asleep or staying asleep. Sleep is more than rest. It's also a time when the body performs critical tasks, including tissue repair and the release of hormones that play important roles in immune function.

Although no one as yet understands precisely how sleep provides its benefits, there are several stages of sleep in which body processes are altered. During REM sleep (an activated state marked by periods of *rapid eye movements*), dreams process the day's memories and, according to experts, restore the mind. During non-REM sleep, muscles relax, heartbeat slows, and blood pressure lowers, perhaps to restore body functions. Most people require 7½ to 8½ hours of sleep a night, but many get by on less or need more. If you are getting the right amount of sleep for your body, you should awake feeling refreshed and be able to function in an alert manner during the day.

Insomnia may be primary, occurring with little or no apparent connection to your psychological condition or to existing health problems. Or it may be secondary, arising as a direct result of a number of diseases or the drugs used to treat them. For example, painful conditions such as arthritis often provoke sleep problems. And some of the drugs used to treat both psychiatric problems (such as certain antidepressants) and physical problems (such as corticosteroids) interfere with sleep. Food and drink are great contributors to insomnia as well. For example, products containing caffeine keep many people from falling asleep, and alcohol, although it may initially promote sleep, triggers frequent awakenings. Shift work and jet lag contribute to sleep problems by upsetting the body's natural sleep-wake cycles. Other sleep disorders, such as sleep apnea, which causes frequent awakenings when breathing stops briefly during the night, also lead to insomnia. And shifts in hormones influence sleep; frequent awakening is very common among menopausal women, for example, who often begin to sleep the night through once they begin hormone replacement therapy. For most people, though, stress, tension, anxiety, worry, and depression are the most common causes of difficulty sleeping.

Whatever the cause, the end result is the same: Chronic sleep deprivation leads to daytime fatigue, impaired clarity of thought, and reduced short-term memory. Joint and muscle pain may occur. In addition, production of interleukins—substances that activate the immune system—is reduced; this may lower resistance to infection. Coordination and reaction time may be affected, leading to increased risk of accidents. And of course falling asleep at the wheel is a major cause of serious accidents and death.

◎ SYMPTOMS

- Inability to fall asleep within a half hour of getting into bed.
- Awaking in the morning much earlier than planned and being unable to fall asleep again.
- Awaking one or more times during the night, unrelated to the need to urinate.

◎ STRATEGIES FOR RELIEF

Even when you remove an underlying cause of insomnia, sleeplessness may have become a learned habit. Sleep experts recommend improving sleep hygiene regardless of other treatments. Try these tips:

- Exercise regularly during the day. However, avoid vigorous exercise in the evening; the workout may have a stimulating effect and make it more difficult to fall asleep.
- Don't eat a big meal a few hours before bedtime. Your body revs up to digest it.
- Similarly, avoid alcohol within a few hours of sleep. It may initially help you to get to sleep but as it wears off you will awaken.
- Use your bedroom only for sex and sleep. Leave stress-producing work, exciting or serious TV programs, and other distractions in other rooms.
- Go to sleep and get up at the same hours every day, even on weekends.
- Check your environment. Your bedroom should be cool but not cold. It should be fully darkened with shades or blinds. It should be quiet. If outside noise is a problem, mask it with neutral sound from a fan, air conditioner, or "white noise" machine. For serious light or noise problems, use a sleep mask and earplugs.
- Make sure your bed is comfortable. Choose a firm mattress for good body support. Treat yourself to bed linens that feel good. Consider smooth percale in summer and fluffy flannel for winter. Choose blankets that are warm but lightweight.
- Take a warm bath about ninety minutes before bedtime. Warm water relaxes your muscles. Try adding a scented oil to the bath. Develop your own aromatherapy for relaxation. In particular, lavender and vanilla may ease stress and promote sleep.

- Establish a nightly routine. Rituals help us relax. Develop your own adult version of the "bedtime story" plan. It may include reading, listening to soothing music or a relaxation tape, drinking hot milk or herbal tea—whatever helps you unwind. Chamomile tea, in particular, has long been known as a sleep-promoting nighttime beverage. Avoid colas, coffee, and chocolate, which contain caffeine.
- Learn progressive relaxation or self-hypnosis techniques to help you prepare for sleep.
- If you can't fall asleep, some experts recommend that you don't turn on the light to read. They say that light only reawakens your brain when it needs to calm down. Especially problematic can be halogen or fluorescent or other "natural light" sources that can disturb your body's natural hormonal sleep-wake cycles. Instead, just try to relax in the dark.
- If you can't fall asleep, instead of thrashing around, get up and go into another room and read for a while. When you grow sleepy return to bed.
- Practice finding a comfortable position and lying perfectly still—resisting all temptation to move even a little—to let your body quiet and relax to sleep.
- When you get up in the morning, go outdoors as soon as possible to expose your body to bright sunlight. That helps normalize your sleep-wake cycle.

Diagnostic Steps

A complete physical checkup may be in order to rule out an underlying disease. It is likely that your doctor will want to discuss your lifestyle, life situation, and emotional experience. For persistent unexplained insomnia, an evaluation in a sleep laboratory may be necessary.

Conventional Treatments

Any underlying condition that is triggering the insomnia must be diagnosed and treated, which will usually clear up the sleep problems. Sometimes, however, sleeplessness gets to be a habit and the insomnia will still need to be treated.

Mild insomnia is often treated with nonprescription drugs, especially antihistamines that are available over the counter. More severe insomnia may be treated with various types of prescription drugs. However, none are really suitable for long-term use for chronic insomnia. Rather, they can help you move past short-term sleeping problems or act as a bridge to better sleep habits (see Strategies for Relief, opposite). None of these drugs should ever be taken with alcohol, which can lead to fatal overdosage.

- *Antihistamines* include diphenhydramine (Nytol; the sleep-inducing ingredient in Tylenol P.M.) and doxylamine (Unisom). Their sedative effect often disappears within a few days. They also may cause dry mouth, blurred vision, urinary retention, or constipation. These problems may be worse in elderly people. Although these are over-the-counter drugs, don't take them without consulting your doctor if you have glaucoma or prostate problems.
- *Benzodiazepines* have been the most commonly prescribed sleeping pills for many years. They include estazolam (ProSom), quazepam (Doral), temazepam (Restoril) and triazolam (Halcion). However, with time, these drugs produce tolerance, so you need ever-increasing doses to get the same benefit. They also may produce physical dependence, so that sleep problems actually worsen when you discontinue them. Some also may cause daytime anxiety, sleep hangovers, and even amnesia, especially among the elderly.
- *Hypnotics.* Two new drugs in this general class promise quick action, no tolerance, and no next-day drowsiness. Zolpidem (Ambien) is effective primarily for helping get to sleep. Its sedating effects last approximately seven hours, so it should not be taken again if you awaken in the middle of the night and have to get up early the next morning. The effects of Zaleplon (Sonata) are so brief that it can be taken in the middle of the night if need be, or both to get to sleep and to return to sleep later. Even these newer drugs may cause temporary memory impairment,

nightmares, and confusion, however, especially at higher than recommended dosages.

Nutraceuticals for Insomnia

Herbal preparations, hormones, and other supplements seem to affect sleep in very different ways from conventional drugs, although much less is known about the ways in which they promote sleep. Nonetheless, they may be better suited for long-term benefits.

■ VITAMINS AND MINERALS

Calcium and magnesium

How they work. It is not known how these minerals promote sleep, but studies have linked mild deficiencies with sleep problems.

Recommended dosages. Take 500 to 600 mg of each an hour or so before going to bed. Take them with a small amount of food and a full glass of water or juice. The supplements should be included as part of the daily requirements.

Possible problems. Very high doses of calcium may promote kidney stones in people who are prone to developing them. Calcium supplements also cause constipation in some people, and magnesium supplements should not be taken by people with kidney disease.

■ NUTRITIONAL SUPPLEMENTS

5-HTP

How it works. 5-HTP (5-hydroxytrytopham) is chemically related to tryptophan, an amino acid that raises levels of serotonin, a brain chemical that enhances mood, calms anxiety, and promotes sleep, among other functions.

Recommended dosages. Start with a relatively low dose of 50 mg taken about thirty minutes before going to bed. If this doesn't help, gradually increase the dosage to 100 mg.

Possible problems. The use of 5-HTP is somewhat controversial because it is very similar to L-tryptophan, which was banned by the Food and Drug Administration in 1989 after several deaths were traced to the supplement. It was later determined, however, that the problem was due to contamination in the manufacture of L-tryptophan, rather than the tryptophan itself. Possible side effects of 5-HTP include nausea and other intestinal upsets and drowsiness. It should not be taken before driving or operating dangerous machinery.

Melatonin

How it works. This hormone, which induces sleep, is normally released by the pineal gland at night. Use of melatonin can help restore the body's normal sleep-wake cycle.

Recommended dosages. Lower doses work better than higher ones. Studies have shown success with 2 or 3 mg, taken before bedtime. As small a dose as 0.5 mg may be effective.

Possible problems. People who have autoimmune inflammatory disorders, such as rheumatoid arthritis and lupus, should not take melatonin; it may increase the risk of a flare-up.

■ BOTANICAL MEDICINES

Valerian (*Valeriana officinalis*)

How it works. Studies in Germany and Britain have documented not only that valerian helps people fall asleep but that it enhances the quality of sleep. It may do this, in part, by easing anxiety by its actions on the brain receptors for gamma-aminobutyric acid (GABA), a nerve chemical (neurotransmitter).

Recommended dosages. As little as 4 mg of valerian has been shown to promote sleep, but a 400-mg dose, taken a half hour before going to bed, is more likely to yield benefits. It can be taken in capsules or as a liquid tincture; it can also be brewed into a tea, using 3 to 5 of the herb per cup. However, the tea and tincture have a bitter taste, which can be disguised by adding honey or lemon balm to the brew.

Possible problems. For occasional use, valerian seems both effective and safe. Herbalists generally recommend not taking it for more than two weeks at a time. Very high doses can cause morning grogginess, nausea, nervousness, and headache.

Kava (*Piper methysticum*)

How it works. For centuries, South Pacific islanders have relied on drinks made from kava roots for both social and medicinal purposes. In Europe, kava is prescribed for its calming and sedating effects, and an increasing number of Americans are also using it to ease anxiety and overcome insomnia. Researchers don't fully understand how kava works, but many believe that one of its main ingredients—kavalactones—acts on the brain's limbic system, the center of emotions.

Recommended dosages. The typical dosage calls for taking 250 mg of kava root extract, standardized to contain 30 percent or more kavalactones, a half hour before bedtime.

Possible problems. When taken in very high doses, kava has an intoxicating effect similar to alcohol. It should not be taken with alcohol or medications—prescription or herbal—that affect the central nervous system. Long-term use increases the risk of side effects, which include an upset stomach and loss of appetite. There have also been reports that taking kava for several months sometimes causes the skin to become dry, scaly, and take on a yellowish tinge. Conjunctivitis and confusion can also occur.

Lavender (*Lavendula augustifolia*)

How it works. Lavender has a sedative effect and is often recommended for restlessness or insomnia. Studies in Britain have shown that elderly people who used aroma therapy with lavender found relief from insomnia.

Recommended dosages. One to four drops of lavender extract may be absorbed into a sugar cube and placed in herbal tea, or an infusion of dried lavender leaves and flowers may be prepared. Or lavender oil may be sprinkled on your bed linens or placed in a bath before bedtime.

Possible problems. No health hazards are known in connection with lavender. However, not all types of lavender are soothing. Some species, especially Spanish lavender, may have a stimulating effect.

IRRITABLE BOWEL SYNDROME

Irritable bowel syndrome, or IBS, is a disorder of the intestinal tract marked by abnormal, uncoordinated muscle contractions in the colon. As a result, contents of the intestines move too rapidly or too slowly, resulting in diarrhea or constipation or alternating between the two.

IBS is extremely common, affecting 10 to 20 percent of the population, and it is much more common among women than men. IBS problems range from annoying to debilitating, and, although the disorder does not cause permanent damage to intestinal tissue, it can interfere with day-to-day life. Previously referred to as "spastic colon," IBS is considered a "functional" disorder, meaning that the intestines function abnormally but no disease process is present. The causes of IBS remain unknown, but stress can certainly trigger flare-ups. A prevailing theory holds that persons with IBS have hypersensitive colons that overreact to particular foods and other stimuli that are normally harmless. Hormones may also play a role; women with IBS suffer more during their menstrual periods.

Diagnostic Steps

The diagnosis of IBS is usually made on the basis of the symptom pattern after ruling out other possible, potentially serious causes. Tests to elim-

⦿ SYMPTOMS
IBS is often characterized by any of the following symptoms, to varying degrees.

- Painful abdominal cramps and bloating.
- Gassiness, which can be frequent and embarrassing.
- Constipation, diarrhea, or alternating bouts of diarrhea and constipation.
- Mucus in bowel movements.
- Possible frequent headaches, depression, fatigue, and nausea.

Chinese herbal remedies have been used for hundreds of years to treat disorders of bowel function. In 1998, a rigorously controlled Australian study, published in the *Journal of the American Medical Association*, reported success in treating IBS with Chinese herbal preparations. After sixteen weeks of taking individualized or standardized Chinese herbal formulations, symptoms were reduced by 40 to 60 percent. (The formulation of 20 Chinese herbs is available in the United States as Calm Colon, marketed by Samra Health and Beauty Inc.)

⊙ STRATEGIES FOR RELIEF

▪ Keep a diary to try to identify any foods, medications, nutraceuticals, and lifestyle factors that trigger IBS symptoms. If you discover a pattern, try avoiding the suspected triggers to see if symptoms abate.

▪ Pay attention to your diet, especially when it comes to foods that provoke bloating and gas. Some IBS sufferers cannot tolerate caffeine and/or alcohol. Cut back on fats, which are hard to digest, and try consuming more frequent, smaller meals rather than three large ones.

▪ Increase your fiber intake (see Psyllium, opposite). High-fiber foods help normalize bowel function and are helpful in combating both constipation and diarrhea. Between 25 and 30 g of dietary fiber daily helps avoid constipation in most people, but you may require less to feel better. Read nutrition labels, and consult the table on page 110 for examples of high-fiber foods.

▪ Try to minimize intestinal gas, one of the most unpleasant and embarrassing symptoms of IBS. Ginger, fennel, cinnamon, and peppermint teas may help. If all else fails, try taking one or two activated charcoal capsules as soon as symptoms appear. However, use charcoal only as needed; taking it on a regular basis can interfere with the absorption of essential nutrients. Simethicone tablets (e.g., Gas-X) are often helpful.

▪ Work to reduce stress, which can trigger an IBS flare-up. Regular exercise, yoga, relaxation exercises, deep breathing, meditation, hypnosis, and biofeedback have all been shown to be effective in calming the symptoms of IBS. Seek support from friends, family, or professional counseling.

inate more serious diseases frequently include stool samples to test for blood; sigmoidoscopy or colonoscopy, in which a viewing tube allows a visual inspection of the lower or complete colon; X rays of the intestines; abdominal ultrasound or scans.

Conventional Treatments

There's no single therapy for IBS, although new medications appear promising. Treatment has conventionally relied on diet and stress reduction (see Strategies for Relief, below) and a variety of medications. Antidepressants are effective in some people, although some may worsen symptoms in various people. Treatment with antispasmodics used to be common, but these have not generally proved effective and usually have distressing side effects. Otherwise, treatment has targeted specific symptoms. Doctors may recommend over-the-counter laxatives when constipation is the chief problem. But laxatives are not entirely benign because they can become habit-forming. For gas, over-the-counter or prescription antacids containing simethicone may be helpful.

New drugs that have been developed specifically for the treatment of IBS have begun to enter the market. Alosetron (Lotronex) in clinical tests leading up to its approval by the FDA has been shown to be effective—in women only—in types of IBS marked by diarrhea. If it lives up to claims, it will reduce the urgency and frequency of bowel movements and lessen pain and discomfort. Other drugs in the testing stage include tegaserod (Zelmac) and prucalopride, which appear to relieve IBS-related constipation.

Nutraceuticals for Irritable Bowel Syndrome

■ NUTRITIONAL SUPPLEMENTS

Psyllium

How it works. Supplementing the diet with psyllium (the ingredient in the laxative Metamucil and an additive in some high-fiber cereals) may help normalize bowel function during a flare-up of IBS. Psyllium husks contain soluble fibers that absorb large amounts of water, causing them to expand and produce soft, bulky stools that are easy to pass. Because it absorbs water, psyllium may also help normalize bowel function when diarrhea is a common problem, especially in people who consume a diet otherwise low in fiber.

Recommended dosages. A typical dose is 1 to 3 rounded teaspoons of psyllium powder, or about 5 to 10 g. Stir it into an 8-ounce glass of fluid, such water, milk, or juice, and drink it quickly before the mixture thickens. Psyllium is also available in capsule and wafer forms, which some people find more convenient to take than the powder. However, these forms must still be consumed with ample water.

Possible problems. Too much dietary fiber can cause cramps and diarrhea; it can also interfere with the absorption of some minerals. When starting psyllium, use a low dosage of 1 teaspoon (or the equivalent amount in capsule or wafer form) and gradually increase the amount to no more than 3 teaspoons. Always take it with a full glass of fluid, and drink it quickly to prevent the fiber from swelling in your throat. In fact, it should not be taken by people who have difficulty swallowing because it can block the esophagus or cause choking. Drink at least eight to ten full glasses of fluid during the course of the day. Without adequate fluid, psyllium (and other high-fiber products) can cause intestinal obstruction.

Acidophilus

How it works. Acidophilus, a strain of lactobacillus, is a type of beneficial bacterium that occurs naturally in the body, including the intestines, where it helps control the populations of other organisms, including gas-producing bacteria. Some studies indicate that acidophilus supplements can aid digestion and combat diarrhea and other IBS symptoms. Acidophilus is often added to cultured milk products, such as yogurt.

Recommended dosages. Take enteric-coated capsules, which are digested in the intestines, in dosages that provide a total of 1 to 3 billion live organisms. Or mix acidophilus powder in water. Follow instructions on the label of the product you see. Alternatively, you can consume one or two 8-ounce servings per day of yogurt containing live acidophilus cultures.

Possible problems. No evidence exists of toxic reactions to acidophilus, although taking extremely large dosages may trigger diarrhea and bloating. If you are taking antibiotics, wait at least two hours before ingesting acidophilus.

■ BOTANICAL MEDICINES

Peppermint (*Mentha piperitia*)

How it works. Menthol is peppermint's primary ingredient, and the one that has been used in human studies of peppermint's ability to soothe. Peppermint oil is an antispasmodic agent that counteracts colonic contractions. At least two double-blind studies indicate that it can calm intestinal spasms, thereby relieving IBS symptoms. Another study found that a two-week course of peppermint oil taken in the form of softgel capsules relieved IBS in forty patients.

Recommended dosages. Taken as tea, a daily dose should be 3 to 6 g of leaves, steeped in hot water for ten minutes. A common dosage of peppermint oil is 0.6 ml in an enteric-coated form (allowing it to pass into the intestines without being digested in the stomach), divided into three doses and taken between meals.

Potential problems. While many people find relief with peppermint oil, some people with IBS find it highly irritating. Large amounts of peppermint oil (more than 2 g) can be toxic; excessive consumption can also cause kidney damage. People with gastroesophageal reflux disease (GERD), gallbladder disease, and severe liver damage should avoid peppermint oil. (See Mint/Peppermint, p. 501.)

Bilberry (*Vaccinium myrtillus*)

How it works. Bilberry, a cousin of blueberries, has long been used in Europe to treat diarrhea and other intestinal upsets. It is rich in tannins and the dried berries contain substances called anthocyanosides, which have an antidiarrheal effect.

Recommended dosages. Dosages range from 40 to 160 mg of bilberry extract, standardized to provide 25 percent anthocyanosides. Or you can brew a tea by pouring a cup of hot water over 1 to 2 tablespoons of dried whole bilberries (2 to 3 teaspoons of crushed berries). Let it steep for ten minutes, strain, and drink up to three cups a day.

Potential problems. Bilberry is safe when taken in the recommended amounts. However, fresh bilberries can cause or worsen diarrhea.

KIDNEY DISORDERS

Shaped like beans and as small as fists, the kidneys filter the blood of waste substances and syphon off extra salt and water to maintain the body's chemical balance. They produce and release hormones into the bloodstream, help regulate blood pressure and red blood cell production, and contribute to bone formation and maintenance.

Most kidney disorders attack the filtering units known as nephrons. Kidney diseases can develop suddenly, as the result of chemical poisoning or a direct blow to one of the organs. More often, however, symptoms appear after kidney function has been declining for years. Common kidney disorders include:

• *Kidney stones.* Kidney stones plague more than a million Americans yearly, most of them men. Stone-forming substances build up in the urine and begin to crystallize. The resulting stones can be the size of small pebbles, and passage can be extremely painful. The most common type of kidney stone contains mostly calcium. Struvite stones, which are less likely, are the result of urinary tract infections (UTIs). Heredity increases kidney-stone risk, as do gout and urinary tract blockages. High doses of vitamin C may increase the risk in susceptible people. Anyone who has passed a stone is likely to do so again in the future.

◉ **SYMPTOMS**
- A decline in kidney function may be marked by any of the following:
- Burning, pain, or other difficulty when urinating.
- Increased urge to urinate, especially during the night.
- Blood in the urine.
- Urine that foams more than normal (due to excess protein).
- Swelling of the feet, legs, or hands, or beneath the eyes.
- Elevated blood pressure.
- Pain in the back or side, just below the ribs.
- Drowsiness and trouble concentrating.
- Muscle cramps.
- Numbness.

• *Nephritis.* Meaning inflammation of the nephrons, nephritis is the third leading cause of end-stage renal disease, when nearly all kidney function is gone and life is at risk. Nephritis may be hereditary, caused by infection, or result from excessive levels of triglycerides in the bloodstream.

• *Kidney failure.* In acute kidney (renal) failure, the kidneys suddenly become unable to filter waste products, which build up in the blood. Burns, severe dehydration, shock, allergic reaction, surgery, medications, poison, and various recreational drugs are among many possible causes.

In chronic kidney failure, function declines slowly over a long period, often because of diabetes, high blood pressure, or another serious disease elsewhere in the body. It leads to end-stage renal disease, which is fatal if not treated. In addition, medications, including long-term use of aspirin-acetaminophen combinations, can precipitate a progressive kidney failure.

Diagnostic Steps

Tiny kidney stones may be discovered in a routine urinalysis. Larger, painful ones may require blood and urine tests, plus imaging procedures to determine their size and location. An intravenous pyelogram involves injecting a contrast material into the blood that allows stones to become visible on X rays.

A wide variety of blood and urine tests are used to diagnose nephritis and other kidney disorders. Blood and urine are monitored for creatinine, a waste product created by normal muscle tissue breakdown; urine may also be tested for its protein content. A high concentration of blood urea nitrogen (BUN) is a marker for disordered kidney function; it means the body isn't properly clearing urea, a by-product of protein metabolism. Collection of urine over a twenty-four-hour-period may be required. Ultrasound, computed tomography (CT scan), and magnetic resonance imaging (MRI) are among the imaging procedures that may be employed. Sometimes a biopsy of kidney tissue may be necessary to rule out cancer.

Conventional Treatments

The majority of kidney stones pass on their own. Physicians usually have patients drink upwards of three quarts of water daily while waiting for the stone to be excreted. Pain may be considerable, and a variety of pain medications may be prescribed. Sometimes ultrasound can be used to pulverize the stones; the process is called extracorporeal shock wave lithotripsy. For stones that are blocking the lower ureter, an endoscope inserted upwards through the bladder may be used for removal. Rarely, surgery is required. Potassium or other medications may be prescribed

Symptoms of kidney stones include:
- Intense, sharp, intermittent pain, usually starting in the area of the kidneys, or in the lower abdomen, possibly radiating to the groin.
- Nausea and vomiting.
- Fever and chills (if infection is also present).
- Blood in the urine.
- Cloudy or foul-smelling urine.

◉ STRATEGIES FOR RELIEF
- Diet is a powerful weapon against kidney conditions. Although individualized dietary regimens are necessary because of the diverse contributions to kidney disease (including diabetes and high blood pressure), consider the following:
- If your urine contains high levels of oxalate, eat the following foods sparingly: spinach, nuts, tea, chocolate, beets, rhubarb, strawberries, and wheat bran.
- Moderate protein intake. Excess dietary protein leads to higher blood calcium levels, which could increase kidney stone risk in those who are vulnerable. Very low protein intake can slow the rate of damage in kidney failure. Meat and dairy products, as well as many soft drinks are high in phosphorus, which must be limited in kidney failure. Unless otherwise advised, limit yourself to the Recommended Dietary Allowance for protein of about 63 grams a day for men, 50 for women. One ounce of meat, poultry, or seafood supplies about 7 grams.
- Be cautious about taking calcium supplements. Most kidney stones are calcium-based, so this mineral may be off-limits in large amounts. After you pass a stone, check with your doctor about its composition and ask whether you should reduce your calcium intake.
- Restrict salt intake. Sodium increases the kidneys' workload. Excess levels leach calcium from bones, causing blood levels to rise. Sodium also promotes the fluid retention so often seen in kidney disorders, and it aggravates high blood pressure in some people. Limit sodium to 3 grams (1½) teaspoons daily, largely by avoiding processed and fast foods.
- Increase your fluid intake. Drinking fluids is as important as diet in the management and prevention of kidney problems. According to the National Kidney Foundation, research shows that people who consume 64 ounces of fluid daily reduce their risk for developing

kidney stones by 38 percent compared with people who drink 32 ounces or less. To prevent kidney stones, the National Kidney Foundation recommends consuming 12 to 16 cups of fluid daily, mostly as water. You need to drink enough fluids to produce at least 2½ quarts of urine every day. Drinking adequate water, milk, or juice typically makes enough urine to dilute any of the substances that could form kidney stones.

• Researchers say coffee (decaf and regular), tea, and wine drinkers may produce more dilute urine that thwarts stone formation. Cola, however, apparently increases the likelihood of stone formation in men.

• Avoid grapefruit juice, which may actually promote kidney stones.

to help dissolve some types of stones. To prevent further formation of some types of stones, allopurinol and potassium citrate may be prescribed. For people with excess calcium in their urine (hypercalciuria), thiazide diuretics may be prescribed. Antibiotics are usually given when struvite stones are found.

Treatment of nephritis and kidney failure vary widely depending on the cause and the degree of illness. Diuretics are often prescribed to help the kidneys excrete water and salt, as are other medications that help to regulate the buildup of toxic minerals. In acute kidney failure, function may return gradually once the body is rid of the toxic substance or recovers from the trauma. In chronic conditions, strict regulation of the diet is essential because the kidneys are no longer able to clear waste materials properly. End-stage renal disease requires dialysis—frequent filtering of the blood with a machine that acts essentially as an artificial kidney—and possibly a kidney transplant. There is no other treatment.

Nutraceuticals for kidney diseases

■ VITAMINS AND MINERALS

Calcium

How it works. Kidney stones typically consist of calcium bound either to oxalate or phosphate. Regulating calcium intake is ordinarily important, as is cutting down on oxalate-containing foods if necessary (see "Strategies for Relief"). Research shows, however, that people with a history of calcium oxalate stones can eat foods containing moderate oxalate levels if they wash it down with milk. It appears that the calcium in dairy foods binds oxalate, preventing its absorption by the body.

Recommended dosages. Study participants drank about 8 ounces of milk daily with each of three meals.

Possible problems. Calcium supplements do not appear to have the same effect on oxalate levels, so stick with dairy foods, but consult your doctor first.

■ BOTANICAL MEDICINES

Cranberry (*Vaccinium macocarpon*)

How it works. Urinary tract infections (UTIs) increase the risk of kidney stones and kidney diseases. Cranberry prevents bacteria from clinging to the walls of the urinary tract, helping to keep urinary tract infections at bay.

Recommended dosages. Drink 3 to 10 fluid ounces of 100 percent cranberry juice daily as a preventative measure, especially if you are prone to UTIs. To treat a current infection, drink 12 to 32 ounces daily. Or take 2 to 4 capsules of supplemental cranberry each day.

Possible problems. Undiluted cranberry juice is very bitter unless mixed with other juices, such as blueberry or apple juice. Diabetics may wish to mix cranberry extract in diet ginger ale, since commercially prepared cranberry juice contains a significant amount of sugar.

Goldenrod (*Solidago species*)

How it works. Goldenrod is a natural diuretic. It is used to reduce inflammation that results from conditions of the urinary tract, and to help pass kidney stones and to prevent their formation or recurrence.

Recommended dosages. Take 6 to 12 grams of goldenrod daily along with at least two quarts of fluid. The dried flowers can also be prepared as tea and drunk several times daily.

Possible problems. Don't take goldenrod if you are suffering from fluid retention as a result of impaired heart or kidney function. Also, some people are allergic to goldenrod; do not take it if the plant provokes hay fever or other allergy symptoms.

Parsley (*Petroselinum species*)

How it works. Like goldenrod, parsley helps you pass kidney stones by flushing the urinary tract, and it's used to prevent their recurrence. It also reduces urinary tract inflammation.

Recommended dosages. Eat a tablespoon of chopped leaves or roots a day. Or take 6 grams of the prepared supplement.

Possible problems. Parsley is not for pregnant women or anyone with kidney inflammation. Don't use it if you are retaining fluid as a result of impaired heart or kidney function. Full-strength essential oil of parsley is toxic and should not be consumed.

LEG CRAMPS AND RESTLESS LEGS

Almost everyone at one time or another suffers from painful muscle cramps in the legs or feet. The most common types develop suddenly after exercise, at the onset of sleep, or while at rest; these usually are not serious. Those that occur as you are falling asleep are likely to be quick, jolting spasms that often end within seconds. Cramps that occur in the thigh, calf, or foot after exercise can last for several minutes. Although they sometimes seem to be related to muscle overuse or stress, doctors know little about the cause of such leg cramps.

Musculoskeletal leg cramps

- Sudden pain occurs at rest, after exercise, or at night.
- Muscle goes into intense contraction.
- Pain disappears within a few seconds to a minute or two.

Circulatory leg cramps (intermittent claudication)

- Beginning as a gradual cramping ache or during exercise, as the condition develops pain may grow severe.
- Pain worsens when walking rapidly or uphill.
- Pain disappears with rest in one to ten minutes.
- Foot may become painful, cold, or numb.
- Skin on the foot and leg may become dry and scaly.
- Hair on lower legs may virtually disappear.

Leg cramps that arise during exercise and abate with rest may be a sign of a serious vascular disease called intermittent claudication. The cramping may first occur in the calf, thigh, or buttocks. In the beginning, the pain disappears after one to five minutes of rest. As the problem worsens, the distance you can walk before pain occurs gradually decreases, the pain itself becomes progressively more severe, and the amount of rest needed for it to abate grows longer. If the condition becomes severe, the poor circulation can cause skin ulcers on the lower leg or foot and, in the worst cases, tissue death and even gangrene.

Some 4 million Americans, most of whom are over age sixty-five, have intermittent claudication. Sometimes called angina of the legs, it is a circulatory disorder usually related to atherosclerosis or hardening of the arteries. Fatty plaque deposits of cholesterol and other substances block the leg arteries, restricting the flow of oxygen-rich blood to muscles. Because muscular requirement for oxygen increases with exercise, pain and cramping result. The risk factors for this problem are the same as those for blockage of the coronary arteries: high blood pressure, high cholesterol, diabetes, smoking, and obesity. The incidence of coronary heart disease leading to heart attacks and strokes is much higher in people who have intermittent claudication.

Other possible problems of leg discomfort include varicose veins (see p. 194), phlebitis, and restless legs syndrome (see box on p. 152).

Diagnostic Steps

If you have any persistent cramps, see your doctor for an evaluation. Musculoskeletal-related cramps usually can be diagnosed based on the description of symptoms and a physical examination. If circulatory problems are suspected, the doctor checks the pulse over the arteries in the leg and ankle. Doppler ultrasonography and a special type of X ray called an arteriogram can identify the precise areas of blocked blood flow. The doctor may request blood tests to check cholesterol levels and, possibly, other tests to evaluate coronary arteries for similar problems.

Conventional Treatments

No particular medical treatment is available for common musculoskeletal leg cramps. However, intermittent claudication is a serious health problem that requires major lifestyle changes (see Strategies for Relief, page 151), medication, and, sometimes, surgery.

Drugs prescribed for intermittent claudication include pentoxifylline (Trental), which has been shown to improve blood flow and enhance tissue oxygenation in the legs. Side effects are uncommon. Vasodilators, drugs that widen (dilate) blood vessels, may be prescribed, although their benefits are variable and unproven. Cilostazol (Pletal), a newer drug, appears to be more effective. Research shows that it improves blood flow, decreases clotting, and decreases the concentration in the blood of triglycerides while increasing levels of the "beneficial" HDL cholesterol.

Angioplasty involves inserting a small balloon into the obstructed artery and inflating it to compress the plaque and widen the vessel. Unfortunately, there is a high incidence of renewed obstruction. Therefore, in some cases, a small metal stent—which looks something like the metal spring in a ballpoint pen—may be left in place to hold the artery open.

Surgery may eventually be needed to bypass the affected arteries. This is similar to cardiac bypass surgery. An artificial blood vessel—or one taken from elsewhere in the body—is attached above and below the blocked areas to normalize blood flow.

Nutraceuticals for Musculoskeletal Leg Cramps

▪ VITAMINS AND MINERALS

Calcium and magnesium

How they work. These minerals play an important role in connective tissue health and are needed for proper muscle contraction and relaxation.

Recommended dosages. Some doctors recommend a total of 1,200 mg of calcium and 750 to 1,000 mg of magnesium daily, divided into smaller doses to enhance absorption.

Possible problems. Very high doses of calcium might contribute to kidney stones. Magnesium can cause diarrhea, but may counteract the constipating effects of calcium. However, magnesium should not be taken by persons with kidney disease.

Nutraceuticals for Intermittent Claudication

Because intermittent claudication is caused by the same types of problems that cause heart disease, the same nutraceuticals that help lower abnormal cholesterol levels and treat atherosclerosis (see p. 68) may help. Those that may be of particular value for leg problems are discussed below.

◉ STRATEGIES FOR RELIEF

Musculoskeletal leg cramps are best treated by simple measures at the time the cramp occurs. Simply stretch the muscle gently in the opposite direction of the contraction.

- For a cramp in the calf, with your ankle being forced down into a ballerina's point, flex your sole upward; or simply stand gently on a flat foot.
- For a cramp in the sole of the foot, with your toes curling under, grasp your toes and gradually stretch them back up.
- For a cramp in the front of your thigh, hold on to a chair for balance, then bend your knees and squat.
- For a cramp in the back of your thigh, sit on the floor with your feet straight out in front of you and stretch your arms toward your toes.

Intermittent claudication requires a heart-healthy lifestyle to slow the progression of atherosclerosis.

- Develop a gradual exercise program in consultation with your physician. At first, you may only be able to walk half a block before pain hits and you must rest. But, over the long term, exercise can help you develop small, collateral blood vessels in your legs. Gradually build up to a regimen of forty-five minutes to an hour daily of such aerobic exercises as walking or jogging.
- If pain also occurs at night, raise the head of your bed by four to six inches, which harnesses the force of gravity to improve blood flow in the leg.
- Wash your feet daily, using lukewarm water, a mild soap, and a gentle touch. If you find any sores or other problems, have them treated by a doctor promptly. Never self-treat corns or calluses.
- Don't wear elastic hose or constricting garters.

RESTLESS LEGS SYNDROME

If you feel an antsy, crawling sensation in your legs when you are trying to go to sleep—unpleasant but not painful—it's probably restless legs syndrome (RLS). It occurs in up to 5 percent of all adults and tends to run in families. Most commonly, the discomfort occurs deep in the calves, although some people also have it in their arms, genital area, or trunk. It most often occurs when sedentary, usually at night, and is relieved by physical activity, such as walking, stretching, rocking, or kicking. Such movement may become uncontrollable. Indeed, you may move involuntarily even during sleep. As the problem becomes more severe, sleep quality deteriorates, and relaxation becomes difficult.

Doctors believe the problem is usually neurological and related to sleep disorders. RLS may also occur in association with other health problems, such as kidney disease, diabetes, and rheumatoid arthritis. When the underlying problem is controlled, the RLS is often reduced or banished. RLS also may occur in association with iron deficiency, and supplements may eliminate the problem. Health practitioners also report benefits with supplements of vitamin E, folic acid, and other B vitamins. In particular, 800 to 1,000 mcg of folic acid daily have been prescribed (see Folacin, p. 237).

Medically, doctors often treat RLS with dopaminergic drugs, such as carbodopa and levodopa, or dopamine antagonists such as bromocriptine and pergolide. These are the same type of drugs used to treat Parkinson's disease, another neurologic disorder. However, these drugs are most likely prescribed for moderate to severe cases, because their benefits may wear off with time, leading to rebound symptoms. Other options include opioids and benzodiazepine drugs taken before sleep.

For mild to moderate RLS problems, simple lifestyle changes may be sufficient. Develop regular sleep habits and practice relaxation exercises, because fatigue and stress exacerbate RLS symptoms. Exercise regularly. In particular, a brief exercise period followed by a massage or hot bath before bedtime may help promote sleep.

VITAMINS AND MINERALS

Vitamin E

How it works. Vitamin E has mild blood-thinning properties, which may help increase flow through narrowed arteries in the legs.

Recommended dosages. Doctors typically recommend 400 to 800 IU a day; look for the natural (dl-alpha) forms, which are more readily absorbed than the synthetic (dl-alpha) forms.

Possible problems. Vitamin E in dosages up to 1,500 IU is considered safe. However, check with your doctor if you are already taking low-dose aspirin or other blood-thinning nutraceuticals or medications such as Coumadin.

NUTRITIONAL SUPPLEMENTS

Grape seed extract

How it works. Grape seed extract is rich in flavonoids—antioxidant substances that protect against cellular damage from unstable molecules (free radicals) released when the body burns oxygen. It also contains substances called proanthocyanidins, which improve blood flow by reducing platelet clumping. It is widely prescribed in Europe to treat various vascular disorders, including impaired blood flow to the legs.

Recommended dosages. Dosages range from 100 to 200 mg a day; look for products that are standardized to contain at least 92 percent proanthocyanidins.

Possible problems. No adverse effects have been reported when taken in the recommended amounts.

BOTANICAL MEDICINES

Ginkgo (*G. biloba*)

How it works. Ginkgo biloba extract (GBE) improves blood flow in the legs, just as it does elsewhere in the body; it also reduces the ability of platelets to form clots. Studies have shown that people using ginkgo can walk 75 to 110 percent farther without pain than before using it.

Recommended dosages. Multiple studies have shown that 40 mg of ginkgo extract taken twice daily provides as much or even more relief than the medication pentoxifylline.

Possible problems. Occasional abdominal distress, headache, or dizziness may occur. GBE should not be taken with Coumadin or other blood-thinning drugs or nutraceuticals because the combination can result in serious bleeding problems.

Garlic (*Allium sativum*)

How it works. The sulfur compounds in garlic have been shown to have blood-thinning properties, making clots less likely to form in the arteries. It may help lower cholesterol, but studies on this aspect have produced mixed results. The most benefit seems to come from fresh or slightly cooked garlic.

Recommended dosages. In one study, patients were given 800 mg of garlic daily and, on average, walked noticeably better by their fifth week of participation.

Possible problems. Some people dislike the taste of raw garlic; it also gives the breath a bad odor. Garlic may increase the effect of other blood-thinning agents, so should be taken with caution by people who are on anti-clotting drugs.

Hawthorn (*Crateagus laevigata*)

How it works. Studies have shown better blood flow and walking in people with intermittent claudication after receiving hawthorn injections, although some practitioners say the same benefits can be obtained with oral dosing.

Recommended dosages. Naturopaths recommend 120 to 240 mg of hawthorn extract taken three times a day. It should be a standardized extract containing 1.8 percent vitexin-4-'rhamnoside or 10 percent oligomeric procyanidins.

Possible problems. Because hawthorn is a powerful heart medicine, it should not be taken without your doctor's approval.

LIVER DISEASES

The liver, which is about the size of a football, is the largest organ in the body. Often referred to as the body's chemical processing plant, the liver performs a host of life-sustaining functions. It neutralizes and destroys toxins and waste products. It helps convert substances in food into chemical compounds that the body can use. It stores sugar in the form of glycogen, which it converts into glucose and releases into the blood for energy when blood sugar levels drop too low. It produces bile, a substance vital for fat breakdown in the intestinal tract. It stores vitamins A and D. Among still other functions, it manufactures new body proteins; oversees the transportation of fat; regulates blood clotting; controls the production and excretion of cholesterol; metabolizes alcohol and other drugs; and helps maintains hormone balance.

◉ LEG CRAMPS DURING PREGNANCY

Many pregnant women suffer from leg cramps, especially in the last trimester. Studies show that calcium supplements—up to 1,500 mg a day taken in three divided doses—provide relief for many women. As with any medication or nutraceutical, be sure to check with your doctor before taking extra calcium.

Liver disorders often go undiagnosed until they reach an advanced or acute stage. Hepatitis is often mistaken for flu or an intestinal upset. Cirrhosis can smolder along for years without any warning symptoms. Fatty liver also may have no symptoms and be detected only when a health care practitioner feels an enlarged liver during a physical examination. But according to the American Liver Foundation, all the following could signal a liver problem:

- Jaundice, a yellowing of the skin and the whites of the eyes.
- Dark urine.
- Fatigue or loss of stamina.
- Persistent unexplained fever.
- Loss of sexual drive or performance.
- Gray, yellow, or light-colored stools.
- Nausea, vomiting, and/or appetite loss.
- Bloody vomit.
- Bloody or black stools.
- Abdominal swelling.
- Prolonged itching, all over the body.
- Unintentional weight loss or weight gain within a two-month period.
- Mental confusion.
- Sleep disturbances.

● STRATEGIES FOR RELIEF

Prevention

Experts say that even if you are disease-free, adopting certain habits can protect your liver for a lifetime:

- Limit alcohol consumption to one or two drinks daily.
- Avoid mixing any medication with alcohol.
- Avoid alcohol completely if you have or are recovering from liver disease.
- Take the lowest dose of medication effective for any condition. Never exceed recommended dosages of acetaminophen-containing medicines, e.g., Tylenol.
- If you are a woman and have been diagnosed with hepatitis or another liver disorder, do not use birth control pills, which increase the risk of liver damage.
- If your job or hobbies require working with chemicals, wear a protective fume mask.
- Practice safe sex to protect against hepatitis.

Although the list of liver diseases numbers over one hundred, only a few are relatively common; these include:

- *Hepatitis,* which is characterized by liver inflammation and swelling. Most hepatitis cases are caused by viruses, although it may also be due to parasites and other infectious agents, excessive alcohol, drugs (abused and prescribed), and poisons. Most of the six different types of viral hepatitis are transmitted by direct contact with infected blood, body fluids, or human waste. About 4 million Americans harbor hepatitis C alone, a potentially serious problem because it increases the risk of liver cancer and cirrhosis, an incurable liver disease.

- *Cirrhosis,* a degenerative disease that destroys the liver by replacing normal cells with scar tissue. In the United States, most cirrhosis is caused by alcohol abuse, although viral infections, toxins, certain drugs, and a blockage of the bile ducts may also be responsible. Among middle-aged people, cirrhosis is the third most common cause of death (following heart disease and cancer).

- *Fatty liver disease,* which is also commonly related to alcohol abuse and often progresses to cirrhosis. The liver swells, becoming tender to the touch; jaundice and other symptoms of liver dysfunction soon develop. Fatty liver disease may also be caused by starvation, obesity, diabetes, a very low protein diet, intestinal bypass surgery for obesity, vitamin A toxicity, various drugs (such as corticosteroids, tetracycline, and methotrexate, among others), or exposure to such chemicals as carbon tetrachloride.

Diagnostic Steps

Indications of liver disease may be observed or felt during a physical examination. Blood and urine tests that evaluate liver function will be performed. Further blood tests may be necessary to determine the presence of a virus. Ultrasound will reveal an enlarged liver. Since the liver may still function normally while areas of the organ are becoming diseased, scanning procedures that use contrast material (radioactive isotopes) will show the interior of the organ and the degree of scarring or other damage. A liver biopsy, in which a thin needle is inserted into the liver to obtain a tissue sample, may be ordered.

Conventional Treatments

Early treatment and abstaining from alcohol and other substances that harm the liver greatly improve the chances for recovery from liver disease. In fact, the liver has a remarkable ability to heal itself although the scarring of cirrhosis is irreversible. Lactulose and neomycin are drugs that control blood ammonia levels, which can accumulate in the bloodstream because of cirrhosis. Supplemental vitamins A, D, and K may be prescribed, since the diseased liver may not be able to absorb them. Even so, frequent liver-function tests are necessary to make sure that these fat-soluble vitamins are not causing further liver damage.

Since most hepatitis is the result of viruses, there are few conventional treatments for it. Interferon treatments, using an immune-system component, are effective in some cases of chronic hepatitis B and C. Researchers are working with combining interferon with antiviral agents such as ribavarin, amantadine, and rimantadine.

A surgical procedure known as shunting may be necessary when scar tissue in the liver blocks the flow of blood from the intestinal tract to the organ, causing portal hypertension (extremely high blood pressure in the vein leading to the liver). Liver transplant is the last resort when all else fails to thwart the progression of liver disease.

Nutraceuticals for Liver Diseases

■ VITAMINS AND MINERALS

Vitamin B-complex

How they work. The B vitamins, especially B_{12} folic acid, and niacin, are essential for many metabolic processes, including those that take place in the liver. B-complex supplements promote healing by easing the liver's workload.

Recommended dosages. Look for B-complex supplements that provide 100 to 150 mcg of folacin (folic acid), B_{12}, and biotin, and 100 to 150 mg of the other B vitamins.

Possible problems. B-complex supplements are generally safe when taken in these amounts.

■ NUTRITIONAL SUPPLEMENTS

Coenzyme Q₁₀

How it works. This substance, which is found in all living organisms, plays a role in many metabolic processes, including those that take place in the liver.

Recommended dosages. The usual dosage is 50 to 60 mg taken twice a day, preferably with food.

Possible problems. Coenzyme Q_{10} is generally safe, although it may cause diarrhea and an upset stomach when taken in very high doses.

Digestive enzymes

How they work. These enzymes help break down fats and other foods, thereby easing the liver's workload. Supplemental enzymes may be derived from animal sources (e.g., pancreatin) or plants (e.g., papain and

---

⊞ STRATEGIES FOR RELIEF (cont.)

- Avoid sharing personal items such as toothbrushes or razors.
- Never use an unsterilized hypodermic needle. If you have an acupuncture treatment, get pierced or tattooed, or become ill in a foreign country and need an injection, always inquire about sterilization practices.
- Take advantage of hepatitis A, B, and D vaccines before traveling or if you are at high risk.

◎ DIET AND LIVER HEALTH

Good nutrition plays a critical role in helping a diseased liver heal itself. A registered dietitian can help devise a diet tailored to individual needs. Dietary advice for anyone with liver disease includes the following:

- Always avoid undercooked or raw animal foods and seafood, which can harbor viruses and bacteria that can infect the liver.
- Rely more on milk and plant sources of protein than on meats; for example, eat soy products and a combination of legumes and grains (e.g., rice and beans). A high-protein diet can lead to a dangerous buildup of ammonia, while inadequate intakes slow the liver's healing process. Animal products, other than dairy sources, contain certain amino acids that produce more ammonia than the amino acids in plant proteins and dairy products.
- Adopt a low-fat diet and use safflower oil in favor of other fats and oils. When the liver is unable to produce adequate bile, dietary fat passes through the body and into the stool (a condition called steatorrhea). Recent studies indicate that safflower oil is easier to digest than other fats and oils.
- Cut back on salt (sodium) intake to reduce swelling.
- When traveling in areas with poor sanitation or high rates of disease, avoid raw foods and drink only bottled water.

bromelain). Naturopaths usually recommend a combination of digestive enzymes (specifically, amylase, protease, and lipase).

Recommended dosages. Dosages vary according to the type of enzymes; look for a multidigestive product and take according to label instructions. Some are taken before eating; others after meals.

Possible problems. These are generally safe when taken according to instructions.

■ BOTANICAL MEDICINES

Milk Thistle (*Silybum marianum*)

How it works. Silymarin is the active ingredient of milk thistle, which protects liver cells from toxins and provokes the production of proteins to aid in liver-cell regeneration. It fights inflammation and seems to improve liver function in people with a variety of liver diseases. In cancer patients taking chemotherapy, milk thistle helps protect them from liver damage.

Recommended dosages. Milk thistle is used in Europe to help treat chronically inflamed liver tissue and cirrhosis. The recommended dose is 450 mg daily of a supplement standardized to 70 percent silymarin. Tea preparations are not recommended for medicinal purposes, since the silymarin is not water-soluble. Take it alone or in a liver complex or lipotropic (fat-metabolizing) supplement, which may also contain dandelion and B-vitamins choline, inositol, and methionine.

Possible problems. When used properly, there are no known side effects.

Licorice (*Glycyrrhiza glabra*)

How it works. The glycyrrhizin in licorice acts as an antiviral, increases production of interferon by the immune system, and appears to aid in the treatment of hepatitis B and C. Licorice also has anti-inflammatory and antioxidant properties.

Recommended dosages. Recommendations vary widely, from less than 1 g to 10 g daily of the powdered root. Because glycyrrhizin has dangerous side effects at high dosages or at any dose over a long period, it is best to stay on the safe side and take no more than 1 g daily of the supplement standardized to 22 percent glycyrrhizin or glycyrrhizinic acid for ten days to a month. (Do not take the DGL form, from which the glycyrrhizin has been removed.) Anyone attempting a higher dose should self-treat for no more than the ten-day limit.

Possible problems. At high medicinal dosages over a short term or at low dosages taken regularly, licorice can raise blood pressure to dangerously high levels, deplete potassium levels, cause fluid retention, alter heart rhythms, cause lethargy, and diminish sexual interest and performance, among other possible adverse effects. Licorice also alters the effectiveness of hormones (such as supplementary thyroid, oral contraceptives, hormone replacement therapy) and steroids. German health authorities caution that medicinal licorice should not be taken beyond four to six weeks. Individuals with kidney disease, heart disease, or hypertension should not take any form of whole licorice. The best advice, especially if you have current liver disease, is to discuss it first with your doctor.

LUPUS

Lupus is an autoimmune disorder in the rheumatic disease family, which means that it is a relative of arthritis. The most common type is systemic lupus erythematosus (SLE), which affects the entire body. Discoid lupus erythematosus is largely limited to the skin. As many as 2 million Americans have lupus. However, it's difficult to know the precise figure because many cases are undiagnosed, while others that are thought to be lupus are actually something else. Women are afflicted with lupus ten to fifteen times more frequently than men.

The cause of lupus remains unknown. But it is likely that one or more environmental factors (such as a disease of the large intestine, a virus, and sun exposure) trigger an inherited genetic predisposition to develop the disease. About 10 percent of lupus patients have a close relative with lupus. The disease is also more common among people of African, Native American, Asian, and Hispanic origin. Doctors also suspect that estrogen—the major female sex hormone—may play some role because so many patients are women, and some women experience a worsening of symptoms before their menstrual periods or during pregnancy.

Whatever the underlying cause, lupus prompts the immune system to become overactive and attack the body's own tissue as if it were a foreign invader. This means that persons with the disease produce antibodies that attack their skin, joints, and other connective tissue throughout the body. While it is usually a lifetime chronic disease, symptoms can come and go—getting worse, which is called a flare, or disappearing, which is called a remission.

Diagnostic Steps

Lupus is difficult to diagnose because it can affect almost any part of the body. Symptoms may be similar to chronic fatigue syndrome, fibromyalgia, and rheumatoid arthritis, for example. Many people have the disease with slowly worsening symptoms for five to ten years before it is diagnosed. There's no single test for lupus. A doctor makes the di-

◉ SYMPTOMS

Discoid lupus erythematosus:
- Rash on the face, neck, and scalp.
- In severe cases, symptoms of systemic lupus

Systemic lupus erythematosus:
- A butterfly-shaped rash over the cheeks and nose.
- Rashes elsewhere on the body.
- Debilitating fatigue.
- Joint and muscle aches and pains.
- Worsening of symptoms after exposure to light from the sun or fluorescent or halogen bulbs.
- Mouth sores that look like canker sores, but are usually painless.
- Dry eyes and mouth.
- Hair loss.
- Anemia and other blood disorders.
- Shortness of breath.
- Heart problems.
- Inflamed kidneys.
- Intestinal upsets.
- Vaginal dryness.
- Mental changes.

Many lifestyle measures can help reduce the impact of lupus on your life; these include the following:

• Get adequate rest. The debilitating fatigue of lupus cannot be ignored. Get plenty of sleep, don't overwork, and rest in bed when you are tired.

• Avoid unnecessary stress, which often triggers flare-ups. Get training in progressive relaxation or meditation and practice it every day. If your work is stressful, consider changing jobs.

• Exercise regularly. It's relaxing and can help you maintain ideal weight if you are on steroids. Exercise also helps prevent muscle weakness and fatigue. Although you should not stress inflamed joints during a flare-up, do as much exercise as you can—at least an hour three times a week.

• Eat a healthy diet. Some research suggests that diets low in animal fat can help reduce the inflammation that causes pain in lupus. Diets high in the cruciferous vegetables—broccoli, cabbage, Brussels sprouts, and kale—may contain a chemical that changes estrogen into a less threatening form for people with lupus. Salmon, sardines, and other fatty fish are also recommended.

• Beware of the sun. Some people with lupus may need to avoid being outdoors between ten A.M. and four P.M. in the spring and summer when the sun is strongest. Always use sunscreen with an SPF of 30 or higher. Also consider a hat and other sun-protective clothing.

• Don't smoke. There's a higher incidence of lupus among smokers—so it may increase your risk of flare-ups.

• Certain foods, especially alfalfa sprouts, can cause a lupus flare-up. Keep a food diary, and avoid those that seem to worsen symptoms.

• Plan pregnancy carefully because you may be at high risk for miscarriage and other complications. Get your lupus under control before getting pregnant. Find an obstetrician experienced in treating lupus patients or one who will work with your rheumatologist.

• Find a support group. Local chapters of the Lupus Foundation of America often can direct you to a group, where you can talk with others who have lupus. Support groups can help counteract the sense of aloneness that comes with a chronic disease.

agnosis based on a detailed history, observing a cluster of symptoms, and lab test results. These include blood tests looking for abnormal antibodies and other factors.

Conventional Treatments

Mainstream medical treatment seeks to reduce symptoms by quieting the inflammation and, if necessary, subduing the overactive immune system. The specific treatment depends on the severity of the disease, which varies widely from one person to another. Medications fall into four broad categories.

• *Nonsteroidal anti-inflammatory drugs (NSAIDs),* such as aspirin, ibuprofen, naproxen, among many others. They are available both over the counter and in prescription strengths. They work by reducing inflammation and, thus, pain and joint swelling.

• *Antimalarial drugs,* such as hydroxychloroquine and chloroquine. These are a mainstay of conventional lupus therapy. It is not known exactly how these drugs work on the immune system, but they are very helpful, at least temporarily, in easing the fever, skin rashes, and joint problems of lupus.

• *Corticosteroid drugs,* such as prednisone, prednisolone, or methylprednisolone. These medications are given to people with moderate to severe lupus. Unfortunately, long-term use of high doses of steroids can cause many problems, including weight gain, bone weakening, and an increased risk of heart disease, diabetes, infection, other autoimmune disorders, cataracts, and other problems. Thus, doctors recommend reducing the dose slowly to the lowest possible level to control the disease.

• *Immunosuppressive drugs,* such as azathioprine, methotrexate, and cyclophosphamide. These drugs, which are reserved for the most severe lupus, are commonly used for patients receiving organ transplants. In lupus, they work by suppressing the overactive immune system.

Nutraceuticals for Lupus

■ VITAMINS AND MINERALS

For starters, take a simple daily multivitamin with minerals. Several studies have shown that people with some types of arthritis have underlying vitamin and/or mineral deficiencies. It's unknown whether this is due to their diets or problems with the way they absorb, metabolize, or excrete nutrients.

Beyond the recommendations below, other research is looking at the potentially positive effect of vitamin B_6 and folacin (folic acid, or folate) on lupus. In particular, folic acid may provide benefits by mechanisms similar to those seen in coronary heart disease, that is, by helping reduce blood levels of homocysteine, a protein that the body produces as a natural by-product of metabolism. High levels of homycysteine can damage the blood vessels, making them vulnerable to a buildup of fatty deposits.

Further, if corticosteroids are prescribed, it's important to take supplements of calcium and vitamin D to help prevent bone loss, which can lead to osteoporosis (see p. 175).

Vitamin E

How it works. Vitamin E can have a powerful anti-inflammatory impact on the body, and studies have shown that people with lupus may have abnormally low levels of vitamin E.

Recommended dosages. A German study of people with rheumatoid arthritis showed that 1,500 IU of vitamin E daily yielded improvements in pain, grip strength, and morning stiffness equal to that of standard doses of diclofenac (a powerful nonsteroidal anti-inflammatory drug)—without the stomach upset of NSAIDs.

Possible problems. Excessive vitamin E is excreted from the body, so doses up to 1,500 IU a day of the natural (d-alpha) form are generally safe. However, many experts recommend lowering the long-term dosage to 1,000 IU.

Vitamin A and beta-carotene

How they work. One study has shown that people with lupus may have abnormally low levels of vitamin A and beta-carotene (which the body converts to vitamin A). These nutrients are powerful antioxidants—substances that help prevent the cell damage that occurs when the body burns oxygen. Vitamin A also stabilizes the outer surfaces of cells, which could help counteract inflammatory reactions that tend to increase when membranes are unstable.

Recommended dosages. Most daily multivitamins contain the RDA of vitamin A, which is 5,000 IU. A higher dosage may be needed to have an effect on lupus symptoms, but high doses should be taken only under the supervision of a qualified nutritionist or other health care professional trained in nutrition.

Potential problems. High doses of vitamin A can be toxic; they can also cause birth defects if taken during pregnancy (see Vitamin A, p 207). High doses of beta-carotene do not appear to carry these risks. Even so, follow the guidance of a qualified nutritionist or doctor with a background in nutrition when taking these supplements.

■ NUTRITIONAL SUPPLEMENTS

GLA (gamma-linolenic acid)

How it works. Several studies have shown benefits from use of supplements containing gamma-linolenic acid, a fatty acid found in seed oils such as evening primrose oil and borage oil. Because abnormal fatty acid levels have been shown in various types of inflammatory arthritis, researchers have tested the benefits of supplements in people with rheumatoid arthritis and lupus—with good results. GLA seems to replace arachidonic acid in the body as a building block for prostaglandins, thus creating a less inflammatory environment.

Recommended dosages. If you want to try it, you must take high doses and be prepared to give it plenty of time to work. Studies showing benefits have used from 525 to 2,000 mg of GLA daily—and it takes four to eight weeks to see an improvement. Some suggest that taking at least 1,300 mg daily is essential for a benefit.

Potential problems. GLA is generally safe. (See Essential Fatty Acids, p. 295.)

DHEA (dehydroepiandrosterone)

How it works. One of the master hormones in the body, DHEA (dehydroepiandrosterone) is broken down into androgens and some estrogens. People with lupus often have low levels of DHEA.

Recommended dosages. Ongoing research has shown benefits with doses of 200 mg daily, although this is much higher than what is usually recommended. It may reduce the need for corticosteroids and alleviates lupus symptoms.

Possible problems. At high dosages (above 50 mg), some women develop acne; it may also promote the growth of estrogen-sensitive tumors. Reducing the dose may continue the antilupus benefits but reduce acne. Since significant side effects are possible, it is advisable to have DHEA levels checked before taking supplements.

MACULAR DEGENERATION

◉ SYMPTOMS

Dry type
- Vision slowly grows hazy.
- Printed words appear blurred.
- A blank spot develops in the center of the field of vision.
- Colors seem dimmer and the world looks grayer.

Wet type
- Straight lines take on a wavy quality, due to excess fluid in the eye.
- A central blind spot develops and vision loss may be rapid.

Macular degeneration—also called age-related macular degeneration (AMD)—is the most common cause of legal blindness among middle-aged and older Americans. It affects the retina, the paper-thin tissue lining the back of the eyeball that is sensitive to light and essential to vision. In macular degeneration, the macula—a tiny area at the center of the retina—becomes diseased, resulting in a loss of sharp, central vision.

There are two types of macular degeneration, "dry" and "wet." The dry form accounts for 90 percent of cases and is marked by slow deterioration of the light-sensing macular cells. Although vision loss is usually not total, it becomes difficult or even impossible to see clearly anything that's directly ahead. Faces, the printed page, TV images, and myriad other objects become blurred images. The wet variety almost always develops in people who already have the dry type. It occurs rapidly when new, fragile blood vessels begin to grow below the macula and leak fluid and blood; deterioration of eyesight is rapid. The toll on quality of life among the largely elderly people who develop macular degeneration can be enormous.

Symptoms of macular degeneration are present in up to 15 million Americans over age fifty. About 10 percent of people over age sixty-five are affected and more than 75 percent of those over age seventy-five. Whites are far more likely to develop macular degeneration than are blacks, and people with light-colored eyes are at greater risk. The causes are unknown, but the disorder tends to run in families. Smoking greatly increases the risk, and long-term exposure to sunlight and high blood cholesterol may be contributing factors.

Diagnostic Steps

Macular degeneration is pain-free, so it may go undetected in its early stages unless you have regular, complete eye examinations. In addition to routine visual acuity tests that assess vision at various distances, and direct inspection of the retina with an ophthalmoscope, doctors may use an Amsler grid to detect changes in vision. This is a chart with lines that may appear distorted or blurred as macular degeneration develops. If signs of the wet form are present, a test called fluorscein angiography is usually performed to detect leaky blood vessels. This is done by injecting a special dye into an arm vein and then taking X rays of the blood vessels in the retina.

Conventional Treatments

There is little to be done for dry macular degeneration to reverse symptoms. For the wet form, laser surgery can slow progression of the disease, especially if the disease is detected early, but rarely restores significant vision. A high-energy beam is used to seal off the leaking blood vessels.

Nutraceuticals for Macular Degeneration

■ VITAMINS AND MINERALS

Vitamin C

How it works. Vitamin C is a powerful antioxidant that protects cells against free radicals, unstable molecules that are formed when the body metabolizes oxygen. Exposure to air pollution, cigarette smoke, and ex-

◉ **STRATEGIES FOR RELIEF**

▪ Low-vision aids can help people with macular degeneration make the most of the vision they have and substantially improve their quality of life. Contact the Lighthouse Information and Resource Service at 1-800-334-5497.

▪ If you smoke, make every effort to stop. Studies confirm the association between lifetime cigarette use and macular degeneration. Smoking constricts the blood vessels that feed oxygen-rich blood to precious eye tissue. Cigarettes also lower the body's levels of vitamin C, increasing the risk to the eyes.

▪ Protect your eyes from the sun by wearing glasses that filter out harmful ultraviolet rays.

▪ Consider other nutraceuticals that are high in bioflavonoids. In addition to bilberries, these include green tea, ginkgo biloba extract, and grape seed extract.

▪ If you do consume alcohol, limit your intake to one drink a day. The best choice is red wine; at least one study has found that a glass of red wine a day may reduce the risk of macular degeneration, but higher alcohol intake damages the eyes and all other body tissues.

cessive sunlight increases production of free radicals. Vitamin C is highly concentrated in the eyes, where it is thought to protect against age-related eye disorders, including macular degeneration. Studies show that high vitamin C intake is associated with a decreased chance of developing macular degeneration as well as cataracts.

Recommended dosages. The current Recommended Dietary Allowance for vitamin C is 75 to 90 mg a day, and at least 100 mg for smokers. One well-controlled, highly regarded vitamin C study suggests that 200 mg of vitamin C is required to fully saturate all parts of the body, including eye tissue. Some experts recommend that persons who have a high risk of macular degeneration or early signs of the disease take 500 to 1,000 mg a day.

Possible problems. High doses of vitamin C (1,000 mg or more a day in pill form) can cause abdominal pain and diarrhea in some people. High doses should not be taken by people with a tendency to form kidney stones or store excessive iron. It may also interfere with the action of anticoagulants.

Vitamin E

How it works. Vitamin E is another antioxidant that appears to protect against macular degeneration, perhaps by helping control blood cholesterol, reducing the risk of clot formation, and increasing the effectiveness of other antioxidants. In one important study involving seventy-one patients with severe macular degeneration, the condition stabilized among those taking vitamin E and other antioxidant supplements, but continued to progress in the control group.

Recommended dosages. Patients in the study cited above took 400 IU of vitamin E a day, along with 20,000 IU of beta-carotene, 750 to 1,000 mg of vitamin C, and 50 mcg of selenium. Choose natural (the d-alpha or RRR-alpha form) vitamin E, which the body absorbs more readily than synthetic (dl-alpha or all rac-alpha) forms.

Potential problems. Vitamin E is an anticoagulant (blood thinner) that can lead to excessive bleeding in people who are taking aspirin or other blood thinners, such as Coumadin or certain botanical medicines, especially ginkgo biloba. High doses may also pose a risk to people who have a genetic tendency to bleed excessively.

Vitamin B-complex

How they work. Some of the B vitamins, especially riboflavin, play an important role in retinal function.

Recommended dosages. A B-complex supplement that provides 50 to 100 mg (or mcg in the cases of folacin [folic acid], B_{12}, and biotin) should be ample, especially if the diet includes the recommended five to nine daily servings of fruits and vegetables and five or more servings of whole-grain or enriched breads, cereals, and other grain products.

Possible problems. B vitamins are closely related and supplements should provide a balance of them all to prevent deficiencies or problems with proper absorption.

Zinc

How it works. Zinc is a mineral essential to the proper functioning of all body cells, including the retina. Studies have found that zinc may help slow the progression of macular degeneration.

Recommended dosages. Many older people are zinc-deficient; the usual dosage is 30 mg a day. Bran and other high-fiber foods hinder zinc absorption, so if you take it with food, make sure it is low in fiber.

Possible problems. Taking high doses of zinc (more than the recommended 30 mg a day for more than two weeks) can interfere with proper immune-system function. Zinc should not be taken at the same time as iron pills or antibiotics; allow at least two hours to elapse before taking the zinc. In addition, zinc interferes with copper absorption; to compensate, take 2 mg of copper a day.

■ NUTRITIONAL SUPPLEMENTS

Lutein and zeaxanthin

How they work. Lutein and zeaxanthin are the two major carotenoids (natural red, yellow, and orange pigments) found in the macula and retina, suggesting that they provide protection for your eyes. This pair of powerful antioxidants has sparked interest, since studies show that foods rich in lutein and zeaxanthin protect against macular degeneration. They may also help filter out damaging ultraviolet rays. Egg yolk and corn supply the most lutein and zeaxanthinin in combination; lutein is concentrated in kiwi, red seedless grapes, zucchini, and pumpkin. Zeaxanthin is concentrated in oranges and their juice, honeydew melon, and mango. Green leafy vegetables are other sources.

Recommended dosages. To consume sight-protecting carotenoids from food, eat at least five servings of fruits and vegetables daily, as well as a varied diet that includes whole eggs. As supplements, sources suggest taking mixed carotenoids that also contain vitamin A.

Potential problems. Large doses may turn the skin orange. (See Beta-Carotene/Carotenoids, p. 270.)

Flavonoids

How they work. The natural pigments known as flavonoids (also known as bioflavonoids) may act as antioxidants while enhancing the action of vitamin C. They appear to protect capillaries, the tiny blood vessels that help bigger vessels transport nutrients to eye tissue and waste products away from them. Flavonoids are bountiful in fruits and vegetables, including apricots, blackberries, broccoli, cantaloupe, grapefruit, grapes, and tomatoes. Coffee, cocoa, tea, and red wine also boast flavonoids.

Recommended dosages. A diet that includes at least five or more servings daily of brightly colored fruits and vegetables should provide ample flavonoids. They also may be taken in supplement form; look for mixed flavonoids combined with vitamin C and follow the instructions on the label.

Potential problems. None are known.

■ BOTANICAL MEDICINES

Bilberry (*Vaccinium myrtillus*)

How it works. Bilberry extract is high in vitamin C and anthocyanosides, flavonoids that are especially beneficial to the retina. Studies indicate that bilberry extract may prevent macular degeneration, or at least slow its progress; it may also protect against cataracts.

Recommended dosages. The recommended preventive dosage for people at high risk of macular degeneration (e.g., smokers or persons with a family history of the disease) is 40 mg of bilberry extract (standardized to provide 25 percent anthocyanidins) taken two or three times a day. A higher dosage, up to 160 mg two or three times a day, may help slow the progression of dry macular degeneration.

Potential problems. No adverse effects have been reported.

MIGRAINE HEADACHES

Also called vascular headaches, migraines cause severe, throbbing pain, usually on one side of the head and face. More than 23 million Americans over the age of twelve suffer from migraines, with women outnumbering men three to one. And the problem is getting worse; according to the Centers for Disease Control and Prevention (CDC), there has been an unexplained 60 percent increase in migraines in the last two decades.

No one knows exactly what causes migraines, but many factors seem to be involved. They tend to run in families, so heredity probably plays a role. For about 70 percent of women sufferers, migraines are linked with the hormonal changes of the menstrual cycle. Women taking estrogen—either in birth control pills or as part of hormone replacement therapy (HRT)—sometimes suffer an increase in migraines. Stress; changes in weather; reactions to certain foods; excessive caffeine, nicotine, or alcohol; too much or too little sleep; allergies; high altitude; bright or flickering lights; noxious fumes; and some medications are among the dozens of migraine triggers in susceptible people.

Regardless of the cause, migraine symptoms are produced by a complex set of responses involving the brain, nerves, blood vessels, blood platelets, and various body chemicals, especially serotonin, an important brain chemical that dulls our perception of pain, and histamines and prostaglandins, body substances that can cause inflammation and pain.

◉ SYMPTOMS

Classic, or migraines with an aura (10 percent of migraines)
- A twenty- to sixty-minute warning period marked by visual distortions (i.e., flashing lights, brilliant zigzags).
- Possible one-sided facial numbness and tingling, garbled speech, dizziness, and feelings of disorientation.
- Onset of headache and other symptoms, such as nausea, vomiting, diarrhea, chills, and hot flashes.

Common, or migraines without an aura (90 percent of migraines)
- Warning (prodrome) phase, lasting hours or even days, marked by mood swings, erratic behavior, fatigue, sensitivity to light and sound, difficulty in thinking clearly, vague feelings of anxiety, loss of appetite, and food cravings, especially for sweets.
- Onset of headache and possible other symptoms.

Recent research implicates a chemical process involving the neurotransmitters (body chemicals that carry nerve messages) that stimulate the release of serotonin. In addition to dulling pain, serotonin also narrows, or constricts, blood vessels. In a migraine headache, the blood vessels in the head are first narrowed, and then widened, resulting in the characteristic throbbing pain of a migraine. Recent research has found that migraine sufferers experience unexplained, periodic drops in serotonin levels that coincide with their headaches. When they are given serotonin injections, the pain stops.

Diagnostic Steps

Doctors can usually diagnose migraines on the basis of symptoms alone. However, a physical exam, basic neurological tests, blood studies, and perhaps a CT or MRI scan should be done to rule out other possible causes. The patient should keep a careful diary for several weeks, noting any headache symptoms along with foods and medications, activities, unusual stresses, and other possible related factors, such as menstruation or abrupt weather changes. This can help pinpoint possible migraine triggers.

Conventional Treatments

Mainstream medicine relies heavily on medications, which fall into one of two categories.

Abortive medications work best when taken at the first warning sign of an impending migraine in the hopes of stopping the headache before it takes hold. These include aspirin, acetaminophen, ibuprofen, naproxen, and other nonprescription painkillers; ergotamin preparations, such as Cafergot, Wigraine, or Ergostat, which are powerful vasoconstrictors (drugs that narrow widened blood vessels); and drugs such as sumatriptan (Imitrex), which affect levels of serotonin, the brain chemical believed to be instrumental in migraines.

Preventive medications are taken daily by people who suffer frequent migraines. They include calcium channel blockers and beta blockers, drugs used mostly to treat high blood pressure and heart problems; antidepressants that also block pain sensations; and Depakene, a drug used more commonly to prevent seizures.

Nutraceuticals for Migraine Headaches

Just as there is no single medication that works for all migraine sufferers, there also is no single nutraceutical that helps everyone. But there are a number of products that produce varying degrees of relief, and they are certainly worth trying.

◉ STRATEGIES FOR RELIEF

Here are proven strategies that work for many migraine sufferers. Try experimenting with one or more to find what works best for you. If the migraines persist or worsen, by all means see a headache specialist. Studies show that even though most migraine sufferers can be helped, two-thirds fail to consult a doctor.

▪ Keep a diary of foods, beverages, and activities and see if any are frequently followed by a migraine. After you have identified possible migraine triggers, avoid them to see if the number of headaches lessen.

For people who suffer only occasional migraines:

▪ When you sense that a headache is coming on, immediately drink a cup of strong coffee (or a caffeinated cola) and take two aspirin, an aspirin-acetaminophen combination, or naproxen or a similar nonprescription painkiller. Then lie down in a quiet, darkened room with an icepack or cool compress on your forehead. This strategy helps abort a migraine in several ways: The caffeine helps prevent the dilation (widening) of the blood vessels, and it speeds the body's absorption of aspirin and similar painkillers. If taken early enough, aspirin and other nonsteroidal anti-inflammatory painkillers block the release of prostaglandins, in addition to blunting pain sensation. Lying down in a darkened room minimizes the unpleasant visual disturbances and sensitivity to light and sound. Finally, the cool compress reduces the coursing blood flow that causes the throbbing pain.

If you invariably suffer from migraines around the time of a menstrual period, try the following:

▪ Take 500 mg of ginger capsules (or about 2 teaspoons of fresh grated ginger) daily during your premenstrual phase. Or brew the dry ginger into a tea. If you feel a headache coming on, increase the ginger to 500 mg every four hours. A word of warning: In some people, ginger is a migraine trigger. Obviously, do not try this strategy if you are sensitive to ginger.

▪ Women taking oral contraceptives who develop migraines during the "off week" should consult their physicians about starting the new cycle of pills several days early. This practice is considered safe and may prevent menstrual migraines.

Riboflavin

How it works. Riboflavin (vitamin B_2) has been used in the treatment of migraines for more than fifty years. It is not known how it works, but a Belgian study found that high doses of riboflavin significantly reduced the incidence of headaches.

Recommended dosages. The Belgian study used a daily dose of 400 mg of riboflavin; improvement was generally noted in three to four months.

Possible problems. High doses are generally safe, although they may interfere with metabolism of thiamin and vitamin B_6.

Magnesium

How it works. Magnesium—a mineral found in leafy green vegetables, legumes, nuts, fortified whole-grain products, and shellfish—has many of the same effects as antimigraine drugs: it inhibits platelet clumping, constriction of blood vessels, and inflammation. In addition, some studies have found that brain concentrations of magnesium fall during a migraine. In one study, three thousand migraine sufferers were given magnesium supplements; about 80 percent reported some improvement. Several smaller double-blind studies have also found varying degrees of improvement among people receiving magnesium.

Recommended dosages. The amounts used in research studies varied from 200 to 600 mg of magnesium per day. (Note: The Recommended Dietary Allowance for magnesium ranges from 280 mg for adult women to 350 mg for men; experts generally recommend 400 to 600 mg as part of an antimigraine program and are contraindicated for kidney patients.)

Possible problems. High doses of 600 mg can cause diarrhea. To avoid this, divide the 600 mg into three 200-mg doses to be taken with meals.

■ NUTRITIONAL SUPPLEMENTS

Omega-3 fatty acids

How they work. These fatty acids—found in rapeseed, evening primrose, and borage oils; walnuts; and salmon, sardines, and other fatty fish—are high in gamma-linolenic acid (GLA), a substance that inhibits platelet aggregation, inflammation, and blood-vessel constriction (vasospasm). These properties may conceivably help prevent or lessen migraines. In one double-blind study, fifteen patients whose migraines were not helped by antimigraine medications took high doses of fish oil, and all experienced reduced headache symptoms. Similar scientific studies using omega-3 fatty acids from plant sources have not been carried out. However, a number of women whose migraines are linked to their menstrual cycle have reported a reduction in headaches when taking evening primrose oil to lessen premenstrual symptoms.

Recommended dosages. Participants in the fish-oil study took 5 g of concentrated oil (MaxEPA) three times a day with meals. The usual daily dosage of GLA to treat migraines is 270 to 360 mg, or the amount in 3 to 6 g of evening primrose oil.

Possible problems. High doses of fish oils can cause diarrhea and other intestinal problems. Persons on low-dose aspirin or other blood thinners may have an increased risk of bleeding problems when taking high doses of GLA. (See Essential Fatty Acids, p. 295.)

■ BOTANICAL MEDICINES

Feverfew (*Tanacetum parthenium*)

How it works. The leaves of this member of the daisy family are rich in parthenolide, a substance that reduces platelet activity and the release of histamines and prostaglandins, thus preventing swelling and inflammation. (Much of the throbbing pain of a migraine headache is due to blood coursing through inflamed, swollen blood vessels in the head.) Parthenolide also helps prevent the ups and downs in serotonin levels that are linked to migraines.

Recommended dosages. Researchers in Canada and Europe have established 250 mcg of parthenolide taken daily as effective in helping to prevent or minimize migraine attacks. This is the amount in 125 mg of dried feverfew leaves or in an extract that contains at least 0.2 percent of parthenolide. To determine how many pills are needed to get the recommended 250 mcg of parthenolide, multiply the milligrams of feverfew (either leaves or extract) by 0.2 percent. For example: 150 mg of feverfew $\times$ .002 = 0.3 mg or 300 mcg, a little more than what is actually needed. But taking more than the recommended 250 mcg is unlikely to be harmful, and because parthenolide tends to be unstable, manufacturers recommend taking extra pills just to be sure.

Improvement should be noted in four weeks. If there is no change, it may indicate that the product does not contain adequate parthenolide. In such cases, it may be prudent to try a different brand.

Note: A new nutritional supplement, called Migra-Lieve, combines feverfew, magnesium, and riboflavin in amounts that have been found effective in preventing migraines.

Possible problems. Some herbal manuals recommend chewing three or four fresh or freeze-dried feverfew leaves a day to prevent migraines. The leaves have a bitter flavor, and about one in five people who chew them develop mouth sores or blisters. People who cannot chew the fresh leaves can try feverfew tea. Brew six to eight fresh or freeze-dried leaves in a cup of boiling water. If even the tea causes mouth sores, stick with pill forms of feverfew.

Ginkgo (*G. biloba*)

How it works. The ginkgolides in ginkgo biloba extract inhibit platelet-activating factor (PAF), the substance that signals these blood components to go into action. Recent research indicates that PAF may play a role in migraine headaches; thus, inhibiting PAF may be helpful.

Recommended dosages. French researchers reported benefits against migraines among patients who took 120 to 240 mg of ginkgo biloba extract a day. However, more research is needed to confirm these results, and it should be noted that some people actually develop headaches after taking ginkgo.

Possible problems. Persons taking blood thinners, especially warfarin (Coumadin), should not take ginkgo biloba extract.

Ginger (*Zingiber officinale*)

How it works. Ginger roots (rhizomes) contain gingerols and shogaols, pungent substances that inhibit inflammation and platelet clumping; they also help quell nausea and are mild painkillers. All of these actions may be beneficial in fighting migraine symptoms.

Recommended dosages. No dosage has been established. However, some experts recommend taking 500 mg to 600 mg of ginger powder mixed with water every four hours, beginning at the onset of warning symptoms.

Possible problems. Ginger actually triggers migraines in some sufferers and they should not try this remedy.

MOUTH SORES

There are several types of mouth sores, but the most common are canker sores, known medically as aphthous stomatitis. These are small ulcers that most often form on the inside of the lip or cheek, and less commonly on the tongue and upper part of the throat. Although they can be exquisitely painful and make eating and even speaking difficult, most canker sores are not dangerous and heal on their own without leaving scars.

There are two types of canker sores: The most common is known as minor aphthae, which are less than a fifth of an inch across, and they have a white center surrounded by a red margin. They generally disappear on their own in ten days or less. In contrast, major aphthae are one-fourth of an inch across or larger, and they can last for weeks and cause scarring. Both types tend to recur, often two or three times a year. Some unfortunate people, however, seem to get them one after another.

Canker sores occur most often in teenagers and young adults, and

⦿ SYMPTOMS
- One or more small, whitish ulcers with bright red margins.
- Localized pain and tingling that worsens when touched or exposed to spicy or acidic foods.
- In severe cases, swollen lymph nodes in the neck, fever, and general malaise.

women are affected more often than men. The cause is unknown, but a combination of factors may be involved. They often appear during times of high stress. Many women develop canker sores at about the time of their menstrual periods, so hormonal changes may play a role. Some studies implicate nutritional deficiencies, especially iron, vitamin B_{12}, and folic acid, as predisposing factors. Some people find that certain foods, especially highly spiced ones, trigger sores, as can an aspirin held against the mouth's delicate mucous membrane. Other common factors include allergies, irritation from ill-fitting dentures or orthodontic braces, a tendency to bite one's lip or cheek, and overly vigorous tooth brushing.

Diagnostic Steps

In general, a doctor should be consulted for any mouth sore that lasts more than two weeks, especially if it is not painful—a possible sign of oral cancer. A doctor or dentist can usually diagnose a canker sore simply by examining it. Sometimes, however, other conditions, such as oral herpes (cold sores or fever blisters) or an infection stemming from badly decayed teeth, should be ruled out.

Conventional Treatments

Treatment is usually aimed at relieving the pain and avoiding further irritation until the sore heals. A doctor or dentist may prescribe lidocaine, a mild anesthetic, that can be used as a mouth rinse or applied directly to the sore. When used before meals, this can ease the discomfort of eating, although it may temporarily dull one's sense of taste. Another approach calls for applying a protective paste, such as Orabase, to coat the sore.

Very painful or slow-healing sores can be relieved by using a silver nitrate stick to destroy the nerve under the sore. A newer approach uses a laser to destroy the sore; this treatment also lowers the incidence of recurrence.

Major or frequently recurring sores may be treated with tetracycline mouthwash. Studies have found that an outbreak can sometimes be prevented if this antibiotic is used when the first warning tingling sensation develops.

Nutraceuticals for Mouth Sores

■ VITAMINS AND MINERALS

Vitamin B-complex

How they work. Some studies suggest that people with mild deficiencies of some of the B vitamins, especially vitamin B_1 (thiamin), folic

◎ STRATEGIES FOR RELIEF

▪ If you suffer frequently recurring canker sores, keep a diary of possible triggering factors (onset of menstruation, certain foods, unusual stress) to confirm whether any coincide with flare-ups.

▪ Have a dentist check for possible irritating factors, such as a loose wire on an orthodontic brace, ill-fitting dentures or bridge, or broken tooth.

▪ Avoid acidic foods and drinks, especially orange juice, and highly spiced foods until the sore is completely healed. If such foods seem to trigger sores, eliminate them from your diet.

▪ Pay attention to possible nervous habits, such as sucking or chewing on the inside of a lip or cheek, that may promote recurring canker sores.

acid, and vitamin B_{12}, are more vulnerable to developing canker sores. The B vitamins have numerous metabolic functions, and how a deficiency might contribute to canker sores is unknown.

Recommended dosages. Megadoses of the B-complex vitamins should not be taken unless specifically recommended by a doctor. However, taking a B-complex supplement that provides a balance of 50 mcg each of biotin and vitamin B_{12}, 400 mcg of folic acid, and 50 mg of each of the other B vitamins is safe and may help prevent recurrences of canker sores.

Possible problems. If you already take a daily multivitamin, check the amounts of the B-complex group—you may already be getting all you need, in which case, taking a separate B-complex supplement is unwarranted.

Vitamin C

How it works. Although rare in developed countries, even a mild deficiency of vitamin C can result in mouth sores. However, vitamin C also helps heal sores from other causes that affect the mouth's mucous membrane.

Recommended dosages. Start with 250 mg a day, and gradually increase to 500 mg. To increase the effectiveness, add 500 mg of flavonoids three times a day.

Possible problems. High doses of vitamin C can cause diarrhea; reduce the dosage if you develop this problem. Do not take large amounts of vitamin C if you have kidney disease or a tendency to develop kidney stones; suffer from hemochromotosis (an abnormal buildup of iron); or are taking blood-thinning medications.

Zinc

How it works. Zinc speeds healing of canker sores and, in small amounts, bolsters immunity.

Recommended dosages. Take one 10- to 15-mg zinc lozenge every two or three hours for three or four days.

Possible problems. Zinc causes mouth sores in some people; stop using the lozenges immediately if you have such problems. Also, intake of more than 100 mg of zinc a day for more than two weeks reduces immunity. Dosages of 200 mg can cause diarrhea, nausea, and other intestinal problems. If zinc is used long-term, take 2 mg of copper to compensate for reduced absorption of this mineral

■ BOTANICAL MEDICINES

Chamomile (*Matricariachamomilla, M. recutita, Chamomilla recutita*)

How it works. Chamomile contains a number of anti-inflammatory ingredients that may soothe and hasten the healing of canker sores.

Recommended dosages. Make a strong tea using 2 to 3 heaping teaspoons of dried herb in 8 ounces of water; cool, strain, and use as a mouth rinse before meals. Hold the rinse in your mouth for two or three minutes, swishing it around every few seconds, before spitting it out. (Some herbalists recommend swallowing the rinse, which is not harmful unless chamomile upsets your stomach.) The rinse can also be made by adding 1 teaspoon of tincture or eight to ten drops of chamomile extract to a cup of water.

Possible problems. People allergic to ragweed, chrysanthemums, daisies, and other members of the aster plant family may react to chamomile.

Goldenseal (*Hydrastis canadensis*)

How it works. At least two compounds in goldenseal—berberine and hydrastine—are astringent and also have mild antibiotic properties. These are the components that are thought to soothe and help heal canker sores.

Recommended dosages. To make the mouth rinse, mix 1 teaspoon of powdered goldenseal in 8 ounces of water, and use three or four times a day. Be sure to hold the rinse in the mouth for two or three minutes; it can then be swallowed or spit out.

Possible problems. Large doses of goldenseal can be toxic, but it is safe when used in the recommended dosage. The demand for goldenseal has led to shortages of the herb. Some products are adulterated with other more common herbs, such as yellow dock, bloodroot, or barberry, which can reduce the desired effects and also increase the risk of problems from the added herbs.

Licorice (*Glycyrrhiza glabra*)

How it works. Licorice contains glycyrrhizin, which reduces inflammation and also bolsters immunity. But even DGL (deglycyrrhizinated licorice) can help because, when taken as a lozenge or wafer, it forms a soothing, protective coating over the sores, allowing them to heal.

Recommended dosages. Take 380 mg of DGL in lozenge or wafer form three or four times a day, or until the sore heals.

Possible problems. Regular use of whole licorice affects the adrenal glands and can raise blood pressure. It should not be taken by anyone with high blood pressure or liver, kidney, or heart disease. It also interacts with diuretics and digitalis. The DGL form, however, does not contain glycyrrhizin and has no adverse side effects. (See Licorice, p. 493.)

Myrrh (*Commiphora molmol*)

How it works. Myrrh is highly astringent and can both lessen the pain and promote healing of canker sores.

Recommended dosages. Add five to ten drops of myrrh tincture to 8 ounces of water and use as a mouth rinse before meals. Use a cotton swab to gently apply a drop or so of the undiluted tincture directly to the sore.

Possible problems. Some people find myrrh causes an intense stinging when applied directly to the sore. If this is the case, use only the diluted mouth rinse.

NAUSEA

Nausea is that queasy sensation in your stomach that makes you feel as if you're going to vomit. When you become nauseous, digestion in the stomach stops. If you vomit, the muscles go into reverse and send food backward from the small intestine, through the stomach, and upward through the esophagus into the mouth. Emptying the contents of the stomach sometimes provides relief. But in some cases, like nausea caused by cancer therapy or pregnancy, relief can be hard to find.

Nausea can be caused by something as innocuous as driving in a car to something as serious as a brain tumor. It can be a side effect of anesthesia, many common medications, and cancer chemotherapy, radiation treatments, and various medications. It commonly occurs during pregnancy; about 50 to 90 percent of pregnant women experience nausea, while 25 to 55 percent experience vomiting (see Nutraceuticals Just for Women, p. 567). It can be a symptom of motion sickness (see opposite), food poisoning, viral infections, digestive disorders, physical or emotional shock, head injury, migraine headaches, gallbladder disease, or gastroesophageal reflux disease (GERD), a common cause of chronic heartburn. Although vomiting itself is usually not harmful, and can sometimes be lifesaving when it rids the body of ingested poisons, it could signal a serious illness.

Extended bouts of nausea accompanied by vomiting can result in dangerous dehydration. Children under the age of six are most at risk for dehydration and should see a pediatrician if vomiting lasts for more than a few hours, if diarrhea also occurs, if there is a fever over 100°F, and if the child goes more than six hours without urinating. In adults, nausea or vomiting that begins shortly after eating may indicate a peptic ulcer. Nausea occurring within eight hours after eating suggests food poisoning, though some foodborne diseases, such as salmonella, can take longer before triggering symptoms. If, however, you begin suffering severe nausea or prolonged (more than one week) nausea after starting a new medication, following a head injury, or for no apparent reason, you'll need to be checked out by your doctor.

◉ SYMPTOMS
- Queasiness and sour stomach.
- Dizziness.
- Excessive salivation.
- Possible shortness of breath.
- Clammy skin.

◉ MOTION SICKNESS
Because of its recurrent nature, motion sickness is a particularly bothersome form of nausea. Whether it be from a car, a boat, a bus, a train, a plane, or a carnival ride, in some people movement causes a disconnect between what their eyes see and what the inner ear registers and sends to the brain. Even astronauts are not immune to these effects. The result is an increased heart rate, dizziness, sweating, clammy skin, headache, nausea, and sometimes vomiting. It's been estimated that nearly 80 percent of people experience motion sickness at one time or another, but for some sufferers even their daily ride across town can bring it on. Over-the-counter drugs such as Dramamine or Bonine can help alleviate nausea in some people, but they often cause sleepiness.

Here are some other tips for minimizing the effects of motion sickness:

- In a car, sit in the front seat. Drive if you can; you're much less likely to get motion sickness if you're driving.
- On a bus, sit close to the front.
- On a plane, sit close to the wing.
- Get plenty of fresh air. If you are on a ship, get out on the deck. If you're in a car, roll down the window.
- Don't read. It can aggravate your nausea.
- Keep your head still.
- Watch where you are going from within the car.

Diagnostic Steps

If the reason for your nausea is obvious, such as pregnancy, a migraine, or motion sickness, no additional diagnosis is necessary. The diagnosis may become clear upon taking a complete medical history. Tracking down the cause may involve additional blood and urine tests, X rays, scans, and ultrasound studies.

Conventional Treatments

Numerous medications, most prominently antacids, are available over the counter and by prescription to combat the symptoms of nausea, even when other conditions are producing these symptoms. If your nausea is caused by GERD or an acid stomach, your doctor may be able to prescribe medications for those conditions, which will keep nausea under control. For cancer chemotherapy, new prescription antinausea medicines can be extremely effective.

Nutraceuticals for Nausea

■ VITAMINS AND MINERALS

Vitamin B_6

How it works. Researchers aren't sure how it works, but pregnant women who take vitamin B_6 supplements experience significantly less nausea than those who don't take it.

Recommended dosages. At least one study has found that 25 mg taken every eight hours is effective.

Possible problems. It is well documented that long-term megadoses (500 mg a day or more) of vitamin B_6 can cause nerve damage to the extremities. Also, check with your doctor, especially if you're pregnant, before taking high doses of B_6 or any other nutraceutical or pharmaceutical product.

■ BOTANICAL MEDICINES

Ginger (*Zingiber officinale*)

How it works. Ginger may be as effective as some prescription drugs for treating nausea due to pregnancy, motion sickness, morning sickness, and chemotherapy.

Recommended dosages. Take 2 to 4 g of the cut rhizome or dried extract per day. As a tea, use 0.25 to 1 g in a cup of boiled water, three times a day. Quanterra is a standardized brand of ginger extract sold in

---

⊕ MOTION SICKNESS (cont.)

▪ Be well rested before you start on your trip. A lack of sleep makes you more susceptible to motion sickness.

▪ Avoid odors like cigarette smoke, which provoke or worsen nausea.

▪ Traveling at night may make you less likely to experience motion sickness, since you can't see the motion of the car, boat, or plane.

▪ Don't drink alcohol to relax. You could just be making the motion sickness worse.

▪ Do not travel on an empty stomach. Eat small, low-fat meals before traveling. Nibble on crackers every few hours.

▪ Try acupressure. Place your right thumb on the inside of your left arm, about three finger-widths above the inside center of your wrist. Take a deep breath, breathe deeply, and press the thumb into the arm firmly for one minute. Then do the same about a half finger-width closer to the wrist crease. Repeat the steps on the opposite arm.

STRATEGIES FOR RELIEF

- Lie down in a quiet place, with your head and shoulders raised.
- Try foods that are easy on your stomach, such as:

  Toast, crackers, and pretzels
  Yogurt
  Sherbet
  Angel food cake
  Bland hot cereals, such as cream of wheat, cream of rice, or oatmeal
  Boiled potatoes, rice, or noodles
  Skinned chicken that is baked or broiled, not fried
  Canned peaches or other soft, bland fruits and vegetables
  Clear liquids
  Ice chips
  Carbonated drinks
  Raspberry leaf tea

- Avoid foods that are:

  Greasy
  Very sweet, such as candy, cookies, or rich cake
  Spicy or hot
  Strong smelling

- Eat small amounts, often and slowly. Eat before you get hungry, because hunger can make feelings of nausea stronger.
- Suck on a lemon or sour candy.
- If nausea makes certain foods unappealing, then eat more of the foods you find easier to handle. Also, foods served cold or at room temperature are not as likely to provoke nausea as those that are hot.
- Avoid eating in a room that's stuffy, too warm, or has cooking odors that might disagree with you.
- Drink less liquids with meals. Drinking liquids can cause a full, bloated feeling and trigger nausea.
- Don't force yourself to eat favorite foods when you feel nauseated. You can develop permanent dislike for those foods.
- Rest after meals, because activity may slow digestion.
- If nausea is a problem in the morning, try eating dry toast or crackers before getting up.
- Wear loose-fitting clothes.
- If undergoing radiation or chemotherapy, avoid eating for one to two hours before treatment. (For other suggestions, see Cancer, p. 51.)

the United States. It comes in 250-mg capsules to be taken thirty minutes before traveling and again every four hours.

Possible problems. Ginger could affect the ability of the blood to clot. Check with your doctor if you're taking any medications, such as aspirin, warfarin, heparin, or naprosyn, or have a medical condition that slows blood clotting. Ginger should not be taken one week before any surgical procedure.

Cinnamon (*Cinnamomum zeylanicum*)

How it works. The volatile oils and other substances in cinnamon may help relieve nausea and other intestinal upsets.

Recommended dosages. Take as a tea (a teaspoon in plain boiling water or in a cup of regular cinnamon) to ease nausea.

Possible problems. There are no problems associated with drinking cinnamon tea. However, cinnamon bark contains volatile oils that can provoke an allergic reaction or cause mouth sores when it is chewed.

Peppermint (*Mentha piperita*)

How it works. Peppermint oil can reduce nausea by aiding digestion and reducing intestinal spasms by relaxing muscles in the digestive tract.

Recommended dosages. Experts recommend drinking a cup of peppermint tea after eating. Alternatively, take a 0.3-milliliter capsule of peppermint oil two or three times a day.

Possible problems. Peppermint is very safe, but it should not be taken by people who suffer from gastrointestinal reflux or heartburn; its muscle-relaxing properties promote the backflow of stomach acid into the esophagus. (See Mint/Peppermint, p. 501)

Goldenseal (*Hydrastis canadensis*)

How it works. Although goldenseal is used primarily to bolster immunity and fight infection, it may also quell nausea associated with intestinal infections by destroying the organisms responsible for the symptoms.

Recommended dosages. Herbalists recommend taking one 125-milligram capsule every four hours as needed to calm an upset stomach. It can also be consumed as a soothing tea.

Possible problems. Very high doses can irritate the delicate mucous membranes of the mouth; they can also provoke diarrhea, nausea, and respiratory problems. In addition, goldenseal should not be taken for more than a few weeks at a time because its effects lessen with prolonged use.

OSTEOPOROSIS

Osteoporosis is a disease in which the bones lose calcium and other essential minerals, causing them to become fragile and easily breakable. Osteoporosis is a major public health threat for more than 28 million Americans, 80 percent of whom are women. In the United States today, 10 million people already have the disease and 18 million more have low bone mass, placing them at increased risk for it.

While osteoporosis can strike at any age, it is most commonly the scourge of the elderly, causing fractures, primarily of the spine, ribs, wrist, and hip. Only half of those who suffer hip fractures ever return to normal activities. For some, it leads to fatal complications. One in two women and one in eight men over age fifty will have an osteoporosis-related fracture in their lifetime. The exact cause of osteoporosis is unknown, but a number of risk factors have been identified. Heredity appears to play a role; the disease tends to run in families, and persons of Northern European or Asian extraction have a higher incidence of the disease than other ethnic or racial groups. Also at greater risk are those who have a thin or small build, smoke, and use excessive amounts of alcohol. Hormones also are a factor; women who enter a premature menopause or those who exercise so much that they have very low levels of estrogen are more likely to develop osteoporosis, and at an earlier age than their counterparts who have normal estrogen levels or who are on estrogen replacement therapy.

Although bone seems rock hard, it is constantly growing. Some cells die and others form to replace it. When this metabolic balance is thrown off, bone strength can decrease. Age-associated loss of mineral and protein components, especially calcium, are the most common underlying cause of loss of bone density. The process is faster in women than in men. It accelerates in the years after menopause because the female hormone estrogen plays a critical role by enhancing the body's absorption of calcium. Demineralization of bone also can be caused by a variety of problems, such as Cushing's disease, liver disease, or the long-term use of corticosteroid drugs, such as prednisone, as is common in people with asthma, lupus, rheumatoid arthritis, and other inflammatory diseases. Certain drugs used to treat epilepsy, endometriosis, cancer, and thyroid diseases also promote bone loss.

Diagnostic Steps

Diagnosis is based on special X rays known as bone scans. The most accurate scans are done by dual-energy absorptiometry (DEXA) machines. These tests involve only a fraction of the radiation used in a chest X ray, for example. Many doctors recommend that women have a baseline scan at menopause, then repeat it six months to a year later, to

⊙ SYMPTOMS
Initial bone loss occurs silently, without symptoms. Later, these may develop:

- Mild back pain.
- Loss of height and dowager's hump due to collapsed vertebrae.
- Fractures that occur spontaneously or with little or no pressure.

⊙ STRATEGIES FOR RELIEF
Lifestyle measures to help build and maintain bone density are important tactics to reduce the impact of age-related bone loss.

- Eat a diet high in calcium. Calcium-rich foods include milk and milk products, dark green leafy vegetables, and seafood. An 8-ounce glass of milk, a cup of yogurt, or a slice of cheese each contains about 300 mg of calcium; unfortunately many adults are unable to properly digest these foods. If you have problems digesting milk, try brands that have added lactase, a digestive enzyme. Alternatively, look for brands of orange juice and other products that have added calcium.
- Include good sources of vitamin D in your diet. Salmon, herring, eggs, mackerel, and liver, as well as vitamin D–fortified breakfast cereals, are good choices. The body also manufactures vitamin D when exposed to the sun. People who live in most areas except the far north can make all the vitamin D they need by exposing a moderate amount of skin (the arms, for example) to the sun for fifteen to twenty minutes two or three times a week.

• Exercise regularly. A sedentary lifestyle contributes to bone loss. Those who exercise regularly in childhood and adolescence are more likely to reach peak bone density than those who are inactive. Those who maintain an exercise regimen in maturity are less apt to suffer severe bone loss. The best exercise for your bones is weight-bearing exercise such as walking, aerobics, dancing, jogging, stair-climbing, and racquet sports. Strength training by lifting weights or working out on weight-training machines also helps build and maintain strong bones.

• Avoid soft drinks containing phosphorus, especially colas and diet products because it causes calcium to be excreted by the kidneys. Similarly, use salt in moderation; it also increases calcium loss.

• Avoid heavy drinking (more than 2 to 3 ounces of alcohol a day); it increases your risk of bone loss.

• Do not smoke. Women who smoke go through menopause earlier than nonsmokers. In addition, studies suggest that smoking itself speeds up bone loss.

help them decide whether or not to take estrogen replacement therapy. Even for women on estrogen, periodic bone scans are recommended to make sure their bones remain healthy. New tests that use ultrasound scanning, which does not utilize X rays, are being developed.

Conventional Treatments

Although there is no cure for osteoporosis, treatment is aimed at slowing and reversing bone loss. Four drugs are commonly used to fight osteoporosis:

• *Estrogen replacement therapy* is used for both prevention and treatment of osteoporosis in postmenopausal women. It decreases the risk of spine and hip fractures by 50 to 70 percent. However, because taking estrogen alone increases the risk of endometrial cancer, it should be taken with progesterone by women who have not had a hysterectomy. (Note: Some practitioners advise against taking synthetic hormones, if possible, in favor of naturally derived estrogen and progesterone.)

• *Bisphosphonates* decrease bone turnover and shift the balance of bone metabolism toward bone formation. Only one of the bisphosphonates, alendronate (brand name, Fosamax) has also been approved for osteoporosis prevention and treatment.

• *Salmon calcitonin (Miacalcin)* is a peptide hormone that interferes with bone resorption. It is given as a nasal spray or injection rather than a pill and is approved only for the treatment of osteoporosis.

• *Selective estrogen receptor modulators* (also called SERMs or "designer estrogens") are the newest class of drugs for osteoporosis prevention and treatment. The first to be FDA-approved is raloxifene (brand name, Evista).

Other treatments under investigation include sodium fluoride, vitamin D metabolites, and parathyroid hormone.

Nutraceuticals for Osteoporosis

■ VITAMINS AND MINERALS

Vitamin and mineral supplementation plays an important role in both the prevention and treatment of osteoporosis.

Calcium

How it works. Calcium is an important mineral in bone metabolism. National nutrition surveys have shown that many women and young girls consume less than half the amount of calcium recommended to grow and maintain healthy bones.

Recommended dosages. Depending on your age, you should be getting between 1,000 and 1,500 mg a day. If you don't get enough calcium from your diet, you may need calcium supplements.

Possible problems. Absorption is an important issue. Calcium, whether from the diet or supplements, is absorbed best by the body when it is taken several times a day in amounts of 500 mg or less, but taking it all at once is better than not taking it at all. Taking digestive enzymes, especially if you are over age thirty-five, helps increase calcium absorption. Calcium carbonate is absorbed best when taken with food. Calcium citrate can be taken anytime.

Calcium supplements may reduce the absorption of the antibiotic tetracycline. Because calcium also interferes with iron absorption, the two should not be taken at the same time, unless the iron is taken with vitamin C or calcium citrate. Any medication to be taken on an empty stomach should not be taken with calcium supplements.

Vitamin D

How it works. Vitamin D is needed for the body to absorb calcium. Without enough, you can't absorb calcium from either food or supplements and your body will have to take calcium from your bones for use in heart, muscle and nerve function.

Recommended dosages. Vitamin D comes from two sources: through the skin following direct exposure to sunlight and from the diet. Doctors recommend a daily intake between 400 and 800 IU per day, which can be obtained from fortified dairy products, egg yolks, saltwater fish, and liver, or by supplement. Some calcium capsules come combined with vitamin D.

Possible problems. Very high doses of vitamin D are toxic because it can build up in the liver and damage that vital organ.

Magnesium

How it work. Magnesium is a mineral that complements calcium. It also helps prevent constipation from large doses of calcium. Magnesium citrate and chelated magnesium are absorbed well. They are often combined with calcium in some capsules.

Recommended dosages. Magnesium should be taken in a 2:1 ratio with calcium. So if you are taking 1,500 mg of calcium daily, take 750 mg of magnesium.

Possible problems. In large doses, magnesium can cause diarrhea; to prevent this, always take it with calcium. Also, magnesium should not be taken by persons with kidney disease.

Soy isoflavones

How they work. Isoflavones are phytochemicals, unique to plants, that share a similar structure to estrogens. Thus, isoflavones such as ipriflavone, genestein, and diadzein are considered to be phytoestrogens, or plant estrogens. Ipriflavone, in particular, seems to inhibit bone resorption in a manner similar to estrogen. It also seems to enhance the body's use of calcium.

Recommended dosages. Ipriflavone has been shown to be safe and effective at doses of 200 mg taken three times a day. An alternative approach calls for taking 25 to 50 g of soy protein a day. This can be bought in powdered form and mixed with other foods. For example, blend one-fourth cup of soy protein with a cup of low-fat milk, fruit juice, or calcium-enriched orange juice for a nutritious breakfast shake or snack.

Possible problems. Absorption is best when ipriflavone is taken with food. (See Soy Products, p 349.)

PSORIASIS

Psoriasis causes a potentially disfiguring rash that recurs at unpredictable intervals. Remissions may last a few weeks or months or be more durable, lasting for years. Sometimes it disappears never to return. It is relatively common, striking more than one out of every one hundred Americans. It is rare in infants and the elderly, usually striking between ages ten and forty, with twenty-eight as the average age of onset. Some people with psoriasis also develop an inflammatory form of arthritis, which can become disabling if not medically treated.

The underlying cause of psoriasis remains unknown, although the immune system is believed to be involved. The disease seems to run in families—more than a third of patients have one or more family members with the disease—and it is most common among Caucasians. For example, 2 to 4 percent of white Americans have psoriasis. Although it sometimes makes its first appearance after a general infection or skin injury, subsequent flare-ups may be triggered by emotional stress, drug reactions (especially to lithium and beta-blockers, among others), or strep throat. Winter weather, sunburn, stress of any kind, and upper respiratory infections are frequent aggravating factors. But attacks can also occur for no apparent reason.

The rash itself is caused by a pileup of skin cells that have reproduced too quickly—about a thousand times faster than the normal rate. Because this rate overwhelms the ability of the body to shed dead skin

◉ SYMPTOMS

- A red, scaly rash appearing most commonly on the knees, elbows, lower back, and scalp, although it can occur anywhere on the body.
- Silver, scaly patches of skin that may or may not itch.
- Flaking of the skin and scalp similar to dandruff.
- Pitted and grooved nails that may separate from the nail bed.

cells, they accumulate on the skin with their characteristic bumps and scales.

Diagnostic Steps

A doctor can usually diagnose psoriasis by examining the characteristic rash. In the early stages, it may be mistaken for dandruff. A sample of the skin (biopsy) may help confirm the diagnosis.

Conventional Treatments

Psoriasis cannot be cured. Therapy is aimed both at normalizing the balance of body chemicals that are responsible for replication of skin cells and at removing the scales and reducing the redness. Topical treatments are most common, and may include:

- *Corticosteroids,* which are anti-inflammatory drugs that are applied to the skin as ointments, creams, or shampoos.
- *Coal tar,* which may be used as ointments or shampoos. These products control scaling for some people.
- *Acid gels or creams,* which are used to remove the skin scales.
- *Topical retinoids,* which are vitamin A acids. These are relatively new drugs that are effective in slowing the turnover of skin cells.

Miscellaneous other treatments include:

- *Phototherapy,* which includes carefully controlled exposure to sunlight or ultraviolet lamps. Care must be taken, however, to avoid sunburn, which can worsen psoriasis.
- *PUVA (psoralen plus ultraviolet A).* These treatments, which are typically scheduled two or three times a week for several weeks, entail taking a psoralen drug, which makes the skin more sensitive to ultraviolet light, and then sitting in a special light chamber for a few minutes.
- *Drugs to suppress the immune system.* These treatments are reserved for the most severe cases or those that include psoriatic arthritis, because they make the person more vulnerable to infection.

Nutraceuticals for Psoriasis

Nutraceuticals are used to supplement nutrients found to be low in people with psoriasis and to reduce the inflammatory environment in the body.

◉ **STRATEGIES FOR RELIEF**
- Avoid medicines available over the counter unless recommended by your physician. Some promise miraculous cures but provide only disappointment. Many are a waste of money and can delay your getting proper treatment. And some make the condition worse.
- Add cold-water fish, such as salmon, mackerel, and herring, to your diet to boost your intake of fish oils.
- Decrease your intake of meat, animal fats, and dairy products, which contribute to the inflammation.
- Learn relaxation techniques and try to lower your stress levels, which may reduce flare-ups of psoriasis.

■ VITAMINS AND MINERALS

Vitamin A

How it works. People with psoriasis often have low levels of vitamin A, which plays a critical role in healthy skin.

Recommended dosages. The amount of vitamin A found in a daily multivitamin, 5,000 IU, is sufficient.

Possible problems. Avoid overdoses of vitamin A, which can be toxic because it is fat soluable and excess amounts are stored in the liver. If long-term doses are required, select products that are mostly beta-carotene which are nontoxic.

Vitamin D

How it works. Some evidence suggests that vitamin D plays a role in controlling cellular replication. Daily topical applications of a synthetic form of vitamin D_3 (a prescription drug sold under the brand name of Dovonex), slows production of skin cells, Another new treatment uses activated vitamin D, which is available only with a doctor's prescription, to reduce psoriasis symptoms.

Recommended dosages. Dovonex is applied twice a day according to a doctor's instructions. Activated vitamin D, which should not be confused with the supplement forms, should be taken only under a doctor's supervision.

Possible problems. High doses of vitamin D can be toxic, causing severe liver damage and other problems.

Zinc

How it works. Levels of this mineral, which plays a role in skin health, also are often found to be low in people with psoriasis. Supplementation with zinc was helpful in a study among people with psoriatic arthritis. If zinc is taken for more than a few weeks however, also take 2 mg of copper to compensate for reduced absorption of this mineral.

Recommended dosages. Most regimens call for 20 to 30 mg a day.

Possible problems. None at this dose; higher doses, however, reduce immunity, impair the production of HDL cholesterol (the "good" kind), and may cause digestive disturbance.

■ NUTRITIONAL SUPPLEMENTS

Omega-3 fatty acids

How they work. Several studies have shown that fish oils and flaxseed oil, rich in eicosapentanoic acid (EPA) and docosahexanoic acid (DHA), help control psoriasis symptoms. These fatty acids create a less inflammatory environment.

Recommended dosages. Some studies have shown improvement with daily supplements of 10 to 12 g of fish oil, providing 1.8 g of EPA and 1.2 g of DHA. A tablespoon of flaxseed oil daily also provides benefits.

Possible problems. You may need to take these supplements for at least eight weeks before seeing any benefit. (See Essential Fatty Acids, p. 295.)

■ BOTANICAL MEDICINES

Licorice (*Glycyrrhiza glabra*)

How it works. Topical licorice seems to have an effect similar to that of hydrocortisone creams in the treatment of psoriasis. In one study, those using licorice creams had an even better response than those using steroids.

Recommended dosages. Apply to the skin two to three times daily.

Possible problems. None when applied topically.

Capsaicin

How it works. When applied to the skin, capsaicin is known to interfere with substance P, a chemical messenger that plays an important role in pain and inflammation. Several studies have found that topical application of capsaicin creams relieves psoriasis.

Recommended dosages. Use a cream with a 0.025 or 0.075 percent concentration of capsaicin. It may take a few weeks for benefits to be evident.

Possible problems. Wash your hands carefully after applying the cream. Remember that capsaicin is the ingredient that gives chili peppers their "bite." Never apply it to broken skin and be extra careful not to get it in your eyes or on mucous membranes. (See Cayenne, p. 411.)

Chamomile (*Matricaria chamomilla, M. recutita, Chamomilla recutita*)

How it works. Chamomile is known for its soothing qualities and is often used topically to reduce inflammation.

Recommended dosages. A topical cream can be applied several times a day.

Possible problems. Avoid chamomile if you have hay fever, because it is a member of the ragweed family and could worsen the symptoms.

TOOTH DECAY AND GUM DISEASES

⊙ **A VACCINE FOR CAVITIES?**

A team of British researchers recently announced that they had developed a vaccine that eliminated decay-causing bacteria from the mouth. Large clinical trials will be necessary to validate the results.

⊙ **SYMPTOMS**

Cavities

It is possible to harbor a cavity for years and never know it. Or you may have these telltale signs and symptoms:

- Nagging toothache or increasing sensitivity to hot and cold foods and fluids.
- Discolored teeth, as the enamel deteriorates and allows the underlying dentin to show through.
- Bad breath.

Periodontal disease

According to the American Dental Association, any of the following can signal periodontal disease, but it's also possible to harbor the condition without experiencing any symptoms:

- Gums that bleed easily or gum tissue that is red, swollen, and tender.
- Gum tissue that has pulled away from the teeth.
- Pus that oozes from between the teeth and gums when pressure is applied to gums.
- Persistent bad breath or bad taste in your mouth.
- Permanent teeth that are loose or separating.
- Any change in the way your teeth fit together when you bite.
- Any changes in the fit of partial dentures.

Tooth decay and gum diseases, such as gingivitis and periodontal disease, are responsible for most tooth loss in the United States. Despite great advances in preventive dentistry, cavities (or dental caries)—the hallmarks of tooth decay—are a growing problem among people of all ages, especially children. In addition, 75 percent of Americans over the age of thirty-five suffer from some form of gum disease.

Bacteria in the mouth that feed on carbohydrate foods are the culprits in tooth decay and gum disease. Everything that contains carbohydrates—fruits, juices, breads, grains, milk, and, of course, sugar—attracts these bacteria. When these foods linger in the mouth, the bacteria feed on the sugars and starches and produce acids that erode the hard outer coating of teeth (the enamel) and cause cavities.

The bacteria also leave behind a sticky substance known as plaque. Frequent brushing and flossing reduces plaque buildup but may not completely remove it, particularly around the gum line. Gingivitis—inflammation of the gums—develops as plaque irritates gums, making them red, tender, and more likely to bleed easily. Gingivitis can usually be controlled by improved dental hygiene and regular professional cleaning.

Plaque that lingers, however, hardens into a mineral coating called tartar that is very difficult to remove. Tartar erodes the gum tissue and eventually leads to periodontitis, which is often difficult to treat. As the disease advances, it causes the gums to recede and pockets form around the teeth. When the roots of the tooth become exposed, they become much more vulnerable to cavities. And when bacteria invade the roots of the teeth and attack the ligaments that anchor the teeth to the bone, tooth loss may result. Recently, researchers have discovered a connection between gum disease and heart disease and stroke. Women with gum disease may be more likely to deliver low-birth-weight babies.

Misaligned teeth, fillings that have become defective over time, and dentures that no longer fit increase the presence of plaque, as do clenching and grinding your teeth. Risks for periodontal disease increase during periods of hormonal change (puberty, pregnancy, oral contraceptive use, and menopause) and with certain diseases, including diabetes, AIDS, and chronic systemic infections. Some drugs also increase the likelihood of gum disease, including corticosteroids and others that suppress the immune system; phenytoin (Dilantin), an antiseizure drug; and nifedipine (Procardia), a calcium channel blocker used to treat high blood pressure and heart disease.

Recent research has identified a genetic mutation that reduces the level of a key enzyme that keeps periodontal disease at bay. Scientists are beginning to believe that this enzyme deficiency could explain why some people who practice good oral hygiene have persistent gum disease. This discovery may lead to new ways to prevent and treat periodontal disease in everyone.

Fluoridation in municipal water systems and improved dental care for children has contributed to a decline in tooth decay among children in middle- and upper-income families. But the battle has not been won. Americans of all ages tend to consume vast quantities of sugary soft drinks, candies, and other sweets, which have a direct effect on dental decay and gum disease.

Diagnostic Steps

During a checkup, a dental hygienist or dentist inspects your mouth for tooth decay and periodontal disease in several ways. Checking for cavities, a dental hygienist or dentist looks for teeth that have taken on a chalky white and grayish white appearance, or have a very clear, open lesion. Then, using a dental probe, he or she locates soft areas on or between teeth. X rays can reveal cavities between teeth.

For gum diseases, visual examination is key, but so is probing for pockets between the gums and teeth. Pockets deeper than 3 mm indicate gingivitis, or worse. Depending on the severity of periodontal disease, you may need X rays to determine the health of the supporting bone and to detect other problems invisible to the naked eye. Your dentist may refer you to a periodontist, a specialist in the diagnosis and treatment of periodontal diseases, for further evaluation and treatment.

Conventional Treatments

The typical conventional treatment for a cavity is a filling. Depending on the extent of the decay, a crown may be required. Sometimes dentists take a cautious watch-and-wait approach when erosion is slight, because decay does not always worsen.

For mild gingivitis, your dentist will thoroughly clean and scale the teeth to remove plaque and tartar from below the gum line. Some will plane the tooth roots to provide a smooth surface for gum reattachment, and may place antibiotic fibers in the pockets to prevent infection and encourage normal healing. To control bacterial growth in the mouth, he or she may recommend antibiotics or mouth rinses with antibacterial properties, such as Peridex. In some cases, antibiotics are prescribed on a short-term basis. Some people require an adjustment in their bite, since misaligned teeth contribute to plaque retention.

In advanced periodontal disease, because larger gaps between gum and teeth cannot be properly cleaned of plaque and tartar, surgery is usually required. The gum is peeled back, and roots of teeth are cleaned and smoothed; gum tissue is then stitched back into a position that makes it easier to clean daily at home. Depending on the severity, per-

STRATEGIES FOR RELIEF

- Along with brushing teeth twice daily with a fluoride toothpaste that has the American Dental Association Seal of Acceptance, daily flossing, and regular dental checkups, a healthy diet is your greatest ally in defeating plaque and preventing dental caries. Avoid consuming large amounts of simple sugars, especially sugary soft drinks and sticky or hard candies.

- If you smoke or chew tobacco, stop now. Smoking not only aggravates periodontal disease, it increases your risk of ever having it. Chewing tobacco substantially increases risk for tooth decay.

- Include dairy products and other high-calcium foods in your daily diet. After meals, nibbling on a small wedge of aged cheese such as cheddar may provide a double benefit: it provides calcium as well as neutralizes the acids created by the mouth bacteria that foster cavity creation.

- Chew gum. Contrary to popular wisdom, some dental researchers now believe that chewing gum—the sugar-free variety—is good for the teeth. Chewing gum stimulates saliva, a natural cleansing agent that also helps strengthen teeth. Gum that contains baking soda also helps neutralize acid produced by bacteria.

- Try swabbing your gums or rinsing with liquid folic acid. Research suggests this treatment helps reduce swelling and bleeding in people with gingivitis.

iodontitis may require bone surgery to rebuild what has been destroyed by bacterial infections; gum grafts may be necessary to replace lost tissue.

Nutraceuticals for Tooth Decay and Gum Diseases

■ VITAMINS AND MINERALS

Calcium

How it works. Calcium is the body's most abundant mineral. It lends strength to bones and teeth. In fact, a significant portion of the body's calcium is stored in teeth, accounting for their toughness. Researchers at the State of University of New York at Buffalo found that men and women who consumed about half the required calcium had increased susceptibility to gum disease.

Recommended dosages. According to the National Academy of Sciences, adults up to age fifty need 1,000 mg of calcium daily; after that, 1,200 to 1,500 mg a day is appropriate. Eight ounces of milk, yogurt, or calcium-fortified juice provides about 300 mg, as does 1½ ounces of hard cheese. If you don't get enough calcium through food, consider calcium supplements to make up the difference. Calcium supplements are absorbed best when taken in small (500 or 600 mg) dosages with meals throughout the day.

Possible problems. The tolerable upper limit for calcium is 2,500 mg a day, according to the National Academy of Sciences. Too much calcium may interfere with the function of certain medications, including the antibiotic tetracycline, and may cause constipation and bloating. Calcium supplements made from oyster shells, dolomite, or bone meal may contain lead. Consult your doctor before taking calcium supplements if you have kidney disease.

Vitamin D

How it works. Vitamin D is calcium's necessary and helpful partner. Vitamin D promotes the body's uptake of calcium and its deposit into teeth and bone. The skin forms vitamin D when exposed to the sun. Being in the sun, without sunscreen, for as little as fifteen minutes a day may be enough to provide all the vitamin D you need, at least for younger people. Food is a relatively poor vitamin D source, with the exception of milk, which is fortified with vitamin D. Margarine and certain breakfast cereals provide vitamin D, but to a much lesser degree. Egg yolks and fatty fishes, such as salmon and mackerel, are natural sources of some, but not all, of the vitamin D you need for healthy teeth.

Recommended dosages. The National Academy of Sciences has determined that adults require 200 IU of vitamin D daily until age fifty-one, when needs double to 400 IU a day until age seventy-one; after age seventy-one, 600 IU are required each day. However, one review of vitamin D studies suggests that about 1,000 IU a day provides better protection for bones and teeth. Eight ounces of vitamin D–fortified milk provides 100. Drinking two glasses a day can satisfy a younger person's vitamin D needs, but in all likelihood, a supplement is necessary to fulfill most people's daily needs, especially if they get little sun exposure or if they are over fifty.

Possible problems. The National Academy of Sciences advises taking no more than 2,000 IU of vitamin D daily. At high doses over long periods, vitamin D can cause liver damage. Doses over 1,000 IU per day for long periods have been linked to heartbeat irregularities and gastrointestinal problems.

Vitamin C

How it works. Vitamin C is a vital component of collagen, the connective tissue found in teeth and bones. It is also needed to keep gum tissue intact. Inadequate vitamin C leads to bleeding and swollen gums, which increases the risk for tooth decay and tooth loss. Food sources of vitamin C include citrus fruits, strawberries, broccoli, cantaloupe, kiwi fruit, and green leafy vegetables.

Recommended dosages. The Recommended Dietary Allowance for adults is 75 to 90 mg a day; 100mg or more if you smoke. But that may not be enough. One study shows that 200 mg a day is necessary to reap the benefits of vitamin C throughout the body, which probably means a supplement is necessary to achieve that mark. Some experts are now recommending taking 200 to 500 mg of vitamin C daily, in addition to eating a diet rich in vitamin C.

Possible problems. Supplements over 1,000 mg a day can cause intestinal distress, including diarrhea and bloating. Large doses may also interfere with the action of anticoagulant medications such as Coumadin. If you're prone to kidney stones, the American Kidney Foundation advises limiting supplemental vitamin C to 60 mg a day, since too much boosts risk for kidney stones in some people. It also increases iron absorption, which can be a serious problem for people with a genetic tendency to store excessive iron.

Fluoride

How it works. Fluoride, a mineral, toughens tooth enamel, making it harder and more resistant to decay. Although fluoride's protective effect is greatest during the time of peak tooth formation—up to age eight—fluoride is effective for people of all ages.

Recommended dosages. The American Dental Association says fluoridated water is the most effective, cost-efficient way to get fluoride. Experts say one part per million of food or water is acceptable, providing about 2 mg a day. Bottled water does not typically contain the fluoride you need, however, and filtering water may remove some or all of its fluoride (check with the manufacturer). Cooking foods in fluoridated water can increase their fluoride content. Drinking tea provides fluoride, since black and green tea are rich sources of the mineral. Fluoride can also be absorbed from toothpastes and other dental products containing this mineral.

Possible problems. Consuming large doses of fluoride, about 20 mg a day, over long periods can result in toxicity and cause bone, kidney, muscle, and nerve problems. Children's teeth take on a mottled appearance when fluoride intake is too high. Drinking several cups of tea per day that is made with fluoridated water may mean getting too much fluoride.

■ NUTRITIONAL SUPPLEMENTS

Flavonoids

How they work. Flavonoids (also called bioflavonoids) act as antioxidants, protecting gums and other tissues from damage from free radicals. In addition, flavonoids strengthen the walls of the blood vessels that supply gum tissue with oxygen.

Recommended dosages. At least one study suggests that taking 300 mg a day of flavonoids plus the same amount of vitamin C will improve gum health in people with gingivitis. Foods rich in flavonoids include oranges, grapefruit, tangerines, apricots, blackberries, black currants, broccoli, cantaloupe, cherries, grapes, lemons, papayas, plums, and tomatoes. Tea, red wine, and nuts also boast flavonoids. Five servings of fruits and vegetables daily will probably provide sufficient flavonoids.

Possible problems. Probably none.

Coenzyme Q_{10}

How it works. Every cell in the body contains coenzyme Q_{10}, which acts in conjunction with several enzymes to provide the energy for healing and many other bodily processes. It is also an antioxidant. Supplemental coenzyme Q_{10} helps to reduce swelling in gingivitis and promote healing.

Recommended dosages. One study suggests that 50 mg per day of coenzyme Q_{10} for three weeks relieves gingivitis symptoms. Consume coenzyme Q_{10} with a small amount of fat—such as oil, margarine, or peanut butter—or with a meal to promote absorption.

Possible problems. Probably none.

Tea

How it works. Tea, particularly black tea, may reduce your chances for gum diseases. Several animal studies show that tea thwarts plaque production, and there's promising human data, too. In one study, subjects who rinsed with a black tea solution inhibited the production of amylase in their saliva. Amylase is an enzyme that breaks down the carbohydrate in starchy foods to a form that bacteria feed on. In reducing amylase, mouth germs are starved and fail to manufacture harmful toxins. Tea also contains fluoride, which fights tooth decay by bolstering tooth enamel, while helping strengthen the bone that secures teeth. Sipping tea also supplies vitamin K, which, along with an array of nutrients, is vital for bone strength, too.

Recommended dosages. No one knows how many cups of tea it takes to treat gum disease; many of the solutions used in the studies were highly concentrated tea extracts. Nevertheless, it can't hurt your gums to exchange coffee or sugary drinks for brewed tea, minus the sweeteners and milk products that feed mouth bacteria.

Possible problems. Tea contains caffeine; the longer you brew it, the more it has. If caffeine bothers you, try decaffeinated tea, which experts say provides similar health benefits. (See Green Tea, p. 312.)

■ BOTANICAL MEDICINES

Chamomile (*Matricaria chamomilla, M. recutita, Chamomilla recutita*)

How it works. Chamomile tea soothes irritated gums and may help prevent gum disease. It contains numerous components, including flavonoids, that have anti-inflammatory and antibacterial effects.

Recommended dosages. Brew for ten to fifteen minutes about 1 heaping tablespoon of dried chamomile flower heads and three-quarters cup boiling water. Pass through a tea strainer. Use this chamomile concoction as a mouthwash three or four times a day between meals or drink it after meals.

Possible problems. Chamomile is related to ragweed. Allergic reactions are possible, although rare.

Sage (*Salvia officinalis*)

How it works. Sage has anti-inflammatory properties that reduce swelling of gums and may prevent gum diseases. It also has antioxidant effects that may help prevent gum damage from free radicals.

Recommended dosages. To soothe irritated gum tissues, brew about 2 teaspoons of the herb in 8 ounces of boiling water. Use it as a mouthwash or drink as tea. Or use two to three drops of sage oil in about 5 ounces of water or 5 g of the alcohol extract in 8 ounces of water.

Possible problems. Sage contains thujones, which are toxic and can cause convulsions in high doses, so it should not be used as your daily tea of choice. It is safest as a mouthwash or gargle. Never ingest purified sage oil, which is only safe when cooked. Medicinal sage oil generally contains lower amounts of thujones but still should be used carefully and only for brief periods.

Bloodroot (*Sanguinaria canadensis*)

How it works. Bloodroot contains sanguinarine, a natural antibacterial substance that can prevent dental plaque from forming.

Recommended dosages. Many natural toothpastes and mouthwashes contain bloodroot. Look for brands that also contain fluoride for added tooth protection.

Possible problems. None when used as directed.

ULCERS

Peptic ulcers, as they are technically known, are open sores in the tissues that are most exposed to stomach acids and digestive juices. Ten percent of all Americans suffer from them, sometimes with serious consequences.

Ulcers of the duodenum, which is the first portion of the small intestine leaving the stomach, are much more common than those of the stomach (gastric ulcer) or esophagus. Normally, the stomach and the duodenum secrete mucus to protect their linings from the erosive effects of digestive substances. Also, under normal circumstances, the caustic excretions produced by the stomach during digestion is buffered by food; any unbuffered acid that makes it to the duodenum is swiftly neutralized by sodium bicarbonate produced by the pancreas. Ulcers occur when, for generally unknown reasons, the natural protections fail. Ulcers occur in the esophagus when acids back up from the stomach in gastroesophageal reflux disease (GERD) (see Heartburn, p. 123).

Stress and spicy foods were once considered the principal causes of ulcers. Although stress and irritants may contribute, the discovery that bacterial infection is the culprit in most ulcer disease has changed the detection, and treatment, of this condition. For the most part, ulcers are attributable to *Helicobacter pylori*, a germ that clings to the lining of the stomach and is the only bacterium that can live in its acid environment. *H. pylori* is responsible for more than 90 percent of duodenal ulcers and more than 80 percent of gastric ulcers.

Chronic consumption of aspirin, ibuprofen, and other nonsteroidal anti-inflammatory drugs (NSAIDs) greatly increase the likelihood of gastric ulcers, which are common in people who take these medications for chronic pain conditions such as arthritis. This type of ulcer will generally heal when the medication is stopped. In smokers, ulcers are less likely to heal, and more likely to cause death, than in nonsmokers. It is believed that smoking may increase the risk of *H. pylori* infection. Chronic stress, too, may lower the body's resistance.

Duodenal ulcers rarely become malignant, but gastric and esophageal

⊙ SYMPTOMS

Ulcers, which usually come and go, have a wide variety of symptoms. Even the symptoms that are considered "typical" may occur in only half or less of people diagnosed with a particular type.

Duodenal ulcer

- Gnawing or burning pain that is felt right below the breastbone.
- Stomach pain that recurs in the middle of the night or after a few hours of not eating (although usually not upon awakening).
- An uncomfortably "empty" feeling accompanying hunger.
- Stomach pain that is temporarily eased by eating or taking antacids.

Gastric ulcer

- A burning, aching, or gnawing pain that occurs after eating.
- Recurrent bloating, nausea, and vomiting after eating.

Esophageal ulcer

- Pain in the upper chest that occurs when swallowing or lying down.

⊙ IMPORTANT WARNING!

Any of the following symptoms indicate a potentially life-threatening situation that requires immediate medical attention.

- Unexplained black, dark, bloody stools.
- Vomiting blood.
- Sudden, intense abdominal pain.

ulcers sometimes do. All types of peptic ulcers have potentially dangerous consequences, however. One complication is perforation, when the ulcer goes completely through the stomach or duodenum, causing infection that can lead to shock and death. Bleeding can lead to anemia and can be life-threatening. Pyloric obstruction, a blocking of the stomach exit, can require a partial removal of the stomach in severe cases.

Diagnostic Steps

H. pylori infection is detected with a blood test or a breath test. Endoscopy can determine the presence of an ulcer as well as *H. pylori* infection via a flexible viewing tube inserted through the mouth into the stomach; a tiny piece of tissue from the stomach and duodenum can also be obtained and examined. Sometimes a GI series—X rays that are taken after the patient swallows an opaque substance (usually barium)—may be ordered to pinpoint the site and size of an ulcer.

Conventional Treatments

Numerous medications are available to treat ulcers; those most commonly used include these:

- *Over-the-counter solid or liquid antacids* neutralize stomach acid. They provide symptom relief and help the ulcers to heal.
- *H2 antagonists* lower the levels of two specific digestive enzymes and reduce stomach acid. Ranitidine (Zantac), cimetidine (Tagamet), nizatidine (Axid), famotidine (Pepcid AC) are some types that are available over the counter or in prescription strength.
- *Proton pump inhibitors*, including omeprazole (Prilosec) and iansoprazole (Prevacid) are potent prescription drugs that stop stomach acid secretion and can completely heal the ulcer. They are taken once or twice a day for two to eight weeks, or longer if needed.
- *Antibiotics* are prescribed when *H. pylori* is present. Often they are given in combination with proton pump inhibitors or antacids. Antibiotics are typically taken for at least two weeks.

Nutraceuticals for Ulcers

Note: The following approaches should not substitute for pharmaceutical treatment if *H. pylori* is found, but they may be used as complementary therapies.

◉ STRATEGIES FOR RELIEF

- If you have a history of stomach or duodenal ulcers and you haven't yet been tested for *H. pylori*, ask your doctor about it. Treating infections greatly reduces the chance of ever being dogged by ulcer pain again, and keeps at bay the more serious long-term complications.

- If you smoke, make every effort to stop. Smoking aggravates an ulcer and delays healing.

- Identify foods and drinks that trigger an attack and limit or eliminate them altogether. In most people, all sources of caffeine, coffee (even without caffeine), and alcohol, all of which increase stomach acidity, will worsen the condition. But spicy foods, including dishes containing hot pepper or ginger—may be tolerated or even helpful.

- Increase your intake of high-fiber foods, such as whole-grain breads and cereals. People who consume large amounts of dietary fiber appear to suffer fewer ulcers.

- Eat small, frequent meals rather than a few large ones that may be harder to digest.

- Avoid aspirin and other NSAIDs, such as ibuprofen and naproxen. If you must take an anti-inflammatory medication for arthritis or other painful condition, talk to your doctor about a COX-2 inhibitor (Celebrex or Vioxx); these drugs are also NSAIDs, but are not as likely to cause gastric irritation as the older medications.

- Consider cabbage juice, an old folk remedy, or glutamine supplements. Cabbage juice is high in the amino acid glutamine, which some naturopaths recommend because it benefits the cells that line the digestive tract. Bananas, too, may have anti-ulcer effects.

- Try to improve your stress-coping techniques. Ulcers are not caused by stress, as once believed; nonetheless, stress may make you more susceptible to the bacteria and may interfere with normal digestive processes. Ulcer attacks are often associated with stressful times of life.

■ VITAMINS AND MINERALS

Vitamin C

How it works. Japanese researchers have found that high doses of vitamin C in animals greatly inhibits *H. pylori* proliferation. Still other studies suggest that vitamin C, which is abundant in citrus foods, strawberries, potatoes, and other fruits and vegetables, may protect against *H. pylori*. Vitamin C also promotes iron absorption, which is important if chronic bleeding has caused anemia.

Recommended dosages. The current Recommended Dietary Allowance for vitamin C is 75 to 90 mg a day for adults, and at least 100 mg for smokers. One well-controlled, highly regarded vitamin C study suggests that 200 mg of vitamin C is required to fully saturate all parts of the body.

Possible problems. Large doses of vitamin C in pill form, upwards of 1,000 mg, can cause abdominal pain and diarrhea. For some people, vitamin C poses a threat of kidney stones and excessive iron buildup. It may also interfere with the effects of anticoagulants.

Iron

How it works. Ulcers can cause blood loss from the intestine that often goes undetected. Iron, a mineral found most abundantly in meat, poultry, seafood, fortified breads, grains, cereals, legumes, and dried apricots, is a constituent of hemoglobin, the pigment in red blood cells that carries oxygen to cells. Chronic blood loss can result in anemia.

Recommended dosages. Women past menopause and all men require 10 mg of iron a day. Premenopausal women need 15 mg daily, 30 mg when pregnant. If iron supplements are necessary, a doctor should determine the appropriate dosage. Remember, too, that vitamin C enhances absorption of iron; coffee and tea hamper it.

Possible problems. Iron pills are known for their constipating qualities and may also upset stomachs. Make sure you consume adequate fiber and water to keep your bowels running smoothly. People who suffer from a genetic disorder called iron overload syndrome (hemochromatosis) should avoid iron supplements altogether.

■ NUTRITIONAL SUPPLEMENTS

Acidophilus and bifidus

How they work. These are two beneficial bacteria, naturally present in the digestive system, that may help control the proliferation of *H. pylori*. Fermented dairy products such as buttermilk and yogurt contain these "good" bacteria, which are also available as supplements. According to a large study of Swedish adults, the greater the consumption of fermented dairy products, the lower the ulcer risk.

Recommended dosages. Include at least one cup a day of reduced-fat yogurt containing live, active acidophilus or bifidus cultures. Follow product labels when using supplements.

Possible problems. In large quantities, they may cause diarrhea or stomach upset.

■ BOTANICAL MEDICINES

Licorice (*Glycyrrhiza glabia*)

How it works. Prescribed in Germany for ulcers, licorice root helps heal ulcers by promoting the production of mucus to protect the lining of the stomach and duodenum. The deglycyrrhizinated (DGL) form, in which a substance called glycyrrhizin has been removed, should be used. Otherwise, the pure form of licorice can raise blood pressure to dangerous levels.

Recommended dosages. Chew DGL licorice wafers or tablets before meals and at bedtime. Recommendations range from 200 to 500 mg or more each time.

Possible problems. Probably none, if you take the DGL form. (See Licorice, p. 493.)

Aloe vera (*A. vera, A. barbadensis*)

How it works. Aloe Vera gel extract promotes healing and also contains astringent compounds that help prevent bleeding.

Recommended dosages. Studies in Germany and elsewhere have found that one-third to one-half cup of aloe vera gel extract taken three times a day (just before eating) eases symptoms. However, it may take two or three weeks to notice improvement.

Possible problems. Use only purified commercially prepared gel extract containing 98 percent aloe, with no aloin or aloe-emodin. Avoid the bitter aloe latex or juice which can cause severe diarrhea.

URINARY TRACT INFECTION

Infections of the urinary tract, also known as UTIs, affect the bladder or the kidneys of both men and women. If left untreated, they can cause permanent damage to the urinary tract.

UTIs are the most common bacterial infection in people of all ages.

◎ **SYMPTOMS**
- Frequent urination, sometimes repeatedly during the night.
- Sudden and severe urge to urinate.
- Pain or a burning sensation during urination.
- Smaller volume of urine than usual.
- Blood in the urine.
- Fever and achy feelings, especially in the back.

- If you have or are prone to UTIs, drink at least 8 to 10 glasses of water and other nonalcoholic fluids daily to help flush out infectious material (bacteria).
- Urinate whenever you feel the urge. Do not delay.
- Always wipe from front to back to avoid getting fecal material into the urethra.
- If you are a woman, urinate before and again after intercourse. This helps assure that any bacteria that have entered the urethra are flushed out with urine.
- Women who have frequent UTIs may be advised to avoid use of a diaphragm for contraception because of its association with increased risk.
- If you have diabetes, you are at greater risk of UTIs. Keeping your blood sugar levels in good control may reduce that risk.
- Try teas made from a combination of nettle, goldenseal, and echinacea. These common botanical medicines may bolster immunity and also increase the flow of urine.
- When taking antibiotics, consume 2 or 3 servings of yogurt made with live cultures or take two acidophilus pills that provide 1–2 billion live organisms daily. This helps prevent an overgrowth of yeast organisms due to a lack of friendly (normal) bacteria in the intestinal and urinary tracts.

They are usually caused by bacteria that enter the body through the urethra, the tube that connects the bladder to the exterior of the body. In adults, UTIs are about fifty times more common in women than men. Women are at such increased risk because the female's urethra is much shorter than the male's, and because it is located so near to the vagina and anus, where it comes in contact with infection-causing bacteria. Sexually active women are most at risk, since sexual contact may accidentally move local bacteria into the urethra.

When UTIs occur in men under fifty, they are usually due to some urologic abnormality. However, after the age of fifty, the incidence increases in men, likely due to prostate disease. Decreased urination may result in poor emptying of the bladder, which allows bacteria to grow. (See "Nutraceuticals Just for Men and Athletes.")

Most UTIs affect the bladder only, a condition commonly referred to as cystitis. The urethra (urethritis) may or may not be involved. If untreated, symptoms may persist or may last only a few days and then disappear. But the infection is not necessarily cured. Rather, bacteria may be doing permanent damage inside the body. Untreated infections may move up the urinary tract to the kidney, causing pyelonephritis—a serious renal infection.

Diagnostic Steps

Doctors will often make the diagnosis based on the symptoms and immediately prescribe treatment, usually a broad-spectrum antibiotic. However, to make the most accurate diagnosis, urine studies, including a laboratory culture, are usually needed. These tests not only confirm that an infection is present but they also identify the type of bacterium causing it, allowing the doctor to prescribe the most effective drug to eradicate it.

Conventional Treatments

A 10- to 14-day course of treatment with antibiotic drugs usually cures cystitis and urethritis. Typically, trimethoprim-sulfamethoxazole (Bactrim or Septra) or a fluoroquinolone—e.g., ciprofloxacin (Cipro), norfloxacin (Noroxin), or ofloxacin (Floxin)—is prescribed. If infection is severe, especially if it has been allowed to spread untreated, hospitalization for examinations to determine the cause and extent of the infection, as well as treatment with more potent antibiotics, may be necessary.

Nutraceuticals for UTIs

The following may be taken as complementary medicines when taking a prescription antibiotic to treat a UTI; they may also be taken to help prevent UTIs in susceptible people.

■ VITAMINS AND MINERALS

Vitamin C

How it works. Vitamin C helps acidify the urine, making the bladder less hospitable to bacteria. It also bolsters immunity, which aids in fighting off the infection.

Recommended dosages. Some alternative practitioners recommend very high dosages of 300 to 500 mg every hour or two until burning and other symptoms abate.

Possible complications. Very high doses of vitamin C can cause diarrhea; used long-term, they may also irritate the urinary tract. Such high doses may also cause significant abdominal pain and bloating.

■ BOTANICAL MEDICINES

Cranberry (*Vaccinium macrocarpon*)

How it works. A study reported in the *Journal of the American Medical Association* showed that certain compounds in cranberry juice, as well as blueberry juice, prevent bacteria from adhering to the bladder walls. Instead, they are washed out of the body in the urine. Both berries also contain arbutin, a chemical that has both antibiotic and diuretic properties that are useful in combating UTIs.

Recommended dosages. Recommend dosages range from 3 to 10 ounces of unsweetened, full-strength juice a day when used on a preventive basis, and 12 to 32 ounces a day (average of 16 ounces) during an active bladder infection.

Possible problem. Cranberries are very tart. Thus, some manufacturers load the juice up with sugar, which can be a problem in terms of calories and for people with diabetes. You can make full-strength juice more palatable by mixing it with apple or, even better, blueberry juice, which are naturally sweet. Another option is cranberry tea. Bring a cup of water to a boil and add 2 tablespoons of dried cranberries, reduce the heat to low, and let simmer for 10 minutes. Strain the cranberries (you can eat them as a fruit) and drink two or three cups of the tea a day. Still another alternative is to take 400 mg of cranberry pills two or three times a day.

Uva ursi (*Arctostaphylos uva ursi*)

How it works. This berry also contains arbutin, giving it antibacterial properties that have been documented in German research.

Recommended dosages. The typical recommended dosage to treat bladder infections calls for 500 mg (or ½ teaspoon of tincture) taken up to four times a day for a week.

Possible problems. Overdosage can lead to inflammation and irritation of the bladder. Drink along with citrus fruit juices to make the urine more alkaline. Or you can add a small amount of baking soda (about 2 teaspoons) to foods during the course of the day. Uva ursi needs an alkaline environment to work. Products containing uva ursi may turn urine green. It should not be used during pregnancy and lactation, and is contraindicated in anyone with kidney disease.

VARICOSE VEINS

Varicose veins are blood vessels in which the tiny one-way valves fail to keep blood flowing in one direction (toward the heart). When a series of valves degenerates, blood collects (pools) at the site, resulting in bulges that give varicose veins their characteristic appearance. They most commonly occur in leg veins that are close to the skin's surface; those that develop in the anus are called hemorrhoids.

Most varicose veins are more of a cosmetic than a medical problem. However, when varicosities develop in deeper, hidden veins of the leg they can become inflamed and result in phlebitis. Varicosities of all kinds are increasingly common with age because of weakening of vessel walls and supporting muscles. In fact, about half of all middle-aged adults have some degree of varicosity. They also often arise in women during pregnancy. Some people, especially those who abuse alcohol, develop esophageal varicosities, which can lead to severe bleeding.

Varicosities tend to run in families. Women are four times as likely as men to develop varicose veins. They are also more common in obese people. Many doctors believe that an underlying incompetence in the valves or weakness in the walls of the veins starts the process going. Contrary to popular belief, they are not more common among people who must stand on their feet for hours on end, such as dentists, barbers, or salespeople. But having a job that requires a lot of standing can exacerbate the condition among people who are predisposed to develop varicose veins. People who have hypertension also may be at greater risk because the higher pressure can strain the valves. The hormonal changes of pregnancy or menstruation may cause symptoms to worsen. Also, the pressure applied to the pelvic veins during late pregnancy may produce varicosities; these often disappear after childbirth.

Although varicose veins usually require no medical treatment, they may increase the risk of infection and hard-to-heal leg ulcers. These can

⊙ SYMPTOMS
- Knotlike, twisting blue bulges on the legs, just below the skin's surface.
- Achiness, fatigue, or a feeling of heat in the legs that eases when they are raised.
- Tenderness or soreness along the veins.
- Feelings of heaviness or dull stabbing pain deeper in the legs.
- Leg cramps at night.
- Itching around the ankles.

be especially serious among people with diabetes or other conditions that interfere with circulation.

Diagnostic Steps

When varicose veins are visually obvious, no special testing is necessary. If they can't be seen but are suspected, your doctor may wrap a band around the leg to prompt the varicosities to become prominent. The doctor also may need to rule out other possible causes of the symptoms. In some cases, special X rays may be needed to determine the severity and locations of weak valves in the veins.

Conventional Treatments

Therapy is primarily designed to relieve symptoms and prevent complications. However, some people seek treatment simply to improve their appearance. The choice of treatment may depend on the severity and location of the problem veins.

• *Sclerotherapy* is injection therapy. With the leg elevated so that the veins are as empty of blood as possible, a solution (usually saline) is injected into the vein to irritate its lining. Then a padding is placed over the area to compress the veins. The padding remains in place for about three weeks, although activity can resume almost immediately.

• *Phlebectomy* is a surgical stripping of the veins, which can usually be done on an outpatient basis. The surgeon makes small incisions in the skin at the upper and lower ends of the distorted vessel. The vein is severed and the problem segment is then pulled out through the opening.

• *Laser therapy* uses intense light beams to destroy the varicosities. Several sessions may be needed, and this approach works best on small varicosities, or spider veins.

• One of the newest treatments, called *closure*, uses high-frequency radio waves. It is an outpatient procedure, lasting about forty-five minutes, in which the physician inserts a catheter into the vein. Inside the catheter are electrodes that send radio-frequency energy to heat and collapse the vein.

Nutraceuticals for Varicose Veins

▦ BOTANICAL MEDICINES

A product called Varicosin contains standardized herbal extracts of the following three herbs that support proper circulation and healthy leg veins.

◉ STRATEGIES FOR RELIEF

Your lifestyle can have a pivotal impact on your comfort and may help prevent worsening of the condition.

• Avoid standing for long periods of time. If your job requires you to do so, take breaks to sit down and elevate your legs. Ideally, legs should be raised above the level of your chest.

• Avoid sitting for long periods, whether at a desk or on a plane or train. Get up and stretch your legs at regular intervals.

• Get regular exercise to help enhance your blood circulation.

• You may need to wear compression hosiery, most commonly recommended for small varicose veins that cause only mild symptoms. These may range from lightweight support stockings to heavier prescription elastic hose.

• If you become pregnant, discuss the use of support stockings with your doctor. Preventive support may be helpful.

• Never wrap your legs in elastic bandages. You run the risk of wrapping them too tightly and interfering with circulation, or even making the varicose veins worse. Even if done properly, such bandages quickly loosen and become useless.

• Do not wear round garters, elastic girdles, or other undergarments that can impair circulation.

• Make sure your diet is high in fiber. A low-fiber diet obliges you to strain during bowel movements, which increases abdominal pressure and obstructs the blood flow up from the legs. A daily supplement of ground psyllium seeds (p. 338) may be necessary to help keep the stool soft.

Horse chestnut (*Aesculus hippocastanum*)

How it works. A study published in the British medical journal the *Lancet* reported that horse chestnut seed extract can be as effective as support hose in relieving varicose vein symptoms. The extract may strengthen the blood vessels by decreasing the size and number of the pores in the capillary walls. The active ingredient in horse chestnut seed seems to be aescin, which also helps improve the tone of the veins.

Recommended dosages. Studies have used extracts standardized to provide 50 mg of aescin.

Possible problem. Side effects are not common, although gastrointestinal upset can occur. Do not take higher than recommended doses for extended periods. Never eat the horse chestnut seeds that fall from trees—they're poisonous and require processing before they can be ingested.

Butcher's broom (*Ruscus aculeatus L.*)

How it works. This extract is standardized for its content of saponins, especially ruscogenin, which appear to have anti-inflammatory and vasoconstrictor effects. Researchers are exploring the impact of ruscogenins on the tone of the venous wall.

Recommended dosages. A dosage of 100 to 150 mg three times a day, of an extract standardized to contain 9 to 11 percent of ruscogenin, is recommended.

Possible problems. Stomach upset, nausea, or a rise in blood pressure occurs in rare cases.

Gotu kola (*Centella asiatica*)

How it works. Gotu kola is traditionally used for the skin and connective tissue. Its clinical benefits for varicose veins seem related to its ability to enhance connective tissue structure and improve blood flow, and to improve the structural integrity of the veins.

Recommended dosages. Studies have used 60 to 120 mg of TECA (titrated extract of *Centella asiatica*), although 200 mg of the standardized extract has also been suggested.

Possible problems. Do not take it if you are also taking drugs to lower cholesterol or oral diabetes medications.

WEIGHT PROBLEMS

Obesity has emerged as the number-one public health problem in the United States, affecting one out of three—or about 58 million—adults. In addition, about one in five American children and adolescents are overweight. Obesity greatly increases the risk of premature death, and it is a major risk factor for developing diabetes, heart disease, high blood pressure, gallbladder disease, arthritis, lung problems, and some of our most common forms of cancer. According to government statistics, obesity and inactivity account for about three hundred thousand premature deaths in the United States each year. The treatment of obesity-related diseases totals more than $40 billion a year; in addition, Americans spend more than $33 billion a year on weight-reduction products and programs.

On the surface, weight control should be a relatively simple matter of eating less and exercising more. But as anyone who has tried to lose excess weight and then keep it off knows, weight control is not so simple. Indeed, doctors know obesity is a complex disorder involving many factors—genetics, age, diet, level of activity, ethnic background, environmental and psychological factors, and perhaps hormonal disorders such as thyroid disease or Cushing's syndrome. Although often difficult, achieving and maintaining a healthful weight is possible, and certainly worth the effort.

Diagnostic Steps

Doctors define obesity as carrying too much body fat—typically 25 percent body fat or more in men and 30 percent or more in women. However, a person can be overweight without being obese; for example, bodybuilders, professional football players, and others who are very muscular and have large bones may be technically overweight without being overly fat. These people will look firm and trim, without the rolls of fat and "beer belly" that are the hallmarks of being overweight and obese.

Degree of obesity is determined by a formula called the body mass index (BMI). This can be determined by dividing your weight in kilograms (your weight in pounds divided by 2.2) by your height in meters squared (your height in inches divided by 39.37 and then squared). Or you can use this formula:

1. Weigh yourself first thing in the morning, naked. Multiply your weight in pounds by 704.5. (For example, if you weigh 150 pounds, your result would be 105,675.)
2. Determine your height, convert it to inches, and square the result. (For example, if you are 5 foot 4 inches, you would multiply 64 by 64, getting 4,096.)

◉ **SYMPTOMS**
- Fat, flabby appearance when inspecting the unclothed body in a full-length mirror.
- Clothes become too tight.
- Development of various obesity-related diseases, including type 2 (adult-onset) diabetes, high blood pressure, osteoarthritis, heart disease, gallbladder disease, among others.

Adopting a more healthful lifestyle is perhaps the most important factor in losing excess pounds and then maintaining ideal weight. There are dozens of effective weight-loss programs; most advise the following:

- Reduce your intake of fatty foods, especially those that are rich in animal (saturated) fats, such as fatty meat, cheese, whole milk and whole-fat milk products, and commercial pastries and baked goods. Avoid fast foods.
- Increase your intake of vegetables, whole-grain products, and other high-fiber foods. Fiber helps prevent overeating by promoting a feeling of fullness.
- Start the day with a good breakfast; studies have found that skipping meals early in the day is likely to result in excessive hunger and overeating later in the day.
- Pay attention to hunger and learn to use snacking to prevent overeating. A small, high-fiber snack at midmorning and again at mid-afternoon can curb your appetite and prevent overeating at lunch and dinner.
- Eat smaller portions.
- Drink at least eight to ten glasses of water and other noncaloric fluids a day. Avoid drinking lots of sweetened fruit juice and sugary soft drinks, which add calories and virtually no nutrition to the diet.
- Abstain from alcohol or restrict intake to no more than one drink a day. Alcohol contains 6 calories per gram, compared to 4 calories per gram of carbohydrate or protein.
- Exercise at least thirty minutes a day. A brisk walk before dinner not only burns extra calories, but also helps curb your appetite and prevent overeating.
- Undertake a weight-lifting or strength-building program. Muscles burn more calories than fat tissue, and even a modest gain in muscle mass makes you look trimmer.
- Above all, avoid fad diets. These typically limit food choices (e.g., the egg and grapefruit diet) and if followed, they do achieve weight loss. But they fail to address the real problem—unhealthy eating and exercise habits. Any pounds that are lost are likely to be quickly regained when you resume your normal diet and lifestyle.

3. Divide the results of step 1 (105,675) by the results of step 2 (4,096). The result, 25.8, would be your BMI.

If your BMI is between 19 and 24.9, you're within a healthy weight range; a BMI of 25 to to 26 is overweight; mild obesity starts at about 27; and severe obesity is defined as a BMI of 30 or above.

Conventional Treatments

Most people can achieve and maintain a healthy weight by reducing calories and increasing exercise, but only a lifelong commitment to healthy eating and exercise habits keeps excess weight off for good. Some people find that commercial weight-control programs give the needed motivation. A doctor or a registered dietitian can help develop a personalized diet and exercise program. There are also numerous self-help books and weight-loss programs ranging from the fad of the moment—which don't work long term and should be avoided—to truly helpful advice on adopting a lifelong healthful eating and exercise program.

People whose obesity poses a major health problem may enroll in medically supervised weight-loss programs that are typically high in protein and very low in calories. Prescription medications may be an option, but they often have a high risk of side effects and are most successful when used in conjunction with adopting a more healthful lifestyle. Otherwise, the lost weight is likely to be regained once the drugs or special diets are stopped. The most extreme treatment involves surgery in which the stomach capacity is reduced to limit food intake. Even this approach will not work unless a low-calorie diet is maintained.

Nutraceuticals for Weight Problems

There are no magic potions that achieve and maintain weight loss, but there are nutraceutical products that can help.

■ VITAMINS AND MINERALS

Chromium

How it works. Chromium is a trace mineral that, among other functions, helps the body use insulin, a hormone essential for the body to metabolize glucose, its major fuel. High insulin levels have been implicated in obesity, so, theoretically, chromium supplements may help control levels of insulin. Chromium is also instrumental in fat metabolism, so is often touted as a fat-burning mineral. Although it may aid in weight control, it is not a magic substance that will burn off stored fat. But chromium supplements may be helpful when taken as part of a sensible weight-loss program that emphasizes a low-calorie, fat-restricted diet and an increase in physical activity.

Recommended dosages. There is no Recommended Dietary Allowance for chromium, although dosages of 50 to 200 mcg are generally considered adequate and safe. Weight-loss plans that utilize chromium generally call for 200 mcg taken two or three times a day.

Possible problems. Very high doses of chromium may hinder the body's ability to absorb iron and zinc. Persons with diabetes who take insulin should check with their doctors before taking chromium.

■ NUTRITIONAL SUPPLEMENTS

Carnitine

How it works. Carnitine is a proteinlike substance that helps the muscles burn fats for energy. The liver makes carnitine from two amino acids (methionine and lysine), and it is stored in the skeletal and heart muscles. Without adequate carnitine, the muscles are unable to utilize fatty acids as a source of energy; studies also indicate that carnitine increases exercise endurance. These functions may foster weight loss when carnitine is used along with a reduced-calorie, low-fat diet and regimen of increased exercise.

Recommended dosages. The typical dosage calls for 1 to 2 g a day.

Possible problems. Some forms of carnitine can cause nausea and vomiting when it is taken on an empty stomach. This can be avoided by taking it with meals. If you have diabetes, heart disease, kidney failure, or any serious or progressive disease, check with your doctor before taking carnitine or ALC.

Psyllium

How it works. Psyllium is a form of soluble fiber that absorbs large amounts of water in the intestinal tract. It promotes weight loss by promoting a feeling of fullness and helping prevent overeating. Psyllium is commonly used to treat constipation; it has also been shown to lower blood cholesterol, a common problem among overweight people. A study involving obese women also found that it may lower the risk of gallstones.

Recommended dosages. Psyllium is available in capsule and wafer forms, but it is usually taken as a powder: 1 to 3 tablespoonfuls are dissolved in a full 8-ounce glass of water, juice, or milk. The mixture must be consumed quickly before it forms a thick gel. (Note: Oat bran, another popular soluble fiber, can be used as an alternative to psyllium.)

Possible problems. Large amounts of psyllium—or any dietary fiber—can cause gas and bloating, especially when it is first added to the diet. To avoid this, start with a small dosage of 1 teaspoon of ground psyllium husks and gradually work up to the recommended dosage. Be sure to drink at least eight to ten glasses of water or other nonalcoholic fluid a day to achieve the desired results and also to avoid possible intestinal obstruction.

5-HTP

How it works. This derivative of the amino acid tryptophan is thought to raise levels of serotonin, a brain chemical (neurotransmitter) that is instrumental in mood, sleep, and numerous other functions. It is not fully understood how 5-HTP may aid in weight reduction, but it may be helpful in controlling appetite. A study involving twenty markedly overweight women found that those who received the 5-HTP lost an average of twelve pounds in twelve weeks, compared with two pounds for women in the placebo group. The women who got the 5-HTP did not experience uncomfortable hunger, even when they were on a low-calorie diet. But even when they could eat as much as they wanted, they consumed fewer calories and lost more weight than women in the control group.

Recommended dosages. The usual dosage is 50 to 100 mg taken three times a day, about thirty minutes before meals.

Possible problems. 5-HTP can cause constipation, gasiness, nausea, and drowsiness. These side effects can be minimized by starting with a low dose and gradually increasing it to the recommended level.

Glucomannan

How it works. Glucomannan is a high-fiber powder made from the tubers of *Amorphophallus konjac,* an Asian plant that is grown mostly in Japan. It absorbs up to two-hundred times its weight in water, so even a small amount swells in the stomach and curbs hunger by promoting a feeling of fullness. It also helps prevent constipation, a problem sometimes encountered by people following a low-calorie weight-loss diet.

Recommended dosages. Glucomannan is sold in capsule form; the typical dosage calls for taking one or two 500-mg capsules with a full glass of water about an hour before a meal.

Possible problems. Like other high-fiber supplements, glucomannan can cause bloating, gas, and intestinal discomfort. Start with a low dose and be sure to take it with plenty of water. Don't combine glucomannan with other fiber supplements, such as psyllium; overloading the body with soluble fiber can result in intestinal obstruction.

▪ BOTANICAL MEDICINES

Gugulipid (*Commiphora mukul*)

How it works. Gugulipid, a gummy resin from the mukul myrrh tree of India, contains substances called guggulsterones that appear to increase fat metabolism and stimulate the liver to break down LDL cholesterol, the harmful type that increases the risk of atherosclerosis and heart disease. Studies in India, where gugulipid is a traditional treatment for obesity and atherosclerosis, have found that the substance not only promotes weight loss, but also seems to be most effective in reducing abdominal fat—the type that is the most metabolically active and instrumental in raising blood cholesterol and increasing the risk of atherosclerosis. Some researchers theorize that gugulipid promotes weight loss by stimulating production of thyroid hormones, which in turn speed up metabolism.

Recommended dosages. The usual dosage is 25 mg taken three times a day.

Possible problems. Standardized gugulipid supplements are generally safe, but there have been reports of nausea and other intestinal upsets. The crude gum can cause diarrhea, stomachache, and other intestinal problems, and should be avoided. (See Guggul, p. 476.)

Ephedra (*E. sinica, E. intermedia, E. equisetina*)

How it works. Also known as ma huang, ephedra comes from a shrub that grows in the arid areas of Asia. The Chinese have used it for centuries to treat asthma and bronchitis; it is also a common ingredient in many herbal weight-loss formulas. Its active ingredients—ephedrine and pseudoephedrine—are powerful stimulants, similar to amphetamines and adrenaline, that speed up metabolism. Some weight-loss products combine ephedra and St. John's wort, and are promoted as natural or herbal fenphen, an alternative to the prescription weight-loss drugs that were removed from the market after reports of cardiovascular side effects.

Recommended dosages. The usual weight-loss dosage starts with 6 mg of ephedrine, or about 100 mg of ephedra. The daily dosage should not exceed 8 mg of ephedrine a day. Be sure to check the labels of nonprescription cold and cough medications; these often contain ephedrine or pseudophedrine and can result in an overdose when taken along with an ephedra product.

Possible problems. Check with your doctor before taking any product that contains ephedra, especially if you have heart disease or another chronic disease. Ephedra can cause a dangerous rise in blood pressure and an irregular heartbeat; it can also raise blood sugar (glucose) levels. Thus, it should not be used by anyone with high blood pressure, heart disease, diabetes, or glaucoma. It can cause difficult or painful urination, similar to that of some cold medications, so it should not be used by men with an enlarged prostate or anyone with a urinary tract disorder. Even low dosages can cause nervousness, insomnia, an irregular heartbeat, dizziness, muscle cramps, headache, and other side effects. If it causes a racing pulse, stop taking the ephedra. Do not use a product that combines caffeine with ephedra. The FDA has received more than 800 case reports of adverse effects (possible fatal heart attack or stroke) with ephedra use.

PART 3

The Top 200-Plus Nutraceuticals

Vitamins

Vitamins and minerals are substances that the body needs—usually in very small amounts—to carry out essential body functions and prevent various deficiency diseases. To date, researchers have identified fourteen essential vitamins and fifteen minerals, as well as a number of vitaminlike substances, such as bioflavonoids and coenzyme Q_{10}. But vitamins and minerals are only the beginning—our foods contain thousands of chemical compounds that our bodies use in various ways to promote good health.

Although ancient healers recognized that certain foods could cure or prevent diseases, it wasn't until the emergence of the biological sciences in the early 1900s that researchers realized that specific, unidentified compounds within foods were critical. This became apparent from laboratory studies in which animals were fed purified diets that provided a single nutrient, such as albumin (a protein) or a starch. The animals consumed adequate calories, but they failed to grow normally, developed strange diseases, and often died. In 1912, Casimir Funk, a Polish biochemist working in London, put forth his theory that beriberi, scurvy, and other deficiency diseases developed when the diet lacked certain "vital amines," which he called "vitamines." They were later renamed "vitamins" after it was learned that the substances were not amines, which contain nitrogen. Instead, most were organic substances that functioned as coenzymes, working in concert with the body's enzymes to carry out the chemical reactions behind all bodily processes.

Vitamin A was the first to be chemically isolated, in 1913, by researchers working independently in Connecticut and Wisconsin. Since then twelve other vitamins have been identified and synthesized. (Many lists of vitamins also include choline—classified as one of the B vitamins—which was actually discovered before vitamin A.)

Discoveries involving the nutritional roles of minerals—chemical elements that are not produced by either plants or animals—paralleled those of vitamins. In the early 1800s, a Swedish chemist named Berzelius analyzed the calcium and phosphorus content of bone; several decades later he identified iron as the substance in hemoglobin that was instrumental in carrying oxygen in the body.

As we enter a new millennium, nutrition research continues to add to our understanding of just how important these nutrients are in maintaining health. Even more exciting are a growing number of reports that certain vitamins and minerals—when taken in optimal doses—may prevent heart attacks, cancer, and other killer diseases. Of course, there is another side of the coin—the indiscriminate use of high-dose vitamins and minerals can, like pharmaceutical agents, produce adverse side effects. As stressed throughout this book, a knowledgeable, commonsense approach is essential to reap the benefits of these and other nutraceuticals while minimizing any risk.

The Issue of Quantities

Vitamins and minerals are referred to as micronutrients because they are needed in very small amounts, especially when compared to the macronutrients—carbohydrates, fats, and protein. The Food and Nutrition Board of the National Research Council has established Recommended Dietary Allowances (RDAs) for thirteen vitamins and the major minerals. Nutrition labels on foods are based on Reference Daily Intakes (RDIs), which refer to average needs over a period of time. Although there are some minor differences, the RDAs and RDIs are pretty much the same. The amounts are calculated at levels higher than what is required to prevent deficiency diseases, and are based on the needs of average, healthy people. They do not take into account individual needs, which may vary according to genetic differences, lifestyle, and environmental factors.

The Role of Supplements

For years, we've been told that we can get all the vitamins and minerals we need by eating a varied diet built around ample fruits, vegetables, and whole-grain foods. There is no question that foods are our best sources of vitamins and minerals, largely because they come packaged with many other compounds that play important roles in nutrition and total health. But vitamin and mineral content varies greatly according to where the foods are grown, when they are harvested, and how they are stored or processed.

In addition, many experts question whether the typical American diet—high in meat, fat, sugar, and refined grains and low in fruits, vegetables, and whole grains—really meets the nutritional needs for many if not most people. For example, nutritionists acknowledge that many Americans—especially teenage girls and weight-conscious young women—do not consume enough calcium-rich foods to help ensure against osteoporosis. People who consume excessive alcohol and/or drink a lot of coffee and tea may develop thiamin deficiency. Shut-ins and people living in the northern lattitudes do not get enough sun during much of the year to make the vitamin D needed to utilize calcium. These are but a few of the reasons that many health care practitioners advise taking a multiple vitamin and mineral supplement. These typically provide 100 percent or more of the RDAs for most micronutrients.

Now, a growing number of experts are questioning whether this advice really meets the needs of most people. Just as it's impossible to buy one-size-fits-all shoes, is it really possible to design a supplement that provides optimal vitamins and minerals for everyone? Not likely, especially in light of the new studies showing that high doses of certain nutrients help prevent many diseases.

This section describes the essential vitamins and minerals, outlines their therapeutic uses and dosages, and highlights special cautions regarding dosages and other factors. The following chapters deal with other nutritional supplements and botanical or herbal medicines.

VITAMIN A

Vitamin A is one of the fat-soluble vitamins stored in the liver. Its widely varied functions include supporting vision, growth and development, and the immune system; building and maintaining healthy skin, mucous membranes, organ linings, bones, and teeth; protecting against certain cancers; and carrying out important metabolic and perhaps hormonal roles.

The term "vitamin A" is somewhat misleading because it implies that the nutrient is a single entity. Actually, there are two major forms of vitamin A: preformed or active vitamin A, referred to as retinols, and precursor forms, most notably beta-carotene. Preformed vitamin A, which comes from animal products, is made when an animal converts beta-carotene and other plant precursors into vitamin A and, depending upon the species, stores it in the liver and other organ meats, egg yolks, milk fat, and fatty tissue or oils. The precursor forms come from plants and are commonly referred to as carotenoids, so named because carrots are a major source of beta-carotene. Our bodies also convert the precursor forms into active vitamin A, so that even strict vegetarians can meet their needs from a diet that includes ample yellow, orange, and dark green vegetables and fruits. (Beta-carotene is also an important antioxidant; see p. 270 for details.)

◉ REQUIREMENTS

The Recommended Dietary Allowance for vitamin A is set at:

375 RE for infants under 12 months
400 RE for children 1 to 3 years
500 RE for children 4 to 6
700 RE for children 7 to 10
1,000 RE for males 11 and older
800 RE for females 11 and older

Note: The RDAs are stated in REs, or retinal equivalents. Many supplement manufacturers, however, continue to use the older designation of IUs, or international units. One RE is equal to 3.33 IU of active vitamin A (from animal sources) or 10 IU from beta-carotene (plant) sources.

- Night blindness or difficulty adjusting to dim light.
- Dry eyes.
- Stunted growth in children.
- Rough, dry, and scaly skin.
- Pitted teeth that are prone to decay.
- Reproduction problems, including difficulty conceiving, abnormal fetal growth, and, in severe cases, fetal death.
- Increased vulnerability to colds, sinusitis, skin abscesses, and other infections.

◉ SIGNS OF OVERDOSE

Prolonged high doses of vitamin A can be fatal; symptoms of toxicity include:

- Loss of appetite.
- Abdominal pain, nausea.
- Headaches, irritability, fatigue.
- Dry, scaly skin and loss of hair.
- Bone and joint pain; and easy fractures; muscle aches.
- Jaundice (yellowing of skin) and severe itchiness due to liver damage.
- Birth defects if large amounts are taken just before or during pregnancy.

◉ SUPPLEMENT FORMS

Vitamin A supplements are available as tablets, capsules, pills, and softgel capsules; cod-liver and other fish oils are also used to boost vitamin A intake.

◉ BEST SOURCES

Vitamin A
Liver and other organ meats
Full-fat milk and cheese
Butter and fortified margarine and low-fat milk
Egg yolks

Beta-carotene (see also p. 270)
Deep green, yellow, or orange vegetables and fruits

The many important functions of vitamin A include the following:

Vision. The retina—a light-sensitive lining at the back of the eye—contains two kinds of light-receptor cells: the rods, which are responsible for vision in dim light, and the cones, which distinguish colors and function in bright light. Both types of cells contain pigments derived from retinol (the active vitamin A), but the rods are especially dependent upon its pigment, called rhodopsin. Even a relatively minor vitamin A deficiency results in poor night vision, which typically starts as a slow adaptation when going from a brightly lit room to one that is dark and can progress to total night blindness.

Another manifestation of vitamin A deficiency includes xerophthalmia, a condition in which the covering (conjunctiva) of the eyes dries out and the cornea becomes red and ulcerated. Although rare in Western developed countries, xerophthalmia is one of the most common causes of childhood blindness in those developing countries in which vitamin A deficiency is common.

Growth and development. All cells require a certain amount of vitamin A to grow and develop properly. Laboratory animals fed a diet lacking vitamin A lose their appetites and stop growing, perhaps because they lose their sense of taste. When vitamin A is restored to their diets, the animals resume eating and grow normally.

Vitamin A is also essential for the normal growth and development of bone tissue, teeth, and epithelial cells, the tissue that makes up the skin and the mucous membranes. Without adequate vitamin A, skin cells harden and are shed prematurely. Similarly, the membranes lining the nose, airways, and internal organs may also become hard and dry. Bones become soft and stunted, and tooth enamel fails to form normally, resulting in pitted teeth that are especially vulnerable to decay.

Immunity. Numerous studies show that vitamin A deficiency results in increased vulnerability to infections, but scientists do not fully understand the vitamin's role in immune function. It appears to have a direct effect on the immune system; some researchers also theorize that a deficiency weakens the mucous membranes and allows invading organisms easier access to the body.

Protection against cancer. A number of studies suggest that vitamin A and its carotene precursor protect against certain cancers, especially those arising in the epithelial tissue (the skin and linings of the mouth, airways, intestines, and hollow internal organs). This protective effect may be due to the role vitamin A plays in building and maintaining healthy epithelial tissue; it may also be related to its strengthening of the immune system. Some studies also show that vitamin A may increase the effectiveness of cancer chemotherapy.

Metabolic and hormonal functions. Vitamin A appears to act as a coenzyme in the synthesis of certain nutrients, such as glycoprotein and glycogen. It may also play a role in proper function of the thyroid gland.

Therapeutic Uses and Dosages

Recent studies indicate that vitamin A dosages in excess of the RDAs may be helpful in the following situations:

Diabetes. Several studies indicate that vitamin A in doses up to 25,000 IU a day (7,575 RE) may improve the body's ability to utilize insulin and normalize blood sugar (glucose) levels.

Chronic bronchitis and asthma. In one study, patients with chronic lung disorders who were given vitamin A doses of 5,000 IU (1,5515 RE) a day showed significant improvement of symptoms when compared to those given a placebo.

Acne. Two acne medications—Accutane and Retin-A—are derived from retinols, but these drugs are chemically different from the active forms of vitamin A. There is no scientific evidence that taking large doses of vitamin A can cure acne, despite reports to the contrary in the popular media. In fact, adolescents who take high doses of vitamin A in hopes of clearing up their acne are likely to end up disappointed, and may risk serious toxicity in the process.

Special Cautions

About 90 percent of vitamin A is stored in the liver; small amounts are also found in the retina, kidneys, and fatty tissue. Overdoses of vitamin A can cause serious liver damage. In general, healthy adults should not consume more than 10,000 IU (3,335 RE) a day from all sources; pregnant women should not exceed a daily dosage of 8,000 IU (2,400 RE). Toxicity can occur with prolonged daily intakes of 50,000 IU, or about 15,000 RE of active vitamin A. Toxicity has been reported in children who consume 20,000 to 60,000 IU (5,700 to 17,100 RE) a day for one to three months; in fact, children should never be given vitamin A supplements unless they are specifically prescribed by a doctor.

Toxicity is almost always due to taking high-dose vitamin A supplements. It is almost impossible to overdose on vitamin A from dietary sources alone; exceptions might include young children who are fed large amounts of liver. In contrast, high doses of beta-carotene do not cause vitamin A toxicity because the body converts only a relatively small amount to the active form. However, prolonged high doses of beta-carotene or very high intake of carrots, tomatoes, and other foods high in carotenoids cause a harmless yellowing of the skin (especially the palms and soles) due to storage of the yellow pigments in the underlying fat.

Preparation and Handling

Varying amounts of vitamin A and its precursors are lost during storage and preparation. Both are rapidly destroyed by exposure to ultraviolet light and rancid fats. Allowing leafy vegetables to wilt quickly destroys carotene; to prevent this, store them in a refrigerator crisper and use as soon as possible after harvesting. Cooking or canning decreases the content of vitamin A precursors by 15 to 35 percent; air-drying results in even greater losses. In contrast, the nutrients are preserved during freezing and freeze-drying.

VITAMIN C (ASCORBIC ACID)

Vitamin C, or ascorbic acid, is perhaps the most familiar and versatile of the water-soluble vitamins. It is a powerful antioxidant, important in preventing the cellular damage that occurs when the body burns oxygen. It helps maintain blood vessels and is involved in hundreds of essential body processes, including the growth and repair of cells, immune function, and the production of connective tissue, certain hormones, blood cells, and other body tissues and chemicals.

Vitamin C deficiency results in scurvy, a potentially fatal disease that starts with easy bruising, bleeding gums, and poor healing; if untreated, it can lead to malformed bones, severe hemorrhaging, and heart failure. Scurvy is now uncommon, but it was a major killer until the eighteenth century, when researchers discovered that the disease could be prevented by eating certain foods, especially citrus fruits.

All animal life requires vitamin C, but most species can synthesize it from glucose and other sugars. Exceptions, which include humans, monkeys, guinea pigs, fruit-eating bats, and a few bird species, must include it in their diets. At least a minimal amount should be consumed almost daily because only relatively small amounts are stored in the body. The vitamin is soluble in water and excessive amounts are excreted in the urine. In addition, vitamin C is highly unstable and it deteriorates rapidly during storage and food preparation.

Why It's Needed

Metabolism. Vitamin C plays key roles in the metabolism of fats, cholesterol, and certain proteins, especially tyrosine, which is needed to make adrenaline and the neurotransmitter dopamine, and tryptophan, which is needed to make serotonin, another neurotransmitter. Vitamin C is also necessary to metabolize folic acid and it increases the absorption of iron.

Making connective tissue. Vitamin C is essential in the formation of collagen, a protein that binds body cells together. Collagen, the most

◉ REQUIREMENTS
30 mg for infants under 6 months
35 mg for infants 6 to 12 months
40 mg for children 1 to 3 years
45 mg for children 4 to 10
50 mg for children 11 to 14
90 mg for males 15 and older*
75 mg for females 15 and older*
95 mg during pregnancy and breast-feeding*

*These RDAs were increased in 2000 by a special National Academy of Sciences panel.

◉ SUPPLEMENT FORMS
Vitamin C is available in tablet, capsule, powder, and liquid forms.

◉ SIGNS OF DEFICIENCY
Early symptoms of latent scurvy include sore, bleeding gums; easy bruising; slow wound healing; and small hemorrhages under the skin. There may also be listlessness, fatigue, loss of weight, joint and muscle pains, and shortness of breath. If the deficiency is not corrected, symptoms of acute scurvy include swollen, ulcerated, and bleeding gums; loose teeth; easy fractures and malformed bones; painful, enlarged joints; large bruises; anemia; and possible severe hemorrhaging and heart failure. The elderly, alcoholics, drug addicts, and the homeless are all at risk for developing scurvy.

abundant tissue in the body, is necessary to build and maintain blood vessels, skin, tendons, ligaments, bones and teeth, joints, muscle tissue, and various organs. It is also essential to repair tissue and heal cuts, fractures, bruises, and other injuries.

Immune function. Vitamin C is thought to bolster the immune system in several ways. It spurs production of lymphocytes, white blood cells that are instrumental in fighting infection, and antibodies, substances that protect against disease-causing organisms. It also enhances the function of phagocytes, immune-system cells that destroy bacteria and other foreign invaders, and supports function of the thymus, a key immune-system gland.

Building sound bones and teeth. Vitamin C is necessary for proper calcification, the process that gives bones their hardness. It is also needed to make the cells that form the dentin in teeth.

Antioxidant activity. Vitamin C helps neutralize free radicals in the blood and other body fluids and protect fat-soluble antioxidants (vitamins A and E) from excessive oxidation. These actions help prevent premature aging and death of cells, and may also protect against cancer and other diseases.

Therapeutic Uses and Dosages

There is no clear agreement as to what constitutes an ideal dosage of vitamin C. Dr. Linus Pauling, a Nobel laureate in chemistry who was the first advocate of high-dose vitamin C, recommended taking 2,000 to 9,000 mg a day. Many experts, however, think that 500 mg is the optimal dosage. Age and the presence of various diseases affect the amounts of vitamin C that the body can use effectively. A UCLA study involving eleven thousand adults aged twenty-five to seventy-four found that a daily intake of 300 mg of vitamin C from food and supplements may increase life expectancy by six years. However, a 1997 report in the *American Journal of Clinical Nutrition* asserted that doses above 200 mg a day do not increase blood levels of the vitamin in healthy people. Very high amounts—e.g., more than 1,000 mg a day—are best taken in divided doses. Taking it with food reduces the risk of stomach upset.

Colds and flu. This remains one of the best-known and perhaps the most controversial uses of vitamin C. In 1970, Dr. Pauling published *Vitamin C and the Common Cold*, in which he contended that very high doses of ascorbic acid could prevent the common cold and flu. Since then, dozens of studies have failed to prove Dr. Pauling's basic premise, but some have shown that daily doses of 1,000 mg (or more) of vitamin C can shorten the duration of a cold or bout of flu if taken when symptoms first appear.

Cancer. Many population studies have linked a low intake of vitamin C with an increased risk of many cancers, especially of the digestive tract. Other studies have found reduced cancer mortality among people whose diets include ample fruits and vegetables—good sources of vi-

◙ SIGNS OF OVERDOSE
The risk of toxicity is low because excess vitamin C is excreted in the urine. However, long-term megadoses (more than 3,000 mg a day) can cause oxalate kidney stones, heart damage from oxalate deposits, and a buildup of excessive iron in the body.

◙ BEST SOURCES
Citrus fruits and juices
Cantaloupe and other melons
Strawberries, currants, and other berries
Red and green peppers
Cabbage, kale, and other green leafy vegetables
Tomatoes and tomato juice
Newly harvested potatoes

◙ A LITTLE HISTORY
▪ In 1747, an English naval surgeon named James Lind treated twelve sailors who had scurvy with various remedies, and discovered that lime juice produced a rapid cure.
▪ Captain James Cook, on two long sea voyages between 1768 and 1775, reported that his sailors avoided getting scurvy by eating sauerkraut and stocking up on fresh fruits and vegetables whenever they went ashore.
▪ In 1795, the British Royal Navy eliminated scurvy as a seafaring disease by providing fresh lime juice for all sailors, giving rise to their nickname of "limeys."
▪ In 1928, a Hungarian-born researcher named Albert Szent-Gyorgy isolated a substance that he called hexuronic acid from oranges, cabbage leaves, and ox adrenal glands.
▪ In 1932, researchers at the University of Pittsburgh isolated vitamin C from lemon juice and proved that it prevented scurvy in guinea pigs. A year later, vitamin C was synthesized by a Swiss scientist, and in 1938, the vitamin was given the chemical name of ascorbic acid.

tamin C as well as beta-carotene and other antioxidants. In a landmark 1990 study, Dr. Pauling and his colleagues demonstrated that patients whose cancers were advancing despite conventional therapy lived much longer when they were given 12,000 mg (12 g) of vitamin C a day, along with high doses of other vitamins and minerals. The mean survival of patients in the control group, who did not receive the supplements, was 5.7 months, compared to 72 to 122 months for the 80 percent of patients considered good responders to the vitamin therapy. Even those who were poor responders lived more than twice as long as the control group. Other studies have found that high doses of vitamin C appear to increase the effectiveness of cancer chemotherapy and reduce the damage to healthy tissue from radiation therapy.

Vitamin C is thought to protect against cancer in several ways. It helps neutralize certain cancer-causing substances, including benzopyrene, a carcinogen in cigarette smoke. It also blocks the formation of nitrosamines, cancer-causing agents that are made from the nitrites and nitrates in cured meats and other foods and certain pollutants. Ascorbic acid applied to the skin has been found to lower the incidence of skin cancer.

Cardiovascular diseases. Many studies have correlated a high intake of vitamin C with a reduced risk of heart attacks and strokes. Low blood levels of vitamin C have been linked to an increased incidence of high blood pressure—a major risk factor for both heart attacks and strokes. A recent study found that 200 mg of vitamin C a day produced a significant drop in blood pressure among patients with mild to moderate hypertension. Other studies indicate that vitamin C, in daily dosages of 500 to 1,000 mg, has a beneficial effect on cholesterol by raising HDLs—the "good" cholesterol—while lowering levels of harmful LDLs. High levels of vitamin C may also help prevent atherosclerosis—the clogging of arteries with fatty deposits—by reducing free-radical damage to the blood vessel walls.

A study involving 119 patients who had undergone angioplasty, a procedure to clear blocked coronary arteries, found that vitamin C may reduce the risk of the vessels becoming clogged again. In this four-month study, 76 percent of patients who took 500 mg of vitamin C a day maintained normal blood flow in their treated blood vessels. In contrast, 43 percent of patients in the control group had a reclogging of their coronary arteries.

Diabetes. Low levels of insulin and high levels of blood sugar (glucose) reduce the body's ability to use vitamin C. Studies have found that persons with diabetes have low blood levels of vitamin C despite the adequate intake of the vitamin. Studies have found that supplements of 500 to 1,000 mg improve blood-glucose control and may also reduce the risk of diabetic complications, including heart attack, stoke, circulatory problems, and cataracts.

Cataracts. Vitamin C is highly concentrated in the eyes—about twentyfold over levels in the blood. A large-scale eye study found a reduced incidence of cataracts among persons with high intake of vitamin C. Other studies suggest that supplements of 500 to 1,000 mg of vitamin C a day may protect against cataracts and other age-related eye disorders, including degeneration of the central (macular) area of the retina.

Asthma. Although results have been mixed, some studies have found that 3,000 mg of vitamin C, taken in three divided doses during the course of a day, may reduce asthma symptoms in adults. Researchers theorize that the protective effect stems from the vitamin's antioxidant activity in the lungs, which may reduce the irritation of inhaled asthma triggers. Other studies have found that taking 2,000 mg of vitamin C before exercise lowers the risk of an exercise-induced asthma attack. A British study involving 1,960 adults found that those with high blood levels of vitamin C had a reduced incidence of bronchitis and other lung disorders, compared to those with low levels.

Wound healing. Studies have found that surgery and burn patients heal faster if they take vitamin C supplements; the typical dosage is 1,000 mg taken three times a day.

Miscellaneous disorders. Recent research indicates that vitamin C supplements may protect against or help in the treatment of arthritis, Parkinson's disease, gum disease, mouth ulcers, chronic fatigue syndrome, and gallstones. Although more research is needed to document these benefits, many doctors now recommend taking 500 to 1,000 mg of vitamin C a day.

Special Cautions

High doses of vitamin C can cause such intestinal problems as stomach cramps, diarrhea, gas, and bloating. Lower the dosage to 1,000 mg or less a day if these symptoms develop. High doses also have a diuretic effect, and may result in excessive urination, increase the effects of diuretic drugs, produce occult blood in the stool, or interfere with the action of anti-clotting drugs. Finally, studies indicate that high doses vitamin C (more than 1,000 mg a day) can have a pro-oxidant effect, meaning that it increases (rather than protects against) oxidative damage from free radicals. High doses can also result in a false positive diabetes test, and affect results of hemoglobin studies. Be sure to tell your doctor if you are taking vitamin C (or any other nutraceuticals).

Persons with a history of kidney stones should use extra caution when taking high doses (more than 100 mg) of vitamin C, which can increase the risk of calcium oxalate kidney stones. High doses also should be avoided during pregnancy.

Preparation and Handling

Vitamin C deteriorates rapidly. To minimize vitamin loss, buy fresh fruits and vegetables when they are in season, store them in the refrigerator, and use them as soon as possible. When preparing fresh foods, wash them quickly and do not let them stand in water. Keep chopping to a minimum and cook them as quickly as possible in a minimal amount of water. Do not use iron or copper pans—these metals destroy vitamin C—and avoid thawing frozen foods before cooking them.

VITAMIN D

⦿ REQUIREMENTS

The Recommended Dietary Allowances for vitamin D are set at:

300 IU for infants under 6 months
400 IU for males and females 6 months to 24 years
200 IU for males and females 25 years
400 IU for males and females 51 to 70 years
600 IU for males and females 71 years and older
400 IU during pregnancy and breast-feeding

⦿ SIGNS OF DEFICIENCY

In children
- Skeletal deformities, including weak bones, bowed legs, knocked knees, a curved spine, and deformed skull.
- Weak muscles.
- Pot belly.
- Overgrowth of cartilage, resulting in enlarged joints.
- Teeth that come in late and decay easily.

In adults
- Boness that soften, become distorted, and fracture easily.
- Muscle twitches and cramps.

⦿ SIGNS OF OVERDOSE

Symptoms of hypercalcemia due to excessive vitamin D include:

- Fatigue, irregular heartbeat, nausea, vomiting, weakness, constipation (perhaps alternating with diarrhea).
- Loss of appetite.
- Excessive thirst.
- Weight loss in adults; growth problems in children.

Vitamin D is a fat-soluble vitamin that functions as a hormone in helping to build and maintain healthy bones. It is often called the "sunshine vitamin" because the sun's ultraviolet (UV) light is essential to make it. Vitamin D_2 is made when ergosterol—a substance in plants—is exposed to UV light. Vitamin D_3, the form found in humans and other animals, is made from a type of cholesterol when the skin is exposed to UV light.

In theory, ten to fifteen minutes of exposure to the midday sun two or three times a week should enable the body to make all of the vitamin D that it needs. However, the sun is not a reliable source because many factors affect its ability to penetrate the skin; these include the use of sunscreens, dark pigment, clothing, and environmental conditions, such as fog, smog, smoke, and dust. Between November and February, the sun's rays in northern latitudes (e.g., north of Chicago) are too weak to stimulate adequate conversion or synthesis of vitamin D. In addition, as we age, our ability to make vitamin D diminishes. This is one reason why numerous studies have found that the elderly—especially shut-ins—are deficient in vitamin D.

Most foods have little or no vitamin D. The best source is cod-liver oil, followed by blue-green algae and fatty fish that feed on plankton—organisms that live near the water's surface where they absorb a lot of sunlight. Milk, margarine, grain products, and certain other foods are fortified with vitamin D during processing to help compensate for the sparse dietary sources.

Why It's Needed

Functions of vitamin D include:

Bones and teeth. Vitamin D is essential in order for bones and teeth to take up calcium and other minerals. Children need it to build strong bones and teeth; in adults it's essential for maintaining them.

Mineral absorption. Without vitamin D, the body cannot properly absorb calcium and phosphorus—minerals essential to build and maintain bones—from the small intestine. Consequently, calcium will be lost in the feces and excessive phosphates will be excreted in the urine.

Inadequate vitamin D also results in low blood levels of citrate, which is needed for proper mineral metabolism.

Additional possible benefits of vitamin D include:

Bolstered immunity. Recent studies indicate that vitamin D may play a role in fostering immunity, but its precise role has not yet been discovered.

Cancer prevention. Population studies suggest that vitamin D provides protection against cancers of the prostate, colon, and breast. Some researchers theorize that these benefits may derive from the vitamin's hormonal functions.

Therapeutic Uses and Dosages

Rickets. This disease, which is now rare in developed countries, is caused by a deficiency of vitamin D or an inability to metabolize the vitamin, and the disease can be prevented by adequate exposure to the sun and/or including 200 to 400 IU of vitamin D in the daily diet.

Osteomalacia (adult rickets). This disease develops when the bones lose excessive calcium and phosphorus, causing them to soften and fracture easily. It also causes chronic pain, especially in the back and legs. As with childhood rickets, osteomalacia is treated—or preferably prevented—by getting at least 200 IU of vitamin D a day.

Tetany. This disease, characterized by muscle cramps, twitching, and perhaps convulsion, is caused by low blood levels of calcium. Although it may be due to vitamin D deficiency, it can also be caused by other disorders that interfere with calcium absorption.

Osteoporosis. This very common disease, in which bones are weakened by excessive loss of calcium and other minerals, occurs with aging. In recent years, a number of new osteoporosis treatments have evolved, but a daily intake of 400 to 800 IU of vitamin D, combined with 1,200 to 1,500 mg of calcium, remains a key element in both treatment and prevention.

Psoriasis. An activated form of vitamin D has been found to improve psoriasis symptoms by slowing the proliferation of skin cells. This type of vitamin D is available only by prescription; it is unlikely that high-dose vitamin D supplements, which can be toxic, are beneficial against psoriasis.

Osteoarthritis. A recent study found that vitamin D may slow the progression of osteoarthritis of the knee; more research is needed, however, to prove this benefit.

Special Cautions

Very high doses of vitamin D (more than 1,000 IU a day) for six months or longer can result in toxicity due to high blood levels of calcium

◉ SUPPLEMENT FORMS

Supplements forms include tablets, capsules, softgel, and liquid, as well as cod-liver and other fish oils.

◉ BEST SOURCES

Liver
Fatty saltwater fish, such as cod, tuna, and halibut
Egg yolks
Vitamin D–fortified milk, cream, butter, and cheese
Vitamin D–fortified margarine, bread, and cereals

◉ A LITTLE HISTORY

- Rickets—a disease caused by a deficiency of vitamin D—became epidemic among London's slum children during the Industrial Revolution of the 1800s.
- In the 1820s, cod-liver oil was shown to be effective in treating and preventing rickets.
- In 1890, an English physician linked a lack of sunshine with rickets.
- In 1918, Sir Edward Mellanby, a British scientist, proved that rickets was due to a nutritional deficiency, but he mistakenly attributed it to a lack of vitamin A.
- In 1922, Dr. McCollum, a Johns Hopkins researcher, isolated what he called the calcium-depositing vitamin, which was later named vitamin D.
- In 1924, researchers at the University of Wisconsin and Columbia University independently identified sunlight as a source of vitamin D.
- In 1952, R. B. Woodward of Harvard became the first to synthesize vitamin D, one of his many achievements that won him a Nobel Prize in 1965.

(hypercalcemia). In time, soft tissues—especially in the heart, kidneys, lungs, and blood vessels—become clogged with calcium deposits, which can be fatal. Excessive vitamin D intake during pregnancy or infancy can result in mental retardation, a narrowing of the heart's aortic valve, and other abnormalities.

Preparation and Handling

Vitamin D supplements in the form of oils or powders are sensitive to light, oxygen, and acids. They should be stored in opaque, hermetically sealed containers. Vitamin D in dry pill form is more stable than the oil or powder compounds but should still be stored properly. Vitamin D in foods, including those that are fortified with the nutrient, is quite stable, and is not destroyed by normal cooking.

VITAMIN E

Vitamin E, another of the fat-soluble vitamins, is a powerful antioxidant. It is actually a group of compounds called tocopherols and tocotrienols. Of these, the alpha-tocopherol is the most abundant and biologically active.

Although researchers are still unraveling the many functions of vitamin E, most are related to its antioxidant properties and include slowing of the aging process and protecting against cancer, coronary heart disease, cataracts, and various degenerative diseases. It appears to bolster the immune system, improve circulation, hasten wound healing, and reduce symptoms associated with prostaglandin activity, such as inflammation and premenstrual syndrome. It also protects vitamins A and C from oxidation and is essential to maintaining healthy red blood cells and muscle tissue.

Vitamin E's antioxidant activity keeps fats from turning rancid and prevents cellular damage that results from the metabolism of polyunsaturated fatty acids. In recent years, Americans have been told to lower their risk of heart disease by cutting down on saturated (animal) fats and increasing their intake of vegetable oils, which are high in polyunsaturated fats. While this is sound advice to improve cardiovascular health, a high intake of polyunsaturated fats increases the damage of free radicals, something medical science oxidative stress. This can be countered by increasing your intake of vitamin E.

Vegetable fats—salad and cooking oils, margarine, and wheat germ oil—are the richest dietary sources of vitamin E. In the body, it is stored in fatty tissue, the liver, and muscles; high amounts are also found in the adrenal and pituitary glands, testicles, uterus, heart, and lungs.

◉ REQUIREMENTS
The RDAs are based on alpha-tocopherol, and stated in either milligrams or IU.

3 mg or 4.5 IU for infants under 6 months
4 mg or 6 IU for infants 6 to 12 months
6 mg or 9 IU for children 1 to 3 years
7 mg or 10.5 IU for children 4 to 10
10 mg or 15 IU for males 11 and older
8 mg or 12 IU for females 11 and older
10 mg or 15 IU during pregnancy
12 mg or 16 IU during breast-feeding

◉ SUPPLEMENT FORMS
Vitamin E is available as oil-filled capsules or softgels, or as an oil-free tablet (vitamin E succinate) that contains a water-soluble synthetic compound that can be taken by people who are unable to absorb fats.

D-alpha-tocopherol—also called RRR-alpha-tocopherol or natural vitamin E—is the most biologically active supplement; studies have found that it is more than twice as potent as the synthetic form—dl-alpha-tocopherol or all-rac-alpha-tocopherol. Although d-alpha-tocopherol supplements are usually more expensive than the dl-alpha supplements, the body's increased ability to absorb natural vitamin E more than compensates for the extra cost. For example, one study found that 100 mg (150 IU) of natural (d-alpha) vitamin E was equivalent to about 300 mg (450 IU) of the synthetic (dl-alpha) form.

Why It's Needed

Antioxidant activity. A tiny amount of vitamin E is found in most body cells, where it provides protection against free radicals, unstable molecules that are released when the body burns oxygen or is exposed to radiation, sunlight, or toxic chemicals, including lead, mercury, benzene, and ozone. Damage from free radicals and toxins that function as free radicals can result in premature cell death or can alter cellular response to hormones and other body chemicals. Free radicals can also damage a cell's genetic material, resulting in cancer-causing mutations. Vitamin E not only "scavenges" free radicals and other cancer-causing agents (carcinogens) as they travel through the body, but it also works with other antioxidants, especially selenium, to increase their effectiveness.

Protection against cancer. Various studies have found that vitamin E, in dosages of 400 to 800 IU a day, appears to reduce the risk of several cancers, most notably those of the lungs, esophagus, and colon. Animal studies have found a protective effect against breast and skin cancers; vitamin E also protects the lungs against damage from air pollution.

Metabolic functions. Vitamin E is instrumental in the synthesis of vitamin C, coenzyme Q_{10}, and DNA.

Circulation. Studies have found that vitamin E increases the life span of red blood cells. It also reduces the tendency of blood to clot, and may increase blood flow to the legs.

Anti-inflammatory effects. Vitamin E appears to inhibit the inflammatory action of the prostaglandins, body chemicals that are instrumental in many body processes.

Therapeutic Uses and Dosages

Heart disease. A number of population (epidemiological) studies have correlated a high intake of vitamin E (and, to a lesser degree, vitamin C and other antioxidants) with a reduced risk of heart attacks. It is well known that a high level of LDL cholesterol greatly increases the risk of atherosclerosis (the clogging of arteries with fatty plaque) and coronary heart disease (the leading cause of heart attacks). Researchers have found that atherosclerosis most likely starts with blood-vessel damage caused by the oxidation of LDL cholesterol. Human studies have shown that daily dosages of 400 to 800 IU of natural vitamin E reduces LDL oxidation. More research is needed to prove that vitamin E can actually prevent atherosclerosis and coronary disease; in the meantime, a growing number of cardiologists and other physicians are advising their high-risk patients to supplement their daily diets with 400 to 800 IU of vitamin E, preferably the d-alpha-tocopherol form. Even higher doses—up to 1,200 IU a day—are recommended for persons with di-

◉ SIGNS OF DEFICIENCY
Vitamin E deficiency is rare, occurring mostly in premature babies or people with cystic fibrosis, celiac disease, and other disorders that interfere with fat absorption. In such cases, vitamin E deficiency may cause anemia due to the premature aging of red blood cells.

◉ SIGNS OF OVERDOSE
The body gets rid of excess vitamin E in the stool, so there is not the danger of toxicity that occurs with some other fat-soluble vitamins. However, very high doses can cause diarrhea, flatulence, bloating, and other intestinal symptoms.

◉ BEST SOURCE
Vegetable salad and cooking oils
Margarine and butter
Wheat germ
Egg yolks
Nuts and seeds
Avocados
Salmon, tuna, shrimp, and lobster
Green leafy vegetables

◉ A LITTLE HISTORY
- In 1922, a group of California researchers discovered what they called factor X, a fat-soluble substance in wheat germ and lettuce, and determined that it was necessary in order for rats to reproduce.

- In 1924, factor X was renamed vitamin E; in 1936, it was renamed tocopherol from the Greek terms meaning to bear offspring, a reference to its importance in reproductive function as demonstrated in early animal studies.

abetes, who have a very high risk of atherosclerosis and heart attacks.

Diabetes. A recent study found that vitamin E—in daily dosages of 800 to 1,200 IU—improves blood-glucose control in patients with type 2 (adult-onset) diabetes.

Dementia and Alzheimer's disease. Researchers theorize that oxidative stress to the brain accounts for much of the age-related decline in mental function. It may also be a factor in Alzheimer's disease and other types of dementia. In one United States study involving 341 patients with Alzheimer's disease, a daily dose of 2,000 IU of vitamin E slowed the progression of the disease more than the drug selegiline (Carbex, Eldepryl, or Atapryl). Other studies have found that high doses of vitamin E—800 to 1,200 IU a day—increases blood flow to the brain and may have some value in mental function.

Cataracts and macular degeneration. Numerous population studies show that low levels of vitamin E and other antioxidants increases the risk of age-related cataracts and macular degeneration. Studies in the United States, Canada, and several European countries all found that high blood levels of vitamin E lowered the risk of cataracts 55 to 60 percent. A multicenter U.S. study involving seventy-one patients with severe macular degeneration found that the condition stabilized within eighteen months among those taking vitamin E and other antioxidant supplements. In contrast, patients in the placebo group continued to lose their central and distance vision. The recommended dosage is 400 IU a day, taken along with 20,000 IU of beta-carotene, 750 to 1,000 mg of vitamin C, and 50 mcg of selenium.

Premenstrual syndrome (PMS) and fibrocystic breasts. One study found that 85 percent of women who suffered fibrocystic breast pain obtained relief when they took vitamin E supplements, and in 38 percent, the cysts disappeared completely. Other studies have found improvement in PMS symptoms after two or three months of taking vitamin E. The recommended starting dosage is 400 IU a day; if improvement is not noted in one or two menstrual cycles, increase the dosage to 800 IU, up to a maximum of 1,200 IU.

Leg pain and cramps. Intermittent claudication—leg pain and cramps due to poor circulation—is yet another condition that may benefit from vitamin E supplements. In one study, patients given vitamin E found they could walk farther without pain than those taking a placebo. The recommended daily dosage is 600 to 1,200 IU.

Special Cautions

Patients taking blood-thinning medication should check with their doctor before taking high doses of vitamin E; the combination may result in bleeding problems. High-dose vitamin E should be stopped before surgery to reduce the risk of excessive bleeding. Similarly, people with high blood pressure should not take high doses of vitamin E, which may increase the risk of a stroke from a ruptured blood vessel. Very high doses of vitamin E—more than 2,000 IU a day—can interfere with the body's absorption of vitamin A.

Preparation and Handling

Processing and exposure to oxygen, light, heat, and alkaline substances destroy vitamin E; it deteriorates rapidly during storage so it should be refrigerated. It is also destroyed by contact with certain trace minerals, especially iron and copper.

VITAMIN K

Vitamin K is a fat-soluble vitamin that is instrumental in blood clotting and the healing of cuts and other wounds. This is why it is routinely given to newborn babies and surgery patients to prevent excessive bleeding. Recent research suggests that vitamin K may also help maintain healthy bones and lower the risk of heart disease and cancer.

There are two forms of natural vitamin K: K_1 is found in many foods, especially dark green leafy vegetables; K_2 is made by bacteria that normally live in the intestines. Vitamin K deficiency is rare, occurring mostly in the first few days of life, or until intestinal bacteria have a chance to establish themselves. Deficiency, although rare, may occur as a result of long-term antibiotic use, which destroys beneficial as well as harmful bacteria; it may also develop among people who are unable to absorb fat or who have severe liver disease.

Why It's Needed

Blood clotting. The liver uses vitamin K to make four proteins—factors II, VII, IX, and X—that are essential to form blood clots. When you cut your finger, for example, vitamin K immediately goes to work to convert precursor proteins into these blood-clotting factors.

Bone metabolism. The role of vitamin K in building bones is not clear, but some studies have found that it may play a role in calcium metabolism, especially among older women who have a high risk of osteoporosis.

Therapeutic Uses and Dosages

Surgery. Vitamin K supplements are sometimes prescribed before surgery or given as an injection immediately after an operation (or child-

◙ **REQUIREMENTS**
5 mcg for infants under 6 months
10 mcg for infants 6 to 12 months
15 mcg for children 1 to 3 years
20 mcg for children 4 to 6
30 mcg for children 7 to 10
45 mcg for children 11 to 14
65 mcg for males 15 to 18
70 mcg for males 19 to 24
80 mcg for males 25 and older
55 mcg for females 15 to 18
60 mcg for females 19 to 24
65 mcg for females 25 and older, including during pregnancy and breast-feeding

◙ **SUPPLEMENT FORMS**
A synthetic form, known as vitamin K_3 or menadione, is available as a supplement in either tablet or injectable form.

◙ **SIGNS OF DEFICIENCY**
Deficiency is rare; when it occurs, symptoms include:

- Easy bruising.
- Prolonged bleeding from minor cuts.

◙ **SIGNS OF OVERDOSE**
Very high doses can cause sweating and flushing.

Vitamin K is made by intestinal bacteria; good food sources include:

Turnip greens, kale, Swiss chard, spinach, and other green leafy vegetables
Broccoli, cabbage, Brussels sprouts, and other cruciferous vegetables
Pork and beef liver
Cheese, butter, and vegetable oils
Eggs

● A LITTLE HISTORY

■ In the late 1920s, a Danish biochemist named Carl P. H. Dam discovered that baby chicks fed a fat-free diet died from internal bleeding, which could be prevented by giving them alfalfa, fishmeal, and other foods. He later extracted a fat-soluble substance from these foods.

■ In 1935, Dam named the substance ko-agulation vitamin, which was later shortened to vitamin K.

■ In 1942, Dam was awarded a Nobel Prize for his work with vitamin K.

birth) to prevent excessive bleeding and to promote incision healing. The dosage varies according to the type of operation and individual needs.

Osteoporosis. In a recent Dutch study, seventy postmenopausal women were given 1,000 mcg of vitamin K a day for three months. Women receiving the vitamin experienced a significant reduction in urinary calcium loss compared to women who did not take supplements. Other studies indicate that the vitamin may hasten fracture healing. Small amounts of vitamin K—for example, 50 to 100 mcg—are now included in several bone-building calcium supplements.

Heavy menstrual bleeding. Supplements of 100 mcg or more a day may reduce excessive menstrual blood loss. However, supplements in excess of the RDA should be taken only under a doctor's supervision.

Special Cautions

Although vitamin K is a fat-soluble vitamin, only small amounts are stored in the body; therefore, toxicity is not a problem. However, persons taking blood-thinning medications such as warfarin (Coumadin) should not take vitamin K supplements. Moderate amounts of foods high in the vitamin are unlikely to be harmful, but check with a doctor if your daily diet ordinarily provides more than one or two servings of greens and other foods rich in vitamin K. Conversely, very high doses of natural vitamin E (more than 1,000 IU a day) can interfere with vitamin K metabolism and increase the risk of bleeding.

Preparation and Handling

Most vitamin K survives ordinary cooking; freezing, however, destroys it. Green tea leaves and extracts are rich sources of vitamin K_1; however, very little is found in ordinary brewed green tea because only a small amount of the leaves are used to make a cup of tea.

VITAMIN B-COMPLEX

Vitamin B-complex is made up of eleven individual vitamins that have similar actions and often work together to carry out their various functions. The nutrients forming the B-complex group are: thiamin (B_1), riboflavin (B_2), niacin (B_3), pyridoxine (B_6), cobalamin (B_{12}), folacin (folic acid), pantothenic acid, biotin, and choline. Two other nutrients—

inositol and para-aminobenzoic acid (PABA)—are generally assumed to be part of the B-complex group.

Although the various B vitamins have their own distinct functions, their similarities are greater than their differences. All are water-soluble and most are not stored in appreciable amounts in the body so they need to be consumed daily. They often occur in the same foods, especially yeast and liver; other good sources of B-complex vitamins include whole grains, eggs, meat, poultry, and a variety of vegetables and fruits. Most of the B vitamins function—often in concert—as coenzymes, which are needed to metabolize the macronutrients (carbohydrates, proteins, and fats) and carry out numerous bodily processes.

Why It's Needed

In addition to their roles as coenzymes in energy conversion and other metabolic functions, the B-complex vitamins are needed to maintain healthy nerves, muscles, skin, and liver. Some, such as riboflavin, niacin, and pantothenic acid, play crucial roles in the synthesis of adrenal hormones, cholesterol, and fatty acids. Vitamin B_{12} is needed to make red blood cells and prevent pernicious anemia. Riboflavin is thought to be important for proper functioning of the eye's retina.

Therapeutic Uses and Dosages

Researchers are constantly discovering new functions of B-complex vitamins. For example, recent research has focused on inositol phosphates, or IP_6, a part of the B-complex family that appears to lower high blood cholesterol and also prevent the uncontrolled cell proliferation that results in cancer. So far, IP_6 has been studied mostly in laboratory animals, but some researchers contend that it has great potential as a cancer preventive and treatment for high blood lipids.

More is known about many of the other B-complex group. For example, niacin helps lower the risk of a heart attack by controlling blood cholesterol levels. Similarly, vitamins B_6, B_{12}, and folacin control blood levels of homocysteine, a metabolic by-product that can damage blood vessels and make them more vulnerable to atherosclerosis. When taken before and during early pregnancy, folacin helps prevent spina bifida, a birth defect marked by a deformed spinal column. Vitamin B_6 has been shown to improve symptoms of carpal tunnel syndrome. During pregnancy, surgery, and times of emotional stress, the body quickly depletes its small reserves of many B vitamins, and B-complex is often promoted to counter stress.

Given these and other benefits, it's understandable that many people are taking high doses of the various B vitamins. Caution is needed, however, because some of the B vitamins compete with each other to be absorbed by the body. Thus, taking very high doses of one B vitamin may result in a deficiency of another, so they should be taken only under the supervision of a qualified doctor or nutritionist.

This is only a brief overview of the B-complex vitamins; see the following sections for a more detailed discussion of the major members of this family of nutrients.

VITAMIN B₁ (THIAMIN)

Thiamin—also known as vitamin B_1 or the antiberiberi vitamin—was the first of the B-complex group to be isolated (in 1927) in its pure form. It is necessary to convert blood sugar (glucose) into energy; it also aids digestion, promotes proper growth, and aids in the normal function of the nervous system and the heart and other muscle tissue.

Humans and all other animal life require thiamin to prevent beriberi, a disease characterized by nerve inflammation and pain (polyneuritis), muscle weakness and poor coordination, waterlogged tissues (edema), and heart failure. Even decades before the discovery of thiamin, researchers had concluded that some sort of dietary deficiency caused beriberi, which is now rare, except in third world countries. At one time, however, it was common in societies where the diets were mostly polished rice and other processed foods.

Small amounts of thiamin are found in many foods, but it is easily destroyed during processing. For example, brown rice and other whole grains provide modest amounts of thiamin, but little or none is found in polished white rice, white flour, and other processed grain products. Since the early 1940s, breads, cereals, and other grain products have been enriched with thiamin (as well as riboflavin, niacin, and iron) to help prevent deficiencies due to food processing.

Why It's Needed

Thiamin is a coenzyme that is essential for many body functions, including:

Energy metabolism. Without thiamin, the body cannot use carbohydrates, its major fuel. Thiamin is also instrumental in converting blood glucose into fat and storing it for future use.

Nerve and muscle function. Thiamin is important in the proper function of the peripheral nerves and maintaining muscle tone. Without adequate thiamin, myelin—the protective tissue surrounding nerve fibers—breaks down. The resulting nerve irritation and inflammation leads to numbness, tingling, pins-and-needles sensations, and pain. The

◉ REQUIREMENTS

0.3 mg for infants under 6 months
0.4 mg for infants 6 to 12 months
0.7 mg for children 1 to 3 years
0.9 to 1 mg for children 4 to 10
1.3 mg for males 11 to 14
1.5 mg for males 15 to 50
1.2 mg for males 51 and older
1.1 mg for females 11 to 50
1.0 mg for females 51 and older
1.5 mg during pregnancy
1.6 mg during breast-feeding

◉ SUPPLEMENT FORMS

Thiamin is available in tablet and capsule forms, and it is included in multivitamin and B-complex products.

◉ SIGNS OF DEFICIENCY

Mild deficiency
Depression, irritability, difficulty concentrating, muscle weakness, and numbness or tingling sensations, especially in the lower legs.

Severe deficiency
Nerve disorders, including nerve pain and paralysis; swelling of the legs and hands; difficulty breathing due to heart failure.

◉ SIGNS OF OVERDOSE

In general, high doses do not cause adverse effects because the excess is excreted in the urine. However, excessive amounts of one B-complex component can interfere with absorption of other members of this vitamin family. Thus, high doses of thiamin may reduce absorption of riboflavin and vitamin B_6.

nerve dysfunction also results in a loss of muscle tone, weakness, poor coordination, and difficulty walking.

Mood and mental attitude. Even a mild thiamin deficiency results in depression, apathy, and mental sluggishness. This aspect of thiamin function is thought to be related to its role in metabolizing glucose, the only form of energy that the brain can use.

Therapeutic Uses and Dosages

Alcoholism. This is the most common cause of thiamin deficiency in the United States and other developed countries. Not only do alcoholics tend to substitute drink for food, but alcohol itself also contains a substance that destroys thiamin. Anyone who consumes more than one or two alcoholic drinks a day should take 50 to 100 mg of thiamin. During detoxification, alcoholics are usually given high doses (e.g., 500 mg) of thiamin (and other B vitamins).

Stress. Any stress—both physical and emotional—quickly depletes the body's meager stores of thiamin. Fever and other manifestations of illness also increase the body's needs for thiamin and other B vitamins. To meet these increased requirements, experts generally recommend a daily thiamin supplement of 100 to 500 mg—given along with the proper balance of other B vitamins—during times of high stress or when recovering from surgery or an illness.

Mood disorders. Studies have found that many persons suffering from mild depression, apathy, anxiety, and other mood disorders have low levels of thiamin. A number of studies have found that thiamin supplements of 50 to 100 mg may improve mood, increase mental alertness, and boost energy. It should be stressed, however, that clinical depression should be treated by a psychologist or other mental-health professional, or by a psychiatrist, who may prescribe pharmaceutical agents. In such circumstances, check with the treating doctor before taking any nutritional supplement to avoid possible interactions.

Congestive heart failure. Thiamin has been shown to improve the heart's pumping action and help reduce the fluid buildup (edema) that causes swollen legs and difficulty breathing. In one study, heart failure patients were given a daily 200-mg thiamin supplement along with a powerful diuretic (water pill). After six weeks, patients in the thiamin group showed a 22 percent improvement over those treated with the diuretic alone.

High-carbohydrate diet. Because thiamin is instrumental in the metabolism of carbohydrates, it follows that the more starches and sugars you consume the more thiamin you need to fully utilize it. People who follow the Food Pyramid eating plan and consume 60 percent or more of their calories from carbohydrates may need to supplement the daily diet with 50 mg of thiamin.

Aging. Many older people have mild thiamin deficiency. In a recent study involving persons over age sixty-five, those taking 50 mg a day for three months had a modest reduction in blood pressure and reported improved sleep and mood; these benefits were not found among persons in the placebo group.

Special Cautions

Because the body stores only enough thiamin to last one to two weeks, it needs to be consumed on a regular basis. Many common foods (especially grain products) are now enriched with thiamin, so severe deficiencies are rare—with one major exception: people who consume large amounts of alcohol. But alcohol is by no means the only source of antithiamin substances; coffee and tea (both regular and decaffinated) also reduce thiamin absorption. Raw seafood and some fish contain thiaminase, an enzyme that inactivates thiamin; cooking destroys thiaminase.

Preparation and Handling

Thiamin is lost during milling of grains and destroyed by irradiation, prolonged exposure to oxygen, high heat, and exposure to sulfites, which are used as food preservatives, and alkaline substances, such as baking soda. Because thiamin is water-soluble, it is leached out of foods during canning and lost if the fluid is then drained off. About 30 to 50 percent of thiamin in meat is lost during cooking.

VITAMIN B₂ (RIBOFLAVIN)

Riboflavin is another of the water-soluble B-complex group that, along with thiamin and niacin, is instrumental in the metabolism of all foods. It is made up of a group of enzymes (flavoproteins) that function as coenzymes essential for normal energy metabolism. In addition, it activates vitamin B_6 and it helps convert niacin to forms the body can use.

Although riboflavin deficiency does not produce distinct diseases in humans, it causes diverse symptoms, including anemia, fatigue, slow healing of cuts and other wounds, mouth sores, eye problems, and patches of oily and crusty skin (seborrheic dermatitis). It is found in many foods; the best sources are milk, cheese, and other dairy products; organ meats, beef, lamb, and the dark meat of poultry; and enriched cereals and other grain products.

◉ REQUIREMENTS
0.4 mg for infants under 6 months
0.5 mg for infants 6 to 12 months
0.8 mg for children 1 to 3 years
1.1 mg for children 4 to 6
1.2 mg for children 7 to 10
1.5 mg for males 11 to 14
1.8 mg for males 15 to 18
1.7 mg for males 19 to 50
1.4 mg for males 51 and older
1.3 mg for females 11 to 50
1.2 mg for females 51 and older
1.6 mg during pregnancy
1.8 mg during breast-feeding

Why It's Needed

The numerous functions of riboflavin include:

Metabolism and release of energy. Riboflavin plays a key role in the conversion of all macronutrients—carbohydrates, proteins, and fats—into forms that the body can use for energy. It is also necessary in order for the body to use niacin and thiamin, which are also instrumental in energy metabolism.

Antioxidant activity. Riboflavin appears to boost the antioxidant function of vitamin E to protect cells from damage caused by free radicals, the unstable molecules that are released when the body burns oxygen.

Hormone production and function. Riboflavin plays a part in thyroid hormone function, thereby increasing its role in how the body uses energy. It is also instrumental in the adrenal glands' hormone production, especially of cortisone.

Vision. Riboflavin is a component of retinal pigment that allows the eyes to adjust to changes in light, and a deficiency results in the eyes becoming light-sensitive, a condition called photophobia.

Immune-system function. Animal studies show that riboflavin deficiency results in reduced production of antibodies, the immune-system components that protect against disease.

Blood manufacture. Riboflavin is needed to make and maintain red blood cells, which deliver oxygen to all the body's cells. Consequently, riboflavin deficiency produces anemia similar to that of iron-deficiency anemia.

Nerve function.

Therapeutic Uses and Dosages

Cataract prevention. Animal studies have found that riboflavin deficiency promotes cataract formation. Although more research is needed, preliminary research indicates that riboflavin supplements ranging from 25 to 100 mg may prevent or slow the progression of cataracts.

Migraines. European researchers recently reported that riboflavin reduced the frequency of migraine headaches among a group of fifty-five patients who suffered two to eight headaches a month. After three months of taking daily 400-mg supplements, the number of headaches dropped by an average of more than one-third per patient—results comparable to prescription migraine drugs.

Carpal tunnel syndrome. Several studies have found that 100 to 500 mg of riboflavin a day improves carpal tunnel symptoms. It should be taken with an equal amount of vitamin B_6.

Skin disorders. Studies show that a relatively low dose of 50 mg of riboflavin may improve rosacea, a skin disorder marked by facial flushing

◉ **SUPPLEMENT FORMS**
Riboflavin comes in capsule and pill form, including time-release formulas.

◉ **SIGNS OF DEFICIENCY**
- Fatigue and possible anemia.
- Cracks and sores around the mouth and nose; chapped and painful lips.
- Slow healing of wounds.
- Swollen tongue with painful cracks (fissures).
- Red, bloodshot eyes and sensitivity to light.
- Oily, crusty skin.

◉ **SIGNS OF OVERDOSE**
There is no toxicity to riboflavin, but prolonged high doses can interfere with the metabolism of thiamin and vitamin B_6.

◉ **BEST SOURCES**
Liver and other organ meats
Lean beef, pork, and lamb
Eggs
Enriched bread, cereals, and pasta
Milk, cheese, yogurt, and other milk products
Raw mushrooms

◉ **A LITTLE HISTORY**
- In 1879, researchers discovered a fluorescent pigment in milk whey, and in the following years, a similar yellow-green substance was found in organ meats and egg whites. The pigment was named "flavin," but its nutritional importance was not recognized.
- In 1932, German scientists isolated a yellow enzyme that they recognized as part of the B complex group, and in the next few years, other German researchers and, working independently, a Swiss group, isolated and synthesized the substance, which the Swiss named "riboflavin."

and an enlarged red nose with skin pustules. It may take three months or more to notice improvement.

Physical and emotional stress. As with other members of the B-complex family, any physical or emotional stress requires extra riboflavin. An extra 100 to 250 mg a day may speed healing and help counter the harmful effects of emotional stress; it should be taken in balance with an increased amount of the other B-complex vitamins.

Special Cautions

Oral contraceptives interfere with the metabolism of riboflavin; women who take "the pill" should take a 100-mg supplement to protect against deficiency.

Many elderly people are deficient in riboflavin, especially if they avoid drinking milk because of lactose intolerance or other digestive problems. Many doctors recommend a daily B-complex supplement that provides 25 mg or more of riboflavin, niacin, thiamin, folacin, and vitamins B_6 and B_{12} for their older patients. Similarly, athletes and others who engage in vigorous exercise need extra riboflavin; supplements of 50 to 100 mg are recommended, especially during periods of heavy training.

Preparation and Handling

Riboflavin is very sensitive to light and quickly destroyed when exposed to it. For example, milk—one of the best sources of the vitamin—loses up to 75 percent of its riboflavin in only a few hours if it is in glass jars and exposed to light. Buy only the milk that comes in opaque glass or plastic bottles or cardboard containers, and do not transfer it to clear glass for storage.

VITAMIN B₃ (NIACIN, NICOTINIC ACID)

Niacin, still another of the B-complex family, functions as a coenzyme that works with thiamin and riboflavin to produce energy within cells. It also promotes healthy skin and nerve function as well as normal appetite and digestion.

There are two preformed forms of niacin—nicotinic acid and nicotinamide, which are found in many high-protein foods. In addition, the body, with the aid of other B vitamins, converts tryptophan (an amino acid) into niacin.

Severe niacin deficiency results in pellagra, a disease that causes diarrhea, inflammation of mucous membranes, and a type of dermatitis in which the skin becomes dark, rough, and flakes away. If untreated it can lead to dementia. Until the mid-1900s, pellagra killed tens of thousands of Americans, especially in the South and Southwest where corn was the dietary staple. The disease was so common that doctors thought it was caused by an infectious agent or perhaps a contaminant in corn. After the discovery of niacin, researchers learned that the niacin in corn is bound in a form that the body cannot use; it is also deficient in tryptophan, the niacin precursor. Interestingly, pellagra was not a problem in Mexico and Latin America, where people soaked their corn in lime water, which releases the bound form of niacin into one the body can use. The Native Americans of the Southwest achieved a similar effect by roasting corn in hot ashes.

Why It's Needed

Niacin is present in all body tissues as a part of two coenzymes; specific functions include:

Metabolism. Niacin, working with other B vitamins, is necessary to release energy from carbohydrates. Minute amounts of niacin are present in all body tissues and are necessary in order for the cells to use oxygen. It also plays roles in the synthesis of protein, DNA, and fatty acids, and is essential for normal growth.

Brain and nerve function. Even mild niacin deficiency has adverse effects on the nervous system; symptoms include weakness, irritability, anxiety, depression, and memory problems. Prolonged severe deficiency results in dementia.

Appetite and digestion. Niacin deficiency causes inflammation of the mucous membranes that line the intestinal tract. Mouth sores and a swollen, painful tongue make eating and swallowing difficult. The inflammation also causes diarrhea and rectal itching and discomfort.

Circulation and blood pressure. Nicotinic acid boosts circulation by helping to relax (dilate) blood vessels, thereby reducing the amount of pressure needed to force blood through them. When taken in large amounts, such as those prescribed to lower blood cholesterol, nicotinic acid can cause a rush of blood to the skin surface, resulting in flushing and dizziness. (This effect does not occur with nicotinamide, but this form has little or no effect on lowering cholesterol.)

Therapeutic Uses and Dosages

Lower blood cholesterol. When taken in high doses—typically 500 to 2,000 mg—nicotinic acid can lower high blood cholesterol as effectively as many pharmaceutical products. However, high-dose nicotinic acid should be used only under a doctor's supervision because it can

◉ REQUIREMENTS

Note: Niacin requirements vary according to the amount of protein—specifically tryptophan—in the diet. In general, it takes about 60 mg of tryptophan (typically, the amount in 60 g of protein) to make 1 mg of niacin.

5 mg for infants under 6 months
6 mg for infants 6 to 12 months
9 mg for children 1 to 3 years
12 mg for children 4 to 6
13 mg for children 7 to 10
17 mg for males 11 to 14
20 mg for males 15 to 18
19 mg for males 19 to 50
15 mg for males 51 and older
15 mg for females 11 to 50
13 mg for females 51 and older
17 mg during pregnancy
20 mg during breast-feeding

◉ SUPPLEMENT FORMS

Niacin is available in capsule or table form. Flushing and other adverse effects of nicotinic acid may be reduced by taking time-release pills or a form called inositol hexaniacinate, in which the nicotinic acid is bound to inositol, another member of the B-complex group.

◉ SIGNS OF DEFICIENCY

- Darkened, itchy skin with excessive flaking.
- Diarrhea and other digestive upsets.
- Mouth sores and a painful, swollen tongue.
- Irritability, anxiety, depression, and other mood changes.
- Loss of memory, confusion, hallucinations, and other symptoms of dementia.

◉ SIGNS OF OVERDOSE

- Skin flushing, especially of the face.
- Itchiness.
- Rise in blood sugar (glucose) that mimics diabetes.
- Liver damage.
- Development or worsening of peptic ulcers.

◉ BEST SOURCES

Liver and other organ meats
Lean meat, poultry, and fish
Whole-grain or enriched breads and cereals
Milk and eggs
Nuts, seeds, and peanut butter

- In 1867, a German chemist isolated nicotinic acid from the nicotine in tobacco. Unfortunately, its nutritional benefits were unknown for many decades, during which many thousands of people died of pellagra.

- In the 1920s, Dr. Joseph Goldberger, an American physician-researcher, and his colleagues concluded that pellagra was caused by a nutritional deficiency and experimented with various foods to treat the disease.

- In 1937, researchers at the University of Wisconsin discovered that nicotinic acid could cure black-tongue disease in dogs, an animal counterpart of human pellagra.

- In 1945, another University of Wisconsin team discovered that tryptophan is a precursor of niacin.

cause flushing, dizziness, and itchiness. Prolonged use may also have adverse effects on the liver and blood glucose levels. Doctors typically start patients on a low dose of 100 to 200 mg, and gradually work up to the amounts needed to lower cholesterol—usually 500 to 1,000 mg. If cholesterol levels remain unchanged after two months of high-dose nicotinic acid, it is unlikely that it is going to work, and a pharmacologic agent should be tried.

Special Cautions

Patients taking high doses of nicotinic acid should undergo liver enzyme tests every three months to monitor for possible liver damage. High-dose niacin can also worsen (or perhaps even trigger) peptic ulcers, diabetes, gout, and glaucoma, so it should be used with great caution by patients who have or are predisposed to developing these disorders.

Preparation and Handling

Niacin is more stable than many of the other B vitamins, but because it is water-soluble, it can be leached out in cooking water.

VITAMIN B₅ (PANTOTHENIC ACID)

Pantothenic acid, or vitamin B_5, is another member of the B-complex family of water-soluble vitamins. Like so many of the other B vitamins, it functions as a coenzyme in many metabolic processes, including breaking down carbohydrates, fats, and proteins. It is especially important in the building of fatty acids; it also helps build red blood cells and antibodies, and plays important roles in the functioning of the endrocrine glands and their hormones.

The name pantothenic is derived from the Greek *pantothen,* meaning everywhere; this refers to the fact that it is found in almost all plant and animal foods. It is also synthesized by intestinal bacteria.

Pantothenic acid deficiency rarely if ever occurs in humans, but it can be induced by using a vitamin antagonist to destroy it or providing a synthetic diet devoid of the vitamin. In such cases, immunity is lowered, and digestion, brain and nerve function, and insulin and glucose (blood sugar) metabolism are impaired.

There is no official RDA for pantothenic acid; the following amounts are estimated to be safe and adequate:

2 mg for infants under 6 months
3 mg for infants 6 to 12 months
3 mg for children 1 to 3 years
3–4 mg for children 4 to 6
4–5 mg for children 7 to 10
4–7 mg for everyone 11 and older

This vitamin is marketed as pantothenate calcium (a combination of 92 percent pantothenic acid and 8 percent calcium) and pantethine, a biologically active metabolite. Supplements are available in pill and capsule forms.

Why It's Needed

The varied functions of pantothenic acid include:

Metabolism. Pantothenic acid is converted to coenzyme A, which is used to transform food into molecules that the body can use for energy or to build fatty acids and certain proteins. Pantothenic acid also plays a role in the metabolism of certain minerals.

Immune function. Pantothenic acid stimulates the formation of antibodies, components of the immune system that protect against disease.

Nerve function. Pantothenic acid is needed to transform choline into the neurotransmitter acetylcholine, a chemical that is instrumental in transmitting nerve impulses.

Hormone function. The adrenal glands, which make adrenaline (epinephrine) and other stress hormones instrumental in the body's fight-or-flight response, require pantothenic acid. The vitamin also plays a role in insulin action, which controls blood sugar metabolism.

Red blood cell formation. Pantothenic acid is needed to form porphyrin, a precursor of heme—the protein that binds with iron to form the blood's oxygen-carrying molecule, hemoglobin.

Therapeutic Uses and Dosages

Possible therapeutic uses of pantothenic acid include:

Lowering blood cholesterol. In one study involving more than one thousand patients with elevated blood cholesterol, a high dose (900 mg) of pantethine—a biologically active metabolite of pantothenic acid—lowered cholesterol and triglycerides, another blood lipid (fat). Many of the study participants also had diabetes, and the researchers theorized that high doses of pantothenic acid may also improve blood sugar control. Other studies using pantethine achieved average reductions of 15 percent and 30 percent in cholesterol and triglyceride levels respectively.

Arthritis. Several studies have found that high doses of pantothenic acid (e.g., 900 mg of pantethine) may improve symptoms of both rheumatoid and osteoarthritis. This benefit may be linked to the role of pantothenic acid in producing cortisone, an adrenal hormone that reduces inflamation.

Lupus. Pantothenic acid may reduce symptoms of discoid lupus, the form of this chronic autoimmune disease that affects the skin. In one study, improvement was noted in thirty of thirty-seven patients who were given very high initial doses of 6 to 10 g. After symptoms abated, the dosages were lowered to 2 to 4 g a day.

Special Cautions

Many claims for pantothenic acid (and especially its metabolite, pantethine) have not been proved; these include preventing hair loss and

◉ SIGNS OF DEFICIENCY

Deficiency does not occur naturally, but when it is induced in humans and laboratory animals, symptoms include irritability, depression, insomnia, and other psychological changes; fatigue, numbness, tingling, muscle cramps, burning pain of the feet, and other neurological problems; indigestion, nausea, and abdominal pain; and headache. There may also be increased sensitivity to stress and low blood sugar levels caused by an increased need for insulin. In laboratory animals, deficiency causes skin lesions and premature graying of hair. However, it has not been proved that pantothenic acid has any effect on hair graying or balding in humans.

◉ SIGNS OF OVERDOSE

Pantothenic acid appears to be nontoxic, even in very high doses of 10 g or more a day. However, these megadoses can cause diarrhea and edema (fluid retention).

◉ BEST SOURCES

All plant and animal foods contain some pantothenic acid; the best sources include:

Liver and other organ meats
Wheat brain, whole-wheat products, and
  brown rice
Mushrooms
Nuts
Chicken and eggs

◉ A LITTLE HISTORY

▪ In 1933, a scientist named R. J. Williams isolated a substance from yeast that he named pantothenic acid; a few years later, he isolated it from liver.

▪ In 1940, pantothenic acid was synthesized by Dr. Williams and researchers working independently in two other laboratories.

graying, boosting athletic performance, detoxifying alcohol, and slowing of the aging process. In addition, panthetine tends to be unstable and is quite expensive.

Preparation and Handling

Processing destroys about half of the pantothenic content of grains, fruits, and vegetables. The substance is also sensitive to exposure to oxygen and very high temperatures. But because pantothenic acid is found in so many foods, and is also synthesized by intestinal bacteria, an ordinary diet provides more than enough of the vitamin.

VITAMIN B$_6$ (PYRIDOXINE)

Vitamin B$_6$, one of the most versatile of all vitamins, functions as a coenzyme in more than one hundred metabolic processes. It boosts immunity and plays important roles in nerve function and the synthesis of red blood cells, serotonin and other brain chemicals, antibodies, and genetic material. Vitamin B$_6$ is also instrumental in preventing heart disease, strokes, and kidney stones, as well as treating carpal tunnel syndrome, premenstrual syndrome, mild depression, insomnia, and some aspects of asthma.

There are three, apparently interchangeable, forms of vitamin B$_6$: pyridoxine, pyridoxal, and pyridoxamine. Of these, pyridoxine—which is often used as another name for the vitamin—is the most abundant in food and the most resistant to damage or loss.

Small amounts of vitamin B$_6$ are found in most foods; for example, most vegetables, nuts, legumes, and whole grains contain varying amounts of pyridoxine, while meat, fish, poultry, and other animal products are good sources of the pyridoxal and pyridoxamine forms. Despite its wide distribution in foods, studies have found that up to one-third of American adults, especially women, do not get adequate amounts of vitamin B$_6$. This may be because the body absorbs rather limited amounts of the vitamin, as well as the fact that large amounts are lost in food processing.

Why It's Needed

The varied functions of vitamin B$_6$ include:

Metabolism. Vitamin B$_6$ plays a role in more than sixty different aspects of protein metabolism; thus, it is essential for proper growth,

◉ **REQUIREMENTS**

0.3 mg for infants under 6 months
0.6 mg for infants 6 to 12 months
1.0 mg for children 1 to 3 years
1.1 mg for children 4 to 6
1.4 mg for children 7 to 10
1.7 mg for males 11 to 14
2.0 mg for males 15 and older
1.4 mg for females 11 to 14
1.5 mg for females 15 to 18
1.6 mg for females 19 and older
1.2 mg during pregnancy
2.1 mg during breast-feeding

◉ **SUPPLEMENT FORMS**

Supplements, which are available in tablet, capsule, and liquid forms, are made up of either pyridoxine hydrochloride or a chemical compound called pyridoxal-5-phospate, or P-5-P. There is some evidence that the body absorbs P-5-P somewhat more readily than pyridoxine, but either supplement form is acceptable.

development, and tissue repair and maintenance. It is also involved in carbohydrate and fat metabolism, including energy production.

Immune-system function. Vitamin B_6 is needed to make antibodies, components of the immune system that are instrumental in protecting against disease. Recent studies have found that vitamin B_6 supplements appear to boost immunity in the elderly, and animal studies have found that B_6 may slow tumor growth. More research is needed, however, to prove these benefits.

Nerve function. Vitamin B_6 helps make serotonin and other brain chemicals (neurotransmitters) that help carry messages from the brain to nerves throughout the body. Neurotransmitters are also important in fostering a sense of well-being, which is why vitamin B_6 helps counter depression. It also helps prevent seizures, and may play a role in treating epilepsy.

Manufacturing blood cells. The body needs vitamin B_6 to convert iron into hemoglobin, the oxygen-carrying pigment in red blood cells.

Controlling homocysteine. High blood levels of homocysteine, a by-product of protein metabolism, makes blood vessels more vulnerable to damage and a buildup of fatty deposits (atherosclerosis). In fact, recent research suggests that homocysteine may be as important as cholesterol in the development of atherosclerosis.

Therapeutic Uses and Dosages

Carpal tunnel syndrome. Studies show that daily supplements of 100 to 200 mg help a large number of patients suffering from hand pain and other carpal tunnel symptoms. However, it may take three months of B_6 therapy before symptoms abate.

Mild depression. Because vitamin B_6 is instrumental in the production of serotonin—a mood-elevating brain chemical—it is logical to assume that supplements may be beneficial in treating mild depression and anxiety. Research to prove this, however, has produced mixed results—some studies have reported improvement in mood among people taking 100 to 500 mg of vitamin B_6 while others have found little or no benefit.

Premenstrual syndrome (PMS). In one double-blind study involving twenty-five women with severe PMS, a daily 500-mg B_6 supplement in time-release form produced significant improvement in twenty of the patients. Symptoms relieved included bloating, irritability, breast tenderness, and headaches. Other studies have found that B_6 supplements alleviated PMS-related nausea and dizziness, and—to a lesser degree—helped against anxiety, depression, and mood swings.

Kidney stones. Studies have found that vitamin B_6 in dosages of 100 to 300 mg a day may help prevent recurrent oxalate kidney stones.

Diabetes. Vitamin B_6 supplements have been found to improve blood sugar (glucose) control in some diabetes patients; it may also help prevent some of the nerve damage caused by this disease. The improved

◎ **SIGNS OF DEFICIENCY**

Infants who are deficient in B_6 may suffer convulsions, muscle twitchiness, and irritability. In adults, deficiency does not appear to cause a specific disease, but it can cause:

- Patches of scaly, oily skin (seborrheic dermatitis) that start on the face and spread to other parts of the body.
- A smooth, red tongue.
- Loss of weight.
- Depression and other mental changes.
- Muscle weakness.

◎ **SIGNS OF OVERDOSE**

Taking 2,000 mg (2 g) of B_6 for more than a few weeks can cause serious nerve damage, and some people have developed problems with prolonged dosages as low as 500 mg. Symptoms include:

- Numbness and tingling of the feet and hands.
- A stumbling gait and poor coordination.

Symptoms usually improve when the high-dose supplements are stopped, but some numbness may be irreversible.

◎ **BEST SOURCES**

Liver and other organ meats
Lean beef, pork, lamb, and poultry
Fish and seafood, especially clams
Rice and wheat bran; whole grains and brown rice
Bananas and avocados
Soybeans, nuts, and seeds
Milk, yogurt, cheese, and other dairy products
Eggs

◎ **A LITTLE HISTORY**

- In 1926, researchers attempting to produce pellagra in rats instead induced severe skin lesions.
- In 1936, a Hungarian scientist found a cure for the skin lesions by feeding the laboratory animals a yeast extract. He determined that it was different from the other known B vitamins, so he named it B_6.
- In 1938, five different research teams working independently isolated B_6, which was synthesized a year later.

glucose control is attributed to enhanced metabolism of tryptophan, an amino acid that plays a role in glucose metabolism. Studies have also found that B_6 supplements during pregnancy may reduce the risk of gestational diabetes; low doses (e.g., 25 mg a day) may also relieve morning sickness. A word of caution, however: Diabetics or pregnant women should not take high doses of vitamin B_6 (or any other nutraceutical product) except under the supervision of a qualified nutritionist or a doctor trained in nutrition.

Tuberculosis (TB). Patients with this disease are often treated with isoniazid, an antibiotic that can cause nerve inflammation and pain. This adverse effect can be prevented by taking 50 to 100 mg of B_6 a day.

Special Cautions

As a general rule, no one should take more than 50 to 100 mg of vitamin B_6 without first consulting a nutritionist or qualified doctor. Even though excess vitamin B_6—as with other members of the B-complex family—is excreted in the urine, prolonged high doses can be detrimental (see Signs of Overdose, above).

Oral contraceptives interfere with the body's absorption of vitamin B_6, which results in abnormal metabolism of tryptophan, an amino acid. Therefore, a daily supplement of at least 5 mg is advisable for women who take "the pill." Although much higher doses are often recommended, studies show that 5 mg is usually enough to restore normal tryptophan metabolism.

High doses of vitamin B_6 interfere with the metabolism of levodopa, a drug commonly used to treat Parkinson's disease. Therefore, L-dopa should not be taken with B_6 supplements.

Finally, studies have found that taking 200 mg of B_6 for more than a month can result in a type of dependency in which deficiency symptoms appear when the supplements are stopped.

Preparation and Handling

Processing destroys 35 to 85 percent of vitamin B_6, depending upon the type of processing. For example, milling wheat into flour destroys more than 80 percent of the vitamin; even so, B_6 is not included in most enriched grain products. Ordinary cooking destroys about half the B_6 in vegetables and fruits; this can be minimized by using minimal water or steaming vegetables.

VITAMIN B$_{12}$ (COBALAMIN)

Vitamin B$_{12}$ is yet another of the water-soluble B-complex group that is essential for proper metabolism of the macronutrients—carbohydrates, protein, and fat. It is also needed to form red blood cells and choline (another B vitamin), maintain nerve tissue, and properly metabolize homocysteine, a naturally occurring substance linked to an increased risk of heart disease.

Vitamin B$_{12}$, the largest and most recently discovered of the B-complex family, has a somewhat checkered history. Ever since the late 1940s, researchers have known that B$_{12}$, or cobalamin, is essential to prevent pernicious anemia, a disease that occurs mostly among older adults. But soon after its discovery in 1948, some practitioners built thriving businesses of administering B$_{12}$ shots, claiming the vitamin possessed remarkable abilities to energize and rejuvenate. Mainstream physicians denounced the B$_{12}$ therapy as quackery and even dangerous. But recent research is turning the tables. While B$_{12}$ is not a magical fountain of youth, it does appear to alleviate a number of neurological and psychological problems and promote a sense of well-being.

Dietary B$_{12}$ is found only in animal products. (The small amounts that are made by bacteria in the human digestive tract do not appear to be absorbed.) About 70 percent of B$_{12}$, when consumed in moderate amounts throughout the day, is absorbed in a complicated, three-hour process that requires intrinsic factor, a substance secreted by the stomach. It is the only B vitamin that is stored in fairly large amounts; on average, an adult's liver has enough B$_{12}$ to last for three to five years.

Deficiency results in pernicious anemia, a potentially fatal disease. It occurs mostly among people with stomach disorders that prevent the production of intrinsic factor; strict (vegan) vegetarians who do not take B$_{12}$ supplements sometimes develop pernicious anemia, but this usually takes a number of years because even vegan foods often contain bacteria and other contaminants that provide small amounts of B$_{12}$.

Why It's Needed

The numerous functions of vitamin B$_{12}$ include:

Metabolism. In the body, vitamin B$_{12}$ is transformed into coenzymes that are needed to properly metabolize carbohydrates and fat. Its role in protein metabolism is not as clearly understood, but researchers have established that the requirements for B$_{12}$ go up or down according to the amount of protein in the diet. In addition, it is necessary to make various enzymes, choline, and genetic material (DNA and RNA).

Maintaining nerve tissue. Vitamin B$_{12}$ is necessary for the synthesis of myelin, the fatty material that forms a protective sheath around nerve

◉ REQUIREMENTS
0.3 mcg for infants under 6 months
0.5 mcg for infants 6 to 12 months
0.7 mcg for children 1 to 3 years
1.0 mcg for children 4 to 6
1.4 mcg for children 7 to 10
2.0 mcg for males and females 11 and older
2.2 mcg during pregnancy
2.6 mcg during breast-feeding

◉ SUPPLEMENT FORMS
Oral vitamin B$_{12}$ is available as pills, capsules, and sublingual tablets that are placed under the tongue to be absorbed into the bloodstream. People who cannot properly absorb B$_{12}$ from the intestinal tract usually require injectable forms, although some may be able to get enough with the sublingual or nasal aerosol forms.

◉ SIGNS OF DEFICIENCY
Symptoms of mild to moderate deficiency include fatigue, weakness, loss of weight, sore tongue, numbness and tingling sensations, back pain, depression, anxiety, and other nerve or psychological problems. Severe deficiency can lead to pernicious anemia, which causes pallor, shortness of breath, easy bruising and bleeding problems, sore tongue, unsteady gait, depression, and other mental disturbances.

◉ SIGNS OF OVERDOSE
There are no symptoms of overdose from oral vitamin B$_{12}$; excessive amounts taken by injection may cause skin problems, which clear up when the injections are stopped or the dosage is reduced.

◉ BEST SOURCES
Liver and other organ meats
Lean meat, poultry, fish, and shellfish
Eggs
Milk, cheese, and other dairy products

- In 1925, a University of Rochester researcher proved that liver cured anemia in dogs. The following year, a team of Harvard researchers proved that liver cured pernicious anemia.

- In 1948, researchers working independently in England and the United States isolated a red pigment from liver that they named vitamin B_{12}. Later that year, a Columbia University researcher demonstrated that injections of the substance cured patients suffering from pernicious anemia—a disease that had been considered incurable and invariably fatal.

- In 1955, researchers at Oxford University and Harvard synthesized vitamin B_{12} from cultures of bacteria and fungi—a method that is still used.

cells. Some researchers theorize that it may also protect against Alzheimer's disease, but more study is needed to establish this.

Making red blood cells. Vitamin B_{12} is necessary in order for red blood cells to mature properly in the bone marrow. Without sufficient B_{12}, the blood is flooded with large, immature cells (blasts), which can cause megaloblastic anemia.

Therapeutic Uses and Dosages

Pernicious anemia. This disease is usually treated with daily injections of 15 to 30 mcg of vitamin B_{12}. After symptoms subside, monthly 30-mcg injections are given. In the rare cases in which vegetarians develop pernicious anemia, a daily oral supplement may be substituted for the monthly injections. There are also new B_{12} supplements that are taken by nasal inhalation or in pills placed under the tongue (sublingual), which allow the vitamin to be absorbed directly into the bloodstream.

Nerve and psychological disorders. Mild B_{12} deficiency results in a variety of neuropsychiatric symptoms, including memory loss, confusion, decreased reflexes, difficulty walking, impaired touch and pain perception, depression, and anxiety. In one study involving elderly patients with such symptoms, daily B_{12} supplements resulted in dramatic improvement in all thirty-nine participants. Recommended dosages range from 100 to 500 mcg. Higher dosages (up to 1,000 mcg a day) may be helpful in alleviating numbness, tingling, and tinnitis (ringing in the ears).

Sprue. This disease, characterized by an abnormality in the small intestine that prevents proper absorption of nutrients, is treated with a combination of vitamin B_{12} and folacin. The precise dosages should be prescribed by a doctor.

Other possible therapeutic uses include:

Fatigue. Even a mild B_{12} deficiency can cause fatigue and apathy—vague symptoms that many alternative practitioners have long treated with B_{12} injections. Although more research is needed to demonstrate the value of such injections, there are thousands of people who maintain that the shots give them renewed vigor, improved appetite, and an enhanced sense of well-being. Many doctors recommend supplements of 500 to 1,000 mcg, especially for older patients who may have an impaired ability to absorb the vitamin. Supplements in these amounts should be taken along with 400 to 800 mcg of folacin.

Allergies. Recent studies indicate that vitamin B_{12} may be helpful in blocking certain allergens, especially sulfites—preservatives that are added to wine and many foods. In one double-blind study, sulfite-sensitive patients were given either 2,000 mcg of sublingual B_{12} or a placebo; seventeen out of eighteen receiving the B_{12} did not develop their usual symptoms (asthma, headache, and nasal congestion or dripping) after ingesting sulfites. Other studies have found that 2,000 to 4,000 mcg (2 to 4 mg) of B_{12} can prevent most sulfite allergy symptoms.

Protection against cancer in smokers. Cigarette smoke contains substances that reduce levels of vitamin B_{12} and folacin in lung tissue. In a recent study, researchers recruited seventy-three men who had smoked a pack a day for twenty or more years. None had lung cancer, but they all had precancerous changes in their bronchial tissue. The men were divided into two groups—those in one were given 500 mcg of B_{12} and 10 mg of folacin a day, while the second group received a placebo. After four months, the men who received the vitamins had significantly fewer precancerous cells than the placebo group. The researchers caution, however, that more study is needed and, even if the vitamins do turn out to be protective, they cannot compete with the long list of benefits gained by not smoking.

Multiple sclerosis. Some preliminary studies indicate that 1,000 mcg of B_{12} a day may help slow the progression of this disease, in which destruction of the myelin results in loss of nerve function.

Special Cautions

High doses of vitamin B_{12} should be matched by comparable amounts of folacin, a member of the B-complex group that works with B_{12}.

Strict vegetarians should not rely on claims that spirulina, sea vegetables, tempeh, miso, brewer's yeast, and other such products provide adequate vitamin B_{12}. Analyses of these products found only traces (if any) of B_{12}, certainly not enough to prevent eventual deficiency. In addition, babies born to vegetarian mothers often have low B_{12} reserves; this can be prevented by taking supplements during pregnancy and breast-feeding.

Preparation and Handling

Ordinary cooking destroys about one-third of the B_{12} in most animal foods. An exception is milk pasteurization, which kills only about 10 percent of the vitamin. Vitamin B_{12} is also destroyed by light; thus, milk should be kept in opaque or cardboard containers. The presence of vitamin C (ascorbic acid) appears to increase vitamin B_{12} heat sensitivity and increase its loss during cooking.

BIOTIN

Biotin, a member of the water-soluble family of B vitamins, is a coenzyme that is essential to transform blood sugar (glucose) into energy. It

There are no official RDAs for biotin; the following amounts are estimated to be safe and adequate:

10 mcg for infants under 6 months
15 mcg for infants 6 to 12 months
20 mcg for children 1 to 3 years
25 mcg for children 4 to 6
30 mcg for children 7 to 10
30–100 mcg for everyone 11 and older

SUPPLEMENT FORMS
Biotin is usually included in B-complex capsules, pills, and tablets. It is also available as an individual nutrient.

SIGNS OF DEFICIENCY
Deficiency is rare, but when it occurs, symptoms may include:

- Itchy, dry skin and hair loss.
- Inflamed, sore tongue.
- Loss of appetite, nausea, and vomiting.
- Muscle pain.
- Depression.

SIGNS OF OVERDOSE
There are no known toxic effects, although long-term high doses can interfere with the absorption of other B vitamins and result in their deficiency.

BEST SOURCES
Kidney, liver, and other organ meats
Mushrooms
Wheat bran and whole grains
Eggs
Nuts, peanut butter, and legumes
Cauliflower
Sardines and salmon

A LITTLE HISTORY
- In 1936, a group of German researchers isolated a substance from cooked egg yolks that they called biotin.
- In 1937, a Hungarian scientist fed laboratory animals a substance that he called vitamin H to prevent deficiency symptoms caused by feeding raw egg whites. The following year, the substance was found to be identical to biotin.
- In 1943, American researchers synthesized biotin.

works closely with pantothenic acid to form fatty acids and carry out numerous body processes.

Biotin is found in many foods; it is also made by intestinal bacteria, but it is not known how much—if any—of this is absorbed by the body. Deficiency is rare, but can be induced by consuming large amounts of raw egg white, which contains a substance (avidin) that binds with biotin and prevents its absorption. Cooking inactivates avidin and releases biotin in a usable form.

Why It's Needed

Metabolism. Like most of the other B-complex family, biotin acts as a coenzyme in the metabolism of carbohydrates, fats, and protein. It is needed to form fatty acids and purines, which are used to make genetic material (DNA and RNA).

Therapeutic Uses and Dosages

Therapeutic doses of biotin are usually given along with pantothenic acid, choline, and thiamin. Possible uses include:

Brittle nails. Swiss researchers found that 1,000 to 1,200 mcg (1 to 1.2 mg) of biotin increased nail thickness by an average of 25 percent in two-thirds of study participants. Allow six months for improvement to occur.

Hair loss. Although biotin cannot cure or slow most balding, it can help restore hair growth in persons whose baldness is related to nutritional deficiencies. Dosages are similar to those used to treat thin, brittle nails.

Diabetes. Some studies indicate that high doses of biotin may improve blood sugar (glucose) control as well as help prevent diabetes-related nerve problems. A nutritionist or physician trained in nutritional diabetes therapy should determine the appropriate dosage.

Special Cautions

Biotin is included in some protein supplements that are promoted to improve athletic performance. There is no proof, however, that these products actually work, and long-term use may result in kidney damage due to their high-protein content.

Preparation and Handling

Biotin is relatively stable and resistant to heat, but it is destroyed by strong acids, alkali, and exposure to oxygen and ultraviolet light. Milling destroys much of the biotin in whole grains.

FOLACIN (FOLATE, FOLIC ACID)

Folacin—another of the essential B vitamins—is actually a group of compounds that include folic acid and similar substances. It is essential for making genetic material (DNA and RNA) and red blood cells, healing wounds, and building muscle tissue. It is also instrumental in a number of metabolic functions, including the synthesis of choline (another B vitamin) and the formation of various amino acids—the building blocks of proteins. It works closely with vitamins B_6 and B_{12} to, among other functions, protect against heart disease by controlling blood levels of homocysteine, a by-product of protein metabolism. In recent years, the critical role of folacin in fetal development has gained widespread public notice.

Folacin is found in many foods, especially organ meats, green leafy vegetables, oranges and orange juice, and whole-wheat bread and cereals. Deficiency can result in megaloblastic anemia, a disorder in which red blood cells fail to mature normally. It most commonly develops in babies and in women during pregnancy.

Why It's Needed

Functions of folacin include:

Metabolism. Folacin coenzymes are necessary for the formation of compounds needed to synthesize DNA and RNA, critical genetic material. It is also instrumental in the metabolism of several amino acids and in controlling levels of homocysteine.

Growth and development. The critical role that folacin plays in the synthesis of DNA and RNA is instrumental to proper cell division, growth, and development.

Fetal development. It is now well known that folacin deficiency in early pregnancy greatly increases the risk of birth defects, especially spina bifida and other abnormalities affecting the brain and nerves. Folacin deficiency also increases the risk of miscarriage and serious pregnancy complications, including pre-eclampsia (toxemia of pregnancy) and placental abnormalities.

Making red blood cells. Folacin is needed to form heme, the protein that contains iron in red blood cells. Thus, folacin deficiency may result in anemia, even in the presence of adequate iron.

Therapeutic Uses and Dosages

Megaloblastic anemia. High doses of folic acid, which may be given with or without vitamin B_{12}, are used to treat this form of anemia, which

REQUIREMENTS
25 mcg for infants under 6 months
35 mcg for infants 6 to 12 months
50 mcg for children 1 to 3 years
75 mcg for children 4 to 6
100 mcg for children 7 to 10
150 mcg for children 11 to 14
200 mcg for males 15 and older
180 mcg for females 15 and older
400 mcg during pregnancy*
280 mcg during breast-feeding*

*Some experts recommend that women take 800 mcg of folacin during pregnancy and 500 mcg when breast-feeding.

SUPPLEMENT FORMS
Folacin is available in tablet, capsule, powder, and liquid forms; it may be sold under other names, including vitamin B_9, folic acid, and folate. Supplements should be taken along with vitamin B_{12} to avoid a situation where the folacin masks a vitamin B_{12} deficiency.

SIGNS OF DEFICIENCY
Severe folacin deficiency causes megoloblastic anemia; symptoms include:

- Fatigue.
- Pallor.
- Shortness of breath and weakness.
- Irritability.

Other deficiency symptoms may include:
- A smooth, red, sore tongue (glossitis).
- Diarrhea and other intestinal upsets.
- Possible depression, memory problems, confusion, and other mental changes.

SIGNS OF OVERDOSE
In general, high doses of folacin are not in themselves toxic, but they may mask vitamin B_{12} deficiency, which can cause permanent nerve damage. Daily dosages should not exceed 1,000 mcg (1 mg).

Liver and other organ meats
Oranges and orange juice
Green leafy vegetables, especially spinach and
   broccoli
Asparagus, celery, and beets
Whole-wheat bread and cereals
Lentils, chickpeas, and other legumes
Nuts

◙ A LITTLE HISTORY

▪ In 1931, a doctor working in a Bombay, India, maternity hospital noted that pregnant women with anemia improved when given yeast extracts. Further research found a group of related vitamins, which was named folacin.

▪ In 1941, a group of Texas researchers found a similar substance in spinach and named it folic acid.

▪ In 1945, folic acid was synthesized and proved an effective treatment for megaloblastic anemia.

▪ In 1998, the U.S. government ordered that a number of common foods be fortified with folacin to help prevent deficiencies, especially among pregnant women and young children.

occurs mostly in infants, pregnant women, and persons taking antiseizure or anticancer drugs that interfere with folacin absorption.

Sprue. In this disease the small intestine is unable to absorb certain nutrients; it is treated with high doses of folacin and vitamin B_{12}

Heart disease treatment and prevention. Preliminary studies indicate that folacin may help prevent coronary artery disease by controlling high levels of homocysteine. Recommended dosages range from 400 to 800 mcg a day, taken with similar high dosages of vitamins B_6 and B_{12}.

Special Cautions

Oral contraceptives interfere with folacin absorption; women taking "the pill" should take supplements of folacin and other B-complex vitamins. Folacin supplements of 400 to 800 mcg a day are especially important for women who stop taking "the pill" with the intention of conceiving.

Alcohol and large amounts of coffee and tea also reduce folacin absorption. So, too, do a number of medications, including corticosteroids, barbiturates, phenytoin and other antiseizure medications, sulfa drugs, some antibiotics and anticancer drugs, and high-dose aspirin, which is sometimes prescribed to treat rheumatoid arthritis. When taking any medication—either prescription or over-the-counter—ask your doctor or pharmacist whether it is likely to hinder your body's ability to absorb folacin and other essential nutrients and what you should do to compensate for the interaction.

Preparation and Handling

Half or more of the folacin in food is lost during processing and cooking. Also, vegetables stored at room temperature can lose 50 to 70 percent of their folacin in only two or three days. Refrigerate fresh vegetables and, whenever possible, eat them raw. Those that must be cooked should be steamed or stir-fried using only minimal water.

Minerals

Minerals are compounds that come from the soil and are neither animal nor plant substances. So far, fifteen minerals have been identified as essential to maintain human health. Some, such as calcium and phosphorus, are present in the body in relatively large amounts and have multiple functions. Others, such as cobalt and iodine, are barely detectable in the body and appear to have single, very specialized roles. Overall, however, minerals are responsible for the following functions:

- They give bones their strength and rigidity.
- They control the body's fluid, biochemical, and acid-base balances.
- They play important metabolic roles by activating enzyme systems and working in concert with vitamins, other minerals, and hormones.

As with vitamin deficiencies, lack of a specific mineral can produce disease symptoms; iron-deficiency anemia is one of the most common examples. Similarly, excessive amounts can result in dangerous toxicity; in fact, iron overdoses are the most common cause of accidental childhood poisoning deaths in the United States.

Historic Overview

Ancient healers recognized various mineral deficiency diseases, and although the substances had not yet been identified, they devised appropriate treatments. For example, a five-thousand-year-old Chinese medical text recommends seaweed and sponges—rich sources of iodine—to treat goiter, a thyroid disease caused by iodine deficiency.

Many cultures learned that adding a rusty nail or piece of iron to vats of beer and wine eased anemia symptoms. It wasn't until the early 1800s, that researchers began to isolate minerals. The first to be discovered, by a British chemist, were calcium, sodium, potassium, magnesium, sulfur, and chlorine. In 1801, a Swedish chemist measured the calcium and phosphorus content of bone, and later discovered that iron was essential to make hemoglobin—the oxygen-carrying molecule in red blood cells.

Throughout the twentieth century, researchers continued to identify the functions of a growing list of essential minerals. The latest to be added to the list (in 1972) were fluorine and silicon. And nutrition scientists think that there are still others waiting to be discovered.

Classification of Minerals

Minerals are generally classified as macro, meaning they are found in relatively large amounts in the body, and micro or trace elements, which are needed in very small amounts. (The essential macro minerals are: calcium, phosphorus, magnesium, sodium, chloride, and potassium. The essential trace elements, or micro minerals are: iron, zinc, iodine, copper, manganese, molybdenum, fluoride, selenium, and chromium.) The body's ability to absorb minerals varies according to need; for example, a person who is anemic will absorb more iron than someone with normal reserves of the mineral.

In general, a balanced and varied diet based on the Food Guide Pyramid should meet normal needs for most minerals, but there are exceptions. During pregnancy, it is difficult, if not impossible, for a woman to get all the iron and calcium that she needs for herself and her growing fetus from diet alone. Because minerals come from the soil, geography also plays a role. Historically, people who lived in inland or mountainous areas where the soil is deficient in iodine tended to develop goiters and other forms of thyroid disease. Such deficiencies are now rare, however, because many common foods are fortified with scarce minerals and modern transportation makes it possible to get food from distant places.

The Question of Supplements

Caution is needed when it comes to taking mineral supplements because even small doses of some are toxic. Multivitamin pills include a few minerals, especially calcium, magnesium, and zinc, typically in amounts of 50 to 150 percent of the Recommended Dietary Allowance. For most people, these supplements are safe. Otherwise, you should consult a doctor before taking any mineral supplement in amounts higher than the RDA. The following section discusses the fifteen minerals that are considered essential for human health.

CALCIUM (CA)

Calcium is the most abundant mineral in the human body, making up about 2 percent of total weight—typically 27 to 32 ounces in adult women and 35 to 45 ounces in males. About 99 percent of this calcium is stored in the bones and teeth, and the remaining 1 percent circulates in the blood and is found in muscles, nerves, and other soft tissue.

Only about 20 to 30 percent of dietary calcium is actually absorbed from the intestinal tract into the bloodstream. (Slightly more is absorbed in times of increased need, such as during pregnancy, a childhood growth spurt, or the healing of a broken bone.)

Why It's Needed

The numerous functions of calcium include the following:

Building bones and teeth. Calcium gives bones their strength and hardness. Although bones appear to be rock hard and static, in reality, bone tissue changes constantly as calcium (and other minerals) move in and out—a process called remodeling.

Controlling muscle function and maintaining the heartbeat. Muscle tissue, especially the heart, requires small amounts of calcium in order to contract and relax normally.

Transmitting nerve impulses. Calcium is needed in order for a nerve cell to transmit its messages to other nerves or to muscles. In addition, calcium inside cells transmits messages to special receptors. Some of these messages are instrumental in controlling blood pressure and other body functions.

Promoting blood clotting and wound healing. Calcium is one of fourteen essential factors that are directly involved in the formation of blood clots and start the process of wound healing.

Miscellaneous other functions include acting as a coenzyme in various metabolic activities, controlling the permeability of membranes to allow nutrients to pass through cell walls, and helping synthesize hormones and enzymes necessary for digestion. Recent research indicates that calcium may also protect against colon cancer.

Therapeutic Uses and Dosages

Calcium supplements are important in preventing and treating osteoporosis, the demineralization of bones that is especially common among older women. Calcium supplements should be taken in dosages of 500 to 600 mg two or three times a day, depending upon how much calcium is obtained from foods. In order to absorb calcium, it's helpful to take

◎ REQUIREMENTS

400 mg for infants under 6 months
600 mg for infants 6 to 12 months
800 mg for children 1 to 10 years
1,200 mg for males and females 11 to 24
1,000 mg for males and females 51 or older*
1,300 mg during pregnancy and breast-feeding

*Many experts recommend 1,500 mg or more for people who have or are at high risk of developing osteoporosis.

◎ SUPPLEMENT FORMS

Calcium supplements are available in tablet, capsule, liquid, and powder forms. Check supplement labels to determine the type of calcium (e.g., carbonate, citrate, gluconate, malate, etc.) and the amount of elemental calcium. Calcium citrate is the most readily absorbed; but calcium carbonate is reasonably well absorbed. Some of the new chewable supplements may be more absorbable than small, hard pills. (To determine the degree of absorbability, place a calcium pill in a half cup of vinegar and stir every few minutes. After thirty minutes, at least 75 percent of the pill should be dissolved.) Do not take more than 600 mg of calcium at a time; instead, distribute intake throughout the day. Take supplements with small amounts of food to increase the flow of stomach acids, which are necessary to dissolve the calcium salts.

◎ SIGNS OF DEFICIENCY

Children who suffer from severe calcium deficiency develop rickets, a disease marked by poor growth and soft, malformed bones; the adult counterpart is called osteomalacia. (Inability to utilize vitamin D can also cause childhood rickets). Long-term calcium deficiency contributes to osteoporosis, which is especially common among older people. Low blood levels of calcium can cause muscle spasms and cramps.

◎ SIGNS OF OVERDOSE

A daily calcium intake of 2,500 mg—from a combination of food and supplements—appears to be safe. However, very high doses may contribute to kidney stones, and calcium carbonate can cause gas and constipation. Long-term calcium overdoses can result in calcium deposits in body tissues, including heart muscle, and cause muscle and abdominal pain.

Low-fat milk, cheese, yogurt, and other milk products
Canned salmon and sardines (with bones)
Broccoli, kale, and collard, dandelion, and turnip greens
Almonds and dates
Cantaloupe, Cassaba, and honeydew melons
Dried beans, lima beans, and other legumes
Tofu, soy milk, and other soy products

■ A LITTLE HISTORY

▪ In 1801, a Swedish chemist named Berzelius analyzed the calcium and phosphorus content of bones.

▪ In the 1840s, a Swiss physician was honored for his studies showing that pigeons grew normally when calcium carbonate was added to their diet of wheat and water.

▪ Calcium's role in muscle and nerve function were not discovered until the early twentieth century, and researchers are continuing to find new functions for this essential mineral.

■ REQUIREMENTS

400 mg for infants under 6 months
600 mg for infants 6 to 12 months
800 mg for children 1 to 10 years
1,200 mg for males and females 11 to 24
800 mg for males and females 25 to 50
1,200 mg during pregnancy and breast-feeding

■ SUPPLEMENT FORMS

Phosphorus is available in capsule, tablet, powder, and liquid forms.

---

200 to 400 IU of vitamin D with each calcium pill (many calcium supplements combine the two). Other factors that enhance calcium absorption include lactose (milk sugar), adequate stomach and intestinal acids, and certain proteins (amino acids), especially lysine and arginine. In contrast, many factors interfere with calcium absorption; these include:

- *Phosphorus imbalance.* Calcium and phosphorus should be consumed in about equal amounts. The balance can be upset by consuming large amounts of meat or phosphorous-containing soft drinks (especially colas and diet soft drinks), resulting in reduced absorption and increased excretion of calcium.
- *Bran and dietary fiber.* The phytic acid in bran and dietary fibers bind with calcium to inhibit its absorption. The oxalic acid in foods like spinach, beet greens, Swiss chard, rhubarb, and cocoa have a similar effect.
- *High-fat intake.* Fats, especially the highly saturated animal fats, reduce absorption by combining with calcium to form a soapy compound.
- *Tea.* The tannins in tea bind with calcium to reduce its absorption. Do not drink tea within two hours of taking a calcium pill.
- *Miscellaneous factors.* that reduce calcium absorption include stress, aging, lack of weight-bearing exercise, and use of antacids that contain aluminum and magnesium.

Special Cautions

Do not take calcium supplements that are made of bonemeal, dolomite, or oyster shells, all of which may be contaminated by lead, arsenic, mercury, and other dangerous metals. Excessive calcium intake can interfere with the body's ability to absorb iron, zinc, magnesium, and other essential minerals.

PHOSPHORUS (P)

Phosphorus is the second most abundant mineral in the body, exceeded only by calcium, making up about 1 percent of average body weight. About 85 percent of the body's phosphorus is bound with calcium to form calcium phosphate, which gives bones their strength and hardness. In addition, the small amounts of phosphorus present in all body cells are essential to many metabolic and body processes.

Phosphorus is found in almost all animal foods, especially milk and meat. Soft drinks (colas) and many processed foods are also high in phosphorus. The body absorbs about 70 percent of phosphorus from the diet, compared with only 20 to 30 percent of calcium.

Why It's Needed

In addition to working with calcium and other minerals to build strong bones and teeth, phosphorus is a part of all body cells; it is also a component of genetic material (RNA and DNA) and phospholipids, compounds that carry cholesterol and other fatty substances in the blood. It is also needed for normal milk secretion during breast-feeding. Its numerous other functions include:

- Strengthening cell membranes.
- Helping to build muscle tissue.
- Helping to maintain the body's normal acid-base and fluid balances.
- Working with various enzyme systems to metabolize energy and form and metabolize proteins.

Therapeutic Uses and Dosages

Supplements are needed only in very unusual circumstances, such as the recovery from severe burns or part of the treatment for kidney and digestive diseases. They should be taken only under the supervision of a doctor or clinical dietitian.

Special Cautions

Phosphorus and calcium should be consumed in about equal amounts—known as the calcium-phosphorus ratio. The average diet provides more than enough phosphorus—about 1,000 to 1,500 mg a day. In fact, many experts believe that Americans consume too much phosphorus, especially those who eat a lot of meat and processed foods and drink large amounts of soft drinks (colas and diet sodas), which tend to be high in phosphorus. Consequently, most Americans consume more phosphorus than they do calcium, an imbalance that causes the bones to release extra calcium and increases the risk of osteoporosis.

MAGNESIUM (MG)

Magnesium is the fourth most abundant mineral in the body. About 60 percent is found in the bones and teeth; 28 percent is in the muscles,

◙ **SIGNS OF DEFICIENCY**

Deficiency is very rare, and is virtually unknown in humans. However, it can be produced in rabbits and other laboratory animals by feeding them a diet of plants grown in low-phosphorus soils. Under these circumstances, deficiency symptoms include:

- Poor growth and abnormal bone formation, resulting in bone pain and rickets.
- Muscle weakness.
- Loss of appetite and weight.

Some experts theorize that strict (vegan) vegetarians who eat only foods grown in phosphorus-depleted soils may also develop phosphorus deficiency, but this has not been proven.

◙ **SIGNS OF OVERDOSE**

Excessive intake of phosphorus interferes with normal calcium metabolism and can accelerate the loss of bone calcium.

◙ **BEST SOURCES**

Most animal products, including meat, poultry, fish, eggs, and milk
Peas, beans, and other legumes, especially when grown in phosphate-rich soil
Soft drinks, including diet sodas
Processed foods, in which various phosphates are used as additives

◙ **A LITTLE HISTORY**

- In 1669, a German alchemist discovered phosphorus in human urine. At the time, the discovery created tremendous interest because before that, phosphorus was known only in its free forms—which glow in the dark or catch fire spontaneously when exposed to air.

◙ **REQUIREMENTS**

The Recommended Dietary Allowances, as established by the National Academy of Sciences, are:

40 mg for infants under 6 months
60 mg for infants 6 to 12 months
80 mg for children 1 to 3 years

120 mg for children 4 to 6
170 mg for children 7 to 10
270 for males 11 to 14
400 mg for males 15 to 18
350 mg for males 19 and older
280 mg for females 11 to 14
300 mg for females 15 to 18
280 mg for females 19 and older
320 mg during pregnancy
366 mg during breast-feeding

◉ **SUPPLEMENT FORMS**
Magnesium is included in some calcium supplements and many multiple vitamin and mineral pills.

◉ **SIGNS OF DEFICIENCY**
Magnesium deficiency severe enough to cause symptoms is usually the result of other disorders, such as kidney disease, alcoholism, malabsorption disorders, and hyperparathyroidism, a hormonal disorder. Consequences of long-term mild deficiency include an increased risk of high blood pressure and heart disease. More severe deficiency may cause:

- An irregular heartbeat.
- Fatigue.
- Painful muscle spasms.
- Jittery nerves, confusion, fatigue, and personality changes.

◉ **SIGNS OF OVERDOSE**
Toxicity is rare because the kidneys excrete excess magnesium. In the presence of kidney disease, however, high doses of magnesium can cause muscle weakness, breathing problems, and lethargy and mental confusion.

◉ **BEST SOURCES**
Peas, beans, and other legumes
Whole-grain breads and cereals
Dark green vegetables
Nuts
Cocoa
Some types of mineral water
Antacids and laxatives that contain magnesium

◉ **A LITTLE HISTORY**
- In 1810, a British chemist named Sir Humphrey Davy isolated magnesium.
- In 1926, a French researcher proved that magnesium is an essential nutrient for laboratory animals, and over the following two decades, other researchers identified deficiency symptoms in both animals and humans.

liver, and other soft tissues; and 2 percent is in the body fluids. It is essential to build bones and teeth and numerous metabolic functions; magnesium is also an ingredient in some antacids and laxatives and is used to prevent premature birth and treat certain types of convulsions and rapid heartbeats (tachycardia). Recent research indicates that magnesium deficiency may be a factor in the development of atherosclerosis and coronary artery disease—the major cause of heart attacks.

Why It's Needed

Magnesium works with calcium and phosphorus to build strong bones and teeth; it also plays roles in the following functions:

Normal metabolism. Magnesium activates many enzymes and works with others to carry out some three hundred metabolic functions, including protein digestion and synthesis, energy production, and the synthesis of insulin.

Proper nerve and muscle function. Magnesium is needed to transmit nerve impulses; it also allows muscles to relax after contraction, a critical factor in heart function.

Stimulating calcium function. By acting as a calcium antagonist, it balances the role of calcium in regulating the heartbeat and other functions.

Preventing dental cavities. Magnesium strengthens dental enamel and makes the teeth less vulnerable to decay.

Miscellaneous other functions include promoting immunity, making DNA, and boosting the actions of potassium and some of the B vitamins. It may also aid in the treatment of asthma, cardiac arrhythmias, high blood pressure, fibromyalgia, and diabetes.

Therapeutic Uses and Dosages

Researchers are constantly expanding the list of conditions that benefit from magnesium. For example, one large-scale study indicates that daily supplements of 400 mg of magnesium significantly reduce the risk of atherosclerosis and heart disease; other studies show that 500 mg a day may help lower high blood pressure and improve insulin metabolism in diabetes. The recommended dosage to treat cardiac arrhythmias and asthma is 400 mg taken twice a day.

Preliminary research indicates that magnesium may be helpful in treating or preventing migraine headaches; one study found that some fibromyalgia patients improved on twice-a-day doses of 150 mg of magnesium combined with 600 mg of malic acid.

Special Cautions

Magnesium supplements should be balanced with an increased intake of calcium to obtain the maximum benefits of both minerals. Dietary factors that reduce magnesium absorption include high intakes of calcium and phosphates, fats, bran and whole grains, and spinach, rhubarb, and other foods high in oxalic acid.

Magnesium supplements reduce the effectiveness of tetracycline, a common antibiotic. Supplements should not be taken by patients with kidney disease unless it is specifically ordered by a doctor.

SODIUM (NA)

Sodium, along with chloride, forms table salt—the major dietary source of both minerals. Sodium, potassium, and chloride are electrolytes—minerals that have electrical properties when they are dissolved in a salty medium, such as the fluid portion of blood. Electrolytes are essential to maintain the proper balance of fluids and body chemicals. The average adult body contains about 100 grams (or about 3.5 ounces) of sodium.

Americans are often cautioned about the risks of our typical high-salt diet, which can worsen high blood pressure and increase the workload of the kidneys and heart. But at one time in human history, salt was scarce in many inland parts of the world. Wars were fought to gain control of salt mines and, in some places, it was actually more precious than gold.

Today, of course, salt is inexpensive and plentiful; next to sugar, it is our most widely used food flavoring.

Why It's Needed

Sodium is found in the fluid surrounding all body cells. Scientists theorize that when living creatures emerged from the world's salty primordial waters to live on land, they carried some of the sea within them in the form of salty body fluids. Sodium's specific functions include:

Maintaining body chemistry. Sodium is necessary to maintain the proper balance of fluids, acids, and bases.

Promoting nerve and muscle function. Sodium is a positively charged ion that is instrumental in transmitting nerve messages and prompting muscles to contract.

Other miscellaneous functions include promoting the proper absorption and metabolism of carbohydrates; sodium is also a component of sweat, tears, bile, and pancreatic digestive juices.

◉ REQUIREMENTS

There are no Recommended Dietary Allowances (RDAs) for sodium; the following are the estimated minimum requirements established by the National Academy of Sciences:

120 mg for infants under 6 months
200 mg for infants 6 to 12 months
225 mg for children 1 to 2 years
300 mg for children 3 to 5
400 mg for children 6 to 9
500 mg for everyone 10 and older

Use one of these formulas to calculate the amount of sodium in salt:

1 teaspoon of salt contains 2.1 g of sodium
2.5 g (2,500 mg) of salt contains 1 g of sodium

◉ SUPPLEMENT FORMS

People who are seriously dehydrated may be given intravenous fluids containing sodium and chloride; otherwise, depleted sodium reserves can be restored by taking ordinary table salt and extra fluids, such as orange juice, which is also high in potassium.

◉ SIGNS OF DEFICIENCY

Symptoms may include:

- Muscle cramps.
- Nausea and/or diarrhea.
- Headache.

In addition to the above, heat exhaustion is marked by reduced sweating, dry lips and skin, very high fever, and possible delirium and loss of consciousness.

Toxicity can develop when large amounts of salt are consumed without adequate fluids. Babies are especially vulnerable to salt toxicity.

BEST SOURCES

Table salt, monosodium glutamate (MSG), and baking soda

Bacon and other salt-cured meats and fish

Frankfurters, luncheon meats, corned beef, and other preserved meats

Pickles, green olives, and other pickled foods

Potato chips, pretzels, and other snack foods

Many breads, cereals, and baked goods

Canned vegetables and soups and soup mixes

Commercial salad dressings

A LITTLE HISTORY

- Although ancient people used salt and other compounds containing sodium, the element was not isolated until 1807 when an English chemist did so.
- In 1918, researchers demonstrated that sodium is essential to maintain health and life in a series of animal experiments.

REQUIREMENTS

Table salt is about 60 percent chloride and 40 percent sodium, so a diet that includes even a little salt provides ample chloride. There are no Recommended Dietary Allowances (RDAs) for chloride; the following are the estimated minimum requirements established by the National Academy of Sciences:

180 mg for infants under 6 months

300 mg for infants 6 to 12 months

350 mg for children 1 to 2 years

500 mg for children 3 to 5

600 mg for children 6 to 9

750 mg for everyone 10 and older

Therapeutic Uses and Dosages

Extra sodium may be needed during times of extreme fluid loss (dehydration), such as prolonged diarrhea and/or vomiting and excessive sweating. People with Addison's disease, a disorder affecting the adrenal glands, excrete excessive sodium in the urine. In these unusual circumstances, extra salt (and perhaps potassium) and fluids are given to restore the body's normal balance. In addition, there are a few people who have abnormally low blood pressure (hypotension) and may experience dizziness and other symptoms when they abruptly shift positions. These people may need to add more salty foods to their diets. Otherwise, sodium supplements are rarely if ever necessary.

Special Cautions

Most Americans consume much more sodium than they need, which can be a serious problem for those who have a genetic predisposition to develop high blood pressure. For them, the excessive sodium intake increases the blood's fluid volume, meaning that the heart must work harder to raise the pressure needed to pump the expanded amount of blood through the body. Untreated high blood pressure greatly increases the risk of a heart attack, stroke, and kidney failure.

CHLORIDE (C1)

Chloride, or chlorine as it is also known, partners with sodium to form ordinary table salt (sodium chloride). As an electrolyte, it works with sodium and potassium to maintain the body's balance of acid-base and fluids. On average, the adult body contains about 100 grams (or about 3.5 ounces) of chloride. The highest concentrations are found in the stomach and the fluid that surrounds the brain and spinal cord (cerebrospinal fluid). As with sodium, it is also a component of the fluids surrounding cells.

Why It's Needed

The functions of chloride closely parallel those of sodium, and include the following:

Maintaining the body's proper chemical and fluid balance. Chloride is a negatively charged ion that works with the positively charged sodium and potassium ions to maintain the body's delicate biochemical balance and regulate osmotic pressure and fluid and acid-base balances.

Promoting red blood cell function. Most of the body's chloride is found in the fluid surrounding cells (extracellular fluid), but it can enter red blood cells to maintain an equilibrium between the cell's contents and the fluid surrounding it. This ability to move in and out of the red blood cells allows the blood to carry large amounts of waste carbon dioxide to the lungs, where it is exchanged for oxygen.

Making stomach acids. Chloride is needed to make hydrochloric acid, which the body needs to activate the enzymes that break down starches. The body also needs hydrochloric acid to absorb vitamin B_{12} and iron.

Protecting against bacteria and other micro-organisms. Hydrochloric acid destroys most of the bacteria and other micro-organisms that make their way to the stomach. Chlorine—a derivative of chloride is a common disinfectant; it is used to purify water in swimming pools, and many cities add it to municipal water supplies.

Therapeutic Uses and Dosages

A diet that includes moderate amounts of salt provides ample chloride. However, supplements may be needed by people who are on a very strict low-salt diet because of heart, liver, or kidney disease. Supplements are usually taken in the form of sodium-free salt substitutes or pills; a doctor or clinical dietitian should determine the appropriate dosage.

Special Cautions

The body's chloride reserves may be depleted by prolonged diarrhea and/or vomiting, overuse of diuretics (water pills), or following a strict low-salt vegetarian diet.

POTASSIUM (K)

Potassium is another mineral that is classified as an electrolyte, a substance that has electrical properties when it is dissolved in the fluid part of the blood. Like sodium and chloride—the other two electrolytes—potassium is involved in maintaining the body's fluid and acid-base balances. It also is essential for proper muscle function and various metabolic processes.

Potassium comprises about 5 percent of the body's mineral content, making it the body's third most abundant element (exceeded only by

◉ **SUPPLEMENT FORMS**
Chloride is available in pill form or as a component of sodium-free salt substitutes. In cases of severe deficiency, chloride may be given as part of intravenous fluids.

◉ **SIGNS OF DEFICIENCY**
A severe chloride deficiency can result in a buildup of alkali in the blood, a condition called alkalosis. Symptoms include:

- Slow, shallow breathing.
- Muscle cramps.
- Loss of appetite and listlessness.
- In extreme cases, convulsions.

◉ **SIGNS OF OVERDOSE**
Toxicity rarely occurs because the kidneys excrete excess chloride.

◉ **BEST SOURCES**
Table salt
Any food prepared with salt (see list under Sodium, p. 246)

◉ **A LITTLE HISTORY**
- In 1774, a Swedish chemist discovered chloride when performing experiments with hydrochloric acid.
- In 1810, an English chemist demonstrated that chloride is an element.

◉ **REQUIREMENTS**
There are no Recommended Dietary Allowances (RDAs) for potassium; the following are the Estimated Minimum Requirements established by the National Academy of Sciences:

500 mg for infants under 6 months
700 mg for infants 6 to 12 months
1,000 mg for children 1 to 2 years
1,400 mg for children 3 to 5
1,600 mg for children 6 to 9
2,000 mg for everyone 10 and older

Supplements come in tablet, liquid, and powdered forms; some salt substitutes are also high in potassium. As stressed earlier, all potassium supplements should be used only under a doctor's supervision.

◙ SIGNS OF DEFICIENCY

Potassium deficiency is rare; when it occurs, symptoms include:

- A rapid, irregular heartbeat.
- Muscle weakness, twitching, and possible paralysis.
- Nausea, vomiting, and diarrhea.
- In extreme cases, cardiac arrest.

◙ SIGNS OF OVERDOSE

It is virtually immmposible to develop potassium toxicity (called hyperkalemia) from food alone, but it can occur when high-dose supplements are used. Babies and people with kidney disease are especially vulnerable. Overdose symptoms include:

- Nausea and vomiting.
- Muscle fatigue.
- Irregular heartbeat and, in extreme cases, cardiac arrest.

◙ BEST SOURCES

Dried fruit, especially peaches and apricots
Blackstrap molasses
Raw or lightly processed fruits and vegetables, especially bananas, tomatoes, oranges, and green leafy vegetables
Soybeans, lima beans, dried peas, and other legumes
Potatoes (cooked with skins on)
Wheat and rice bran
Nuts and seeds

◙ A LITTLE HISTORY

- In 1807, the English chemist Sir Humphry Davy isolated potassium. He gave it its name and the chemical symbol K, for *kalium,* the Latin term for alkali.
- In 1938, researchers using laboratory animals demonstrated that potassium is essential to maintain life.

calcium and phosphorus). About 98 percent of the body's potassium is found inside the cells, but as part of its normal action, it briefly changes places with the sodium that circulates in the fluid surrounding cells. It can also leak through the cell membranes, which have a very efficient pumping system to carry it back into their interior. This pumping action is important because if all the body's potassium suddenly surged into the bloodstream, it would stop the heart.

Deficiencies are rare, but the body's stores can be gradually depleted by prolonged diarrhea and vomiting, the use of certain diuretics, and an extreme semifasting diet of 800 calories or less a day. Profuse sweating over a period of several days can theoretically reduce potassium stores, especially if the person consumes mostly salty, highly processed foods. This can be prevented by increasing your intake of high-potassium foods and fluids, such as orange juice or sports drinks. Rehydration formulas, which are sold in most pharmacies, are designed to replace fluids and electrolytes lost through prolonged diarrhea.

Why It's Needed

Potassium works closely with sodium to maintain the body's proper balance of fluids and acid-base; specifically, potassium controls the amount of fluid inside the cells while sodium maintains the balance of fluid outside the cells. Other functions include:

Conducting nerve impulses and regulating muscle function. The positively charged potassium ion helps carry nerve messages to the muscles. It then prompts the muscles to relax following a contraction.

Regulating the heartbeat and blood pressure. Potassium regulates the heartbeat by allowing the heart muscle to relax after calcium stimulates it to contract. It is not fully understood how potassium helps control blood pressure, but studies have found that people whose diet provides ample potassium have a reduced risk of hypertension, stroke, and heart attacks.

Aiding in energy metabolism. Potassium is needed to help convert blood sugar that is not needed immediately into glycogen, a form of stored energy in the liver and muscle tissue. It is also instrumental in the secretion of insulin, the hormone that regulates glucose metabolism. Potassium's other metabolic functions include protein synthesis, carbohydrate metabolism, and various enzyme actions.

Therapeutic Uses and Dosages

Potassium supplements are rarely needed because a varied diet based on the Food Guide Pyramid provides all that the body needs. A possible exception involves people taking certain diuretics to treat high blood pressure. Supplements are sometimes needed if the diet does not provide adequate potassium to replace that washed out by the diuretics. The type and dosage should be determined by a doctor.

Special Cautions

Potassium supplements should be consumed with food to avoid stomach upset. Care must be taken not to get too much potassium. For example, patients whose doctors prescribe a potassium supplement risk an overdose if they also take a high-potassium salt substitute. Potassium supplements should not be taken by patients with kidney disease or those taking ACE inhibitors (e.g., captopril or enalapril) for heart disease or high blood pressure.

Preparation and Handling

All living cells—both plant and animal—contain potassium, so it is found in many foods. However, it can be lost during processing, so the best sources are raw or lightly processed fresh fruits and vegetables.

IRON (FE)

Perhaps the most familiar and most studied of all the trace elements, iron is essential to make hemoglobin, the molecule in red blood cells that gives them their color and, more importantly, carries oxygen to all the cells in the body. Iron is also a component of many enzymes that are involved in energy metabolism.

The average male body contains about 4 grams of iron, compared with 2.5 grams in females, with hemoglobin containing about 70 to 80 percent of the total. Iron is also present in myoglobin, the components of muscle cells that absorb oxygen. Any iron that is not needed immediately is converted to ferritin and hemosiderin and stored in the liver, bone marrow, and spleen.

On average, the body absorbs only about 10 percent of the iron in foods, and perhaps more when the body's iron stores are low. Heme iron—the kind found in meat and other animal products—is two to five times more absorbable than the nonheme iron from plant foods. Absorbability of nonheme iron can be increased, however, by combining high-iron foods with citrus fruit or other good sources of vitamin C. In contrast, the tannins in tea, oxalic acid in spinach and certain other foods, and the phytates from bran and other whole-grain products reduce iron absorption.

◉ **REQUIREMENTS**

The Recommended Dietary Allowances, as established by the National Academy of Sciences, for iron are:

6 mg for infants under 6 months
10 mg for infants and children 6 months to 10 years
12 mg for males 11 to 18 years
10 mg for males 19 and older
15 mg for females 11 to 50
10 mg for females 51 and older
30 mg during pregnancy
15 mg during breast-feeding

◉ **SUPPLEMENT FORMS**

Ferrous sulfate is the least expensive and most common form of iron supplement. Many people find, however, that it causes an upset stomach and constipation. Other supplement forms, such as ferrous fumarate or ferrous gluconate, are less likely to cause these problems. Time-release pills also may be gentler on the stomach.

- Paleness of the skin and mucous membranes.
- Persistent unexplained fatigue.
- Shortness of breath.
- Rapid heartbeat and dizziness.
- Increased sensitivity to cold.
- Tingling of the fingers and toes.
- Cravings for ice chips or eating clay.

⊙ SIGNS OF OVERDOSE

There are about two thousand cases of iron poisoning in the United States each year. As little as 3 g of iron can be fatal to a two-year-old child; the lethal dosage for an adult is 200 to 250 mg per kilogram of body weight.

A more common problem involves persons who are genetically inclined to absorb and store too much iron—a condition called hemochromatosis. This can lead to liver and heart damage, cardiac arrhythmias, diabetes, and zinc deficiency.

⊙ BEST SOURCES

Liver and other organ meats
Red meat, dark poultry, and other muscle meats
Shellfish and fish
Iron-fortified breads and cereals
Dried apricots, raisins, and other dried fruits
Egg yolks
Soybeans and other legumes
Tomatoes and other acidic foods cooked in cast-iron pots

⊙ A LITTLE HISTORY

- Hippocrates and other ancient healers prescribed iron-rich tonics to treat fatigue and other symptoms of anemia.
- The use of cast-iron cooking pots was a major source of iron for primitive cultures that consumed only limited meat.
- In 1867, experiments carried out by a French chemist demonstrated the human need for iron.
- Recent research indicates that iron overload is a more serious and widespread problem than previously thought, and may be partly responsible for the high incidence of heart disease in developed countries where people consume a lot of meat.

The body is very efficient in recycling its own iron from worn-out red blood cells. This is why blood loss—for example, heavy menstrual bleeding, hemorrhaging from a wound or surgical incision, or small steady losses from a bleeding ulcer or tumor—often results in iron-deficiency anemia.

Why It's Needed

The major functions of iron include:

Transporting oxygen. Iron (heme) combines with a protein (globin) to form hemoglobin, the molecule in red blood cells that transports oxygen through the body.

Energy metabolism. Iron is a component of many enzymes that are involved in converting food into energy.

Therapeutic Uses and Dosages

Iron supplements should be taken only under the close monitoring of a doctor or clinical dietitian. Iron supplements are recommended for most women during pregnancy to meet the needs of the developing fetus and also support the increased blood volume. They are prescribed for people suffering from iron-deficiency anemia, the most common nutritional deficiency in the United States. They may also be prescribed for patients undergoing surgery that entails blood loss. The typical dosage calls for 20 to 30 mg of iron to be taken two or three times a day.

Special Cautions

Never take iron pills unless they are specifically recommended by a doctor. Be especially careful to keep them out of the reach of young children; iron pills are the leading cause of accidental childhood poisoning in the United States. Check the label of multiple vitamin pills; chances are you should avoid those with iron, especially if they provide more than 10 mg.

When iron supplements are needed, taking them on an empty stomach increases absorption, but can cause an upset stomach. If so, try taking the iron with a small amount of food; good choices are orange juice or other foods high in vitamin C, which increase absorption. Or iron can be taken with a small amount of meat, which also boosts iron absorption. Time-release iron pills may be gentler on the stomach than regular forms.

ZINC (ZN)

Zinc is a micromineral that plays important roles in immunity, wound healing, normal growth and development, reproduction, and various metabolic processes. Recent research indicates that it may help fight the common cold and other infections; it may also be useful in treating fibromyalgia, osteoporosis, and rheumatoid arthritis.

Every cell in the body requires tiny amounts of zinc, with the largest amounts concentrated in the liver, kidneys, pancreas, bones, skin, eyes, and the prostate gland. It is found in the drinking water of many areas and a variety of foods, especially those that are also high in protein. Although only very small amounts are needed, studies indicate that many Americans don't get enough zinc.

Why It's Needed

Zinc is involved in well over one hundred metabolic process and body functions, which include the following:

Normal growth and development. Zinc plays important roles in bone growth and mineralization and the development of reproductive organs.

Maintaining healthy skin and bones. Zinc deficiency is linked to various skin disorders, including eczema, acne, and excessive flaking similar to what occurs in psoriasis. Hair becomes dull and lifeless looking.

Metabolic processes. Zinc is a component of various enzyme systems, and it is essential for the synthesis and metabolism of proteins and genetic material. The red blood cells also need zinc for the proper transfer of carbon dioxide.

Healing and immune function. Zinc promotes the healing of burns and wounds; it also bolsters the immune system to fight colds and other common infections.

Taste and smell. Zinc's role in these senses enable a person to distinguish the taste of different foods.

Therapeutic Uses and Dosages

The typical zinc dosage is 30 mg a day. To shorten the duration and severity of a cold, 10- to 15-mg zinc lozenges may be taken every two to four hours, to a maximum of 150 mg a day. Do not, however, take this high dosage for more than a week at a time.

◉ **REQUIREMENTS**
The Recommended Dietary Allowances (RDAs) for zinc, as established by the National Academy of Sciences, are:

5 mg for infants under 12 months
10 mg for children 1 to 10 years
15 mg for males 11 and older
12 mg for females 11 and older
15 mg during pregnancy
19 mg during breast-feeding

◉ **SUPPLEMENT FORMS**
Zinc is available as tablets, capsules, lozenges, and in liquid form.

◉ **SIGNS OF DEFICIENCY**
Symptoms of long-term deficiency include:

- Loss of appetite.
- Stunted growth in children and delayed sexual development and hypogonadism (low levels of testosterone and small sex organs) in males.
- Skin and hair problems.
- White spots in the fingernails.
- Loss of the ability to taste and smell normally.
- Slow healing of wounds.

◉ **SIGNS OF OVERDOSE**
Toxicity can cause nausea and vomiting. Long-term high doses can lower immunity and cause anemia due to impaired copper absorption.

◉ **BEST SOURCES**
Oysters
Liver
Meat and poultry
Nuts and peanut butter
Wheat bran and wheat germ
Various spices

■ Animal studies in the 1920s showed that zinc was essential for proper growth and sexual development.

■ In the 1960s, clinical studies demonstrated that zinc is also essential for humans.

● REQUIREMENTS

The RDAs for iodine, as set by the National Academy of Sciences, are:

40 mcg for infants under 6 months
50 mcg for infants 6 to 12 months
70 mcg for children 1 to 3 years
90 mcg for children 4 to 6
120 mcg for children 7 to 10
150 mcg for males and females 11 and older
175 mcg during pregnancy
200 mcg during breast-feeding

● SUPPLEMENT FORMS

In addition to adding iodine to table salt, the mineral is included in many multivitamin pills.

● SIGNS OF DEFICIENCY

In addition to goiter, iodine deficiency can cause:

■ Coarse hair and dry skin.
■ Unexplained weight gain.
■ Easy fatigue, lethargy, slowed reflexes, and difficulty thinking clearly.
■ Rise in blood cholesterol levels.
■ Constipation.

● SIGNS OF OVERDOSE

Very high doses—for example, 45 mg—can result in:

■ A metallic taste in the mouth.
■ Mouth sores.
■ Diarrhea and vomiting.
■ Swollen salivary glands.
■ Difficulty breathing.
■ Overgrown thyroid gland (also a sign of deficiency).

Special Cautions

Long-term use of high doses of zinc—for example, 100 mg a day—can actually impair rather than enhance immune function. High doses of zinc also impair copper absorption; if it is taken for more than a month, 2 mg of copper should be added to the regimen.

Zinc is best taken on an empty stomach, either an hour before or two hours after a meal. Zinc interferes with the absorption of some antibiotics, so it either should be avoided or taken at least two or three hours after taking these drugs.

IODINE (I)

Iodine has only one, highly critical function in the body—making thyroid hormones. The average adult body contains only about 25 mg of iodine, of which 10 mg are concentrated in the thyroid gland. When the thyroid does not get enough iodine, it enlarges in an attempt to increase its hormone production. This enlargement, which appears as a growth at the front of the neck, is called a goiter.

As with all minerals, iodine comes from the soil. In the past, iodine deficiency was common in parts of the world where it was lacking in the soil; these include the Great Lakes and Pacific Northwest of the United States, large sections of South America, the Thames Valley of England, and the Alps, Himalayas, and other mountainous areas. To reduce the risk of goiter and other consequences of iodine deficiency, the element is now added to table salt.

Why It's Needed

As a substance essential for proper thyroid function, iodine plays an indirect role in the hundreds of thyroid hormone activities. Among other functions, these hormones regulate the metabolism of all nutrients and are essential for proper growth, mental development, nerve and muscle function, and reproduction.

Therapeutic Uses and Dosages

Iodine supplements are rarely needed because a half teaspoon of iodized salt provides more than the Recommended Dietary Allowance. Babies born to iodine-deficient mothers require immediate supplements to prevent a severe form of retardation and growth abnormalities (cretinism). This is why the iodine levels of newborn babies are now routinely tested.

Special Cautions

Some foods—especially kale, cauliflower, and other members of the cabbage family—contain substances called goitrogens; these block the action of thyroid hormones and, in time, promote growth of a goiter. This can be prevented by making sure the diet provides adequate iodine.

◎ **BEST SOURCES**

In addition to iodized table salt, sources include:

Kelp and dried seaweed

Shrimp, clams, and other shellfish and seafood

Vegetables grown in iodine-rich soil

Eggs and milk products (provided the animals are fed adequate iodine)

◎ **A LITTLE HISTORY**

▪ More than five thousand years ago, Chinese healers treated goiter with seaweed and sponge—rich sources of iodine.

▪ In the fourth century B.C., Hippocrates adopted similar treatments for goiter.

▪ In 1811, a French chemist isolated iodine from seaweed.

▪ In 1914, a Mayo Clinic researcher isolated iodine from the thyroid gland, work that won him a Nobel Prize and led to the movement to add iodine to table salt.

COPPER (CU)

Most people are aware of the importance of iron in preventing anemia, but few know that copper, another trace mineral, also plays a critical role. Without small amounts of copper circulating in the body, iron cannot be absorbed from the intestinal tract or released from its storage sites in the liver and elsewhere. Copper is also necessary to make hemoglobin, the iron-protein molecule in red blood cells that carries oxygen to all the body's cells.

The body contains about 75 to 100 mg of copper, making it the third most abundant of the trace elements. Deficiencies severe enough to produce symptoms are rare, but many nutritionists contend that a large number of Americans do not consume enough copper to reap its full benefits. In fact, researchers are constantly learning new areas in which copper may make a difference; these include helping prevent osteoporosis, high blood pressure, heart disease, and cancer.

Why It's Needed

In addition to facilitating the body's ability to use iron, copper is instrumental in the following body processes:

◎ **REQUIREMENTS**

Recommended Dietary Allowances (RDAs) have not been established for copper, but the National Academy of Sciences has set the following as Estimated Minimum Requirements:

0.4–0.6 mg for infants under 6 months

0.6–0.7 mg for infants 6 to 12 months

0.7–1.0 mg for children 1 to 3 years

1.0–1.5 mg for children 4 to 6

1.0–2.0 mg for children 7 to 10

1.5–2.5 mg for children 11 to 18

1.5–3.0 mg for everyone 19 and older

◎ **SUPPLEMENT FORMS**

Copper is included in many multivitamin and mineral supplements; it is also available in tablet and capsule forms of copper aspartate, citrate, or picolinate.

◎ **SIGNS OF DEFICIENCY**

Copper deficiency is rare and occurs mostly in premature infants or babies fed only milk (either cow's or breast) for more than the first year of life. Deficiencies may also develop in people with severe intestinal disorders that prevent copper absorption. Symptoms include:

- Anemia.
- Skeletal deformities.
- Nerve degeneration similar to that of multiple sclerosis.
- Loss of hair and skin color.
- Infertility.
- Heart defects.

⊛ **SIGNS OF OVERDOSE**

Severe copper toxicity is rare, although there have been reports of liver damage and even deaths among pesticide workers exposed to very large amounts of copper. A dosage of 10 mg can result in nausea and stomach and muscle pain.

⊛ **BEST SOURCES**

Raw oysters
Black pepper
Blackstrap molasses
Brazil nuts and other nuts and seeds
Lobster and other shellfish
Wheat bran and wheat germ
Soybean flour
Avocados and green olives

⊛ **A LITTLE HISTORY**

- In 1925, researchers at the University of Wisconsin discovered that small amounts of copper were essential for the body to utilize iron.
- In 1931, copper was shown to be more effective than iron alone in treating anemia in milk-fed babies. Ongoing research is uncovering numerous other roles of copper.

⊛ **REQUIREMENTS**

Recommended Dietary Allowances (RDAs) have not been established for manganese, but the National Academy of Sciences has set the following as Estimated Minimum Requirements:

0.3–0.6 mg for infants under 6 months
0.6–1.0 for infants 6 to 12 months
1.0–1.5 mg for children 1 to 3 years
1.5–2.0 mg for children 4 to 6
2–3 mg for children 7 to 10
2–5 mg for everyone 11 and older

Metabolism. Copper is a component of several enzyme systems that are instrumental in energy metabolism. It is also a component of at least fifteen proteins (amino acids).

Maintaining the skin. Copper is instrumental in the formation of collagen, the protein building block of connective tissue, skin, and bones. It is also involved in making melanin, the pigment that gives skin and hair their color.

Nerve health. Copper is needed to build and maintain myelin, the protective sheath surrounding nerve fibers.

Wound healing. Copper plays a role in clot formation and promotes healing of cuts, burns, and other wounds.

Building and maintaining various organs. Copper is required to form and maintain the skeleton (bones, tendons, and connective tissue), cells of the brain and spinal cord, and blood vessels.

Therapeutic Uses and Dosages

Supplements of 3 mg a day, plus including high-copper foods in the diet, will meet the body's basic needs and perhaps confer other benefits. For example, a study of women aged forty-five to fifty-six found that those taking 3 mg of copper per day had no loss of bone mass, while those taking a placebo showed significant osteoporosis. A study involving middle-aged men found a link between low copper levels and significantly elevated LDL cholesterol, the type that leads to coronary artery disease and heart attacks.

Special Cautions

Zinc supplements hinder the absorption of copper; if you take zinc for more than a month, also take 2 mg of copper a day. To reduce the risk of stomach upset, take copper with a meal, preferably at about the same time each day to maintain even blood levels.

MANGANESE (MN)

Manganese is an essential trace element that is a component of a number of enzymes needed for metabolism; the body also uses it to build bone tissue and connective tissue and carry out various other functions. Manganese has an antioxidant effect that protects against tissue damage from burning fats. Most manganese is concentrated in the bones, liver, pancreas, and brain.

Why It's Needed

Body processes that require manganese include:

Metabolism. Manganese is a component of enzymes involved in breaking down carbohydrates and synthesizing cholesterol and genetic material (DNA and RNA).

Insulin action. Without manganese, the body cannot fully utilize insulin, thereby interfering with glucose (blood sugar) metabolism.

Cartilage formation. Manganese activates enzymes that are necessary to form cartilage and connective tissue in bones and skin.

Blood clotting. Manganese works with vitamin K to promote proper clotting and wound healing.

Therapeutic Uses and Dosages

Manganese may be useful as part of the treatment for epilepsy, osteoporosis, and disorders affecting the tendons and joints. However, dosages have not been established.

Special Cautions

Excessive calcium and phosphorus hinder the absorption of manganese.

◉ SUPPLEMENT FORMS
Manganese is added to some multivitamin pills; it is also available as manganese gluconate. Dried kelp and alfalfa leaf meal are sometimes marketed as manganese supplements.

◉ SIGNS OF DEFICIENCY
Not much is known about manganese deficiency in humans; in animals, a lack of the mineral results in:

- Abnormal bone and cartilage formation.
- Retarded growth and brain abnormalities.
- Reproductive problems and birth defects.
- Abnormal glucose metabolism.
- Increased risk of convulsions.

In addition, low manganese levels have been found in certain groups, including children with birth defects affecting joints and bones, osteoporosis, multiple sclerosis, epilepsy, and Lou Gehrig's disease (amyotrophic lateral sclerosis). It is not known, however, whether low-level manganese deficiencies contribute to these disorders.

◉ SIGNS OF OVERDOSE
Toxicity from high dietary doses of manganese have not been reported, but problems have developed in miners and other workers who inhale large amounts of airborne manganese or those who drink manganese-contaminated water. In such cases, the manganese builds up in the liver and central nervous system, producing symptoms similar to those of schizophrenia and Parkinson's and Wilson's diseases.

◉ BEST SOURCES
Brown rice and rice bran
Nuts and sunflower seeds
Pineapples
Whole-grain products, especially those made with oats and wheat
Soybeans, peanuts, dried beans, and other legumes
Molasses
Certain spices
Potatoes

◉ A LITTLE HISTORY
- In 1774, a Swedish chemist became the first to recognize manganese as a distinct element, and a year later a colleague succeeded in isolating it.
- In 1931, University of Wisconsin researchers demonstrated that manganese is essential for laboratory animals and concluded that it is also necessary for humans.

REQUIREMENTS

Recommended Dietary Allowances (RDAs), as established by the National Academy Sciences, are:

15–30 mcg for infants under 6 months
20–40 mcg for infants 6 to 12 months
25–50 mcg for children 1 to 3 years
30–75 mcg for children 4 to 6
50–150 mcg for children 7 to 10
75–250 mcg for everyone 11 and older

SUPPLEMENT FORMS

Molybdenum is added to some multivitamin and mineral supplements, but a varied diet provides enough to meet ordinary human needs.

SIGNS OF DEFICIENCY

Molybdenum deficiency is very rare, occurring mostly as a consequence of other serious disorders or a buildup of copper and/or sulfate. Symptoms include breathing problems and neurological disorders.

SIGNS OF OVERDOSE

Toxicity has been observed in cattle who graze in pastures with molybdenum-rich soil. Excessive molybdenum has been linked to copper deficiency in animals, resulting in anemia, diarrhea, weight loss, and fading of hair color. Among humans, intakes of 10 to 15 mg a day have been linked to an increased incidence of goutlike symptoms due to a buildup of uric acid.

BEST SOURCES

The molybdenum content of food varies depending upon the soil's mineral content. In general, however, the following foods are good molybdenum sources.

Lima beans and other legumes
Wheat germ, cereals, and other grain products
Eggs
Organ meats
Spinach and other green leafy vegetables

A LITTLE HISTORY

- In 1778, a Swedish chemist recognized molybdenite as the ore of a new element and in 1782, another Swedish researcher succeeded in isolating molybdenum. He derived its name from the Greek term for lead, *molybdos.*
- In 1953, researchers established that molybdenum is an essential human nutrient.

Molybdenum is a trace mineral that is a component of three enzyme systems. Thus, it is involved in numerous metabolic functions. It is also needed to build strong tooth enamel and it may help prevent dental decay.

Only small amounts of molybdenum—less than 10 mg—are stored in the body, mostly in the liver, adrenal glands, kidneys, and bones. It is not known whether a lack of molybdenum causes symptoms in humans, but growth abnormalities and metabolic problems have been noted in molybdenum-deficient animals.

Why It's Needed

Metabolism. As a component of various enzyme systems, molybdenum plays essential roles in the metabolism of carbohydrates, fats, proteins, amino acids that contain sulfur, iron, and genetic material. Molybdenum also helps control levels of uric acid, a by-product of the metabolism of prunes (substances found in legumes, aged cheese, cured meats, beer, wine, and other foods).

Building strong teeth. Molybdenum is a component of enamel, the hard material that forms the tooth surface and protects against decay.

Therapeutic Uses and Dosages

Multimineral supplements may contain molybdenum, but most diets provide adequate amounts.

Special Cautions

Molybdenum metabolism is reduced by excessive copper, sulfate, and tungsten, an environmental substance. In addition, high intakes of molybdenum reduces the body's reserve of copper by increasing its excretion in the urine.

FLUORIDE (F)

Fluoride, or fluorine, is a trace mineral that is essential for forming and maintaining healthy bones and teeth. Its usefulness has been amply demonstrated by a 50 percent reduction in dental decay among children living in areas where fluoride is now added to the drinking water. Still, the routine fluoridation of municipal water is not without controversy. Despite extensive public health and medical studies showing the safety of minute amounts of fluoride—typically 0.5 to 1.0 parts per million (ppm)—a number of groups contend that the mineral increases the risk of everything from hyperactivity and behavior problems to lead poisoning and cancer.

The adult human body contains only about 1.4 mg of fluoride, and most of this is in the bones and teeth. Although the amount is small, fluoride helps make bones and teeth strong and hard. But this is definitely one case in which a little is good and too much is bad; excessive fluoride causes bones to become soft and porous, tooth enamel to become dull and chalky, and the teeth themselves to wear down too fast.

Why It's Needed

Fluoride helps make bones and teeth strong and hard. During bone and tooth mineralization, a crystal called hydroxyapatite is formed from calcium and phosphorus—the body's two most abundant minerals. Fluoride enters the picture by replacing the hydroxy part of the crystal, hardening the bones and teeth. In addition, fluoride increases resistance to dental decay by reducing the destructive acids produced by oral bacteria.

Studies have found that populations who have adequate fluoride, along with calcium and vitamin D, develop increased bone mass and suffer fewer fractures. Researchers theorize that this building of increased bone mass at a young age lowers the risk of later osteoporosis, but more research is needed to demonstrate that fluoride actually prevents this disease.

Therapeutic Uses and Dosages

The American Academy of Pediatrics recommends supplementation, starting at six months, for babies whose drinking water provides less than 0.3 ppm of fluoride. The dosages are 0.25 mg for ages six months to three years, 0.50 mg for children three to six years, and 1 mg after age six. The recommended supplements for children in areas where the local water provides 0.3 to 0.6 ppm is 0.25 beginning at age three and continuing to age six, and then increasing to 0.50 mg. No supplements

◉ REQUIREMENTS
Recommended Dietary Allowances (RDAs) have not been established for fluoride, but the National Academy of Sciences has set the following as Estimated Minimum Requirements:

0.1–0.5 mg for infants under 6 months
0.2–1.0 for infants 6 to 12 months
0.5–1.5 mg for children 1 to 3 years
1.0–2.5 mg for children 4 to 6
1.5–2.5 mg for children 7 to 18
1.4–4.0 mg for everyone 19 and older

◉ SUPPLEMENT FORMS
Most municipal water is now treated with 0.5 to 1 ppm of fluoride. In addition, fluoride supplements, available as prescription liquid drops, are recommended for infants. Fluoride is also added to toothpaste and some mouthwashes, and dentists sometimes apply it to the teeth of young children.

◉ SIGNS OF DEFICIENCY
Excessive tooth decay is the most common sign of fluoride deficiency.

◉ SIGNS OF OVERDOSE
Excessive fluoride can cause fluorosis, in which the teeth become mottled and wear away unevenly. Other signs of fluoride toxicity include deformed teeth and bones and an increased risk of osteoporosis due to bone demineralization.

◉ BEST SOURCES
In addition to drinking water, which may be either naturally or artificially fluoridated, dietary sources include:

- Dried seaweed
- Tea
- Canned sardines and salmon (with bones), shrimp, and mackerel

◉ A LITTLE HISTORY
- In 1886, a French researcher isolated fluoride and derived its name from the Latin term *fluo*, which means "to flow," in recognition of its historic use in metallurgy.
- In 1945, the first water fluoridation program was implemented to increase the concentration to 1 ppm.

are recommended for children in areas where the water provides 0.6 ppm or more.

Some older people with osteoporosis are given fluoride along with calcium, vitamin D, and perhaps other minerals. A doctor should determine the appropriate dosage.

Special Cautions

Fluoride is 100 percent absorbable when taken on an empty stomach, preferably at bedtime. Most bottled water does not contain fluoride, and water filters remove it from tap water. If you rely on these sources for your drinking water, you may be robbing your bones and teeth of a necessary mineral, and may want to consider supplements.

SELENIUM (SE)

Selenium is a component of an antioxidant enzyme called glutathione peroxidase. In the body, it teams up with vitamin E, another important antioxidant. There is mounting evidence that selenium plays an important role in preventing several types of cancer, heart disease, cataracts, and fertility problems, among other disorders.

Selenium comes from the soil and is found in small amounts in many animal and plant foods. However, the soil in some parts of the United States—most notably west of the Rocky Mountains and east of the Mississippi River—contains very little selenium, and crops and livestock produced in these areas are selenium-deficient. In contrast, there are areas in some of the Plains states where the soil is so loaded with selenium that plants grown in it are toxic to animals and humans alike.

Why It's Needed

Researchers are only beginning to define the many functions of selenium, but it appears to play an important role in the following functions:

Protecting the cells' genetic material. As a component of an antioxidant enzyme, selenium helps protect cellular DNA against free radicals, the unstable molecules released when the body burns oxygen. Free radicals also develop when the body is exposed to excessive sunlight, pollution, tobacco smoke, and other cancer-causing agents.

Detoxifying certain poisons. Selenium binds with arsenic, mercury, cadmium, and other toxic metals to reduce their toxicity. Selenium is also added to shampoos and topical medications used to treat dandruff and fungal infections.

◉ **REQUIREMENTS**

Recommended Dietary Allowances (RDAs) for selenium have been set at the following:

10 mcg for infants under 6 months
20 mcg for children 1 to 6 years
30 mcg for children 7 to 10
40 mcg for males 11 to 14
50 mcg for males 15 to 18
70 mcg for males 19 and older
45 mcg for females 11 to 14
50 mcg for females 15 to 18
55 mcg for females 19 and older
65 mcg during pregnancy
75 mcg during breast-feeding

◉ **SUPPLEMENT FORMS**

Selenium is available in capsule and tablet forms.

◉ **SIGNS OF DEFICIENCY**

Specific symptoms of selenium deficiency have not been established, but some researchers think that an increased risk of cancer, heart disease, cataracts, and other diseases may be due to inadequate of selenium (and perhaps vitamin E as well).

Protecting against cancer. Population studies show that people living in selenium-deficient areas have higher rates of certain cancers, including those of the breast and prostate. Some researchers theorize that selenium protects against cancer by counteracting free radicals and other toxic substances that cause cell mutations. Others believe it may work by stimulating the body's immune defenses against cancer cells, or perhaps a combination of the two.

Helping prevent heart disease. Laboratory studies have linked selenium deficiency with an increased incidence of serious heart defects in large animals, such as cattle, sheep, and monkeys. Even moderate stress seems to cause sudden death in these animals. Analyses of these animals' heart tissue often finds abnormally low levels of coenzyme Q_{10}, a substance critical for energy metabolism in the heart and other muscle tissue. Some researchers think these findings may apply to humans, and that deficiencies of selenium and vitamin E—substances needed to maintain adequate coenzyme Q_{10} may be responsible for many of the sudden cardiac deaths that strike down thousands of apparently healthy people each year.

Boosting immune function. Selenium is thought to bolster immunity by strengthening the disease-fighting properties of phagocytes, the white blood cells that destroy invading micro-organisms.

Preventing cataracts. Laboratory studies show that selenium deficiency can lead to cataracts in rats, and human studies have found that lenses affected by cataracts have only about one-sixth the normal amounts of selenium. While it has not been proved that selenium deficiency actually causes cataracts, some researchers think it may be a contributing factor.

Preventing fertility problems. Again, the evidence comes from animal studies, which have linked selenium deficiency with sperm abnormalities and an increased risk of early pregnancy loss.

Protecting newborns against sudden infant death syndrome (SIDS). Babies fed cow's-milk formulas have a higher incidence of SIDS than those who are breast-fed. Cow's milk contains half the selenium and a small fraction of the vitamin E found in breast milk, which has led some researchers to theorize that selenium deficiency may be a factor in SIDS. This correlates with the increased incidence of sudden death among selenium-deficient calves and lambs. Other researchers, however, think that allergic reactions to cow's milk is a more likely explanation for human SIDS.

Therapeutic Uses and Dosages

In one study, a group of men from the Southeast, where soil is selenium-deficient, were given 200 mcg of selenium a day. Researchers found they had a significantly lower incidence of cancers of the prostate, lungs, and colon compared to a control group that did not take the supplements. Some ongoing cancer prevention studies are using dosages up to 400 mcg, but the safety of these high doses has not been established.

◙ **SIGNS OF OVERDOSE**
Selenium toxicity can cause:

- A garlicky breath odor.
- Irritability, jittery nerves, and depression.
- Nausea and vomiting.
- Loss of hair and peeling fingernails.
- Excessive tooth decay.

◙ **BEST SOURCES**
Selenium content varies greatly according to the region in which plants and animals are grown. In areas where the soil contains adequate selenium, good sources include:

Fish flour; smelt, lobsters, and other seafood
Butter
Wheat germ and whole-wheat products
Brazil nuts
Brewer's yeast and blackstrap molasses
Pork and lamb
Soy flour, kidney beans, and other legumes

◙ **A LITTLE HISTORY**
- Selenium was discovered in 1817 by a Swedish chemist while he was experimenting with sulfur and sulfuric acid.
- In the 1950s, researchers in the United States, Germany, and elsewhere undertook animal studies with selenium and vitamin E and demonstrated their importance in preventing various diseases.
- In 1973, researchers at the University of Wisconsin discovered the complementary antioxidant actions of vitamin E and selenium by demonstrating that the mineral is a cofactor of glutathione peroxidase, a substance that breaks down toxic substances formed during the oxidation of fats.

Special Cautions

As little as 900 mcg of selenium can be toxic. Experts caution against long-term use of more than 200 mcg a day until the safety of higher dosages is established. Short-term use of up to 600 mcg to fight an infection may be safe, but this much selenium should not be taken for more than a few days, especially if the diet also provides foods high in the mineral.

CHROMIUM (CR)

Chromium, another of the essential trace minerals, works with insulin to metabolize blood sugar (glucose), the body's major fuel; it is also essential for proper fat and protein metabolism. Chromium is widely distributed in body tissue, with the highest concentrations in the liver, kidneys, spleen, and bones.

The body absorbs only small amounts of dietary chromium, and many factors further reduce its absorption. For example, absorption decreases with aging, a possible reason why many older people have low chromium levels. A diet that emphasizes highly processed foods and sugar depletes chromium reserves; a high-fat diet reduces chromium absorption.

One form of the mineral—chromium picolinate—is widely promoted as a weight-loss and muscle-building aid. However, results of research attempting to document these benefits have been mixed: some people taking chromium picolinate lose weight and increase muscle mass, while for others, it does not seem to have any effect.

Why It's Needed

Chromium is a component of a hormonelike substance called glucose tolerance factor (GTF), which is released into the blood when there are high levels of blood sugar and insulin. It works with insulin to metabolize protein, fatty acids, and carbohydrates, and it promotes metabolism of nutrients within the cells. Other functions of chromium include:

Activating various enzymes. In this role, chromium helps metabolize energy; it also activates trypsin, a digestive enzyme.

Protecting genetic material. Chromium, along with several other minerals, helps stabilize DNA and RNA. Some researchers theorize that it helps prevent genetic mutations, and thus may help prevent cancer.

Building fatty acids and cholesterol. Chromium stimulates the synthesis of these substances in the liver.

◉ REQUIREMENTS

Recommended Dietary Allowances (RDAs) have not been established for chromium, but the National Academy of Sciences has set the following as Estimated Minimum Requirements:

10–40 mcg for infants under 6 months
20–60 mcg for infants 6 to 12 months
20–80 mcg for children 1 to 3 years
30–120 mcg for children 4 to 6
50–200 mcg for everyone 7 and older

◉ SUPPLEMENT FORMS

Chromium is available in capsule, tablet, softgel, and liquid forms; it is also included in many multivitamin and mineral pills and in some weight-loss products. Brewer's yeast is sometimes taken as a chromium supplement.

◉ SIGNS OF DEFICIENCY

A lack of chromium results in a rise in blood sugar and diabeteslike symptoms. It also raises blood levels of harmful LDL cholesterol and lowers levels of the beneficial HDL cholesterol, thereby increasing the risk of coronary artery disease and heart attacks. Other disorders linked to chromium deficiency include:

- Cataracts.
- Retarded growth in children.
- Sexual dysfunction.
- Reduced resistance to infection.
- Various neurologic disorders, including numbness and tingling sensations characteristic of diabetes.
- Unexplained weight loss.

Therapeutic Uses and Dosages

The typical dosage for healthy adults is 200 mcg a day; 200 mcg twice a day is recommended for weight loss; and 200 mcg three times a day may help persons with diabetes improve their insulin metabolism. Because chromium supplements can cause stomach irritation, it should be taken with food and/or a full glass of water. Taking chromium with orange juice or other foods high in vitamin C increases its absorption.

Special Cautions

If you have diabetes, check with your doctor before taking chromium; it may interact with insulin and other medications prescribed to treat this disease. Taking chromium with calcium or antacids containing calcium carbonate reduces its absorption. Stress appears to increase chromium needs.

Preparation and Handling

There is some evidence that cooking acidic foods such as tomatoes in stainless steel pots leaches out small amounts of chromium. It is doubtful, however, that this adds significant amounts to the diet.

◙ **SIGNS OF OVERDOSE**
Chromium, even in high doses, does not appear to cause symptoms, but supplements may reduce the absorption of zinc and iron.

◙ **BEST SOURCES**
Liver
Brewer's yeast
Whole grains
Nuts and peanuts
Cheese
Fresh or minimally processed fruits and vegetables

◙ **A LITTLE HISTORY**
▪ In 1797, a French chemist discovered chromium, but it took nearly two hundred years to recognize its role in human health.
▪ In 1959, two German researchers working in the United States found that chromium salts normalized glucose metabolism in laboratory animals. They later demonstrated that chromium functioned as a cofactor of insulin.

Other Important Minerals

Researchers have identified a number of other trace minerals that they think are important to human health, but not as much is known about them as those described in the preceding section. There are other trace minerals that are consumed in a typical diet that either have no obvious benefits or are toxic if taken in large doses. These include aluminum, arsenic, cadmium, and lead. The following table summarizes trace minerals that are assumed to be important or perhaps essential.

MINERAL	POSSIBLE FUNCTIONS	POSSIBLE HAZARDS	GOOD SOURCES
Boron	May play a role in bone development and protect against osteoporosis.	Safe when consumed as part of diet.	Grains and many other plant foods.
Bromine	May play a role in sleep cycle, but this has not been proved.	Dietary sources are not toxic.	Grains, nuts, fish.
Cobalt	Essential component of vitamin B_{12}.	None are known.	Cobalt is found in many foods, but humans absorb only that found in vitamin B_{12}.
Lithium	Used to treat the mania phase of manic-depression; animal studies indicate it may be needed for normal reproduction.	Excessive lithium can cause muscle weakness, tremor, drowsiness, upset stomach, and clouded thinking; severe toxicity can cause convulsions, coma, and death.	Eggs, milk, fish, potatoes, and many vegetables, processed meats.
Rubidium	Needed for normal growth of some animals; may have similar function in humans.	Dietary sources are nontoxic.	Coffee, tea, fruits, asparagus and many other vegetables, poultry, fish.
Silicon	Needed for normal growth of some laboratory animals; may have similar functions in humans.	Silicon found in food is safe, but nondietary forms can cause serious lung disease (silicosis).	Whole grains, organ meats, muscle meat.
Sulfur	Component of several amino acids; needed to make hair and nails.	Sulfur salts are toxic; food sources are safe.	Wheat germ, legumes, beef, clams.

Nutraceutical Supplements

The products reviewed in this section are neither vitamins nor minerals nor botanical medicines. Many have distinct medicinal effects; in fact, researchers have found that some are as effective and often safer than their pharmaceutical counterparts. They are widely available in pharmacies, supermarkets, health food stores, and various other outlets, where they are sold as nutritional supplements.

ACIDOPHILUS

Probiotics, an umbrella term meaning "for life," is often used to describe the beneficial bacteria and other micro-organisms that live in the human intestinal tract, the vagina, and other parts of the body. Of the four hundred or more different micro-organisms inhabiting our bodies, perhaps the most beneficial are *Lactobacillus acidophilus* and *Bifidobacterium bifidum,* which are also found in fermented foods, such as yogurt, kefir, and tempeh, and are available as nutritional supplements.

In popular usage, the term *acidophilus* generally refers to many strains of probiotic bacteria, which differ greatly in their ability to survive the acid environment of the stomach and provide potential health benefits. These include aiding in digestion, manufacturing vitamin K and certain other essential nutrients, helping keep cholesterol in check, bolstering the immune system, preventing an overgrowth of yeast and other potential harmful organisms, and perhaps protecting against colon cancer.

Role as a Supplement

Lactobacillus acidophilus is taken either as a supplement or as a component of fermented milk or soy products to help prevent and treat a number of minor as well as serious conditions. For example, acidophilus supplements are used to prevent and treat traveler's and antibiotic-induced diarrhea, vaginal yeast infections, and urinary tract infections. People who are lactose intolerant—meaning they are unable to digest the sugar found in milk—can often tolerate yogurt and other fermented milk products because acidophilus predigests lactose.

To qualify as a probiotic, a microorganism must be able to survive the acidity of the stomach during digestion, which some strains of acidophilus are able to do. The intestinal tract is an integral part of the exquisitely complex human immune system. When probiotics survive passage through the stomach, the strongest bacteria colonize in the intestinal tract and, through a cascading series of events, boost the production of important immune factors such as phagocytes and antibodies. This in turn helps the body fight infections and helps prevent and treat diarrhea caused by invasive bacterial infections.

When you take an antibiotic, the drug indiscriminately kills the beneficial intestinal bacteria along with the harmful ones causing the infection. This upsets the normal intestinal flora and often results in diarrhea and other symptoms. (It can also result in vaginitis and other yeast infections when the yeast that are normally kept in check by bacteria are allowed to proliferate out of control.) Acidophilus supplements can help prevent these adverse effects, or if diarrhea and/or a yeast infection has already developed, help stop it by restoring the normal bacterial balance.

Probiotic bacteria, such as *L. acidophilus,* may inhibit colon cancer, but the exact mechanism of how this occurs is not known. However, researchers have offered several possible explanations including: (1) enhancing the body's immune response, (2) suppressing the growth of intestinal bacteria thought to produce carcinogens and cancer promoters, (3) binding potential carcinogens, (4) producing antitumor compounds in the colon, (5) altering physiologic conditions, such as pH in the colon, that affect the metabolic activity of intestinal bacteria, and (6) altering the action of bile acids.

Though some studies have shown milk products fermented with *L. acidophilus* can aid lactose digestion in those suffering from lactose intolerance, others have not. Other strains of probiotic bacteria, such as *Lactobacillus bulgaricus* and *Streptococcus thermophilus,* which are also used in live yogurt cultures, have proven to be even more beneficial in aiding lactose digestion.

Probiotic bacteria may also play a role in controlling blood cholesterol. In 1974, researchers discovered that Masai warriors, who typically drink about two quarts of fermented milk every day, had low cholesterol levels, and credited probiotic bacteria with this finding. Laboratory studies have since shown that some types of *L. acidophilus* may take up cholesterol, and some researchers theorize that probiotic bacteria may also increase cholesterol excretion in humans.

Evidence of Efficacy

Decades of research suggest that regular consumption of milk products fermented with probiotic bacteria benefit overall health. For example, population studies in the United States and France have correlated a decreased incidence of several kinds of cancer and regular consumption of fermented milk products. But most studies involving acidophilus and other probiotics have been done in the laboratory or with animals. Long-term studies examining large numbers of human subjects under standardized conditions can provide more conclusive evidence of the health benefits of probiotics.

Sources

Acidophilus and other probiotics are found naturally in fermented milk and soy products or foods to which bacteria cultures have been added. However, not all yogurts contain *L. acidophilus.* Yogurts are required only to contain the starter cultures of *S. thermophilus* and *L. bulgaricus.* Check labels to see which bacterial cultures a product contains.

Forms and Usual Dosages

Supplements of *L. acidophilus, L. bifidus,* and other probiotic bacteria are available as powders, capsules, tablets, and liquids. The usual dosage to restore intestinal bacterial balance calls for taking one or two capsules or other supplements containing at least 1 billion live organisms.

There is little agreement about how much probiotic bacteria a healthy person needs to maintain a healthful balance of probiotics. However, some studies have shown lowering of cholesterol with less than a cup a day of acidophilus milk and reduction in the recurrence of vaginal infections with 5 to 6 ounces a day of yogurt fermented with *L. acidophilus,* plus other bacterial cultures. For any source of *L. acidophilus* to provide long-term benefits, however, it must be taken or consumed on a regular basis to maintain a healthy balance of bacteria in the intestinal tract.

Potential Problems

As the body adjusts to increased consumption of acidophilus, there may be some gas and bloating, but there are no such problems with consuming foods or supplements containing acidophilus on a regular basis.

What to Look For

There is no standardization with supplements and they can vary greatly in their acidophilus counts, so opt for a trusted brand name and follow dosing instructions on the label. To choose a fermented milk product, read labels to be sure it contains *L. acidophilus*. A mixture of probiotic bacteria is probably best. And make sure the product is fresh. The longer a fermented milk product sits on the grocery shelf, the fewer live organisms it contains.

See Also

Cancer
Diarrhea
Diverticular Disease
Inflammatory Bowel Disease
Irritable Bowel Syndrome
Ulcers

BEE POLLEN

Bee pollen—the most widely used of a group of bee products marketed as nutritional supplements—are pellets of compressed pollen that are collected from hives. In addition to pollen from seed-bearing plants, the pellets contain varying amounts of bee saliva and flower nectar. (Other supplements derived from bees include royal jelly, a type of saliva produced by worker bees to nourish the queen bee, and propolis, a resin that bees collect from pine trees to repair their hives.)

Role as a Supplement

Bee pollen enthusiasts tout it as a "perfect food" that is loaded with protein, vitamins, and other nutrients. It is marketed as a general health tonic to boost immunity, increase athletic prowess and muscle strength, and improve stamina. It is also promoted as a remedy for numerous ailments: eczema and other skin problems, hay fever and other allergies, anemia, menstrual disorders, and bleeding problems, among others. Propolis and bee pollen extracts are added to salves and ointments used to soothe and soften dry skin and treat eczema and skin lesions.

Evidence of Efficacy

There is little or no convincing evidence to support most of the claims for bee pollen. An exception might be in the treatment of hay fever and other allergies. There is some evidence that taking small amounts of bee pollen can, over time, desensitize a person against pollen allergies, perhaps in much the same manner as allergy shots. However, the types and amounts of pollen vary from one product to another and also according to the area in which they are harvested. So it is not as reliable as the carefully controlled dosages used in allergy shots.

Although bee pollen does contain some protein, carbohydrates, vitamins B and C, certain minerals, and digestive enzymes, there are hundreds of equally (or more) nutritious foods that are much less expensive. Royal jelly, which is even more costly than bee pollen, may provide all the nutrition that a queen bee needs, but there is no scientific evidence that what's good for a queen bee is equally valuable for humans.

Most of the studies on bee pollen have been done in China, where it has been used as a general health tonic and natural medicine for centuries. In recent years, Chinese researchers have reported results of animal studies indicating that bee pollen slows the aging process, inhibits benign prostate overgrowth, and lowers cholesterol and other blood lipids. There is no evidence, however, that humans derive the same benefits.

Claims that bee pollen enhances athletic performance and stamina appear to stem from research conducted in the former Soviet Union and Eastern Europe. Controlled studies involving American weight lifters, swimmers, and other athletes have found no difference between bee pollen and a placebo. It also should be noted that some propolis products have been found to contain large amounts of lead.

Sources

True bee pollen, royal jelly, and propolis are harvested from beehives.

Forms and Usual Dosages

Bee pollen is marketed as a powder and as tablets, capsules, and in softgel forms. It is also added to salves and ointments; royal jelly is sold as a liquid or softgel. There are no established dosages; some labels recommend taking 1 to 3 teaspoons of powdered bee pollen a day.

Potential Problems

People who are allergic to bee venom should avoid bee pollen and other supplements derived from bees and bee parts. There have been reports of fatal allergic reactions (anaphylaxis) to bee pollen and other bee products among people who are hypersensitive to bee venom. Asthmatics whose disease is aggravated by pollen allergies may suffer a flare-up of symptoms when taking bee pollen. Although bee pollen is sometimes used as an alternative to allergy shots by hay fever sufferers, the pollen dosage varies greatly from one product to another, and can provoke allergy symptoms if too much is ingested.

What to Look For

Some supplements labeled bee pollen are actually pollen collected by humans, not bees. If bee pollen is to be used as a desensitizing agent, some experts advise looking for a locally produced product, which is more likely to contain the allergens that provoke your symptoms.

BENECOL

Benecol is a brand of canola-based margarine spreads and salad dressings that contain tasteless and odorless plant (phyto) chemical compounds called sterol esters. These esters, which are derived from pine trees, have been shown to lower blood cholesterol. Benecol has been available in Finland for the last five years. It was so popular when first introduced there that sales had to be limited to one pound per customer.

Role as a Supplement

In practical use, Benecol is more of a functional food than a supplement. Studies have found that when it is used on a daily basis, Benecol lowers both total blood cholesterol and LDL cholesterol, the harmful component that fosters the buildup of fatty plaque in the arteries (atherosclerosis).

Evidence of Efficacy

Nearly two dozen studies in Europe and the United States have documented Benecol's safety and effectiveness in lowering blood cholesterol levels. It works by blocking absorption of dietary cholesterol. It has been shown to lower cholesterol even in people already following a low-fat, low-cholesterol diet. One study, done by Mayo Clinic researchers, found that after two weeks of regular use of Benecol spread (1 tablespoon three times a day), a group of men and women experienced an average 9.4 percent drop in total cholesterol and a 14 percent drop in harmful LDL cholesterol. In contrast, levels of the beneficial HDL cholesterol were unaffected.

Sources

Benecol is available at most supermarkets under the Benecol brand name as a margarine spread and salad dressings.

Forms and Usual Dosages

Benecol margarine spread and salad dressings containing sterol esters have been shown to provide optimal lowering of cholesterol in people eating three servings a day. A serving of the spread is 1 tablespoon; it comes in regular and reduced-calorie (lite) versions. A serving of the salad dressing is 2 tablespoons.

Potential Problems

No safety problems have been discovered with the regular consumption of Benecol products. The products do, however, contain fat and calories. For those trying to control their weight, the products should be incorporated into a daily eating plan as part of an overall heart-healthy, low-fat, low-cholesterol diet and used as a substitute for an equivalent number of calories from other, less healthful foods. For example, a serving of regular Benecol is equivalent to a tablespoon of butter or other animal fat.

What to Look For

Look for Benecol brand margarine spreads and salad dressings in the supermarket. It costs about two to three times as much as regular margarines or salad dressings, but is still less expensive than many cholesterol-lowering drugs.

See Also

Cholesterol Disorders and Atherosclerosis

BETA-CAROTENE/ CAROTENOIDS

Beta-carotene, a precursor of vitamin A, is a carotenoid, a family of some 600 nutrients made up of yellow and orange plant pigments. (In addition to beta-carotene, other important carotenoids include alpha-carotene, cryptoxanthin, lutein, lycopene, and zeaxanthin.) Beta-carotene and the other carotenoids are important antioxidants—substances that protect the body against free radicals, unstable molecules that are released when the body burns oxygen.

Role as Supplements

Beta-carotene is also referred to as provitamin A because the body can convert it to vitamin A as needed. Unlike vitamin A from animal sources, beta-carotene does not accumulate in the liver and other body tissues; hence it does not carry the risk of toxicity found in high doses of vitamin A. In the body, it acts as a potent antioxidant; it also bolsters the immune system. Other carotenoids appear to be more organ-specific than beta-carotene. For example: Lycopene seems to protect against prostate and intestinal cancers; alpha-carotene, lutein, and zeaxanthin have been shown to reduce the risk of lung cancer; lutein has a special affinity for eye tissue; cryptoxanthin and alpha-carotene are thought to lower the risk of cervical cancer.

Evidence of Efficacy

A growing number of studies document the antioxidant effects of beta-carotene and other carotenoids. The medical literature cites scores of studies correlating reduced risks of cancer with diets high in the fruits and vegetables that are rich sources of carotenoids.

Sources

Beta-carotene is found in carrots and other yellow, orange, and red fruits and vegetables. It is also found in broccoli, spinach and other leafy, dark green vegetables. These foods are also rich in other carotenoids, but the most concentrated sources vary according to specific carotenoid. Carrots and pumpkin are the richest sources of alpha-carotene; watermelon, tomatoes, and red grapefruit are high in lycopene; dark green vegetables and red peppers are rich sources of lutein and zeaxanthin; and peaches, mangoes, oranges, apricots, and other bright orange fruits are high in cryptoxanthin.

Forms and Usual Dosages

Beta-carotene and other carotenoids are available in individual pills, tables, softgels, and capsules; they are also combined into single supplements of mixed carotenoids. The typical dosage calls for 25,000 IU, or 15 mg, of mixed carotenoids. People at high risk of cancer are often advised to take 50,000 IU once or twice a day. Even higher doses may be recommended for people with specific disorders, such as poor night vision. Carotenoid supplements, even at very high doses, appear to be safe although they may temporarily cause the skin to take on a yellow/orange hue.

What to Look For

For overall support of the immune system, look for supplements that contain the six leading carotenoids. For specific problems, select supplements containing the carotenoid most likely to benefit the organ in question. For example, for vision disorders, make sure the supplement provides beta-carotene and lutein.

See Also

Cataracts
Macular Degeneration

BETA GLUCAN

Beta glucans are molecules—specifically polysaccharides—that are found in a variety of substances, especially mushrooms, baker's yeast, oats, and barley. The specific type of beta glucan is determined by the number of glucose molecules that branch off the basic structure. The type that has excited considerable excitement among researchers in recent years is beta 1,3/1,6 glucan, which is extracted from baker's yeast and certain types of mushrooms. It appears to be a potent enhancer of the immune system and may also help lower blood cholesterol.

Role as a Supplement

In addition to bolstering the immune system to fight and prevent disease, beta glucan is also used to treat inflammatory and infectious skin disorders. It works by stimulating macrophages—a type of white blood cell that circulates through the body to destroy disease-causing organisms and mutant cells that may develop into cancer.

Researchers have long known that beta glucans act as a powerful immune modulator to protect plants, fungi, and laboratory animals against infection and tumor development. Supplements for human use are being used to bolster immunity, help lower cholesterol, and as a topical application to treat eczema, dermatitis, and other skin inflammations and to promote healing of skin ulcers.

Beta glucan is also important in some types of agribusiness. The Norwegian salmon farm industry has come to rely on the beta 1,3/1,6 glucan as an alternative to antibiotics to protect farmed fish from bacterial infections. It may find similar uses in other areas of meat and poultry production, thereby reducing the use of antibiotics and the consequent development of antibiotic-resistant strains of bacteria.

Evidence of Efficacy

For thousands of years, the Chinese and Japanese have used mushroom extracts to prevent disease. It was only in recent decades, however, that scientists have succeeded in identifying beta glucan as a major active ingredient in mushroom extracts. In the 1940s, researchers at a number of centers reported that crude preparations of baker's yeast cells appeared to increase disease resistance and limit tumor growth in laboratory animals. Again, beta glucans were identified as the active ingredients, and further study mapped the chemical structure as beta 1,3/1,6 glucan. Subsequent studies have been done using beta 1,3/1,6 glucan at several European centers, as well as at Harvard, Baylor, and Tulane Universities, and indicate that it is superior to other beta glucans in enhancing immunity. Clinical studies using beta 1,3/1,6 glucan as an add-on to cancer chemotherapy and other cancer treatments are underway at several centers. It is also undergoing clinical study as a possible cholesterol-lowering agent. Preliminary results of a small European study involving fifty-seven patients with elevated blood cholesterol levels show promise in this area. The study found an average 12 percent drop in total cholesterol and a 27 percent decrease in triglycerides after one month of taking a beta 1,3/1,6 glucan product made from mushroom extracts.

Sources

Most commercial beta 1,3/1,6 glucan products are made from mushroom or yeast extracts. One product, Norwegian Beta 1,3/1,6 Glucan, made by Biotec ASA, is made using a patented monocloning technique.

Forms and Usual Dosages

Beta glucan is available in pills or capsules that are taken orally and in liquid forms that can be applied topically to promote healing of skin infections and ulcers. Dosages vary from one product to another. The recommended dosage of the Norwegian Beta 1,3/1,6 Glucan calls for 750 mg a day—an amount that has been used in clinical studies. Other products use somewhat smaller dosages.

Potential Problems

Beta glucan is safe when used as directed.

What to Look For

Look for products that are labeled beta 1,3/1,6 glucan and that were made either by a cloning process or based on mushroom or yeast extracts. The beta glucans in oats and barley have not been shown to enhance immunity.

BREWER'S YEAST

Brewer's yeast is a nonleavening yeast (*Saccharomyces cerevisiae*) that is marketed as a nutritional supplement. It should not be confused with baker's yeast, which is used to leaven breads and rolls. Instead, brewer's yeast is a bitter-tasting supplement that is usually obtained as a by-product of brewing beer or it can be specifically cultivated and grown for use as a supplement. It's the ingredient that gives beer its unique flavor. Although brewer's yeast products vary greatly in nutrient content, some are quite rich in protein, minerals, and several of the B vitamins. Some vitamin and mineral products are innoculated with brewer's yeast cultures and an emulsion of active yeast is "grown" with specific vitamin-rich properties. Tablets made from the resultant powders have been shown to be more bioavailable than standard supplements.

Role as a Supplement

Naturopaths and other alternative practitioners often recommend brewer's yeast as a remedy or supportive treatment for a wide variety of ailments, including diabetes, fatigue, eczema, cancer, high blood cholesterol, and constipation. Some brewer's yeast products are rich in amino acids, thiamin, riboflavin, niacin, folic acid, vitamins B_6 and B_{12}, chromium, copper, zinc, and selenium.

Evidence of Efficacy

There is no scientific evidence that brewer's yeast provides unique health benefits over and above what you would expect from a vitamin/mineral supplement containing the same nutrients.

Sources

Brewer's yeast is either a by-product of beer production or the product of cultivating and growing yeast specifically for use as a nutritional supplement.

Forms and Usual Dosages

Brewer's yeast comes in tablet, flake, and powder forms. Because of its bitter taste, tablets may be the most palatable way to take it. However, in tablet form, the dosage may be as high as six to twelve tablets a day. Flakes work well when added to shakes and other dishes. But too much can overwhelm the flavor of the food, so it works best when added to strongly flavored foods. There are debittered brewer's yeast products, but the process used to debitter the yeast can remove some nutrients. As a result, some products are fortified with nutrients. Debittered yeast is sometimes called "nutritional yeast" and is somewhat more palatable than regular brewer's yeast.

Potential Problems

Brewer's yeast can cause gas, bloating, and diarrhea, so start off with a small amount of brewer's yeast (about ⅛ to 1 teaspoon a day), and build up slowly to 1 to 2 tablespoons a day. Some people may also experience allergic reactions, but it should be noted that brewer's yeast is unrelated to *Candida albicans,* an organism that causes yeast infections.

What to Look For

The nutrient profiles of brewer's yeast and nutritional yeast products vary greatly. Read nutritional labels and choose a product that provides the most B vitamins and minerals for the lowest dose. If traditional brewer's yeast is too bitter, opt for a product that has been debittered.

See Also

Hypoglycemia

BROMELAIN

Bromelain is a natural enzyme found in fresh pineapple. It is capable of digesting protein, but it is destroyed during cooking and processing, so it is not found in canned pineapple. The bromelain extract that is sold as a nutritional supplement is usually obtained from the pineapple stem. Originally marketed mostly as an alternative to papain, a more expensive enzyme derived from papayas, bromelain is an ingredient in some meat tenderizers and facial creams. As a nutraceutical, bromelain is promoted mostly as an anti-inflammatory medication to treat minor burns and sports injuries, such as bruises and sprains. Because it helps break down protein, it is sometimes used as a digestive aid. It is also added to some multivitamin and herbal medicines.

Role as a Supplement

Bromelain appears to inhibit production of the prostaglandins that cause inflammation, swelling, and pain. Some studies have found that bromelain may reduce symptoms of arthritis, bronchitis, and other inflammatory disorders. It reduces the ability of blood platelets to form clots, and some naturopaths recommend it as an alternative to low-dose aspirin because it is less likely to cause an upset stomach and other adverse side effects. There is also some evidence that bromelain thins mucus, which may ease symptoms of bronchitis and asthma.

By helping break down and more fully digest protein, it may aid in preventing allergic reactions to food by reducing the number of allergens that are absorbed from the small intestine. Ointments or salves containing bromelain are promoted to speed healing of minor burns, bruises, and sports injuries. Other possible uses include treatment of arthritis, bronchitis, and other inflammatory disorders.

Evidence of Efficacy

There is little firm evidence that bromelain is an effective treatment for any of these conditions. However a few small, older studies and clinical trials did find it to be effective for a variety of conditions including urinary tract infections and to relieve the pain, swelling, and tenderness of some sports injuries. It's also been suggested that it may be helpful in the treatment of lupus, an autoimmune disorder in which a person's own immune system begins to target and destroy the body's connective tissues.

Sources

Bromelain is found in fresh (not canned) pineapple and in some dietary supplements and digestive aids.

Form and Usual Dosages

The activity of supplemental bromelain is measured by either MCU (milk-clotting units) or GDU (gelatin-digesting units). One GDU is equal to 1.5 MCU. A 500-mg tablet that contains 2,000 GDU per gram would provide 1,000 GDU per tablet. Some herbalists and other practitioners recommend as much as 6,000 GDU a day, but much of the research has studied smaller doses of about 1,300 GDU a day. When used as a digestive aid, it is best taken with or just before meals.

Potential Problems

Bromelain is generally considered to be safe, when taken as directed. However, there have been reports that it may cause a rapid heart rate in persons who have high blood pressure. It may increase stomach irritation of ulcer patients. There have also been reports of high doses causing nausea, diarrhea, and other intestinal upsets.

What to Look For

Look for 500-mg tablets of bromelain that provide at least 1,000 GDU per tablet.

See Also

Carpal Tunnel Syndrome
Gout

CAFFEINE

Caffeine, which is a central nervous system stimulant, is the most widely consumed drug in the world. More than 80 percent of American adults consume caffeine-containing foods and beverages every day. While caffeine has been the subject of thousands of studies, its safety is still sometimes called into question. When consumed in large amounts, it has been periodically linked to an increased risk of heart disease, high blood pressure, osteoporosis, birth defects, and cancer.

Despite the occasional health warnings linked to caffeine, there has not been a decline in its use. The continued popularity of caffeine-containing beverages—especially coffee, tea, and colas—is usually attributed to the fact that caffeine improves mental alertness and athletic performance. It is, in fact, a restricted drug in some athletic competitions.

Role as a Supplement

Caffeine is added to supplements for its ability to enhance alertness, boost energy, and prevent sleep. It is also added to some combination painkillers to increase their effectiveness.

Evidence of Efficacy

There is no doubt that caffeine improves mental alertness. Indeed, many people have difficulty getting started in the morning without a jolt of caffeine in the form of a cup of strong coffee. Others use it to ward off drowsiness. Several studies have found that caffeine enhances physical performance in runners, cyclists, and cross-country skiers. But not all studies have found caffeine to be beneficial. The lack of an effect in some studies could be due to the differing doses of caffeine used in studies, the regular consumption of caffeine of the people prior to the study, and differences in their overall diets. There is less research regarding caffeine as an energy booster. But a few studies show that people who are deprived of sleep report feeling an increase in energy after doses of 200 to 600 mg of caffeine. There is research showing that caffeine can improve performance of attention-demanding tasks like driving a car. And a recent study, conducted at the University of Hawaii reported in the *Journal of the American Medical Association,* found that the higher the concentration of caffeine in coffee drinkers, the lower the incidence of Parkinson's disease. More study is needed, however, to document this benefit.

Sensitivity to caffeine varies greatly from one person to another and

COMMON SOURCES OF CAFFEINE

Substance	Caffeine (mg)
Coffee, Starbucks, grande (16 oz)	550
Coffee, Starbucks, Americano tall (12 oz)	70
Coffee, brewed, drip method (6 oz)	110–150
Coffee, instant	40–108
Black tea, brewed 3 minutes	20–46
Black iced tea (12 oz)	12–36
Sweet/dark chocolate (1 oz)	20
Chocolate bar (3.5 oz)	12–15
Soft drinks (6 oz)	36–100
Weight-loss aids (per dose)	140–200
Cold remedies (per dose)	0–65
Stimulants (per dose)	75–200

older people are more sensitive to its effects than younger people. Over time, people develop a tolerance for caffeine so that a regular caffeine consumer may feel no effect from an extra cup of coffee, while a non-consumer of caffeine might feel edgy and nervous after a single cup.

Sources

Caffeine is found in coffee, tea, many soft drinks, and chocolate. It is also found in drinks that contain guarana and often an ingredient in weight-loss and energy-boosting supplements, sports drinks, and some herbal preparations and painkillers. For example, Excedrin—a nonprescription headache and pain remedy—is made up of aspirin, acetaminophen, and caffeine.

Forms and Usual Dosage

Coffee, tea, and soft drinks are the most commonly consumed sources of caffeine. Doses in supplements, drinks, and over-the-counter medications vary greatly (see accompanying table). Experts generally recommend limiting caffeine intake to about 300 mg a day.

Potential Problems

In large amounts (more than 400 mg a day) caffeine can cause nervousness, insomnia, rapid and irregular heartbeats, elevated blood sugar, excess stomach acid, and heartburn. It can also create caffeine dependence. One study found that people who consume about 235 mg a day (the equivalent of about two cups of coffee) experience withdrawal symptoms, including headache, fatigue, lack of energy, and muscle pain, if they stop abruptly. Some people who consume only about 100 mg of caffeine a day may experience some withdrawal upon stopping. To avoid withdrawal symptoms, caffeine consumption should be tapered off slowly. Because of the diuretic effect of caffeine, moderate to high doses should not be used when exercising in a hot, humid environment. Weight-loss supplements that contain caffeine combined with other stimulants such as ephedrine (ma huang) can cause severe, sometimes fatal reactions and should be avoided. Pregnant women should consume caffeine only in moderation (no more than 300 mg a day).

What to Look For

Limit caffeine consumption to caffeine-containing beverages and avoid or minimize the use of supplements and over-the-counter preparations, especially diet pills, that have caffeine as an added ingredient.

CARNITINE

Carnitine, also referred to as l-carnitine, is a proteinlike substance that is made from two amino acids, methionine and lysine. It can be made in the liver; good dietary sources include muscle and organ meats, fish, and milk products.

Carnitine is important for its role in transporting fatty acids to the muscle cells, including those of the heart, where they can be converted to energy. Carnitine is important in preventing a buildup of fatty acids in the heart, liver, and skeletal muscles, and helps keep blood levels of cholesterol and triglycerides, another fatty substance, in check. It also appears to boost the antioxidant effects of vitamins C and E.

The body's stores of carnitine are concentrated in the skeletal and heart muscles. A carnitine derivative—an ester called acetyl-l-carnitine (ALC)—is concentrated in the brain and is thought to slow the aging of brain and other nerve cells. Carnitine is also found in sperm, and may be instrumental in male fertility.

Carnitine deficiency is rare, but some studies have found low levels in patients with liver, heart, and kidney disorders. Vegetarians whose diets are deficient in the amino acids needed to make carnitine may be mildly deficient in the substance. Some drugs, including those used to treat AIDS, increase loss of carnitine in the urine; patients on kidney dialysis may also become carnitine-deficient. Symptoms include fatigue, chest pain, muscle weakness, and confusion.

Role as a Supplement

Carnitine supplements are promoted as an athletic supplement to increase performance, muscle strength, and endurance; as a weight-loss aid; and to treat chronic fatigue syndrome. Possible medical uses of ALC include treatment of heart-muscle disorders, such as congestive heart failure; high blood levels of cholesterol and triglycerides; male infertility; age-related dementia, Alzheimer's disease, and depression; nerve disorders, including diabetic neuropathy; and bolstering immune-system function in AIDS patients.

Evidence of Efficacy

Reports of improved athletic performance and endurance are based mostly on anecdotal evidence, although some studies have found reduced muscle soreness among some athletes taking carnitine. Similarly, there is only modest scientific evidence to support claims that carnitine or ALC is effective in treating chronic fatigue syndrome.

Many of the carnitine and ALC studies have been done abroad, especially in Italy where carnitine is used to treat angina, heart failure, and other forms of heart disease and has been used experimentally to treat Alzheimer's disease and other nerve and brain disorders. A number of these preliminary studies indicate that ALC may slow progression of Alzheimer's disease; other studies have found that ALC improved mood and other symptoms in a group of elderly patients suffering from clinical depression. Studies involving both humans and animals with diabetes have found that ALC injections improved nerve function and reduced nerve pain. Although some of the results appear promising, more research is needed before carnitine and ALC become accepted therapies.

Sources

The body can make all the carnitine that it needs provided it has sufficient lysine and methionine, amino acids that are abundant in meat and other animal products, along with adequate vitamin C and some of the B vitamins. Carnitine supplements are available in health food stores, usually in sections devoted to athletic supplements.

Forms and Usual Dosages

L-carnitine is available as chewable wafers, tablets, and capsules; it may also be given by injection to treat diabetic neuropathy. It is also available as an oral solution. The typical oral dosage is 1 a day. ALC dosages used in clinical studies involving Alzheimer's ranged from 1.5 to 3 a day.

Potential Problems

ALC may cause nausea and vomiting, especially when it is taken on an empty stomach. Experts recommend taking it with meals. Otherwise, carnitine and its derivatives appear to be safe and well tolerated. However, if you have diabetes, heart disease, kidney failure, or any other serious chronic or progressive disease, check with your doctor before taking caritine or ALC.

What to Look For

Check the labels for carnitine or ALC content. For some disorders, L-carnitine is preferred, and for others, ALC appears to be more effective.

See Also

Alzheimer's Disease and Memory Loss
Chronic Fatigue Syndrome
Weight Problems

CHLOROPHYLL

Chlorophyll is the compound that gives green plants their dark green hue. Plants rely on chlorophyll to store light energy collected from the sun's rays. They then use that energy to convert carbon dioxide and water to carbohydrate for food and release oxygen into the air. It is also a potent antioxidant and an effective deodorizing agent.

Role as a Supplement

Traditionally, chlorophyll has been used to help heal wounds, fight infections, and "cleanse" the blood. But it is also promoted as an antioxidant and an anticancer agent; it is also said to fight anemia by boosting hemoglobin synthesis. This notion is based on the fact that hemoglobin and chlorophyll have similar chemical structures, but contrary to popular belief, chlorophyll does not play a role in hemoglobin synthesis, so it is doubtful that it is of value in treating anemia.

Evidence of Efficacy

There are few clinical studies demonstrating long-term benefits of chlorophyll or supplements that contain it. Some animal experiments have suggested that it may reduce inflammation, and laboratory experiments indicate it may block the formation of some cancer-causing compounds; these include heterocylcic amines in cooked meat, polycyclic hydrocarbons in cigarette smoke, and aflatoxins in peanuts and moldy grains. It's been shown to reduce the ability of carcinogens to cause gene mutations that can lead to cancer. Generally, studies have shown that the more chlorophyll a vegetable or plant contains, the greater the protection against carcinogens.

Sources

All green vegetables, including sea vegetables like kelp and nori, are rich in chlorophyll, as are several dietary supplements, collectively called "super green foods," such as algae, chlorella, spirulina, and barley and wheat grass.

Forms and Usual Dosages

Chlorophyll is available as a supplement or as a component of green food supplements in powders, tablets, or juices. No recommended dosage has been established. Chlorophyll tablets are generally a more concentrated source of the compound. For example, one brand of wheat grass provides 18.5 mg of chlorophyll per teaspoon of powder or seven tablets. In contrast, a single tablet of chlorophyll concentrate derived from alfalfa provides 60 mg.

Potential Problems

There have been no reports of adverse reaction to chlorophyll.

What to Look For

A diet rich in dark green vegetables should provide a healthy dose of chlorophyll. For a supplement, choose one of the green food supplements that have been grown under tightly controlled conditions. Some "naturally harvested" algaes have been found to be contaminated with environmental toxins, including bird droppings.

CHOLINE

Choline, a component of lecithin and commonly listed as a member of the B-complex family, is a substance that the body needs to build and maintain cell membranes and metabolize fats. The body also uses choline to make acetylcholine, a brain chemical (neurotransmitter) that is necessary to transmit impulses along nerve pathways, especially to the muscles. It is needed in order for muscles to contract properly, a function that is especially important in heart function. It also plays a role in memory and other mental functions.

Choline is thought to play a role in preventing heart disease. It works with other B vitamins, especially folacin (also called folate or folic acid), to metabolize homocysteine, a by-product of protein metabolism that increases the risk of atherosclerosis when too much circulates in the blood. Choline may also protect the liver against accumulation of excessive fat, cirrhosis, and cancer.

Choline, along with the closely related lecithin, is important in reproduction and fetal development. Choline easily passes across the placenta to reach the developing fetus; in addition, breast milk is very rich in choline. The body can make choline, but perhaps not enough to meet its needs, especially during pregnancy and breast-feeding when needs are increased.

Role as a Supplement

Choline is a component of lecithin supplements; it is also promoted as a separate supplement to increase athletic performance and fight fatigue. Studies have found that body reserves can be significantly reduced during prolonged exercise, such as long-distance running.

Evidence of Efficacy

As with lecithin, many of the claims made for choline are based largely on animal studies, and its precise roles in human health are largely theoretical. An exception may be in the area of physical performance. Blood studies document drops of up to 40 percent in blood choline levels as a result of running a marathon, competing in a triathlon, and other endurance sports. Other studies have found improved performance and endurance among athletes who take choline supplements before competition. In one study, for example, long-distance runners shaved an average of five minutes off their times in a twenty-mile race.

Animal studies have clearly demonstrated that choline given during pregnancy has beneficial effects on brain development and memory in the offspring. Some researchers theorize that choline works with folacin to foster normal fetal brain and nerve development and plays an important role in memory and other mental function. However, human studies in which patients with Alzheimer's disease were given choline supplements showed no memory improvement. Researchers suggested that the disappointing results may have been due to the fact that the Alzheimer's was already advanced when the choline was given, or that sufficient amounts of choline failed to cross the blood-brain barrier, and that its real value may be preventive—that is, increasing choline intake while still healthy may help prevent the disease from ever developing.

Evidence that choline protects against fatty liver disease and other liver disorders are also based mostly on animal studies. But at least one human study in which healthy volunteers were fed a diet devoid of choline developed early signs of liver disorders, and people on long-term artificial feeding (total parenteral nutrition) develop fatty liver disease—a forerunner of cirrhosis—if they are not given choline supplements.

Choline deficiency results in atherosclerosis and heart disease in rats, apparently due to high blood levels of homocysteine. This can be prevented by feeding the animals diets with adequate choline and lecithin.

Sources

Foods high in choline include egg yolks (by far the best source of choline in the human diet), organ meats, and soybeans. It is also found in lecithin supplements.

Forms and Usual Dosages

Cholide supplements are available as choline chloride, bitartrate, and dihydrogen citrate, which are marketed as pills and capsules. The phosphatidylcholine form of lecithin supplements is about 15 percent choline. The usual dosage for healthy people calls for 3 to 5 g of lecithin, which will provide ample choline. If plain choline is used, the standard dosage is 1,500 mg, divided into three doses during the course of a day. Studies that showed improved athletic performance used about 2 g of choline, which was taken about two hours before an endurance event, such as running a marathon.

Potential Problems

Choline supplements are generally safe, although the Food and Drug Administration (FDA) cautions against taking doses exceeding 16 to 20 g a day; this is about thirty times the amount provided in an ordinary diet. Side effects of high doses may include nausea, sweating, loss of appetite, a fishy body odor, and cardiac arrhythmias.

What to Look For

Studies indicate that taking choline in the form of a lecithin derivitive, such as phosphatidylcholine, increases absorbability of the choline and is less likely to cause a fishy body odor than, for example, choline chloride.

CHONDROITIN SULFATE

Chondroitin sulfate is a building block of cartilage, the tough gristle that covers the ends of bones and cushions joints; it is also found in the tissue lining blood vessels and the bladder. Chondroitin plays an important role in maintaining cartilage by allowing water, nutrients, and other molecules to enter the tissue; a critical role because cartilage lacks blood vessels. In the blood vessels, it helps prevent abnormal clotting and also prevents blood and other fluids from passing through the vessel walls.

Chondroitin is structurally similar to glucosamine, another constituent of cartilage; both are classified as glycosamineoglycans (GAGs), and as supplements to treat osteoarthritis, they are most effective when taken together.

Role as a Supplement

In the past, chondroitin was taken to treat atherosclerosis (never shown to be effective in controlled scientific studies), the clogging of arteries with fatty plaque, but more recently, it has emerged as a major treatment of osteoarthritis—the wearing away of cartilage that is especially common among older people.

Evidence of Efficacy

Scores of studies abroad and a growing number in the United States support the effectiveness of chondroitin in slowing or preventing cartilage deterioration. With increasing age, natural production of chondroitin declines, allowing destructive enzymes to destroy the cartilage. Researchers now believe that this is a major factor in the development and progression of osteoarthritis.

Recent studies have demonstrated that taking chondroitin supplements inhibits destructive enzyme action, slows progression of osteoarthritis, alleviates pain and other symptoms, and—when taken along with glucosamine—may even foster a regrowth of deteriorated cartilage. In one well-regarded placebo-controlled study involving 93 patients with osteoarthritis of the knee, the group receiving glucosamine and chondroitin for four to six months showed significant improvement over the placebo group. Another study involving thirty-four U.S. Navy volunteers reported similar positive results for the glucosamine-chondroitin group.

Sources

Chondroitin is extracted from animal cartilage, specifically cow trachea; it is also a component of shark cartilage, which may explain why this supplement seems to help some people with arthritis.

Forms and Usual Dosages

Chondroitin is available in pill and capsule form as a separate supplement or in combination with glucosamine. The typical dosage calls for starting with 400 to 500 mg of chondroitin taken three times a day, preferably with a similar amount of glucosamine. After a few weeks, the dosage can be lowered to two doses a day. Higher amounts of chondroitin—up to 3 to 5 g a day have been attempted—to treat atherosclerosis.

Potential Problems

Chondroitin is generally safe, with no reports of serious side effects. However, very high doses can cause nausea.

What to Look For

A recent University of Maryland analysis of eleven popular chondroitin products found a wide range of the actual amount of chondroitin compared to label claims. Four products contained less than half the stated amount, and one had less than 10 percent. Only five provided 100 percent of the stated amount. The Arthritis Foundation recommends checking which product has been used in favorable clinical studies, and then buying that one.

See Also

Arthritis

COENZYME Q_{10}

Coenzyme Q_{10} (CoQ for short) is a naturally occurring compound that is essential for energy production in the body's cells, especially the heart, which contains a dense concentration of mitochondria—energy-producing components of cells. CoQ also helps preserve vitamin E, which is thought to prevent oxidation of cholesterol. (Oxidized cholesterol damages artery walls and may be a factor in initiating atherosclerosis, the buildup of fatty deposits that raises the risk of a heart attack or stroke.)

Levels of CoQ drop with age and are lower in people with heart disease. In fact, the more severe the heart disease, the lower CoQ levels are thought to be. Moreover, some commonly prescribed medications, such as lovastatin prescribed for high cholesterol, and beta-blockers, such as propranolol for high blood pressure and angina, can lower CoQ levels in the body as well. People who take these medications should consult with a health care provider to see if CoQ supplementation is advisable.

Role as a Supplement

Supplemental CoQ may help raise the body's reserves that have dropped due to age, illness, or medications. Although CoQ has been promoted as a wonder supplement for everything from increasing endurance to reversing aging, it holds the most promise for the heart. It appears to be especially helpful in treating heart-muscle disorders (cardiomyopathy) and congestive heart failure, a disease in which the heart is unable to pump out enough blood. This results in blood collecting in the lungs and pooling in the legs and other body tissue. Studies indicate that CoQ may also lower high blood pressure, steady an erratic heartbeat, lessen attacks of angina, and reduce the formation of blood clots, a major cause of heart attacks and strokes. Some people with Raynaud's disease—reduced circulation to the hands and feet—report that CoQ lessens symptoms.

CoQ is also a powerful antioxidant and may help prevent free-radical damage to tissues throughout the body. There is also some evidence that it may slow the progression of such nerve disorders as Parkinson's disease.

Evidence of Efficacy

Several well-regarded studies indicate that adding CoQ supplements to the conventional regimen for treating cardiomyopathy and congestive heart failure show more improvement than with medications alone. In a study involving more than 2,500 heart patients in Italy, 80 percent experienced reduced symptoms (shortness of breath, swelling of the legs and feet, difficulty sleeping) after three months of taking CoQ. It is also a standard treatment of congestive heart failure in Japan. However, the American Heart Association and the American College of Cardiology do not advocate CoQ as a treatment for heart disease. In any event, CoQ should not be taken as a substitute for prescribed medication to treat heart failure or any other cardiovascular disease, and if you do take it as part of an overall treatment program, be sure to tell your doctor that you are using it.

Several studies are currently under way to investigate whether CoQ may help slow the progression of degenerative nerve diseases, such as Parkinson's and Alzheimer's, as well as fibromyalgia, a disorder characterized by diffuse muscle pain and chronic fatigue syndrome.

Though claims abound concerning CoQ's ability to slow aging, reduce fatigue and improve the quality of life for AIDS patients, promote healing of periodontal disease, and even aid weight loss, more study is needed to document whether it really works in these disorders.

Sources

CoQ occurs naturally in the body and is also found in a wide variety of foods, but is especially rich in organ meats.

Forms and Usual Dosages

CoQ typically comes in tablet or pill form, but it is also available as a liquid or softgel capsule. It's even found in some skin creams. Doses thought to be effective for heart disease range from about 100 to 360 mg a day. One small study found that people with cardiomyopathy who took 100 mg a day of CoQ, in addition to regular therapy, showed significant improvement compared to those who received a placebo. In another study, a significant number of patients given CoQ were able to reduce the number of heart medications they were taking.

Potential Problems

There have been no reports of side effects from taking CoQ supplements.

What to Look For

Look for CoQ supplements that contain oil, which aids in its absorption. It should be taken with food, which also increases its absorption.

See Also

Chronic Fatigue Syndrome
Heart Disease
Liver Diseases
Tooth Decay and Gum Diseases

CREATINE

Creatine is a combination of amino acids that are stored in the skeletal muscles. These muscles can use one of its derivatives—creatine phosphate—to sustain a muscle contraction when the usual fuel—a substance called ATP (adenosine triphosphate)—has been exhausted. In simplified terms, here's an example of how it works: When you lift a heavy weight, the muscles of your arms contract, or shorten, to provide the needed strength and resistance. The energy for this contraction is derived by converting ATP to ADP (adenosine diphospate). When the muscles' reserves of ATP are exhausted, creatine comes to the rescue by giving over its phosphate molecule to make more ADP. High reserves of creatine phosphate allow the muscles to work longer and harder.

Role as a Supplement

The body makes creatine by combining certain amino acids, the building blocks of protein, and then storing it in the muscles. Creatine supplements are marketed as muscle builders and athletic performance enhancers.

Evidence of Efficacy

The scientific evidence backing creatine-supplement efficacy is mixed, at best. There is some evidence that creatine supplements may help muscles hold more water, and theoretically, creatine-rich fluid might supply extra fuel in times of need. A few studies have linked creatine supplements with modest increases in muscle mass and strength among athletes; but many have found no apparent effects. Most of the impetus for its use has been based on testimonials by bodybuilders and professional athletes who claim that creatine has given them a competitive edge. These testimonials have prompted millions of young athletes to take creatine supplements, often as a safer alternative to anabolic steroids. Scientists stress, however, that no supplement alone will increase muscle mass and strength; instead, it is increased muscle use that accomplishes these objectives. In other words, it's working out—not creatine—that builds those bulging muscles that weight lifters and other athletes like to display.

Sources

The body makes all the creatine that it ordinarily needs from high-protein foods—muscle meat, fish, poultry, egg whites, milk and milk products, soybeans, and combinations of legumes and grains.

Forms and Usual Dosage

Supplements are available in several forms including creatine monohydrate, a crystalline powder that is sold in sports shops, health food stores, and other outlets. It can be mixed with a full glass of water or simply sprinkled on food. Be sure to drink plenty of water during the course of the day, but avoid coffee, colas, and other caffeinated drinks. Caffeine has a diuretic effect, which may counteract any beneficial effect of creatine by drawing fluids out of the muscle tissue.

Proponents of creatine supplements recommend starting with a relatively high loading dose of 1 teaspoon (5 g) four or five times a day for the first five to seven days, and after that cutting back to 1 teaspoon twice a day every other day, or no more than five days a week. Some experts recommend limiting daily use to three weeks a month, with a full month off after two months of taking the supplements. Some athletic trainers recommend taking creatine as part of the preseason conditioning, and then discontinuing it during the competitive season, although there is no scientific evidence to support such recommendations.

Potential Problems

High doses—for example, 5 g a day for more than a few weeks—can cause nausea, dizziness, diarrhea, and possibly muscle cramps. Long-term use of supplements may harm the kidneys. Even in the absence of kidney problems, creatine supplements can result in misleading blood tests. This occurs when tests show elevated blood levels of creatinine, a metabolic by-product of creatine. Ordinarily, elevated creatinine points to a kidney problem. Even so, it can pose problems for someone taking an insurance or preemployment physical exam.

Doctors also caution against teenagers taking creatine supplements because its long-terms effects on the kidneys and liver are unknown.

What to Look For

Look for supplements labeled creatine monohydrate. If you don't notice any increase in muscle mass or strength after two weeks of a loading dose, it is unlikely that further use of creatine supplements will be of any benefit.

DHEA

DHEA, or dehydroepiandrosterone, is a hormone that is made from cholesterol by the adrenal glands, which are situated on top of the kidneys. The body can convert DHEA into many other steroid hormones, especially testosterone, the major male sex hormone, and estrogen, the major female hormone. DHEA is often touted as the "mother hormone" because the body appears to use it as a building block for so many other hormones. It is also dubbed the "fountain of youth" hormone, a reference to the fact that blood levels start to rise just before puberty, peak in the third decade of life, and then decline with increasing age. By age seventy, blood levels are only a small fraction of what they were at age twenty.

Some studies indicate that people who maintain relatively high levels of DHEA as they grow older also have somewhat higher levels of sex hormones than persons with low levels. This has been said to influence libido and mood. There is some evidence that men with high levels of DHEA and testosterone have a reduced risk of heart disease; it is not known, however, whether women reap similar benefits. Other functions attributed to DHEA include:

- Reduction of the ability of blood platelets to clump and form clots, which may reduce the risk of heart attacks and strokes.
- Lower blood cholesterol levels.
- Maintain normal blood pressure.
- Bolster immunity.
- Treat certain autoimmune diseases, especially lupus.
- Improve blood sugar control in the treatment of diabetes.
- Reduce the effects of aging and protect against numerous age-related disorders, including Alzheimer's and Parkinson's diseases.

Role as a Supplement

DHEA supplements are very controversial. Promoters and marketers of DHEA tout it as an elixer of youth and a superhormone that can benefit virtually everyone, while prominent researchers have called it "the snake oil of the '90s" and "a disaster in the making." As with any hormonal product, DHEA should be used only under close medical supervision. A leading DHEA researcher, Dr. Peter Hornsby at the Baylor College of Medicine, has urged that "DHEA be classified as an investigational drug and used only in clincal resarch until we figure out what it does and its side effects."

Evidence of Efficacy

Although DHEA is widely promoted as a miracle supplement that can do everything from bolstering flagging libido, controlling weight, and improving mood to preventing or treating many of our most lethal diseases, there is little or no evidence that it can do any of these things in humans. Most of the research to date has been done in animals, and human studies involved only small numbers of volunteers. Still, some of the results have been intriguing and hold promise that DHEA may eventually live up to some of its hype. For example, Dr. Samuel Yen, professor of reproductive medicine at the University of California, San Diego, divided eight men and eight women, aged fifty to sixty-five, into two groups: one group received a placebo and the other 100 mg of DHEA a day for three months, after which the two groups were switched to the opposite regimen. Within two weeks, blood levels of DHEA in those receiving the supplement rose to what would be expected in a young adult. As the study progressed, those receiving the DHEA noted modest increases in muscle strength and lean body mass and a decline in fatty tissue; there was also improvement in immunity. Other human studies have found that DHEA may decrease lupus symptoms; improve insulin metabolism; and lower levels of triglycerides, a blood fat, in postmenopausal women. Researchers emphasize, however, that these studies have involved only a few dozen people and were of relatively short duration. Thus, long-term benefits and risks have not been measured. Claims that DHEA can prolong life and reverse the effects of aging are based mostly on animal studies, so it is not known whether these benefits apply to humans as well. In short, researchers know very little about what DHEA actually does in the human body.

Forms and Usual Dosages

DHEA is marketed as a nutritional supplement and is available in tablet, capsule, and cream forms. The usual recommended dosages range from 5 to 25 mg a day. Originally, DHEA was sold mostly as a nonprescription weight-loss aid. In the late 1980s, the Food and Drug Administration ordered that DHEA be classified as an unapproved drug that could be obtained only by prescription or participation in a clinical study. In 1994, it was reclassified as a nutritional supplement that could be sold in health food stores and other outlets.

Potential Problems

High doses of DHEA can raise testosterone levels and cause acne in both men and women. It can also cause virilization in women, resulting in abnormal hair growth, deepening of the voice, increased muscle mass, irregular menstrual periods (among younger women), and mood changes. Some researchers caution that DHEA may spur the growth of hormone-dependent cancers of the breast in women and prostate in men. Animal studies have found that it may also raise the incidence of liver cancer, but it is not known if humans face the same risk.

What to Look For

If you want to try DHEA, it is best to do so under a doctor's guidance with a prescription product.

See Also

Lupus
Menopause

DMSO AND MSM

DMSO (dimethyl sulfoxide) is a sulfur compound that occurs naturally in the body and is found in soil; it is also a by-product of wood-pulp processing. In the body, DMSO is a potent scavenger of free radicals, the unstable molecules responsible for much of the cellular damage in the body. Proponents of its medicinal use say it can relieve the pain and inflammation of arthritis and is effective in treating other conditions that cause inflammation.

MSM (methylsulfonylmethane) is a metabolite of DMSO that occurs naturally in the blood and is a component of hair, nails, and metabolic enzymes. It is also found in sulfur-containing foods such as milk, meat, and broccoli. As a supplement, it is sold in capsule form. Like DMSO, MSM is said to relieve arthritis pain, but without the strong sulfur odor. It is an approved veterinary medicine and is commonly used in cream form for the treatment of muscle injuries and soreness in horses.

Role as Supplement

DMSO has been approved by the Food and Drug Administration (FDA) as a prescription drug to treat interstitial cystitis, a painful inflammatory bladder disorder that causes pressure, frequent urination (sometimes thirty or more times a day), and scarring of bladder tissue. It is administered as a sort of bladder wash or given intravenously. No other prescription use of DMSO is recognized by the FDA.

Because DMSO is easily absorbed through the skin, it can be rubbed on the skin to ease muscle and arthritis pain. MSM, on the other hand, is taken orally in supplement form. Although it is mainly used for the treatment of arthritis, its proponents claim it is effective for the treatment of a wide variety of ailments, including headaches, muscle pain, fibromyalgia, carpal tunnel syndrome, and allergies.

Evidence of Efficacy

Most of the studies with DMSO have been done abroad, and it is currently used as a therapeutic agent in over one hundred countries worldwide. During the 1970s, numerous research studies were submitted to the FDA in an effort to have DMSO approved as a prescription drug in the United States. However, approval was denied for its use in treating anything other than interstitial cystitis.

As of this writing, only two clinical studies using MSM have been conducted. Both found that 2 to 6 g of MSM were effective in relieving arthritis pain, but neither study has been published in the medical literature. Thus, most of the evidence that MSM works is based on reports of individuals' success stories and the experiences of Stanley W. Jacob, M.D., of Oregon Health Sciences University and Ronald Lawrence, M.D., Ph.D., of the UCLA School of Medicine, the chief proponents of MSM.

Sources

Any food that is rich in sulfur, such as broccoli, eggs, meat, garlic, onions, and milk, contains some DMSO and MSM. DMSO is sold as an industrial solvent that is not intended for human use. MSM is available as a nutritional supplement in health food stores.

Forms and Usual Dosage

DMSO comes in liquid form and is rubbed onto the skin to relieve arthritis pain and inflammation. MSM comes in capsule form. Drs. Jacob and Lawrence suggest starting with 1 g a day and working up to a maximum of 6 to 8 g, whichever dose brings relief. They also point out that it can take four to six weeks to become fully effective.

Potential Problems

For DMSO, the main concern is getting a pure grade that is free of contaminants (see What to Look For, below). However, there have been no safety studies in the United States showing that even pharmaceutical-grade DMSO is safe for long-term use when rubbed on the skin. It has a strong sulfur odor that has been described as smelling like fish, oysters, garlic, and rotten eggs; it can become incorporated into sweat and saliva, causing body odor and bad breath. It can also cause skin irritation at the site of application.

Animal toxicity studies have been done with MSM and it was found to be safe. It is a nontoxic compound, even at high doses. However, it can have a mild blood-thinning effect and shouldn't be taken with non-prescription blood thinners like aspirin, ginkgo biloba, high doses of vitamin E, prescription blood thinners like Coumadin, or other drugs or supplements that reduce clotting.

What to Look For

DMSO comes in three grades or degrees of purity. If you decide to try DMSO, opt for the highest degree of purity you can get. Pharmaceutical grade has been purified and sterilized, but a prescription is required to obtain it. Spectral grade is used for analytical laboratory work. Though it is also pure, it has a slightly greater risk of contamination. Industrial or solvent grade DMSO is sold in hardware stores and is likely to contain harmful contaminants and should not be used medically. Because DMSO is readily absorbed through the skin, the contaminants are carried along with it. Several brands of MSM supplements are available, most of which comes from two suppliers in the United States.

See Also

Gout

ESSENTIAL FATTY ACIDS

Essential fatty acids, or EFAs for short, are fats that the body needs but cannot manufacture and therefore must obtain from the diet or from supplements. Examples include linoleic acid, an omega-6 fatty acid, and alpha-linolenic acid (ALA), an omega-3 fatty acid that the body partially converts to DHA and EPA (the healthy fats found in fish oils). Essential fatty acids are vital for brain development, the production of hormones, and maintaining the health of all the body's cells.

Some experts believe the American diet provides plenty of these essential fatty acids, while others contend that it falls far short of what is needed for optimal health because of its emphasis on foods high in hydrogenated fats—the type used in commercial baked goods, margarine, and other processed foods—which lack EFAs. In addition, the typical American diet provides far too many omega-6 fatty acids and not enough omega-3s. While both types of fatty acids are essential, too much omega-6s and not enough omega-3s may increase the risk for a host of illnesses including heart disease, cancer, diabetes, asthma, and even depression. The current dietary balance is somewhere between 10:1 and 20:1 in favor of omega-6s. Experts recommend that the balance be shifted closer to a ratio of 4:1, or 4 g of omega-6s for every 1 g of omega-3s. It's important to get both DHA and EPA as well as their parent fatty acid, alpha-linolenic acid, since the body is able to convert only about 10 percent of ALA to DHA and EPA.

Role as a Supplement

Supplementing the diet with omega-3 fatty acids, as well as cutting back on dietary omega-6 fatty acid intake, can shift the EFA balance to a healthier direction.

Evidence of Efficacy

Hundreds of studies have investigated the theory that regular intake of fish or fish oils may reduce the risk of heart disease. Several have found that people who regularly eat fish have a lower incidence of heart disease, including sudden cardiac death, than those who don't eat fish. The strongest evidence for fish oil supplements has been for lowering triglyceride and cholesterol levels in the blood. Several studies have also found that doses of about 2.5 to 5 g of DHA and EPA a day may help reduce the pain and stiffness associated with rheumatoid arthritis. Recently, researchers at the National Institutes of Health found evidence that omega-3 intake may help fight some types of mental illness, including depression. Studies have also found that diets rich in ALA—the parent compound of DHA and EPA—may help prevent arthritis, heart disease, and stroke.

Gamma-linolenic acid (GLA), an omega-6 fatty acid, has also been studied as a treatment for rheumatoid arthritis. It's been suggested that it may help suppress the production of compounds that cause inflammation. But it has not been studied as much as the omega-3s. And taking supplements would only further shift the EFA balance in the wrong direction.

Sources

The essential omega-6 fatty acid, linoleic acid, is found in vegetable oils (corn, safflower, soybean, and sunflower), and gamma-linolenic acid (GLA), a derivative of linoleic acid, is found in borage, black currant, and evening primrose oils. The omega-3 fatty acid alpha-linolenic acid is found in green leafy vegetables, flaxseed oil, canola oil, walnuts, and Brazil nuts. ALA is partially converted in the body to the omega-3 fatty acids DHA and EPA, which are found naturally in salmon, sardines, and other fatty cold-water fish. (See also Fish Oils, p. 298).

Forms and Usual Dosages

There is no official recommended intake for EFAs. However, some experts recommend a daily intake of 6 g of omega-6s, 1 g of DHA and EPA combined, and 0.5 g of ALA to provide a healthy 4:1 ratio of omega 6s to omega-3s. Supplements are available as gel cap, capsules, and liquids.

Potential Problems

Fish oil supplements can cause a fishy aftertaste and cause belching that tastes and smells like fish. Some have been found to contain environmental toxins such as heavy metals. People with asthma should not take fish oil supplements unless they do so under a doctor's supervision. Ironically, while fish oil supplements may help some people who suffer from asthma, they may actually aggravate the condition in others. People with diabetes should limit fish oil supplementation to no more than 3 g a day, since higher doses could affect blood sugar levels.

People who take either over-the-counter blood thinners, like aspirin, high doses of vitamin E, or ginkgo, or prescription blood thinners, like Coumadin, should check with their health care provider before taking fish oil supplements, since omega-3 fatty acids may have a blood-thinning effect as well. However, no adverse effects have been seen in studies giving 3 to 8 g daily of omega-3s from fish oil. Supplements of evening primrose oil, black currant seed oil, and borage oil are rich in gamma-linolenic acid (GLA), and high doses of these oils are often taken to reduce inflammation, but when used long-term, they may have the opposite effect. (See Evening Primrose, p. 447). Studies indicate that increasing the intake of the omega-3s may be more effective than GLA in reducing levels of the prostaglandins that cause inflammation. Also, evening primrose oil tends to be expensive and there have been reports of environmental contaminants being found in some borage oil.

What to Look For

Look for "odorless" fish oil supplements that contain DHA (docosah-exaenoic acid) and EPA (eicosapentaenoic acid). The amounts of DHA and EPA combined range from about 300 to 800 mg per 1,000 mg capsule. The higher the concentration of these omega-3 fatty acids, the fewer capsules are required. DHA supplements are also available.

See Also

Arthritis
Cholesterol Disorders and Atherosclerosis
Dermatitis/Eczema
Diabetes
Gout
Heart Disease
Inflammatory Bowel Disease
Lupus
Migraine Headaches
Psoriasis
Sexual Dysfunction

FISH OILS

Fish oils are high in a type of polyunsaturated fats called omega-3 fatty acids, which come from the plankton that fish feed on. Salmon, mack-erel, tuna, and other fish that thrive in very cold water are especially rich in two fatty acids that appear to protect against heart disease. These acids—EPA (eicosapentaenoic acid) and DHA (docosahexanoic acid)—also appear to counteract inflammation and bolster immunity. A third type of omega-3 fatty acid, ALA (alpha-linolenic acid) is found in flax-seed oil and some green leafy vegetables; while it also is beneficial, it does not appear to be quite as effective as fish oils.

Role as a Supplement

Fish oil supplements are promoted to reduce the risk of heart disease and stroke; they may also lower high blood pressure and help prevent cardiac arrhythmias. Because they have an anti-inflammatory effect, they may help prevent the blood-vessel inflammation that is thought to pro-mote atherosclerosis, the clogging of arteries with fatty plaque. They may also be helpful in treating psoriasis, rheumatoid arthritis, lupus, and inflammatory bowel disorders such as Crohn's disease. They may also ease symptoms of fibrocystic breast disorders and perhaps protect against cancers of the breast and colon.

Evidence of Efficacy

In the 1970s and 1980s, researchers studying heart disease in various population groups noted that Greenland Eskimos had a very low incidence of heart attacks despite the fact that their diet was very high in fat. As they further analyzed the Eskimo diet, the researchers found that its fats came mostly from cold-water fish. Further studies documented that the omega-3 fatty acids in fish oils worked in several ways to protect against heart disease. They inhibit the tendency of blood platelets to clump and form clots. Sticky platelets aggravate injuries to the artery walls and promote development of atherosclerosis, the clogging of blood vessels with fatty plaque. The risk of heart attack and stroke is further reduced by inhibiting clot formation. In addition, omega-3s lower blood levels of triglycerides, the most abundant blood fat (lipid).

A controlled study involving patients with Crohn's disease, an inflammatory intestinal disorder, found that fish oil supplements relieved symptoms for nearly 70 percent of patients, compared with 28 percent of the placebo group. Animal studies indicate that fish oil may lower the risk of breast cancer. A number of studies suggest that a diet high in omega-3 fatty acids improves rheumatoid arthritis and perhaps lupus.

Sources

Cold-water fish is the best source of EPA and DHA fatty acids; it is also found in breast milk. The body can convert about 10 percent of consumed linolenic acid—found in canola, soy, walnut, and wheat-germ oils—into EPA and DHA.

Forms and Usual Dosages

Fish oil supplements are available as softgels and capsules; EPA and DHA can also be obtained by eating oily cold-water fish, such as salmon, tuna, trout, mackerel, and sardines. Several studies indicate that having two or three servings of these fish a week is more beneficial than taking supplements.

If supplements are used, the recommended dosages range from 3 to 6 g a day. The Crohn's disease study, for example, used 3 g a day. Higher doses, up to 5 or 6 a day, have been shown to reduce inflammation and pain in rheumatoid arthritis patients.

Potential Problems

Very high doses can cause a fishy body odor. Some people experience nausea, diarrhea, bloating, and intestinal gas, especially when starting the supplements. These side effects can be minimized by taking the capsules with meals and by starting with a low dose and gradually increasing it to the recommended level. The supplements should be used cautiously, if at all, by diabetic patients; some studies indicate that large amounts of fish oil may interfere with blood sugar control.

Omega-3 fatty acids have a blood-thinning effect; check with your doctor if you are also taking an anticoagulant medication such as low-dose aspirin, Coumadin, ginkgo biloba extract, or high doses of vitamin E. Some fish oil supplements have been found to be contaminated with heavy metals and other environmental toxins.

What to Look For

To avoid problems of fish oil supplements going rancid, check the date on the bottle, buy only small amounts—for example, lots of fifty or one hundred capsules or softgels—and store them in the refrigerator. If you find one brand causes gas, bloating, and other side effects, you might want to stop taking it and try another; some people who are unable to tolerate one brand have no problems with another. (See also Essential Fatty Acids, p. 295.)

See Also

Arthritis
Cholesterol Disorders and Atherosclerosis
Dermatitis/Eczema
Gout
Heart Disease
Inflammatory Bowel Disease
Migraine Headaches
Psoriasis
Sexual Dysfunction

5-HTP

Short for 5-hydroxytryptophan, 5-HTP is promoted as an alternative to a chemical cousin, L-tryptophan, an amino acid supplement that has been barred by the Food and Drug Administration. The body makes 5-

HTP from tryptophan, a common amino acid that is found in meat, poultry, fish, and milk products. In the body, 5-HTP raises levels of serotonin, a brain chemical (neurotransmitter) that is instrumental in regulating mood. Low levels of serotonin are implicated in many disorders, including depression, sleep problems, eating disorders, migraine headaches, and obsessive-compulsive disorder and other behavior problems. Supplements of 5-HTP are promoted to treat these and other disorders and as an alternative to Prozac and other selective serotonin reuptake inhibitors (SSRIs). These drugs increase serotonin levels by blocking the nerve's reuptake of the substance. In contrast, 5-HTP works by increasing the body's production of serotonin.

Role as a Supplement

The 5-HTP molecule is small enough to pass through the protective blood-brain barrier where it is readily converted into serotonin. As a supplement, it is promoted to relieve many of the disorders treated by L-tryptophan before it was banned; these include depression, insomnia, migraine headaches, and obesity. It may also be helpful in relieving the muscle pain of fibromyalgia.

Evidence of Efficacy

5-HTP has been used for decades in Europe, where most of the studies on its effectiveness have been conducted. Swiss researchers conducted a multicenter controlled study comparing 5-HTP and an SSRI. The two were found to be equally effective in relieving clinical depression, but participants taking 5-HTP reported it was better tolerated than the SSRI. Another study, this one involving twenty obese patients, found that those taking 5-HTP for twelve weeks lost an average of twelve pounds, compared to two pounds among patients in the placebo group. It works by suppressing the appetite.

Sources

Supplements marketed in the United States are derived from the tryptophan in the seeds of an African plant, *Griffonia simplicifolia*.

Forms and Usual Dosages

5-HTP is available in pill and capsule forms. In obesity studies, 50 to 100 mg of 5-HTP was given thirty minutes before meals. The recommended dosages for depression range from 50 to 100 mg taken two or three times a day. Insomnia may be relieved by taking 100 mg about thirty minutes before going to bed. Migraine headaches are treated with 100-mg doses taken up to three times a day.

Potential Problems

Side effects may include drowsiness and various intestinal upsets, including nausea, gas, and constipation. These can usually be avoided by starting with a low (50-mg) dose and gradually increasing it to 100 mg, if needed.

As a general rule, 5-HTP should be used only under a doctor's supervision, especially by persons who have a long list of chronic diseases: heart disease, cancer, multiple sclerosis, lung or liver disease, AIDS, and such autoimmune disorders as rheumatoid arthritis and lupus. The supplements should not be taken with many pharmaceutical drugs, including SSRIs and other antidepressant drugs, barbiturates and weight-loss medications, antihistamines and cold remedies, antibiotics, and cancer chemotherapy. It also should not be taken with alcohol, which interferes with the metabolism of 5-HTP.

What to Look For

Many brands of 5-HTP are available; many of these contain various herbs, vitamins, and other supplements. Check the labels and select a product that contains only 5-HTP to avoid taking additional ingredients that you may not need or want unless you specifically require the other elements.

See Also

Insomnia
Weight Problems

FLAVONOIDS

Flavonoids, also known as bioflavonoids, make up a group of hundreds, if not thousands, of related chemicals found in many plant foods and herbs. These substances, formerly referred to erroneously as vitamin P, are powerful antioxidants and may play a role in fighting cancer and heart disease. Some enhance the action of vitamin C and other antioxidants. The more common groups of flavonoids include flavones, flavonols, flavanones, and isoflavones. Among the most studied flavonoids are quercetin, catechins, proanthocyanidins, glycosides, and silymarin. Some are responsible for giving foods like berries their red or blue color, while others give a bitter taste to the food that contains them. Quercetin is the major flavonol in the Western diet.

Role as Supplements

Anyone who consumes at least five servings of fruits and vegetables a day is likely to get enough flavonoids from natural sources. But there is mounting evidence that larger, supplemental amounts of some flavonoids can help prevent many diseases in high-risk persons (see below).

Evidence of Efficacy

Laboratory and animal studies have shown flavonoids to have antibacterial and anti-inflammatory properties; they also help prevent allergic reactions, protect cellular genetic material against mutations, fight viruses, prevent abnormal blood clotting, and promote good circulation by opening (dilating) blood vessels. Many flavonoids have antioxidant properties and appear to increase the levels of enzymes that protect cells against cancer-causing substances (carcinogens). Population studies have linked consumption of foods rich in flavonoids with a decreased risk of heart disease and cancer. For example, two large-scale studies of Finnish men and women found that those whose diets were richest in flavonoids had the lowest risk of cancer and heart disease. Flavonoids found in red wine may be responsible for the connection between moderate wine consumption and a reduced risk of heart disease—the so-called French paradox that some researchers theorize explains the low incidence of heart disease in France, despite a rich, high-fat national diet. A recent Japanese study compared the effects on blood fats (lipids) of beer, red and white wine, and grape juice, and found that red wine significantly lowered blood levels of the harmful LDL cholesterol. Isoflavones, which are high in plant estrogens, may reduce the risk of osteoporosis in older women.

Sources

Flavonoids come from plants; a few examples include:

- Anthocyanins, found in blueberries, strawberries, cherries, cranberries, raspberries, grapes, and black currants.
- Catechins and polyphenols, found in black and green tea.
- Isoflavones (daidzein and genistein), found in soybeans.
- Naringin, found in grapefruit.
- Proanthocyanidins, found in red wine and grape seeds.

- Quercetin, found in many fruits, vegetables, and grains, including onions, kale, broccoli, red grapes, cherries, French beans, apples, and tea.
- Rutin and hesperidin, found in citrus fruits.

Herbs that are especially rich in flavonoids include milk thistle, hawthorn, bilberry, grape seed extract, and ginkgo biloba.

Forms and Usual Dosages

There is no recommended intake for flavonoids. Neither is there a standard dosage. However, in the two Finnish studies, average intakes of about 4 mg a day were associated with a decreased risk of disease. Dozens of supplements provide any number of flavonoids alone or in a variety of combinations, with or without other nutrients. Many come in combination with vitamin C. For people who seldom eat fruits and vegetables, a flavonoid supplement might be in order.

Potential Problems

No adverse reactions or side effects have been documented in people taking flavonoid supplements in the recommended amounts. However, while many of these compounds appear to provide health benefits when consumed in foods, laboratory studies suggest that some of them might actually be harmful if taken individually and in large doses.

What to Look For

There are many combinations of flavonoid supplements in health food stores, but little is known about which one might be best. The blends of citrus flavonoids are the least expensive and most widely available; unfortunately, they may also be less effective than products containing only one type of flavonoid. Soy protein, often sold as a supplement for athletes, is high in genistein (an isoflavone), which mimics the effects of estrogen and is promoted as an alternative to postmenopausal estrogen replacement therapy (ERT).

See Also

Dermatitis/Eczema

GLUCOMANNAN

Glucomannan, also called konjac or konjac mannan, is a low-calorie, high-fiber powder that can swell up to two hundred times its volume as it absorbs water in the stomach and intestinal tract. As it swells, it forms an insoluble gel that curbs hunger inducing a sense of fullness.

Role as a Supplement

Glucomannan is marketed as a diet aid; it is also said to lower total blood cholesterol, especially the harmful LDL cholesterol that is implicated in heart disease. It slows the release of blood sugar (glucose), which may aid in the control of diabetes.

Evidence of Efficacy

The Food and Drug Administration maintains that there is little scientific evidence to support glucomannan as a weight-loss product. There are, however, some studies that seem to back its value in weight control. One study, published in the *International Journal of Obesity*, described an eight-week, double-blind study involving a group of obese patients. The researchers found that those taking glucomannan lost a mean of five and a half pounds. In addition, total cholesterol dropped a mean of 21 points, and LDL cholesterol fell 15 points.

Other studies have found that glucomannan can lower total cholesterol by about 10 percent in four weeks; most of this decline is in the harmful LDL cholesterol, while the beneficial HDL cholesterol levels remain unchanged. Still other studies, in both humans and animals, have found that glucomannan can lower fasting blood glucose by 7 percent within a half hour of taking it. The medical literature also contains several reports of studies in which glucomannan has been used to treat childhood obesity.

Sources

The basic ingredient in glucomannan is derived from dried *Amorphophallus konjac*, an Asian tuber that is often referred to simply as konjac. It is cultivated in Japan, where it has been used as a flour for more than two thousand years.

Form and Usual Dosage

Glucomannan is marketed as a capsule; the usual dosage calls for taking one or two 500-mg capsules with a full glass of water or juice about an hour before a meal. One study found that people who took two capsules before each meal (a total of 3 g a day) lost an average of five to seven pounds in two months.

Potential Problems

Glucomannan is generally safe with few side effects. However, it decreases absorption of important vitamins, especially the fat-soluble vitamins A, E, and D, as well as beta-carotene, a precursor of vitamin A. Although glucomannan appears to be safe for children, any weight-loss program for children under age sixteen should be undertaken only under close medical supervision. The capsules should not be taken by people who have swallowing problems; the powder swells almost immediately when it comes in contact with fluids and can cause choking if a person is unable to swallow a capsule quickly.

What to Look For

Most of the supplements sold in the United States come from Japan. Look for 500-mg glucomannan capsules that contain mostly *Amorphophallus konjac.*

See Also

Weight Problems

GLUCOSAMINE SULFATE

Glucosamine is a building block of glycosaminoglycans (GAG), the main components of cartilage—the hard, smooth substance that coats the ends of bones and helps cushion the joints. It works with another substance, chondroitin sulfate (see p. 285), to help build and repair cartilage, tendons, and ligaments. Under normal circumstances, the body makes all of the glucosamine and chondroitin it needs. But for unknown reasons, as they age, people stop making enough glucosamine to maintain healthy cartilage. In time, their cartilage becomes thin and pitted, resulting in osteoarthritis.

Role as a Supplement

Glucosamine, used either alone or in combination with chondroitin, is taken primarily to relieve the pain and other symptoms of osteoarthritis and to help prevent further deterioration of cartilage. Most people who take glucosamine supplements suffer from arthritis symptoms; however, a growing number of runners and other athletes are also taking it in the hopes of preventing joint problems later in life.

Evidence of Efficacy

Veterinarians have used glucosamine for years to relieve arthritis symptoms in animals, with many reports of improvement. As for humans, many clinical studies conducted abroad, most notably in Germany, have shown that glucosamine improves arthritis symptoms in 50 to 80 percent of patients.

So far, only a few randomized clinical studies have been reported in the United States, but these have generally been favorable. In one study, for example, 155 patients with osteoarthritis were given injections of either 400 mg of glucosamine or a placebo twice a week for six weeks. A significantly higher percentage of the patients who received the glucosamine showed improvement when compared to the placebo group.

Sources

There are no food sources for glucosamine; the supplements are made from chitin, a component of the hard, outer shells of shrimp, lobsters, crabs, and other marine animals.

Forms and Usual Dosage

Glucosamine is available as glucosamine sulfate, glucosamine hydrochloride, and N-acetyl-glucosamine (NAG). Experts generally recommend glucosamine sulfate as the preferred form—it is well absorbed, and its sulfur molecule appears to also promote the health of cartilage and other connective tissue. Many products combine glucosamine with chondroitin; some combinations also contain manganese, a trace mineral, and other ingredients. There is some concern that prolonged use of large amounts of manganese can cause nerve damage; so far, this has not been reported with any of the glucosamine products containing manganese.

The typical dosage calls for starting with three 500-mg capsules a day and, after a month or two, reducing the dosage to two capsules a day. Improvement is generally noted after two to three weeks; if there is no change in that time, it may be prudent to try another brand because the quality varies greatly from one product to another. Also, some studies indicate that the combination of glucosamine and chondroitin works better than either supplement alone.

Potential Problems

Glucosamine is generally safe, and few adverse effects have been reported, most commonly mild intestinal upsets, such as heartburn and diarrhea. These can be minimized by taking glucosamine at mealtime. Diuretics may decrease the effectiveness of glucosamine; increasing the dosage from two 500-mg capsules a day to three capsules may avoid this.

Persons with diabetes should check with their doctor before taking glucosamine; there have been some reports of glucosamine interfering with glucose metabolism in people with diabetes.

What to Look For

As with any nutraceutical product, it's best to buy an established brand product from a reputable pharmacy, health food store, or other proven outlet.

See Also

Arthritis

GLUTAMINE

Glutamine is an amino acid, one of twenty or so building blocks of protein; it is classified as nonessential because the body can make all it needs without dietary sources. It is the most abundant amino acid in muscle tissue and blood plasma.

In the body, glutamine has many important metabolic functions. It can be used by cells as a source of energy when glucose reserves are low, such as during sustained exercise. This is important because it helps prevent catabolism, the breakdown of muscle tissue for energy. It is thought to be important in immunity; it can pass through the protective blood-brain barrier and may promote mental alertness and improve mood and memory. Glutamine also helps maintain the cells lining the intestinal tract.

Role as a Supplement

Glutamine is used mostly as an athletic supplement, especially by weight lifters and others who engage in intense anaerobic exercise. It is promoted as a muscle builder and as a performance enhancer. Glutamine supplements may also be important for persons who are unable to eat normally and are getting their nutrition via intravenous (parenteral) feeding. Glutamine supplements may also play a role in protecting against the intestinal damage of Crohn's disease, colitis, and other inflammatory bowel disorders.

Other possible roles include treatment of depression, prevention of muscle loss (wasting) in advanced cancer, and protection of liver tissue against damage from cancer chemotherapy and drugs such as acetaminophen (Tylenol), a common nonaspirin painkiller.

Evidence of Efficacy

Medical researchers have found that glutamine supplements help prevent depletion of this and other amino acids from muscles and other tissues during times of stress, such as during intense athletic training. Researchers have found that glutamine supplements improve nitrogen balance in weight lifters and bodybuilders who take them before an intense workout. A number of human and animal studies have documented the protective effect of glutamine supplements for patients undergoing intravenous feeding. One study involving forty-five bone marrow transplant patients found that adding glutamine to the nutritional formulas significantly reduced their risk of infection. In another study, ten AIDS patients who had lost at least 10 percent of body weight found that 30 to 40 g of glutamine a day reversed the losses, and all regained 2 percent or more of their normal weight.

Animal studies indicate that glutamine protects the liver against damage from anticancer drugs and overdoses of acetaminophen. A preliminary study in Belgium indicated that glutamine supplements were as effective as antidepressant drugs in treating children suffering from clinical depression. An earlier study had found that glutamine also benefited adults suffering from depression. These benefits are thought to be due to glutamine's role as a precursor of GABA, an important brain chemical (neurotransmitter).

Sources

Glutamine is found in meat and other animal products as well as soybeans and other legumes. It is also synthesized in the body.

Forms and Usual Dosages

Glutamine, or L-glutamine as the supplements are usually labeled, is available in powder, pill, and capsule forms; it is also included in the high-protein athletic bars and formulas. There is no standard dosage; experts generally recommend 4 to 10 g a day as a sports supplement, although some advise taking 20 g or more. Up to 20 g day may be given intravenously for surgery and trauma patients.

Potential Problems

Glutamine supplements should not be taken by persons with kidney or liver disease; in these patients, it may increase the risk of a buildup of urea and ammonia. Otherwise, glutamine appears to be safe.

What to Look For

Check athletic supplements and meal replacement products for content of glutamine (or L-glutamine); many of these products provide 1 to 5 g or more of glutamine per serving. The typical nonvegetarian diet provides 10 to 12 g of glutamine a day.

GRAPE SEED EXTRACT

Grape seeds are rich in substances called procyanidolic oligomers, or PCOs, antioxidant compounds that are removed, purified, and concentrated to make grape seed extract. These antioxidant compounds, said to be more powerful than vitamins C or E, are believed to help protect cells from the oxidative damage caused by free radicals. These unstable molecules are released when the body burns oxygen or is exposed to tobacco smoke and certain other pollutants, excessive sunlight, and other harmful substances. Free radicals damage cellular genetic material and are thought to be instrumental in causing cancer, aging, and many degenerative diseases, including atherosclerosis and heart disease.

Role as a Supplement

PCOs, like other potent antioxidants, protect blood fats (lipids) from a process known as peroxidation, a forerunner to the blood-vessel damage that leads to atherosclerosis, the clogging of arteries with deposits of fatty plaque. These benefits may reduce the risk of heart attacks and strokes. PCOs also inhibit enzymes responsible for damaging the structure of blood vessels and help prevent the precancerous changes caused by such cancer-causing compounds as sunlight and tobacco smoke.

In many Western European countries, grape seed extract is widely prescribed to treat or prevent vascular disorders, such as varicose veins and numbness or tingling sensations due to poor circulation, a very common complication of diabetes. The PCOs in grape seed extract may protect vision by preventing diabetes-related damage to tiny blood vessels in the eye; it is also used to halt or slow progression of cataracts and macular degeneration—leading causes of vision loss among older people. Other miscellaneous uses of grape seed extract include:

- Preserving collagen, the key component of skin and connective tissue. It is added to some cosmetic products to make the skin more supple and reduce fine wrinkles.
- Inhibiting the release of some prostaglandins, body chemicals that produce inflammation and pain. Thus, grape seed extract may ease symptoms of such diverse disorders as rheumatoid arthritis, menstrual cramps, and endometriosis.
- Blocking the release of histamines, substances that are instrumental in allergic reactions.
- Inhibiting blood platelet function and reducing clot formation. Preliminary studies using Pycnogenol, a patented compound that contains the same PCOs as grape seed extract, found that it was as effective as low-dose aspirin in reducing blood clots, but it did not cause the stomach irritation that many people experience with aspirin. (See also Pycnogenol, p. 341.)

Evidence of Efficacy

Several studies, mostly from France and Italy, have been published suggesting that grape seed extract is effective in treating peripheral vascular disorders, such as poor circulation to the hands and feet, and slowing the progression of cataracts and macular degeneration.

Sources

Much of the grape seed extract found in supplements is a by-product of the European wine industry. Any seeded grape will provide the same compounds found in grape seed extract, but those used in commercial products come mostly from the red grapes. Seedless grapes contain some PCOs in the skin, but lack the higher concentrations found in the seeds.

Forms and Usual Dosages

Several standardized grape seed extract supplements, many from Europe, are available in the United States, and are available in tablet or capsule form. When used therapeutically to treat a circulatory or vision problem, recommended doses vary from 200 to 300 mg a day. For preventive use as an antioxidant, lower doses of 50 to 100 mg a day are considered sufficient.

Potential Problems

No adverse reactions or side effects have been documented in people taking grape seed extract; animals studies have also found PCOs to be well tolerated with no toxic side effects.

What to Look For

Look for supplements that are standardized to provide 92 to 98 percent PCOs.

See Also

Cancer
Cholesterol Disorders and Atherosclerosis
Circulatory Problems
Dermatitis/Eczema
Heart Disease
Leg Cramps and Restless Legs

GREEN TEA

Tea drinking dates back almost five thousand years, making it one of the world's oldest beverages. All of the more than three thousand different types of tea consumed the world over come from the leaves of the tea plant, *Camellia sinensis*. There are three basic types of tea—black, oolong, and green; the difference lies in the method of processing.

Tea leaves are rich in polyphenol flavonoids, mainly a catechin called epigallocatechin-3-gallate (EGCG), as well as an enzyme known as polyphenol oxidase. After tea leaves are harvested, this enzyme transforms the naturally existing EGCG to another form, altering the color and the chemical composition of the leaves. This chemical reaction is prevented in green tea leaves by steaming or pan-firing the leaves, inactivating the enzyme. The catechin EGCG is believed to be responsible for most of green tea's disease-preventing abilities. Regular consumption of green tea has been associated with a wide range of health benefits, including reducing the risk of heart disease and cancer. Regular black and oolong tea also appear to protect against certain cancers and heart disease, but not to the same degree as green tea.

Role as a Supplement

To reap the full benefits of green tea, a strong, rather bitter-tasting brew is needed—not the pale, weak type that is served in many Asian restaurants. Many people are not tea drinkers—and even many who are—dislike the bitter taste of full-strength green tea. Supplements made from green tea extract allow them to derive the health benefits of the tea without having to drink it. Some extracts provide as much polyphenols as four cups of green tea in a single capsule.

Evidence of Efficacy

Many population studies have found that green tea drinkers have lower rates of cancer of the colon, stomach, pancreas, and esophagus. Laboratory and animal studies back up those findings, showing that the catechins in tea inhibit tumors. It's been suggested that green tea may delay cancer by preventing damage to DNA. And a group of Swedish researchers recently discovered that EGCG may help prevent cancer by stopping the development of new blood vessels that promote tumor growth. Moreover, at least one study is currently looking at the possibility of tea also acting as a therapy for people already diagnosed with cancer. Several studies in China have found that precancerous lesions in the intestinal tract regress and may even disappear when patients are given green tea extract. Population studies attribute a reduced incidence of cancers of the pancreas, stomach, rectum, and possibly the colon to moderate consumption of green tea.

Other studies indicate that regular consumption of green tea may lower cholesterol and reduce the risk of heart attack and stroke. Animal studies suggest that green tea prevents platelet clumping, which can contribute to atherosclerosis and raise the risk of a heart attack or stroke. Green tea also appears to reduce levels of harmful LDL cholesterol and lower blood pressure. However, it is not known whether supplements of green tea extract confer the same health benefits as drinking the actual tea. Green tea provides a complex mixture of polyphenols. The extraction process may filter out important health-promoting compounds in tea that haven't been identified yet. For example, green tea is high in fluoride—a mineral that strengthens bones and protects against tooth decay; this is not found in the extract.

Sources

Green tea and green tea extracts are the best sources of polyphenol flavonoids, which are believed to help prevent cancer and provide other health benefits.

Forms and Usual Dosages

A cup of green tea contains 40 to 90 mg of EGCG. Standardized green tea extracts come in tablet or capsule form and generally contain between 50 and 97 mg of polyphenols, particularly EGCG. Extracts from decaffeinated tea may not contain as many polyphenols, since the decaffeination process tends to remove them along with the caffeine. While some studies have shown health benefits begin with consumption of as little as one cup of tea a day, others suggest it takes much more, maybe ten times more, to see disease-preventing effects. Limit supplementation to the polyphenol equivalent of five cups of green tea a day.

Potential Problems

There are no documented side effects from drinking green tea or taking green tea supplements. The only known side effect is that drinking a lot of green tea can cause insomnia and nervousness due to the caffeine content, which is about half that of coffee.

What to Look For

The first choice should be gunpowder or other traditional Chinese green teas, which are sold in Asian and specialty markets. But for those who don't care for the taste of green tea, there are supplements of green tea extract. Read the label and limit dosage to between 400 and 500 mg of polyphenols per day, the equivalent of about five cups of brewed green tea.

See Also

Cancer
Cholesterol Disorders and Atherosclerosis
Diarrhea

KELP

Kelp is a type of brown seaweed that grows along ocean shores. Some Pacific Coast kelp can grow up to 120 feet; Atlantic kelp is much smaller. Kelp is used in a variety of food products and nutritional supplements and is high in iodine, potassium, calcium, and other minerals as well as many vitamins. Algin, a gel made from kelp, is used as a filler in ice cream and other dairy products.

Role as a Supplement

Kelp is widely used in Asian countries as a good source of calcium, an essential mineral that may be lacking in Asian diets that are low in dairy products. Traditionally, kelp pills—a rich source of iodine—were used to prevent goiter and other thyroid disorders in areas where the soil lacked this mineral.

In recent years, a number of health claims have been made for kelp supplements. These are now promoted as treatments for inflammatory arthritis, psoriasis, circulatory and kidney disorders, constipation, and indigestion. It is also marketed as a weight-loss aid and is said to foster healthy hair and nails.

Evidence of Efficacy

The nutritional value of kelp is relatively easy to establish by chemical analysis of its components. Aside from preventing goiter in iodine-poor areas, most of the therapeutic claims for kelp are unproved or theoretical. For example, the weight-loss claim for kelp is based on the fact that its iodine may improve thyroid function, indirectly helping to control weight.

Sources

Most of the kelp harvested for human consumption is of the *Alaria esculenta* species. Typically, the kelp tops are cut, leaving the bottoms to regrow. Some seaweed is consumed in salads, soups, and other dishes. More often, however, the harvested plants are dried and ground into a powder that is used as a food additive or nutritional supplement.

Forms and Usual Dosage

Kelp can be taken as capsules, pills, or powders. A typical dosage calls for taking one or two 500-mg capsules a day, providing that the dosage does not exceed the RDA of 150 to 200 mcg of iodine.

Potential Problems

Too much iodine from kelp supplements and other sources (including iodized salt) can provoke flare-ups of acne; excessive iodine can also interfere with proper thyroid function. Also, be sure to consume at least eight to ten glasses of water or other fluids a day to absorb the gel.

What to Look For

Check the labels for iodine content, as well as amounts of other minerals and vitamins.

See Also

Constipation

KOMBUCHA MUSHROOMS

The kombucha mushroom, also known as Manchurian mushroom, is not a true mushroom (it has no spores and reproduces by vegetative sprouting), but instead is a yeast culture that thrives on sugar and black tea. The young culture is flat and light gray; as it grows and ages, the culture becomes increasingly darker shades of brown. When the culture digests the sugar and tea, it gives off a somewhat sour or bitter fluid that smells like fermented cider.

New kombucha cultures can be propagated from a mature culture in much the same way that new sourdough starters are obtained. The starter is placed in a clear glass container, fed a mixture of sugar and black or green tea brewed with purified or distilled water, and kept in a dark place. The kombucha cultures use friendly bacteria to digest the sugar and tea, and the resulting liquid—the kombucha or red tea—is said to contain various vitamins, minerals, and healing compounds.

Role as a Supplement

Folk healers in Russia, Manchuria, and Eastern Europe have used kombucha cultures and the tea they produce for hundreds of years. The kombucha tea, which is a waste product produced by the yeast cultures and bacteria, is promoted as a general health tonic and a treatment for everything from infections, inflammatory arthritis, lupus, diabetes, and high blood pressure to depression and other emotional illnesses. The kombucha fad that swept the country in the mid-1990s has died down, but there are still many users who swear by it and credit it with numerous health benefits.

Evidence of Efficacy

There are no scientific studies to back the many health claims for kombucha tea, but anecdotal accounts of improvement of symptoms—often where pharmaceutical medications have been ineffective—abound. Doctors maintain that these benefits are probably due to a placebo effect, but alternative practitioners who recommend kombucha tea feel that it has distinct healing properties.

Sources

Kombucha cultures can be obtained from Asian health outlets; they also can be grown by vegetative propagation, which entails taking a starter from a mature culture and growing it in a new container and a medium of sugar and tea.

Forms and Usual Dosage

Small amounts of the reddish or dark brown liquid surrounding a kombucha culture is drained off and consumed as a tea. Some people drink it as is; others dilute it in water to make it less bitter. Dosages range from 4 to 16 ounces a day; users recommend starting with a low dose and gradually increasing it until the desired benefits are achieved.

Potential Problems

Contamination of a kombucha culture poses a possible health risk. A moldy culture and its tea should be discarded; there have been reports of aspergillus contamination of some kombucha cultures. This fungus can cause a life-threatening infection in people with weakened immune systems. Very old cultures, which are almost black and leathery, should also be discarded.

Some people experience nausea, vomiting, and other intestinal upsets from drinking kombucha tea. It may also interact with prescribed medications, especially drugs used to treat AIDS and other immune-system disorders. If you are taking any medication, or have a chronic disease, check with your doctor before trying kombucha tea.

There have been several media reports linking kombucha tea with unexplained deaths. However, according to the Food and Drug Administration and Centers for Disease Control, autopsies performed in these cases later exonerated kombucha as a possible contributing cause of death. Kombucha appears to be safe so long as proper sanitary precautions in growing the cultures and brewing the tea are followed.

What to Look For

Kombucha cultures are living organisms and are not as easy to grow and propagate as media hype would lead you to believe. The age of a culture, type of sugar and tea it is fed, and even the kind of water used to brew the tea are said to make a difference in the health-giving properties of kombucha tea. If you decide to try growing kombucha mushrooms, seek a culture from an experienced grower and ask for written instructions on how to feed and maintain the culture.

L-ARGININE

L-arginine is one of the twenty amino acids found naturally in protein. Among other things, the body uses it to manufacture a compound called nitric oxide. Researchers only recently discovered the importance of nitric oxide for relaxing blood vessels and allowing blood to flow more freely to and from the heart. In fact, it is the most potent natural vasodilator discovered. It has also been found to help prevent formation of fatty plaque, the substance that clogs the coronary arteries and other blood vessels in people with atherosclerosis. People with high levels of cholesterol tend to have low levels of L-arginine in their blood. A lack of nitric oxide can also contribute to high blood pressure.

Role as a Supplement

Supplemental L-arginine provides the raw material the body needs to produce more nitric oxide and help keep arteries relaxed and blood flowing freely. It also keeps platelets and white blood cells from sticking to artery walls, reducing the risk of atherosclerosis and blood clots, which often lead to a heart attack and/or stroke. It also improves blood flow to the legs, which can reduce the pain of peripheral artery disease, a condition known as intermittent claudication.

Evidence of Efficacy

Researchers discovered only in the last decade that L-arginine is the precursor to nitric oxide. This has led to a great deal of research, mostly in the laboratory and with animals. Much of it showed positive results with L-arginine supplementation. Though there have not been a large number of human studies done with L-arginine, the ones that have been done are promising. One double-blind randomized study of twenty-six men and women suffering from coronary artery disease found that taking 6 g of L-arginine a day significantly improved their circulation after only one week. In another study, using a product (see Forms and Usual Dosage, below) that provided 6 g of L-arginine a day, researchers found that after only two weeks patients suffering from leg pain caused by peripheral artery disease could walk pain-free 66 percent longer than those who received a placebo.

Sources

L-arginine is found in all protein-rich foods, such as beef, pork, fish, and poultry, but soy and pumpkin and squash seeds are also rich sources. However, it is difficult if not impossible to get the therapeutic dosage of 5 or 6 g from food alone.

Forms and Usual Dosage

A dose of 5 to 6 g a day, over and above what's in the diet (which also averages about 5 g a day), has been shown to have a beneficial effect. L-arginine is available in capsules, usually containing 500 or 1,000 mg. Thus, getting the recommended dose requires taking five to twelve capsules a day. It is also available as an ingredient in a nonprescription medicinal health bar which is sold in pharmacies.

Potential Problems

The studies done so far have found supplemental L-arginine to be safe for people with heart disease or diseases of the blood vessels. It has not, however, been tested on people with other medical conditions. It can cause mild diarrhea and trigger a herpes outbreak in those infected with the virus. Some researchers warn that there is a theoretic possibility that L-arginine may increase blood flow to hidden tumors, prompting them to grow faster.

What to Look For

For capsules, opt for 1,000-mg doses, which require only five to six capsules a day to reach the recommended intake. The Heart Bar is another option, but each bar contains 190 calories. With a recommended dose of two bars a day, that adds up to an extra 380 calories a day. To prevent weight gain, the Heart Bar should replace other, less healthful foods—for example, cookies, candy, and other sweets—with the same number of calories.

See Also

Circulatory Problems

LECITHIN

Lecithin, one of a family of fatty compounds called phospholipids, is essential for building the membranes of every cell in the body. These membranes protect cells' interior structures and also control the passage of nutrients and other substances in and out of cells. Without lecithin, the membranes would harden and the cells die.

Lecithin is also found in the protective sheaths surrounding nerve cells (neurons) and muscles. It also carries out essential metabolic functions, especially in helping to break down cholesterol and other lipids. It acts as an emulsifier, a substance that helps fats mix with water and other fluids. Lecithin helps disperse cholesterol and other fats in body fluids so that they can be removed from the body rather than collect in clumps of fatty plaque in the artery walls. Lecithin is also a component of high-density lipoproteins (HDLs), the benefical form of cholesterol that lowers the risk of heart disease.

Lecithin is a major component of bile, the digestive juice that breaks down fats; low levels of lecithin in the bile have been linked to an increased risk of gallstones. Lecithin is a rich source of choline, a chemically similar substance that is often classified as a B vitamin. Like lecithin, it is essential for maintaining cell membranes, and it is also used to make acetylcholine, a chemical (neurotransmitter) that carries nerve messages.

Role as a Supplement

Ironically, some of the best dietary sources of lecithin—eggs, organ meats, and animal fats—have been implicated as culprits in heart disease, obesity, and other health problems. So as Americans reduce their intake of these foods, lecithin supplements may be needed to compensate for the dietary shortfall. Lecithin supplements are also rich in choline (see p. 283), and these two closely related substances are promoted to lower blood cholesterol levels and to treat liver and gallbladder disease. Lecithin may also protect against heart disease by reducing the risk and severity of atheroslerosis—the clogging of coronary and other arteries with fatty deposits. It may also play a role in preventing age-related memory loss and slow progression of Alzheimer's disease.

Evidence of Efficacy

Although lecithin is an essential component of all body cells, many of the health claims made for lecithin supplements are unproved, at least in humans. But some animal studies have involved closely related primates, with promising results. For example, an eight-year study using baboons indicated that lecithin may protect against alcohol-induced cirrhosis (progressive scarring of the liver). Both groups of animals were fed diets high in alcohol—the major cause of cirrhosis in humans. About 80 percent of the baboons who did not receive lecithin developed the liver disease, compared to none of those getting the supplements.

Human studies also indicate that lecithin may increase the effectiveness of some cholesterol-lowering drugs, such as clofibrate. It also seems to protect the stomach and intestines against damage from aspirin, ibuprofen, and other nonsteroidal anti-inflammatory drugs (NSAIDs). In one study involving twenty patients who suffered heartburn and stomach pain from NSAID, fifteen achieved complete relief of symptoms when they took lecithin along with the painkillers.

Sources

Soybeans and egg yolks are rich in lecithin; it is also added to ice cream, mayonnaise, salad dressing, spreads, and many other processed foods to prevent fats and fluids from separating. Other dietary sources include liver and other organ meats, muscle meat, wheat germ, and peanuts.

Forms and Usual Dosage

Most lecithin supplements are a mixture of phospholipids obtained from soybeans. Forms of the supplements include capsules, softgels, pills, powders, granules, and liquid. The powder and granules can be sprinkled on foods or added to shakes. The typical dosage calls for 3 to 5 g of lecithin a day.

Potential Problems

Lecithin is generally safe, although very high doses may cause bloating, diarrhea, nausea, and other intestinal symptoms.

What to Look For

Check the labels for a high content of phosphatidylcholine or phosphatidylserine, lecithin derivatives that are the active ingredients.

See Also

Gallstones

LIPOIC ACID

Lipoic acid, also known as alpha-lipoic acid (ALA), is a substance found naturally in small amounts in the body and in a variety of foods. Although it has some vitaminlike functions, it is not classified as a vitamin because the body can make all that it normally needs.

Lipoic acid is a powerful antioxidant that protects cells against the damage of free radicals, unstable substances that are released when the body burns oxygen or is exposed to certain pollutants, such as tobacco smoke. It also helps preserve or "recycle" other antioxidants, including vitamins C and E and glutathione, a naturally occurring antioxidant in the body. It also works within the body's cells to convert sugars into energy, so it helps lower blood sugar levels. While most compounds are soluble in either water or fat, ALA is soluble in both, a characteristic that makes it especially adept at protecting against free-radical damage both inside and outside the body's cells.

Role as a Supplement

Supplemental ALA may be helpful in the prevention of cataracts; it may also help in the treatment of diabetic neuropathy, the nerve pain or tingling or numbness in the hands and feet that is common among people with diabetes. It may be especially important for vegetarians, since meat is the richest dietary source of ALA. Because the body generally produces less lipoic acid as you age, a supplement may be of help in middle age and beyond. Studies have also found that AIDS patients may benefit from lipoic acid supplements.

Evidence of Efficacy

In the laboratory, the ability of cells to utilize glucose is greatly improved by the addition of ALA to a cell culture. Animal studies show that supplementation with ALA improves the ability of older animals' cells to use oxygen and reduce free radical levels. In pregnant diabetic rats, ALA supplements significantly reduce the risk of birth defects. (Women with diabetes have an increased risk for giving birth to children with birth defects.) And it appears to reduce the effects of stress that results from exercise. Several human studies have found that ALA supplements, given to patients suffering from diabetic neuropathy, significantly relieves the pain and discomfort of the condition, actually regenerating a small amount of nerve tissue in some cases. ALA is approved in Germany as an effective prescription drug for diabetic neuropathy.

Recent studies indicate that ALA inhibits HIV, the virus that causes AIDS, from replicating itself. This benefit is attributed to ALA's ability to raise levels of glutathione, which reduces viral replication.

Sources

Red meat and organ meats are the richest dietary sources of lipoic acid. But it is also present in very small amounts in a variety of vegetables, including potatoes, carrots, yams, beets, broccoli, and spinach.

Forms and Usual Dosages

There are several brands of ALA standardized to deliver 50 to 100 mg of lipoic acid per tablet. Studies that have found ALA to be effective in treating diabetic neuropathy and improving blood glucose metabolism have used doses ranging from 100 to 1,200 mg a day. Doses of 300 to 600 mg a day have been found safe and free of side effects. Studies involving AIDS patients have used 150 mg three times a day. Otherwise, experts generally recommend a daily dosage of 50 to 100 mg a day.

Potential Problems

Ironically, the only reported side effect, low blood sugar, can pose a risk for the very people it may help, namely, patients with diabetes, if their insulin dosage is not adjusted accordingly. The long-term effects of taking lipoic acid supplements are not known.

What to Look For

Look for a standardized preparation of ALA that contains 100 mg per tablet. While ALA is also available in 50-mg tablets, these make it necessary to double the number of tablets to reach the recommended dosage.

See Also

Cataracts

MELATONIN

Melatonin is a hormone that is made in the pineal gland, a tiny organ that lies buried in the brain. Although its existence had long been suspected, researchers isolated melatonin as a distinct hormone only in 1958.

Melatonin regulates the body's circadian rhythms—our internal clock that governs the sleep-wake cycle, release of certain hormones, and numerous other body functions. Its secretion is closely linked with the day-night cycles of light and dark; blood levels start to rise just after dark and peak during the early morning hours. This pattern exists not only in humans, but also in other animal species that sleep at night and are awake and active during the day.

In addition to regulating circadian rhythms, melatonin is thought to play a role in immune function. Because its production declines with advancing age, there has been speculation that melatonin supplements may slow the aging process. It also functions as an antioxidant, protecting cells against damage from free radicals. Thus, it may protect against cancer, heart disease, cataracts, and other degenerative disorders. Some studies also suggest that melatonin may protect against such nerve disorders as Parkinson's and Alzheimer's diseases.

Role as a Supplement

Although melatonin has been touted as a wonder supplement that can prolong life and prevent cancer and heart disease, among other claims, it seems to be most beneficial in treating insomnia and preventing jet lag.

Evidence of Efficacy

Numerous studies show that melatonin supplements can help a person fall asleep and may also improve the quality of sleep. Melatonin can also help restore normal sleep patterns in workers who switch from day to night shifts. Finally, studies have found that melatonin can help travelers who cross several time zones adjust to the time at their destination. This benefit is especially useful for pilots and frequent business travelers who often do not have the time to allow their bodies to adjust naturally to jet lag.

Although melatonin is promoted as an antiaging supplement, the evidence for this comes from animal, not human, studies. In a study conducted in the Netherlands, researchers reported that melatonin may protect against some forms of breast cancer by inhibiting the effects of estrogen. A 1997 Italian study found that melatonin may protect against stroke and heart attacks by protecting arteries against the damage at the root of atherosclerosis. More studies are needed, however, to determine whether melatonin supplements can really produce these diverse benefits.

Forms and Usual Dosages

Melatonin is usually taken in tablet or lozenge form. Some tablets are placed under the tongue so the melatonin can be quickly absorbed into the bloodstream. The typical dosage calls for taking a small dosage—usually 1 to 3 mg—about thirty minutes before going to bed. It usually produces drowsiness in thirty to forty minutes, and the effects last at least three to four hours.

To prevent or treat jet lag, take 1 to 3 mg at bedtime on the day before travel, and a similar dosage at bedtime for the first two or three days after arrival. In addition, force yourself to stay awake during daytime hours after you arrive; to fight the urge to sleep, engage in exercise and try to spend as much time in bright daylight as possible.

Shift workers can reset their biological clock by taking 1 to 3 mg of melatonin about thirty minutes before the time they want to go to bed. For example, someone working a night shift who sleeps during the day may want to take the supplement at 7:30 A.M. to fall asleep by 8 A.M.

Another potential use of melatonin supplements involves treatment of winter depression, or seasonal affective disorder (SAD). A University of Oregon study found that a very small dose, 0.1 mg, taken in the afternoon, improved mood.

Potential Problems

Melatonin may interact with some drugs, including Prozac and other antidepressants, steroids, and other sleep-inducing drugs. Because melatonin causes drowsiness, it should not be taken before driving, operating machinery, or engaging in other activities that require mental alertness. Occasionally, though, melatonin causes a paradoxical reaction, such as agitation and insomnia. Always take the smallest available dose and observe how your body responds.

Product purity is an issue, since several brands were found to contain contaminants including benzodiazepines, such as Xanax. Otherwise, melatonin appears to be safe, although long-term studies of its effects have not been done.

What to Look For

Most supplements are safe and effective; a possible exception are products synthesized from animal glands, which may contain impurities.

See Also

Insomnia

MUSHROOM EXTRACTS

In traditional Chinese medicine, mushrooms are more than tasty, low-calorie foods; they are also sources of important natural medications. There are hundreds of different mushrooms, or fungi. Along with molds and yeasts, they are classified as lower organisms because they reproduce through spores rather than seeds. What we commonly call the mushroom is actually the fungus's fruiting body, and it represents the reproductive phase of its life cycle.

Mushrooms grow worldwide and there are thousands of different varieties. Some are parasitic, existing on living plants and other hosts. Many form symbiotic relationships with their hosts; for example, some of the mushrooms that grow on or near trees provide minerals and water for their hosts in exchange for other nutrients. The fruiting bodies of some mushrooms last for only a few hours, while others persist for months or even years. Some, such as the familiar button mushrooms, are easily cultivated, but many of the most desirable can grow only in the wild. Since ancient times, humans have gathered wild mushrooms, using them for food and medicines. Of course, not all wild mushrooms are safe to eat; in fact, many are highly poisonous. Some of these poisons, such as the ibotenic acid in the *Amanita muscaria* species, are used as recreational hallucinogens—a practice that can be risky indeed.

The mushrooms used most often for medicinal purposes are the *Cordyceps sinensis,* shiitake (*Lentinula edodes*), reishi (*Ganoderma lucidium*), maitake (*Grifola frondosa*), silver-ear (*Tremella fuciformis*), and hoelen (*Poria cocos*).

Role as a Supplement

Since ancient times, various mushroom extracts have been used medicinally. In modern times, some of our first antibiotics were extracted from fungi. Cyclosporin, a drug that is given to transplant patients to suppress the immune system and prevent rejection of the new organ, was originally derived from a fungus that uses insects as a host.

Today, mushroom extracts are said to bolster immunity and help prevent cancer or inhibit tumor growth. Common disorders and the mushroom extracts that are said to be effective in treating them include the following:

- Anti-inflammatories: Reishi and silver-ear.
- Asthma and bronchitis: Cordyceps, reishi, and silver-ear.
- Cardiovascular disorders: Cordyceps, shiitake, reishi, and silver-ear.
- Cholesterol-lowering extracts: Cordyceps, shiitake, reishi, and silver-ear.
- Diabetes: Maitake and silver-ear.
- High blood pressure: Cordyceps, shiitake, reishi, maitake, and silver-ear.
- Improved kidney function: Cordyceps and reishi.
- Liver disorders: Cordyceps, shiitake, reishi, maitake, silver-ear, and hoelen.
- Stress reduction: Cordyceps and reishi.
- Viral infections: Cordyceps, shiitake, reishi, and hoelen.

Evidence of Efficacy

More than 280 reports of scientific studies related to the medicinal uses of mushroom extracts have been published in recent years. Most of these studies have been conducted in Asia and Europe, but there is growing interest in mushroom extracts in the United States. Studies conducted here and abroad have documented the antibiotic properties of certain mushroom extracts. Recently, there has been increasing interest in using mushroom extracts to bolster immunity, especially among people who are HIV-positive. A number of researchers are also investigating the antitumor properties of some mushrooms with hopes of developing anticancer drugs. In fact, mushroom extracts are widely used as adjuncts to cancer treatments in Japan and China. More research is needed, however, to prove these various health benefits, and to develop effective drugs from mushroom extracts.

Sources

The most widely used mushroom extracts are obtained from the species listed above. They may be obtained from health food stores and outlets specializing in traditional Asian medicines.

Forms and Usual Dosages

Mushroom extracts are available in liquid, powder, and pill forms. Dosages vary according to the usage; follow label instructions. Some experts, including Dr. Andrew Weil, the noted proponent of integrative medicine, advocate including a variety of mushrooms in the diet.

Potential Problems

As noted, many wild mushrooms are poisonous, and because so many mushrooms look alike, it's a good idea to leave gathering wild mushrooms to the experts. Some mushroom extracts may interact with pharmaceutical medications; check with your doctor before taking them, especially if you are being treated for a chronic disease.

What to Look For

Take only extracts that are made from edible mushrooms, and buy them from reputable outlets.

OAT BRAN

Oat bran, the outer covering of the oat seed, is one of the most nutritious parts of the grain. About 50 to 80 percent of the minerals in grains are found in the bran, as well as several important disease-preventing phytochemicals, including lignans, tocotrienols, and phenolic compounds.

The bran also contains soluble dietary fiber—a substance that dissolves in water to form a gel, but passes through the human intestinal tract without being digested and absorbed. (Insoluble fiber passes through the intestinal tract pretty much intact without dissolving.) When oats are milled and refined into flour, most of the nutritious bran is lost.

Role as a Supplement

Oat bran is rich in soluble fiber, specifically beta glucan, which when eaten regularly as part of a low-fat, low-cholesterol diet, can lower blood cholesterol levels. Numerous studies show that oat bran is important in controlling blood sugar levels among people with diabetes. It also helps prevent (or treat) constipation because the soluble fiber absorbs large amounts of water as it passes through the intestinal tract, thereby forming a soft, bulky stool that is easier to pass. Oat bran and other high-fiber foods are important in helping control weight by promoting a feeling of fullness and preventing overeating.

Evidence of Efficacy

Dozens of studies have found that both oat bran and oatmeal can help lower blood cholesterol. That's because the soluble fiber found in oats helps the body rid itself of excess cholesterol. It also helps regulate blood sugar by slowing absorption of glucose following a meal. A recent study in Texas clearly demonstrated that a high-fiber diet that supplied 25 g each of soluble and insoluble fiber a day afforded better blood-glucose control than the standard American Diabetes Association diet, which provides 8 g of soluble and 26 g of insoluble fiber a day.

Sources

Oatmeal and other whole-oat cereals are good sources of dietary oat bran; it is also used as an ingredient in multigrain cereals and added to high-fiber breads and other foods. However, several products, including some muffins, chips, and even doughnuts, that claim to contain oat bran, actually provide very little oat bran and may be high in fat and sugar.

Forms and Usual Dosage

As a supplement, oat bran is available in tablet form. However, each tablet typically provides less than 1 g of oat bran. Even taking several tablets a day would provide far less than the dose needed to lower cholesterol and control blood sugar.

Oat bran and oatmeal are found in the cereal section of the supermarket or health food store. Several studies have found that eating 25 to 100 g of oat bran a day can cause a significant drop—6 to 12 percent—in total cholesterol and a reduction of up to 16 percent in the harmful LDL cholesterol.

Potential Problems

Abruptly increasing fiber intake can cause some bloating, gasiness, and other gastrointestinal problems for some people. The best approach is to increase oat bran consumption slowly until you reach an effective, cholesterol-lowering level. Be sure to drink at least eight to ten glasses of water and other nonalcoholic fluids a day because oat bran requires ample fluids to move through the intestinal tract. And keep in mind that oat bran has been proven effective as a way to lower cholesterol only when eaten as part of an overall low-fat, low cholesterol diet.

What to Look For

Look for 100 percent oat bran cereal products, or products that list oat bran as the first ingredient. (Ingredients are listed according to the amount in the product, so if oat bran is listed first, it is the main ingredient.)

See Also

Heart Disease

PERIWINKLE EXTRACT (VINPOCETINE)

Vinpocetine is a dietary supplement derived from an extract of the *Vinca minor* periwinkle plant and other sources, which has been shown to enhance memory and mental function, which often begin to decline in middle age (Unfortunately, it does not appear to work against Alzheimer's disease, the devastating form of dementia that is especially common among the elderly.)

Researchers have identified a number of areas in which vinpocetine exerts a protective effect on brain cells. For example, it protects against damage from normal metabolic changes as well as against a toxic agent called veratridine, which raises the sodium and calcium levels in nerve endings, thereby reducing the transmission of chemical messages within the brain. Other specific mechanisms in which vinpocetine benefits brain function include:

- Increased cerebral blood flow.
- Increased brain metabolism of energy and oxygen.
- Speeds the brain's uptake of glucose, its major fuel.
- Increased production of neurotransmitters, brain chemicals such as serotonin, acetylcholine, and dopamine, which carry messages from one nerve cell to another.

In addition to boosting memory, vinpocetine appears promising in the treatment and prevention of a number of disorders that involve brain circulation: stroke, vertigo, sleep disorders, Meniere's syndrome, ringing in the ear (tinnitus), migraine headaches, certain menopausal symptoms, convulsions, and depression, and other mood disorders. It is also used to improve visual acuity in people with macular degeneration and other eye disorders.

Role as a Supplement

Vinpocetine supplements have been shown to improve short-term memory and to enhance learning and recall, especially among older people. People who have a high risk of stroke, such as those who have had transient ischemic attacks (TIAs or ministrokes) or who have atherosclerosis, can benefit from vinpocetine as a stroke preventive because it appears to inhibit the formation of blood clots in the brain—the leading direct cause of strokes. Young people, such as students taking exams, may also benefit from vinpocetine. Finally, it has been shown to benefit people suffering from such diverse disorders as ringing in the ears, migraine headaches, nerve-related hearing loss, and macular degeneration.

Evidence of Efficacy

Vinpocetine has been subjected to more than 100 clinical studies, involving more than 20,000 patients, at medical and research centers around the world. Many of these have been double-blind crossover studies in which vinpocetine has been matched against a placebo or other supplements or pharmaceutical products. Its benefits have been more pronounced than those of ginkgo biloba extract.

Sources

Vinpocetine is derived from vincamine, an alkaloid extract of the *Vinca minor* periwinkle plant. Vincamine is also derived from Voacanga seeds and the Crioceras longiflorus plant.

Form and Usual Dosages

Vinocetine is available in tablet form. The dosages used in clinical studies ranged from 10 to 40 mg a day. The typical recommended dosage for memory support and improved mental function calls for 15 mg a day, taken in 5 mg pills three times a day.

PHENYLALANINE

Phenylalanine is an amino acid—one of the building blocks of protein—that is abundant in meat and milk products. It is a precursor of another amino acid—tyrosine—and together these two substances are instrumental in making important hormones. These include thyroxine, which is secreted by the thyroid gland, and epinephrine and norepinephrine, adrenal hormones that are secreted during times of stress. In addition, phenylalanine teams up with tryptophan, another amino acid, to control the release of cholecystokinin, an intestinal hormone commonly called CCK. It plays an instrumental role in controlling appetite by signaling the brain when the stomach is full, thereby turning off the hunger signals that can lead to overeating.

Phenylalanine is capable of passing through the brain's protective blood-brain barrier and acting directly on brain chemistry. For example, because it is a precursor of tyrosine, phenylalanine can help synthesize important chemical messengers (neurotransmitters), including dopamine, epinephrine, and tyramine. It is thought to play roles in memory and alertness. Phenylalanine is also thought to prevent the breakdown of the brain's natural painkillers.

Role as a Supplement

Phenylalanine is promoted to treat depression, alleviate pain, and control appetite. It may help overcome alcoholism and other addictions; there have also been reports that it increases libido in persons with a low sex drive.

Evidence of Efficacy

Several studies have documented the value of phenylalanine in treating clinical depression and some pain syndromes, including chronic back pain, migraines and other headaches, and menstrual pain. Claims that it can boost sexual drive, suppress appetite, overcome alcoholism, and improve memory are based mostly on anecdotal accounts and studies of substances with similar chemical properties.

Sources

Phenylalanine is an essential amino acid that cannot be made in the body. It is found mostly in meats and milk products, especially cheese. Lesser amounts are found in wheat germ and oats.

Forms and Usual Dosages

Phenylalanine comes in three forms: L, which is primarily a nutritional supplement; D, which is used primarily to alleviate pain and depression; and DL, a fifty-fifty mixture of the two. Phenylalanine supplements, in any of its forms, should not be taken for more than two or three weeks at a time. One study found that dosages of 100 to 500 mg of DL-phenylalanine completely eliminated symptoms of depression within two weeks. Another study involving patients with manic-depression (bipolar disorder) found that 500 mg of L-phenylalanine given along with 100 mg of vitamin B_6 twice a day worked best. The recommended dosage for pain calls for 500 to 750 mg of the DL form two or three times a day, up to a maximum of 2,400 mg (2.4 g) a day for a maximum of three weeks at a time.

Potential Problems

High doses of more than 2.4 g of phenylalanine a day can cause anxiety and headaches. Because phenylalanine boosts levels of norepinephrine and epinephrine, it may raise blood pressure and should not be taken by anyone who has high blood pressure or a propensity to develop it (for example, a person whose pressure readings fall into the high normal range or who have a family history of it). Some experts recommend that even persons with normal blood pressure monitor their readings when taking phenylalanine, and stop the supplements or reduce the dosage if blood pressure rises. In addition, phenylalanine interacts with antidepressants or high-blood-pressure drugs containing MAO inhibitors, and should never be used by anyone who is taking these medications.

Although there are reports that phenylalanine helps some migraine sufferers, it may have the opposite effect for persons whose headaches are triggered by high levels of the substance. Obviously, phenylalanine supplements should not be taken if they seem to provoke rather than relieve these headaches.

Phenylalanine in any dosage should not be taken by anyone with PKU (phenylketonuria), a genetic defect that prevents them from metabolizing phenylalanine. Some studies suggest that phenylalanine may speed the growth of some cancers, especially melanoma, and should be avoided by anyone with cancer.

What to Look For

Tailor the form of phenylalanine to the target problem. For example, D-phenylalanine is promoted for treating chronic pain and bipolar depression, activities that are enhanced by adding vitamin B_6 to the regimen. The L or DL forms of phenylalanine are said to be more effective in treating the affective type of depression, which is characterized by a consistently sad mood.

See Also

Depression

PHOSPHATIDYLSERINE

Phosphatidylserine, or PS for short, belongs to a special category of fat-soluble substances called phospholipids. It is a natural compound that is found in the membranes of all the body's cells, where it is essential for normal functioning. PS is especially highly concentrated in brain cells, where it helps regulate neurotransmitters, the chemical messengers that carry nerve impulses to and from the brain.

Role as a Supplement

Phosphatidylserine may be helpful in supporting mental function. Studies indicate that taking supplemental PS may improve concentration and memory in people suffering from age-related memory loss, dementia, and Alzheimer's disease.

Evidence of Efficacy

Most of the research with PS has been done in Europe, where researchers report that taking 300 mg a day can significantly improve memory and cognitive function (the ability to think, reason, and concentrate) among people who have suffered a decline in their normal mental abilities. The best results have been found when people were given PS in the early stages of dementia and Alzheimer's disease. Although mental-function tests show significant improvements in Alzheimer's patients, researchers caution that it's generally not enough to make a real difference in the ability to function on a day-to-day basis.

Less research has been done on the benefit of PS among people suffering from normal age-related memory loss, but it is thought to be helpful. PS has not, however, been shown to improve a young, healthy person's ability to think or remember facts. In contrast, older people seem to benefit from the supplements. In one study of fifty-one subjects over seventy-one years of age, those given PS for twelve weeks showed improvements in their abilities to maintain concentration and to recall names of familiar people, the location of misplaced objects, and details from the previous day and the past week, and also improvements in their ability to concentrate. Follow-up studies showed that the benefits may last for several months after PS supplementation stops.

Sources

Originally, PS was extracted from cattle brains, but the scare over mad cow disease had researchers scrambling for a new source. PS now comes from soy, which is a naturally rich source. At least one study found PS from soy to be just as effective as that extracted from cows' brains.

Phosphatidylserine is found in only trace amounts in a typical diet, with lecithin providing very small amounts. However, the body manufactures what it needs from phospholipid building blocks.

Forms and Usual Dosage

PS is available in capsule form and as a chewing gum. The recommended dosage is 300 mg a day, divided into three doses, for three to four weeks. Once improvement is noted, a maintenance dose of 100 mg a day is recommended. Capsules typically provide 100 mg each, whereas two pieces of gum provide about 85 mg a day.

Potential Problems

No side effects associated with phosphatidylserine have been reported, although one expert has suggested that taking PS at night may affect sleep.

What to Look For

Look for PS derived from soy in capsule form. It takes at least six or more pieces of gum a day to deliver the amount of PS found in three capsules.

See Also

Alzheimer's Disease and Memory Loss

PHYTOESTROGENS

Phytoestrogens are plant compounds that have effects similar to those of estrogen, the major female sex hormone, in the body. They can be divided into two main groups: isoflavones, which are found in soybeans, red clover, kudzu root, among others; and lignans, substances that are found in flaxseed, whole grains, and some fruits and vegetables. Soy is a unique dietary source of the much-studied isoflavones called genistein and daidzein.

Phytoestrogens are thought to compete with natural estrogens for estrogen receptors on cells. By binding to the receptors, phytoestrogens prevent estrogen from stimulating certain tissues and theoretically lower the risk of developing cancers that are spurred by estrogen. Isoflavones are much more potent than lignans when it comes to interacting with estrogen receptors in the body.

Although they compete for the same binding sites on cells, phytoestrogens do not act exactly the same way natural estrogens do. Chemically, for example, isoflavones are only about one-thousandth as potent as natural estrogens. But in some of the body's tissues, phytoestrogens mimic the action of estrogen and may alleviate the symptoms of menopause in older women; in other tissues, they block the action of estrogen and thereby lower the risk of developing some kinds of cancer, especially of the breast.

Role as a Supplement

Phytoestrogen-rich soy supplements and isoflavone supplements in pill form are promoted as alternatives for estrogen replacement therapy (ERT) in menopausal women.

Evidence of Efficacy

Population studies have found a link between soy-rich diets and a low risk of breast and endometrial cancer in women and prostate cancer in men. The research that has attracted the most attention has compared Asian women to American women and found that Asian women who eat traditional diets that contain a lot of soy have a much lower risk of breast cancer and rarely experience hot flashes and other menopausal symptoms. These protective effects are attributed to the phytoestrogens found in soy. Several controlled studies have found that giving either soy-supplemented diets or isoflavone supplements extracted from red clover results in a decrease in the frequency of hot flashes experienced by menopausal women.

Laboratory and animal studies show that phytoestrogens can inhibit tumor growth. Studies with cultured human breast cancer cells, leukemia cells, and prostate cancer cells have demonstrated the ability of phytoestrogens to slow tumor growth.

Research has also shown that phytoestrogens can inhibit the oxidation of the harmful LDL (low-density lipoprotein) cholesterol, a step believed to trigger the formation of fatty plaque in arteries. The Food and Drug Administration reviewed the scientific evidence and was convinced enough of the cholesterol-lowering abilities of soy to allow a cholesterol-lowering health claim on soy-containing foods. Specifically, foods that contain at least 6.25 g of soy protein per serving can carry the health claim. Soy experts believe that phytoestrogens are partly responsible for the cholesterol-lowering effects seen with soy protein. Research has also found that isoflavone supplements extracted from red clover increased the ability of arteries to stretch and allow blood to flow freely—a function called arterial compliance—in postmenopausal women.

There is also some research to suggest that phytoestrogens may help prevent osteoporosis. For example, population studies indicate that phytoestrogens may protect against bone loss in older women, including those whose diets provide less than the recommended amounts of calcium. Asian women, for instance, consume very little milk and milk products; they also tend to be thin and small-boned— factors that theoretically would increase their risk of osteoporosis. Yet their incidence of this disease is somewhat less than that of American women, even though Americans generally consume more calcium than Asians. The soy-rich Asian diet is credited with the reduced risk of osteoporosis.

Sources

Phytoestrogens are found naturally in soy, legumes, flaxseed, whole grains, fruits and vegetables, and red clover. Soy protein and whole soy foods like tofu, roasted soybeans, and soy milk are especially good sources.

Forms and Usual Dosages

Isoflavone supplements extracted from either soy or red clover are available in pill and capsule forms. A number of phytoestrogen supplements sold in health food stores contain a mixture of isoflavones and extracts of wild yam, dong quai, and kudzu root—herbal sources of phytoestrogens—along with various vitamins and minerals. Soy protein is available in powdered form, which can be mixed with milk or juice.

The recommended intakes of isoflavones vary considerably, but many experts point to the average Asian intake of about 25 to 50 mg a day as a safe and possibly effective dose. However, some high-potency phytoestrogen supplements provide higher doses of isoflavones of 500 mg or more.

Potential Problems

Some experts are concerned that taking high doses of phytoestrogens could backfire, actually increasing the risk for some kinds of cancer. One group that could possibly be at risk are postmenopausal women with undiagnosed estrogen-dependent breast cancer. Most experts believe that a daily dosage of 50 mg of phytoestrogens is safe for most people, including men. But, it is not known if higher doses taken on a regular basis could cause problems.

What to Look For

Opt for whole soy foods and flaxseed as a natural source of phytoestrogens. If you decide on a supplement, limit your daily dose to 50 mg of phytoestrogens.

PSYLLIUM

Psyllium seed, also known as the plantago seed, is one of the most popular bulk-producing laxatives. As a supplement or laxative, it is made of the cleaned, dried ripe seed of the *Plantago psyllium* plant, which is grown mainly in India. The outer covering or husk of the seeds contains a thick, gel-like material—soluble fiber—that is not digested by humans. When this soluble fiber comes in contact with water, it swells, providing both bulk and lubrication to the mass of food as it moves through the intestinal tract. The increased bulk stimulates the rhythmic waves of intestinal contractions (peristalsis) that move the stool through the colon. This shortens transit time and further prevents or relieves constipation by forming a soft stool that is easy to pass. People who suffer from hemorrhoids and anal fissures often report a lessening of pain, itching, and other symptoms after a few days of taking psyllium.

Psyllium also alters the bacterial balance in the lower intestine, fostering an increase in beneficial bacteria over time. These beneficial bacteria produce substances called short-chain fatty acids (for example, acetic, butyric, and propionic acids), which may help lower blood cholesterol, boost the immune system, and reduce the risk of colon cancer. One study involving obese patients indicated that psyllium may help prevent gallstones, a common problem, especially among women and overweight people.

Role as a Supplement

Psyllium is an excellent source of soluble fiber, which helps prevent and treat constipation as well as lower blood cholesterol. As noted, it also modifies the bacterial balance in the intestinal tract, causing an increase in beneficial bacteria. Finally, it may help control weight by delaying the emptying of food from the stomach and fostering a sense of fullness, which lessens the urge to overeat.

Evidence of Efficacy

Several well-controlled studies have proved that psyllium is an effective bulking agent and laxative. Research also shows that about 10 g of psyllium per day can reduce total cholesterol by about 5 percent and levels of the harmful LDL cholesterol by about 9 percent in people with high levels. Based on the research available, the Food and Drug Administration approved the use of a health claim on psyllium-containing products that states: "The soluble fiber from psyllium seed husk in this product, as part of a diet low in saturated fat and cholesterol, may reduce the risk of heart disease." To qualify for the health claim, a product must contain at least 1.7 g of soluble fiber from psyllium per serving.

Sources

Several over-the-counter bulking laxatives, such as Metamucil, contain psyllium. It is also an ingredient in some herbal products. And it can also be found in a few breakfast cereals, such as Kellogg's Bran Buds.

Forms and Usual Dosage

Psyllium is generally available from health food stores in prepackaged or bulk form; it is also marketed as capsule and wafers. A typical dose is 1 to 3 tablespoons of the ground psyllium a day. However, check the label for instructions; some products are concentrated, and require a lesser amount. Mix the ground psyllium into a full 8-ounce glass of water, juice, or milk; it must be drunk quickly before the mixture thickens into a gelatinlike substance. Improvement in constipation and hemorrhoid symptoms are usually seen within one to three days; it may take a month or more to achieve a significant lowering of blood cholesterol levels.

Potential Problems

Psyllium, like other bulk laxative agents, can cause increased gas production and bloating. Constipation may actually worsen during the week or so of taking psyllium regularly. To reduce potential bloating and gas, start with half the recommended dose and gradually increase it. Gas production should return to normal once a new bacterial balance in the intestine has been established.

Psyllium, as with all bulking agents, must be taken with plenty of water or other fluids—a full glass with the powder itself and at least six to eight additional glasses during the course of the day. Because it can delay the absorption of drugs and other supplements, allow at least two hours to lapse after taking a medication, vitamin, or other supplement before taking the psyllium. Although psyllium is quite safe for most people, an inadequate fluid intake can lead to esophageal or bowel obstruction. Psyllium should not be taken with medications that slow the normal movement of the intestinal tract. Nor should it be taken by anyone with swallowing problems, such as persons with Parkinson's disease; it is also contraindicated for persons with diabetes.

Although rare, psyllium can trigger allergic reactions in some people, especially those who are frequently exposed to psyllium dust, such as health care workers employed in nursing homes where many patients are given ground psyllium as a laxative.

What to Look For

Products that carry the psyllium health claim contain a significant amount of psyllium. But more than one serving a day is needed to be effective as a laxative or to lower blood cholesterol. Over-the-counter laxative bulking agents that contain psyllium or herbal preparations or fiber supplements that contain psyllium are equally effective if psyllium is present in adequate amounts. Read labels to check for psyllium content and dosing schedules; do not exceed 30 g of psyllium in the course of a day.

PYCNOGENOL

Pycnogenol is an extract made from the bark of the maritime pine tree (*Pinus pinaster*), which grows in the south of France. Though originally a generic term used to describe a group of proanthocyanidins—natural bioflavonoids found in concentrated amounts in grape seeds and peanut skins—Pynogenol is now a trade name for a single supplement. It is a composite of about forty natural ingredients that are biologically active. Pine bark extract has been used in folk medicine for centuries; the modern Pycnogenol nutraceutical was first introduced in Europe in the 1950s as an over-the-counter drug to treat circulation problems.

Role as a Supplement

Pycnogenol is claimed to improve or treat a wide variety of diseases and conditions. Specifically, it is said to stimulate blood circulation, improve vision, increase flexibility, reduce bruising, fight inflammation, improve skin smoothness, alleviate symptoms of chronic fatigue syndrome, and increase exercise endurance. It is also said to reduce the risk of heart disease, cancer, stroke, diabetes-related eye problems (diabetic retinopathy), and clotting problems, including phlebitis. It is also said to slow the aging process and protect the skin against sun damage.

Evidence of Efficacy

The most promising studies involve circulatory disorders. Bioflavonoids, including catechins, phenolic acids, and mainly proanthocyanidins, which have antioxidant powers, are credited with its action. Laboratory studies have found it to have greater antioxidant activity than vitamins C or E.

Most clinical studies have been done in Europe, where positive results have been found in the treatment of many diverse disorders, including arthritis, hay fever and other allergies, bronchitis, asthma, bruises and athletic injuries, varicose veins, macular degeneration, and circulatory problems in people with diabetes. Research suggests it may help relieve circulatory problems by keeping blood vessel walls strong. It has also been found to reduce platelet clumping, a forerunner of a tendency of the blood to clot and exacerbate atherosclerosis. In fact, one researcher reported that Pycnogenol has an anticoagulant effect five times that of aspirin. It also seems to help preserve levels of vitamins C and E in the body.

A recent study by an Oklahoma psychologist who specializes in treating attention deficit hyperactivity disorder (ADHD), found that Pycnogenol was as effective as Ritalin and other stimulant drugs in calming children and adults with ADHD. However, the study involved only thirty subjects, and more research is needed to document whether Pycnogenol really is effective against ADHD. Otherwise, the majority of Pycnogenol studies have been done either in the laboratory or in animals; there are relatively few clinical studies involving humans.

Some of the European antiaging skin creams contain Pycnogenol. In addition to restoring skin elasticity and smoothing fine lines, Pycnogenol skin products are marketed as a psoriasis treatment and to protect skin from sun damage.

Sources

Almost identical phytochemicals are found in grape seed extract, which is less expensive than Pycnogenol, and at least one product used in clinical studies (Proanthenol's Bio-Complex) combines pine bark and grape seed extracts. Pycnogenol contains slightly fewer proanthocyanidins than grape seed extracts. Foods containing small amounts of proanthocyanidins include citrus fruits, tea, onions, blueberries, and apples.

Forms and Usual Dosages

The manufacturer of branded Pycnogenol recommends a dose of about 1 to 1.5 mg per pound of body weight for seven to ten days. After that, doses can be reduced to one-half that amount or less. The dose typically recommended for healthy people is 50 to 100 mg a day. Doses used in studies have been as high as 200 mg a day. It is typically available in tablets of 25, 50, 75, and 100 mg.

Potential Problems

No side effects have been reported with taking Pycnogenol; however, it might be a problem for people who are allergic to pine. It generally appears to be safe, even in large doses.

What to Look For

The original French product, which is marketed as Pycnogenol in Europe, is available in the United States as Proanthenol's Bio-Complex, and the name of the original inventor, Dr. Masquelier, appears on the label. This is the product used in European clinical and laboratory studies. (See also Grape Seed Extract, p. 310.)

See Also

Cancer
Cholesterol Disorders and Atherosclerosis
Circulatory Problems

RED RICE YEAST (CHOLESTIN)

Red rice yeast is a traditional Chinese health food and medicine. Also known as *Monascus purpureus,* or by its traditional Chinese name, hong qu, it is made from red yeast grown on rice. It has been used in China for more than two thousand years as a treatment for indigestion, diarrhea, and abdominal pain. An ancient Chinese book of pharmacy records use of the yeast to promote cardiovascular health. Ironically, one of the natural compounds found in red rice yeast supplements is the same active compound found in the prescription cholesterol-lowering statin drug Mevacor. For that reason, in 1997 the Food and Drug Administration ruled that red rice yeast was an unapproved drug and banned it. Later, however, a federal court reversed the FDA ruling, saying red rice yeast was a nutritional supplement, not a drug.

Role as a Supplement

Red rice yeast has been proven to significantly lower blood cholesterol levels. Like some prescription statin drugs, such as Mevacor, it inhibits the action of HMG-CoA, an enzyme found in the liver that regulates the body's production of cholesterol.

Evidence of Efficacy

Two of the more than two dozen clinical studies using red rice yeast were done in the United States; the rest have been done in China. Taken as a whole, the studies have found that red rice yeast can lower cholesterol by 16 to 26 percent as well as lower triglyceride levels and raise levels of the beneficial HDL cholesterol. A recent study found that red rice yeast lowered blood cholesterol an average of 40 points over a twelve-week period compared to just 5 points in people who only made dietary changes. Benefits are greatest in people with total cholesterol levels above 200, the cutoff point of desirable cholesterol set by the American Heart Association.

Sources

Cholestin is the brand of red rice yeast seen most often in the United States. Although there are other brands of red rice yeast available, Cholestin is also the only one that is standardized and that has been scientifically studied.

Form and Usual Dosages

The standard dose is two 600-mg capsules twice a day. It is sold in capsule form at pharmacies and health food stores, and it costs only a fraction of what prescription statin drugs cost. Red rice yeast is recommended for people with borderline-high cholesterol levels (200 to 240) and no other risk factors for heart disease. A low-fat diet is also recommended while taking the supplement. To avoid stomach upset, it should be taken with food or fluids.

Potential Problems

There have been no serious side effects reported from taking red rice yeast. Some of the minor side effects have included heartburn, bloating, and dizziness. There are no known drug interactions with red rice yeast. However, because of its similarity to statin drugs, which should not be taken with niacin, erythromycin, cyclosporin, fibrates, or other statin drugs, the same cautions should be applied to red rice yeast. In theory, red rice yeast could cause some of the same side effects as the statin drugs, including elevated liver enzymes, damage to skeletal muscle, and a possible increased risk of cancer. Pregnant and nursing women should avoid red rice yeast as should those with severe liver or kidney disease. No one under the age of twenty should take red rice yeast. In short, check with your doctor before taking red rice yeast.

What to Look For

Cholestin is the only red rice yeast product that is standardized and that has been proven effective in clinical trials.

See Also

Cholesterol Disorders and Atherosclerosis

SAM-E

SAM-e is the popular name for S-adenosylmethionine, a substance that is produced naturally by the body from methionine, a sulphur-containing amino acid, and adenosine triphosphate (ATP), an energy-producing compound. It is found in all the body's tissues, where it is involved in the synthesis, activation, and metabolism of several important compounds, including certain hormones, neurotransmitters, nucleic acids (found in DNA), proteins, and phospholipids. It is also instrumental in the detoxification of drugs and harmful compounds.

SAM-e was first discovered in 1952, and first made commercially available in Europe in 1976. As a supplement, SAM-e is used to treat depression and arthritis. SAM-e is approved by health authorities in Germany as a first-choice prescription drug to treat osteoarthritis. In Italy, Spain, and Russia, it is used to improve liver function, and in Italy and Russia, it is used to treat depression. In many European countries, SAM-e is a prescription medication, but in the United States it is available as a nonprescription nutritional supplement.

Role as a Supplement

SAM-e may help preserve the gel-like, shock-absorbing cartilage, which wears away in people with arthritis. There is also evidence that SAM-e promotes repair and regrowth of damaged cartilage, making it especially valuable in the treatment of osteoarthritis. SAM-e has also been proven effective in the treatment of depression and may help promote liver health.

Evidence of Efficacy

Supplementation with SAM-e has been shown to enhance mood, promote joint mobility, and help maintain liver health. Clinical studies indicate that benefits are evident after one to two weeks of use.

A large analysis of several studies looking at its effectiveness in treating depression, including more than one thousand patients, showed that those receiving SAM-e experienced 17 to 38 percent more improvement than those taking a placebo. The improvement was comparable to, and in some cases exceeded what is expected from some prescription antidepressants. SAM-e is also faster-acting than many prescription antidepressants.

One long-term, multicenter clinical study of arthritis sufferers in Europe found that relief from pain and an improvement in joint health may begin as early as the first few weeks of supplementation and continue for up to two years. Laboratory studies have found that SAM-e has the ability to maintain and restore normal structure and function to liver cells, but to date, it is not known whether this benefit applies to humans as well as laboratory animals.

Sources

SAM-e is present in all living organisms. Significant amounts, however, are not available through food. It is sold as a nonprescription supplement in pharmacies, health food stores, groceries, and other outlets.

Forms and Usual Dosages

SAM-e is available as 200-mg pills; the recommended doses range from 400 to 1,600 mg a day. The lower doses are used to treat arthritis; somewhat higher doses may be needed to treat depression. The pills are enteric coated so that they do not dissolve until they reach the small intestine, where the substance is maximally absorbed. It is best taken on an empty stomach, about an hour before meals.

There are two forms of SAM-e; the preferred form is 1-4-butanedisulfonate, which is more stable than the older toluensulfonate (tosylate) form.

Potential Problems

SAM-e is well tolerated with few side effects. However, some people may experience nausea, heartburn, and diarrhea when it is taken at the higher doses. Enteric-coated tablets should alleviate heartburn. People suffering from bipolar disorder (manic-depression) should avoid SAM-e; the supplement could exacerbate or unmask manic phases of the disorder.

What to Look For

Look for enteric-coated 200-mg tablets that contain S-adenosylmethionine 1,4-butan edisulfonate, the form that has been used in most clinical studies.

See Also

Arthritis
Depression

SHARK CARTILAGE

Cartilage is a tough, somewhat elastic tissue found mainly in the joints of many animals, including humans. The skeleton of a shark, however, is made entirely of cartilage, rather than bone. Supplements of shark cartilage became popular mainly in response to a book entitled *Sharks Don't Get Cancer,* which claimed that shark cartilage possessed an anticancer substance that protected them against the disease.

As it turns out, sharks actually do get cancer. But it is true that shark cartilage possesses a compound that, in the laboratory at least, has anticancer effects. The growth of any tumor requires the creation of new blood vessels to feed it—a biological process called angiogenesis. Anything that blocks the blood supply to the tumor stops the tumor from growing and eventually kills it. It's believed that shark cartilage contains glycoprotein compounds that have an anti-angiogenesis effect.

Role as a Supplement

Shark cartilage is purported to ease the pain and inflammation of arthritis, but it is best known as an alternative treatment for cancer. It is said to slow the growth of existing tumors and prevent new cancers from developing.

Evidence of Efficacy

Chondroitin sulfate, a compound that has shown promise on its own as an arthritis remedy, is found in significant amounts in shark cartilage, and may explain its role in easing the pain and inflammation of arthritis. More recently, a group of Canadian researchers found that a preparation of shark cartilage, used on the skin, had an anti-inflammatory effect. An animal study conducted in Brazil found that shark cartilage had a pain-relieving effect.

In the 1970s, laboratory studies found shark cartilage to have anti-cancer properties. But human studies have not shown much promise. Most of the evidence of its effectiveness is based on testimonials, rather than scientific research. The most highly publicized study was of sixty patients with several types of advanced cancer who were given daily doses of powdered shark cartilage for twelve weeks. Five patients died during the study and none showed any reduction in the size of their tumors. One large clinical study involving patients from the M. D. Anderson Cancer Center in Texas and the Mayo Clinic in Minnesota is currently underway to test the effectiveness of shark cartilage in combination with conventional cancer therapies.

Claims that shark cartilage is effective against viral diseases, especially HIV and herpes infections, have not been scientifically proved. Many researchers maintain that shark cartilage, when taken orally, is digested by stomach acids and unlikely to be of much benefit.

Sources

Shark cartilage comes from sharks that are caught for food or from non-endangered species such as the spiny dogfish shark. However, some ecologists are concerned that widespread killing of sharks is depleting their numbers worldwide.

Forms and Usual Dosages

Most shark cartilage is taken from the fins and head. It is dried and ground into a powder that is made into capsules and tablets in doses of 250 to 800 mg each. It is also available as a powder and a liquid, and in some countries, it has also been given as an injection. Because shark cartilage is not standardized, the amount of glycoprotein compounds likely varies greatly from product to product. In fact, some products have been found not to contain any shark cartilage at all or have been diluted with bovine (cow) cartilage, which is also being investigated as a possible anticancer agent. To get the dosage used in the research studies, it would take forty or more capsules a day of products available over the counter. Some experts say that the active compounds in shark cartilage may not even be effective when taken by mouth.

Potential Problems

Side effects are not common with shark cartilage, though some people have experienced a bad taste in the mouth, gastrointestinal upset, fatigue, and nausea. Because it is supposed to act by preventing the growth of new blood vessels, it could be harmful if it is taken during pregnancy or by children, surgery patients, or anyone who has sustained a recent injury that has not fully healed.

What to Look For

While it's no guarantee of effectiveness, the best bet is to opt for brands that specialize in shark cartilage, such as Cartilade, whose maker has sponsored at least one clinical cancer trial. It must be emphasized, however, that shark cartilage is not an alternative to conventional cancer treatments.

SOY PRODUCTS

Soybeans and soy products are dietary staples in many parts of the world. Soy protein provides almost as many of the essential amino acids (building blocks of proteins) as meat and other animal products. Tofu and other soy foods are good sources of all the B vitamins except B_{12}, which is found only in animal products, and many minerals, especially calcium, potassium, and zinc. Ounce for ounce, soy provides more protein and iron than beef, more calcium than milk, and more lecithin than eggs. In addition, soy foods are rich in many compounds with medicinal properties. These include isoflavones, which function as plant (phyto) estrogens. The most studied isoflavones are genistein and daidzein, which are also powerful antioxidants that are thought to protect against cancer and cellular damage from unstable molecules (free radicals).

Role as a Supplement

Soy protein is marketed as an alternative to hormone replacement therapy for women going through menopause. The phytoestrogens in soy isoflavones are taken up by the body's estrogen receptors, but they are much weaker than the human hormone, so they probably do not increase cancer risk by stimulating breast and uterine tissue. Thus, women who have a high risk of these cancers, or who cannot take estrogen replacement therapy, can often get adequate relief from hot flashes and other menopausal symptoms by using soy supplements. A manufactured substance called ipriflavone (IF) is marketed as a synthetic isoflavone and is used in many countries abroad to prevent osteoporosis. (A natural IF is found in bee propolis.)

Other benefits of soy supplements—or increased intake of tofu, soy milk, and other soy foods—include reduction of high blood cholesterol levels, pregnancy support, and regulation of hormones during perimenopause—the years before actual menopause when estrogen levels begin to decline. There is considerable evidence that soy also protects against heart disease and some cancers.

Evidence of Efficacy

In one study involving more than fifty menopausal women who were suffering from frequent hot flashes, researchers found that soy supplements reduced the incidence of hot flashes by 40 percent. A pooling of results in some forty studies found the soy lowered total cholesterol by a mean of 23 points. A large body of animal research indicates that soy reduces cancer risk, especially of the prostate, breasts, and uterus. This protective effect is attributed to the estrogenlike activity of soy isoflavones. And when cancer does develop in these organs, a high soy intake appears to slow tumor growth and prevent its spread to other parts of the body (metastasis).

Laboratory studies have also found that soy reduces the oxidative damage that leads to atherosclerosis, the buildup of fatty plaque in the coronary arteries and other blood vessels. A number of population studies indicate that soy may help prevent osteoporosis, the thinning of bones that is so common among older women. A study of postmenopausal women who had early osteoporosis found that 40 g of soy protein a day actually increased their spinal bone density. More than sixty clinical studies abroad have demonstrated the effectiveness of ipriflavone in slowing the progression of osteoporosis in postmenopausal women. Some studies also indicated that IF may enhance the bone-protective effects of estrogen replacement therapy.

Sources

Soy can be added to the diet in the form of tofu, tempeh, miso, soy milk, soy flour, textured vegetable protein, and cooked soybeans or roasted soy nuts. It can also be taken as powdered or pill supplements.

Forms and Usual Dosages

Soy supplements are marketed as powdered soy protein or isoflavone pills or capsules. The typical Asian diet provides between 25 and 200 mg of soy isoflavones a day; most of the clinical research has used dosages of 25 to 50 g of soy protein or 50 to 150 mg of soy isoflavones.

Potential Problems

A few people are allergic to soy protein. For the most part, however, soy foods and supplements are safe, even when consumed in large quantities. An exception may be the synthetic isoflavone ipriflavone. A recent study linked IF supplements with a decreased number of lymphocytes, a type of white blood cell involved in fighting infections and cancer. The women with reduced lymphocytes did not show an increased incidence of cancer or infections, but the findings indicate that women taking it should have their white blood cells monitored every three months or so.

What to Look For

Tofu cakes that are kept in pans of water are easily contaminated with bacteria and may be a source of food-borne illness. Look for tofu in sealed and dated packs. Miso and soy sauce are high in salt, which may be a problem for people susceptible to high blood pressure. Soy protein is often mixed with other vegetable or animal proteins; look for products that are 100 percent soy.

See Also

Cancer
Cholesterol Disorders and Atherosclerosis
Osteoporosis
Menopause
Benign Prostate Enlargement

SPIRULINA

Spirulina, a type of blue-green alga, is a microscopic organism that grows in water; the types used in nutritional supplements are usually harvested from freshwater lakes, ponds, and man-made tanks. Blue-green algae are primitive organisms that have many plantlike characteristics but are technically classified as bacteria. There are more than 1,500 known species of blue-green algae, and their chemical makeup varies somewhat from one variety to another. However, all are rich in protein and beta-carotene, an antioxidant and precursor of vitamin A. Depending upon the species, spirulina may also provide useful amounts of vitamin D, B-complex vitamins, iron and other minerals, chlorophyll, enzymes, and various other nutrients. Some species are also rich in gamma-linolenic acid (GLA), a substance that counters inflammation, helps lower cholesterol, and appears to protect against heart disease.

Role as a Supplement

Spirulina and other forms of blue-green algae have been consumed by humans in many parts of the world for hundreds of years and are touted as a highly nutritious super seaweed that boosts immunity and wards off numerous diseases, including heart attacks and cancer. Some promoters claim that spirulina is a natural antibiotic that can ward off numerous infections, and may also help fight HIV, the virus that causes AIDS. As a source of GLA, spirulina is said to alleviate arthritis, premenstrual syndrome, and eczema. It is promoted to "cleanse the colon" and promote the growth of beneficial (probiotic) bacteria in the large intestine. Spirulina supplements are marketed as a nonanimal source of vitamin B_{12} for strict vegetarians (see Potential Problems, below).

Evidence of Efficacy

Most of the claims for spirulina are unproved or based on laboratory rather than human studies. One exception is a report by the World Health Organization, which attributed a decreased incidence of blindness due to vitamin A deficiency among malnourished children in India when 1 g of spirulina was added to their diets. A recent study, reported in the *Journal of the American Nutraceutical Association,* found that one type of blue-green alga, *Aphanizomenon flos-aquae* (AFA), increased the surveillance activity of certain immune-system cells. These findings are considered important because the AFA did not stimulate the immune systems to go into action and attack normal body tissue, which is a danger that may occur when immune surveillance is increased in the absence of disease or some other real threat. The researchers concluded that AFA may play a role in preventing cancer by boosting immunity against the mutant cells that can lead to the disease. In another study, researchers at the Massachusetts General Hospital demonstrated that the polyunsaturated fatty acids in AFA lowered blood cholesterol levels in rats. More research is needed, however, to determine whether humans achieve similar benefits.

Sources

Blue-green algae thrive in lakes and ponds that have a high mineral content; they can also grow in salt water, where they cluster inside a gel-like sheath. The spirulina used in supplements may be grown under controlled conditions in outdoor tanks or harvested from lakes and ponds. The AFA used in supplements, for example, is harvested wild from Upper Klamath Lake in Oregon.

Forms and Usual Dosage

Supplements are available in powder, flake, capsule, and pill forms; they are also added to some "power" snack bars and drinks. The typical dosage calls for taking 1 g a day with each meal. The dosage may be increased to treat or prevent specific diseases.

Potential Problems

Some wild spirulina products may be contaminated by environmental toxins, bird droppings, bacteria, and other potentially harmful substances. Aside from possible health risks, critics contend that, based on current scientific evidence, most spirulina and/or blue-green alga supplements simply do not live up to their hype. For example, the supplements are promoted as an inexpensive source of high-quality protein; in reality, traditional high-protein foods (meat, poultry, eggs, dairy products, and soybeans and other legumes) are equal or better dietary sources of protein and much less expensive than spirulina and blue-green alga pills.

Spirulina is also promoted as a nonanimal source of vitamin B_{12}. While it's true that spirulina does contain B_{12}, a Food and Drug Administration analysis of at least one popular spirulina product found that much of its B_{12} was actually contaminated from various insects and animal products. The B_{12} from the spirulina itself is in a form that the human body cannot absorb. In addition, according to a Mayo Clinic report, the B_{12} in spirulina may actually block the body's assimilation of regular B_{12}.

What to Look For

AFA supplements used in the immune system research are available as blue-green algae products grown in Klamath Falls, Oregon.

Botanical Medicines

Worldwide, substances derived from various plants are by far the most used medicines. Even many of our pharmaceutical products are based on substances derived from plants. Indeed, many researchers believe that as-yet-undiscovered plant substances may give us cures for cancer and many other diseases. Teams of pharmacologic researchers are constantly combing the world's remaining rain forests in search of new botanical medicines. In the meantime, there is renewed interest in botanical, or herbal, medicines that traditional healers have been using for centuries. This section highlights some of the most common and effective of these botanical substances.

AGRIMONY (*AGRIMONIA EUPATORIA*)

Agrimony is a perennial herb that produces spikes of spicy-smelling yellow flowers. It originated in Europe, but now can be found in many parts of the United States and parts of Asia. Gargling with agrimony tea is said to soothe the throat and refresh the voice, and many singers and actors still keep a bottle of agrimony water handy to use before going onstage. Herbalists also prescribe gargling with agrimony to treat a sore throat; in Europe it a favorite natural remedy for diarrhea and various intestinal disorders.

Common Uses

- Soothe a sore throat, mouth ulcers, and inflamed mucous membranes.
- Treat diarrhea.
- Ease symptoms of inflammatory bowel disease and hemorrhoids.
- Stop bleeding from minor cuts and promote healing of skin ulcers and other skin sores.
- Ease muscle aches.
- Treat mild yeast infections such as oral thrush or vaginitis.

How It Works

Agrimony is high in tannins, which have astringent properties that tighten and dry the skin. These actions may explain why agrimony helps stop bleeding and oozing of skin ulcers. In addition, tannins soothe inflamed and irritated mucous membranes, such as the tissue lining the throat and intestinal tract, and help stop mild diarrhea.

Agrimony also contains substances that have mild antibiotic and antifungal properties, so applying a compress soaked in agrimony to a minor cut or skin ulcer may prevent infection and promote healing. An agrimony mouthwash may help clear up oral thrush, and applying a compress soaked in agrimony to the pubic area sometimes helps alleviate the itching and irritation of mild vaginitis due to an overgrowth of yeast. (Some herbalists recommend treating vaginitis by douching with an agrimony solution, but doctors generally advise against any douching.) A warm agrimony compress or poultice may also ease minor muscle aches.

Evidence of Efficacy

German health authorities have approved agrimony to treat sore throats and mild diarrhea. Although scientific studies have not been done to verify the effectiveness of agrimony in treating sore throats and irritated mucous membranes and healing minor skin sores, European and Asian herbalists have successfully used agrimony for these purposes for hundreds of years.

Laboratory studies have identified antibiotic and antifungal compounds in agrimony, but their effectiveness against infections in humans has not been studied. Researchers have also found that agrimony helps control blood sugar levels in diabetic mice; more study is needed to determine whether the herb is a useful in treating human diabetes.

◉ A LITTLE HISTORY

Agrimony has been used for hundreds of years to heal wounds and soothe a sore throat. But during the ages it has been combined with some rather strange ingredients. For example, an ancient herbal recipe to treat internal bleeding specified that agrimony be mixed with pounded frog and human blood. During the Middle Ages, it was mixed with vinegar and mugwort to treat backaches. Sprigs of agrimony placed under a pillow were said to ensure a good night's sleep.

Forms and Usual Dosages

Agrimony is available as a tincture or dried leaves that can be made into a tea or poultice. The typical dosage to treat diarrhea uses 1 teaspoon of leaves steeped for five to ten minutes in a cup of boiling water. The tea is strained, and up to three or four cups may be consumed during the course of a day. The tea can be cooled and used as a gargle or mouthwash; or soak a compress in it and apply it directly to a skin irritation. To make a poultice, cover 3 or 4 tablespoons of dried leaves with hot water, strain, and put the wet leaves between two layers of cheesecloth.

Potential Problems

Agrimony is generally safe when used in moderation and as directed. However, the leaves do contain substances that may increase sun sensitivity. To be safe, cover any parts of the skin that have been treated recently with agrimony before going into the sun.

ALFALFA
(*MEDICAGO SATIVA*)

A member of the pea family of legumes, alfalfa is thought to have originated in southwestern Asia. It was brought to the United States by Spanish explorers in the mid-nineteenth century and is now grown worldwide. Alfalfa is a remarkably hearty plant, sending its roots deep into the soil, which allows it to withstand extremes of drought and making it one of farmers' most productive crops. It also enriches the soil, thereby increasing farmers' yields for subsequent crops. In the United States, some 70 million metric tons are harvested annually for hay and about sixty thousand metric tons for seed. It is used to feed farm animals and increases the vitamin content of prepared foods for humans.

Alfalfa sprouts germinating from the seeds are a popular and nutritious addition to salads and other foods, and its three-leaflet clusters and pale blue, purple, or yellow flowers, dried and blended into herbal supplements, are used to treat a variety of ailments.

A LITTLE HISTORY

Alfalfa is believed to have originated in southwestern Asia. It was first cultivated in Persia and from there taken to Greece in the fifth century B.C. and to Spain in the eighth century A.D. Spanish explorers brought it to North and South America. Its cultivation in the United States began in 1854 when it was introduced in San Francisco from Chile. Over the years its culture has spread with the development of hearty varieties and the use of better fertilizing and soil-management techniques. The medicinal uses of alfalfa date to the ancient Chinese physicians and the Ayurvedic practitioners of India. These healers prescribed alfalfa leaves and flowers to treat stomach and digestive disorders. Native American healers also used alfalfa to treat intestinal problems, especially jaundice and liver disorders.

Common Uses

- Relieve digestive tract disorders, including indigestion, heartburn, and loss of appetite.

- Treat urinary tract infections and kidney, bladder, and prostate disorders.
- Rid the body of excess fluids.
- Help control diabetes.
- Ease menopausal symptoms.
- Soothe bee stings and insect bites.

How It Works

Alfalfa, a legume, contains eight essential amino acids, the building blocks of proteins. The leaves are rich in minerals, including calcium, magnesium, potassium, iron, and zinc, as well as beta-carotene, the precursor of vitamin A, and vitamins E and K. It is also a major source of chlorophyll.

The active medicinal ingredients in alfalfa include isoflavones, sterols, and other plant (phyto) estrogens; saponin glycosides (2 to 3 percent), which, together with the plant's natural fiber, are thought to have cholesterol-lowering properties; and derivatives of coumarin, an antiplatelet substance that reduces blood clotting and may protect against atherosclerosis, the buildup of fatty plaque along the artery walls.

Alfalfa seeds, ground up into a poultice, have been used to ease the pain of bee stings and insect bites; this effect may be due to antiinflammatory substances in alfalfa seeds. These substances may also explain why alfalfa helps some people with arthritis.

Evidence of Efficacy

Most of the evidence supporting the medicinal claims for alfalfa are either anecdotal or based on animal studies. For example, laboratory studies have shown that alfalfa can lower blood cholesterol levels in animals, but it is not known whether this effect applies to humans.

Forms and Usual Dosages

Dried alfalfa leaves are available as a bulk herb and in tablets and capsules. It is also available in liquid extracts. Some experts recommend 500 to 1,000 mg of the dried leaf per day, usually drunk as a tea, or 1 to 2 ml of tincture.

Potential Problems

Although moderate use of dried alfalfa leaves is believed to be safe, some people are allergic to it and cannot tolerate any amount of it. People who have lupus or a family history of this disease should not consume alfalfa in any form, as it can provoke a severe flare-up of symptoms. This is thought to be due to canavanine, a compound found in alfalfa. Alfalfa sprouts, as with many other sprouted legumes, are susceptible to contamination with *E. coli*: and other disease causing organisms. Thus, they should not be consumed raw by people with lowered immunity.

Animal studies have shown that high doses of saponins, in the amounts needed by the body to lower cholesterol, can damage red blood cells.

ALOE VERA (*ALOE VERA, A. BARBADENSIS*)

Aloe is a succulent plant with fleshy leaves that have small spikes along their edges. Although aloe is a subtropical plant that cannot withstand temperatures much below 40°F, it is very easy to grow as a houseplant. Indeed, many people keep a potted aloe plant on a kitchen windowsill so a leaf can be snipped off when the need arises.

Aloe leaves contain two different fluids—the inner portion is filled with a clear gel, and the thick aloe skin (epidermis) contains a bitter yellow juice or latex. In general, the gel is used externally, and the latex is dried and used in oral drugs, mostly laxatives. There is also a standardized aloe extract, derived from freeze-dried aloe gel, that is taken internally.

Common Uses

Aloe is most often used externally, often by simply applying fresh gel to:

- Treat minor burns, scalds, or sunburns.
- Hasten healing of cuts and other minor wounds.
- Help prevent scarring.
- Reduce tissue damage from frostbite.
- Relieve skin irritation and inflammation; for example, from insect bites and stings.
- Treat external hemorrhoids.
- Moisturize and soften dry, itchy, or rough skin.

The aloe latex or juice is taken internally to treat:

- Constipation.

The powdered aloe gel extract is taken internally to:

- Treat ulcers and other intestinal problems, including diverticulitis and inflammatory bowel disease.
- Bolster immunity.

How It Works

Researchers do not fully understand how aloe works, primarily because its gel is a very complex substance made up of many bioactive ingredients. These include polysaccharides (complex carbohydrates), various sugars, enzymes, amino acids (proteins), vitamins, minerals, antibiotic and antifungal agents, steroid hormones, salicylic acid (an aspirinlike substance), and other compounds—some seventy-five in all.

When used externally, the aloe gel is applied directly to the skin to relieve pain and promote healing of minor burns, sunburns, scalds, and cuts. It also eases skin inflammation and irritation, helps prevent infection, and speeds healing of minor wounds. Some herbalists recommend applying the gel directly to external hemorrhoids to promote healing and soothe anal itching and irritation.

When taken internally to treat constipation, aloe latex—the bitter-tasting juice from the leaf's skin—increases bowel motility and also loosens the stool. These actions derive from compounds in the aloe resin, called anthracene derivatives, which stimulate bowel contractions and also help increase the amount of intestinal fluid, resulting in a more watery stool that is propelled rapidly through the colon.

The aloe gel extract, a powdered form made from freeze-dried slices of the aloe plant, is sometimes used as an ulcer remedy. It is said to form a protective coating over the ulcer, allowing it to heal. Other ingredients in the gel may also promote ulcer healing. The aloe extract is also used to treat diverticulitis, inflammatory bowel disease, and other inflammatory intestinal disorders. Recent studies indicate that it also bolsters the immune system.

Evidence of Efficacy

Numerous studies in the United States and abroad confirm that aloe gel speeds the healing of minor burns and skin wounds, with little or no scarring. It is also an effective skin moisturizer. But caution is needed. Many commercial products labeled "aloe" do not contain enough aloe to be of much value.

There have been reports that ingested aloe extract products may strengthen and stabilize the immune system and may prove useful in treating intestinal inflammatory disorders, rheumatoid arthritis, AIDS, cancer, and a host of other diseases. However, more study is needed to confirm whether aloe, or nutraceutical products derived from it, can indeed confer these wide-ranging benefits.

Forms and Usual Dosages

Many experts recommend simply cutting off several inches of an aloe leaf and slitting it lengthwise so you can easily scoop out the clear gel, which is then applied directly onto a *minor* cut, burn, sting, or other skin irritation. Note the emphasis on minor—some studies have found that aloe may actually impede the healing of a major wound. As the aloe gel dries, it forms a protective coating over the wound. Fresh aloe can be applied three or four times a day, or as needed to soothe itching and irritation. Make sure that the area has been cleaned with an antiseptic solution, such as alcohol or hydrogen peroxide, before applying the gel. If you elect to use a commercial aloe product, look for one that lists aloe vera gel as the main ingredient. Be aware, however, that some experts believe that aloe quickly loses its healing properties and advise using fresh gel obtained directly from a plant leaf.

The typical dosage to treat peptic ulcer is 1 teaspoon of gel (it can be added to milk, water, or juice) three times a day. It should be stressed, however, that many experts do not recommend any internal use of fresh aloe and only very sparing use, if any, of commercial products (see Potential Problems, below).

Taking aloe as a laxative, which is made from the dried latex, is quite problematic because aloe juice is very irritating to the intestinal tract and kidneys. Many aloe laxatives also contain other phyto laxatives, such as senna. In any event, aloe laxatives—available as pills or capsules—should be taken in small doses of 50 to 200 mg a day, and for no more than ten days. Drink several glasses of water throughout the day.

Potential Problems

When taken internally, aloe juice (the bitter yellow latex) can cause severe abdominal cramps, intestinal irritation, and kidney inflammation. Long-term use can result in laxative dependency. Indeed, most experts advise against taking aloe laxatives—there are many effective and safer alternatives.

External use of aloe to treat dry skin and minor skin irritations, wounds, and burns is generally safe. A few people, however, may be allergic to aloe. Discontinue use if it causes skin redness, itching, or swelling.

See Also

Constipation
Diverticular Disease

Heartburn
Inflammatory Bowel Disease
Ulcers

ANISE (*PIMPINELLA ANISUM*) AND STAR ANISE (*ILLICIUM VERUM*)

Anise and star anise are two different plants, but they are used in the same way. Anise is an annual that originated in Greece and Egypt and is now grown worldwide. Its greenish seeds have a taste similar to licorice and are the part that is used medicinally and as a flavoring spice. Star anise is native to southeast Asia and its common name is derived from its star-shaped seeds. Both types of anise are popular digestive aids and remedies for the congestion and coughs that accompany colds and flu.

Common Uses

- Reduce nasal and lung congestion and suppress coughs.
- Aid digestion and treat indigestion.
- Reduce gas and nausea.
- Sweeten bad breath.
- Flavor various medications, candies, and alcoholic beverages.

How It Works

Anise contains anethols and other ingredients that are effective in helping clear airway and nasal congestion by loosening mucus and making it easier to cough up. Many cough drops, syrups, and other medications, as well as nasal inhalants, contain anise.

Anethols also appear to aid digestion and calm intestinal spasms that can cause colicky stomach cramps and nausea. That's the reason many after-dinner cordials and teas are anise-flavored. These substances are thought to help reduce gas production and lessen flatulence. Anise tea is also used to lessen morning sickness, but—as with any pharmaceutical

◉ A LITTLE HISTORY

Anise enjoys a long and colorful history. In ancient times it was cultivated for its fragrance and flavor as well as its medicinal qualities. Pliny, the Roman scholar and writer, recommended chewing it upon awakening to get rid of morning breath; he also advised keeping it near the bed at night to stave off bad dreams. The Romans also used it as a form of currency to pay their taxes. Hippocrates used anise to treat coughs, but it was undoubtedly used by healers long before him. In the sixteenth century, Europeans discovered that mice were attracted to anise, and—in addition to its many medicinal and culinary uses—they baited their mousetraps with it.

or nutraceutical product—a pregnant woman should check with her doctor before taking anise.

The volatile oil in anise seeds has been found to kill or repel some insects, which might explain the traditional use of anise to get rid of scabies and body lice. However, it is seldom used for these purposes today because more effective antiparasitic products have been developed.

Traditional herbalists have long recommended anise to reduce hot flashes and other menopausal symptoms. It contains the compounds dianethole and photoanethole, which are chemically similar to estrogen, which may account for these benefits.

Evidence of Efficacy

Most of the evidence supporting the use of anise as an expectorant and digestive aid comes from its long tradition of use for these purposes. Researchers have found that anethols do stimulate the cells of the bronchial passages that are responsible for clearing them of mucus. How anise aids digestion is unknown, but it has been used for this purpose since ancient times. More recently, German health authorities approved anise seeds and their essential oil as treatments for lung congestion and mild digestive disorders.

Forms and Usual Dosages

Anise is usually taken as a tea made from its crushed or powdered seeds. It is also available as a tincture and an essential oil that can be used in aromatherapy or diluted and applied to the skin. Many of the Chinese herbal blends contain star anise.

The dosage varies according to the form and condition being treated. A popular digestive aid calls for using 1 teaspoon of crushed seeds per cup of water to drink after each meal. Nasal and bronchial congestion is treated by either inhaling steamy vapors that contain the essential oil (which should never be ingested in its full strength) or taking 1 to 2 ml of the tincture two or three times a day. It is sometimes combined with eucalyptus oil and rubbed onto the chest.

Potential Problems

Anise tea appears to be safe if taken as directed, but care is needed not to exceed the recommended therapeutic dosages. Full-strength anise oil can cause vomiting and seizures; as with most essential oils, it should not be ingested. Instead, it is inhaled or diluted with other oils and applied to the skin as aromatherapy. Some people have an allergic reaction to anetholes and can develop a reaction to topical applications. Because of its possible estrogenic effects, pregnant women are advised not to take medicinal anise preparations during pregnancy, although it appears to be safe when used as a weak tea or cooking spice.

ASHWAGANDHA (*WITHANIA SOMNIFERUM D., W. COAGULANS*)

Ashwagandha, also called winter cherry, is a member of the nightshade family and grows in India and parts of Africa. Its roots are widely used in India's traditional Ayurvedic medicine. In fact, ashwagandha is often referred to as Indian ginseng and, like Asian ginseng, it is classified as an adaptogen—a panacea tonic that is reputed to restore health regardless of the nature of the underlying illness or stresses. Thus, ashwagandha is recommended for a wide variety of disorders; it is also promoted as an immune-system booster and a tranquilizer to help counter the effects of stress.

Common Uses

As an adaptogen, ashwagandha is said to:
- Increase energy and restore vigor.
- Promote endurance and strength.
- Bolster immunity.
- Normalize bodily functions.
- Improve emotional well-being and mental function.

Specific diseases that ashwagandha is used to treat include:

- Chronic fatigue syndrome and fibromyalgia.
- AIDS and other immune-system disorders.
- Alzheimer's disease and other age-related disorders.
- Various infectious diseases.

How It Works

Ashwagandha contains compounds called withanolides, which are thought to have actions similar to steroidal hormones. These compounds are credited with reducing the pain and inflammation of fibromyalgia and other disorders. Researchers in India attribute ashwagandha's calm-

◉ A LITTLE HISTORY

Ashwagandha has been used for hundreds of years by India's Ayurvedic physicians as a general tonic; in parts of Africa, traditional healers recommend it for fevers, arthritis, and various inflammatory disorders.

In India, the ashwagandha shoots and seeds are used to thicken milk and are also consumed as food. According to legend, ashwagandha is an aphrodisiac—a somewhat contradictory use because it is also claimed to induce sleep. In fact, part of its Latin name, *somniferum,* means "to sleep."

ing effects to its direct action on brain chemistry—they report that it lowers levels of glutamic acid, a chemical (neurotransmitter) that has an excitatory effect, and at the same time functions much like GABA, an inhibitory brain chemical.

Ashwagandha also contains powerful antioxidants that protect cells, including those in the brain, from free radicals. Antioxidants are credited with bolstering the immune system and protecting against infection and numerous diseases, including cancer. In theory, at least, antioxidants also help slow the aging process and may protect against Alzheimer's disease and other age-related disorders.

Evidence of Efficacy

Laboratory studies on ashwagandha have been carried out mostly in India and have involved animals rather than human subjects. In one study, reported in 1999, researchers treated suppressed immunity in mice by giving them cyclophosphamide, a drug used to prevent rejection of transplanted organs. The animals that were given ashwagandha extracts showed significant improvement in their immune response, compared to mice that did not receive the extracts. In another study, ashwagandha extracts were found to be effective in destroying cultures of cancer cells. Much more study is needed, however, to determine whether ashwagandha is effective against cancer in humans.

Forms and Usual Dosages

Ashwagandha is consumed in capsule, liquid extract, tincture, or tea form. The typical daily dosage calls for two 300-mg capsules, 1 to 2 g of whole root, or 2 to 4 ml of tincture or fluid extract. To make the tea, boil 1 to 2 g (about 1 to 2 teaspoons) of the whole root for fifteen minutes in three cups of water; strain, cool, and sip the tea throughout the day.

Potential Problems

Ashwagandha is generally considered safe, although there have been some reports of upset stomach and intestinal cramps from taking high doses. Its safety during pregnancy and breast-feeding has not been established, so to be safe, it should be avoided.

ASTRAGALUS
(A. MEMBRANACEUS)

Astragalus originated in northern China, and there are now more than two thousand species worldwide, including some four hundred in North America. However, the medicinal variety is found only in central and western Asia, and it has been extensively tested, both chemically and pharmacologically.

A member of the pea family, astragalus is a hairy-stemmed perennial that can grow to about two feet. A yellow core in the center of the sweet-tasting black root is the medicinal substance. That color contributes to its Chinese name, which is huang qi or "yellow leader." It has been used in China for thousands of years as a tonic herb to strengthen qi (pronounced "chee"), the body's life force and protective energy. In Western terminology, strengthening qi implies bolstering the immune system. European botanists first wrote about its medicinal qualities in the 1700s.

Common Uses

Astragalus is taken internally to:

- Strengthen the immune system, especially in persons who are HIV-positive.
- Bolster the immune system, especially during cancer chemotherapy.
- Ward off and help treat colds and other infections.
- Improve heart function, especially after a heart attack.
- Improve memory and learning.
- Temporarily increase urinary output.
- Possibly treat fibromyalgia, stress, chronic fatigue syndrome, viral infections, and promote healing of burns and skin sores.

How It Works

Astragalus appears to have a positive effect on resistance to diseases and infections, helping the body ward off and heal more quickly from disease. The herb theoretically helps you cope with physical and emotional stresses that increase your susceptibility to illness. It contains numerous active compounds that could contribute to the benefits reported, including flavonoids, which protect cells against unstable molecules (free radicals); polysaccharides, which bolster immunity; and various amino acids and trace minerals. The polysaccharides appear to be especially important because they seem to stimulate white blood cell production;

◉ A LITTLE HISTORY
The name of the astragalus family of plants derives from an ancient Greek word meaning "anklebone." These bones were once used as a form of dice. Some historians think that the name was chosen because the rattling seed-pods of the Mediterranean variety of astragalus sound like rolling dice.

spur the activity of killer T cells, the body's defenders against invading viruses and bacteria; and increase production of interferon, a natural protein that stimulates production of other proteins that help prevent and fight viral infections.

Evidence of Efficacy

Although most of the Chinese studies of the herb have been done in the laboratory or on test animals, their findings do support immune supportive benefits for astragalus, especially in chronic rather than acute health problems. They also suggest it may have some promise as an anticancer agent and a heart tonic. Studies involving human subjects have usually used a combination of herbs, making it difficult to tease out the actual contribution of astragalus to benefits seen.

The effectiveness of astragalus was put to the test in a study of cancer patients undertaken at the M. D. Anderson Cancer Center in Houston in the early 1980s. An astragalus extract was given to nineteen cancer patients and fifteen healthy people and appeared to have a restorative effect on immune-system function in the majority of the patients. In some cases, it made the cancer patients' immune systems resemble those of the healthy subjects by restoring T-cell counts (a type of white blood cell that is part of the lymphocyte family) to relatively normal ranges. Although the results were evaluated only in blood samples, not in the patients themselves, the researchers concluded that astragalus contains a potent immune stimulant.

In another study, heart attack patients given astragalus suffered less angina and had a greater improvement in their EKG test results and other measurements than patients given standard heart drugs, such as nifedipine. Chinese researchers report that the herb improves function of the heart's left ventricle after a heart attack, which they theorize may derive from its antioxidant effects. Other Chinese researchers found heart-protective effects in people with Coxsackie B virus, which can cause viral myocarditis.

Studies indicating that various formulations of the herb may improve learning and memory suggest that it may be useful for people with Alzheimer's disease. Astragalus also may be useful as a diuretic because it seems to increase urine output.

Forms and Usual Dosages

Bins of sliced or whole astragalus root, sometimes labeled as huang qi, can be found in health food stores. It can be boiled in water to create a decoction. Chinese herbal textbooks recommend drinking astragalus tea made with an equivalent of 9 to 15 g of the crude herb daily. However, capsules and tinctures yield more exact dosages. Two to three 500-mg capsules or 3 to 5 ml of tincture three times per day are usually recommended.

Potential Problems

Centuries of use suggest that astragalus has no known side effects when used as recommended. However, it has yet to be fully evaluated in Western clinical trials.

See Also

Cancer
Chronic Fatigue Syndrome
Common Cold and Flu

Barberry
(*BERBERIS VULGARIS*)

Barberry is a perennial shrub that originated in Europe and is now common in the northeastern United States. It can grow up to ten feet tall and in the fall it produces red or black berries that are used to make jams and jellies. The berries are rich in antioxidants, especially vitamin C and various bioflavonoids. Medicinally, however, it is the upper root (rhizome) bark, which is rich in alkaloids, that is used. Barberry—also called sowberry—is closely related to the wild Oregon grape (*Berberis aquifolium*), which is now more popular in botanical medicine than its European cousin.

Common Uses

- Soothe sore throat and mouth ulcers.
- Relieve digestive upsets, including ulcers, heartburn, and intestinal inflammation.
- Lower high blood pressure.
- Ease coughs and airway congestion.
- Treat various skin disorders, including psoriasis and minor infections.

⊙ A LITTLE HISTORY

In ancient Egypt barberry was mixed with fennel seed, boiled into a syrup, and ingested in an effort to prevent the plague. In the Middle Ages, Europeans used medicines made with barberry as antiseptics, purgatives, and tonics. Native Americans prepared a decoction from the root bark and drank it to overcome fatigue and improve appetite.

How It Works

Barberry contains a number of alkaloids, especially berberine, that are effective against bacteria, fungi, and other organisms that can cause diarrhea and skin, urinary tract, and vaginal infections. Berbamine, another of barberry's alkaloids, appears to bolster immunity. Scientists have also discovered sedative and anticonvulsant properties in some of barberry's components, as well as substances that may help lower blood pressure and reduce muscle spasms.

In the digestive system, barberry appears to stimulate the flow of bile, the digestive juice made by the liver that is instrumental in digesting fats. Barberry also contains substances that reduce intestinal inflammation. When taken in small amounts, barberry bark extract helps treat diarrhea; in larger amounts, it has a mild laxative effect that can counter constipation.

Evidence of Efficacy

Although scientists have identified a number of active ingredients in barberry, there are no studies proving barberry's effectiveness in treating human ailments. However, many of the properties of the alkaloids contained in barberry have been studied in laboratory cultures or animals. Even so, the German health authorities have not approved barberry for any human ailments. In many parts of the world, however, herbalists use it to treat the various disorders listed above.

Forms and Usual Dosages

Barberry is available as powdered or whole root bark, extract, and tincture. It is often combined with other bitter herbs, such as wild yam, dandelion, and licorice root, as a treatment for digestive conditions. For a decoction, boil 1 teaspoon of the root bark in one cup of water. Let stand for ten to fifteen minutes and then strain. To promote digestion, herbalists recommend drinking small amounts—2 to 5 ml—of the decoction or taking a similar amount of barberry tincture, standardized to contain 5 to 10 percent alkaloids, before meals. To treat skin sores and psoriasis, the typical dosage calls for applying an ointment, made from 10 percent barberry extract, three times a day. Alternatively, soak a compress in barberry tea and apply it directly to the affected skin.

Potential Problems

High doses of barberry can result in nausea, headaches, and low blood sugar. Because of alkaloids' action on the heart and uterine muscle, pregnant women and anyone with heart disease should not take barberry.

Although many herbal manuals recommend barberry eyewashes, doctors caution against the danger of infection from using possibly contaminated herbal substances in the eyes.

See Also

Heartburn

BARLEY
(HORDEUM VULGARE)

Barley is one of the world's oldest grains, originating more than nine thousand years ago, probably in parts of southwest Asia where wild strains still grow. Barley is now cultivated worldwide, and its production is exceeded only by wheat, corn, and rice. The grain is used to make breads, cereals, groats, malt, beer, whiskey, and brewer's yeast.

Through the ages, barley and barley grass have also been used as botanical medicines to treat digestive disorders. More recently, barley has been discovered to contain substances that may bolster immunity, lower cholesterol, and even protect against cancer.

Common Uses

- Treat diarrhea and other intestinal upsets.
- Help control blood sugar levels in diabetes.
- Lower blood cholesterol.
- Soothe a sore throat and mouth ulcers.

How It Works

Barley water—the liquid left over after cooking Scotch or pearl barley or from soaking barley seeds for a few hours—is high in starches and soluble fiber. It is an ancient remedy for an upset stomach and mild diarrhea; when used as a gargle or mouthwash, it can also soothe throat and mouth inflammations. Barley also contains beta glucan, a type of fiber that may help lower blood cholesterol and regulate blood sugar in diabetes.

Barley grass, which is a popular ingredient in juice supplements, is touted as a rich source of chlorophyll, a reputed energy booster, and

◉ A LITTLE HISTORY

Barley is thought to be the oldest cultivated grain, originating in either southern Asia or the highlands of Ethiopia. Although barley was a staple grain food of the ancient world, it was also a popular source of alcohol. In fact, a Babylonian tablet dating to about 2800 B.C. contains a recipe for barley wine. Today, brewers use barley to make beer and malt whiskey.

In ancient Rome, the gladiators were fed barley to give them extra strength. At about the same time, Greek healers discovered that barley water soothed a sore throat and a type of barley porridge could cure diarrhea, and early Chinese physicians treated digestive problems with barley.

antioxidants that may bolster immunity. German researchers have found that sprouted barley seeds contain alkaloids that may also have therapeutic value.

Evidence of Efficacy

Controlled studies have found that the soluble fiber in barley can help lower blood levels of the harmful LDL cholesterol without affecting levels of the beneficial HDL cholesterol. Other studies compared the effects of various grains on insulin and blood sugar levels and found that breads made with barley flour were more effective in controlling glucose levels than products made with wheat and other grains. Studies in Europe have also found that barley products have less impact on raising blood sugar than wheat or corn. Further study is needed, however, to determine the potential benefit of barley in helping to control diabetes.

Animal studies indicate that barley may help protect against cancer, especially colon cancer. It is not known, however, whether this benefit also applies to humans. There is no scientific evidence to back claims that barley enhances immunity.

Forms and Usual Dosages

Barley can be consumed in the form of breads, cereals, malt, and peeled (Scotch or pearl barley) grains cooked as porridge or added to soups. Groats, a type of crushed barley, is popular in many ethnic cuisines. As a botanical medicine, barley grain is available as tea and barley water; the grass is marketed in capsule and powdered forms; it is also sold fresh at juice bars and some health food stores. Follow package instructions for the recommended dosages.

Potential Problems

Humans have consumed barley as a dietary staple for thousands of years, so its safety is well established. In fact, commercial barley cereal is often one of the first solids to be introduced into a baby's diet. However, people who have celiac disease—a disorder in which they are unable to digest gluten, a protein in certain cereal grains—should avoid barley products. Also, if you normally consume a low-fiber diet, suddenly adding large amounts of whole barley grain to your diet can cause bloating and gas. This can be avoided by gradually increasing your fiber content. Also, be sure to drink eight glasses of water, juice, or other nonalcoholic fluids a day to reduce risk of intestinal blockage.

BASIL
(OCIMUM BASILICUM)

Basil, one of our most revered culinary herbs, is an easy-to-grow annual that originated in Africa and Asia and is now cultivated worldwide. A member of the mint family, it comes in dozens of varieties, each with a distinctive aroma and flavor; its colors range from pale green to deep purple.

Although most people associate basil more with pesto, tomato sauce, and other favorite dishes than with botanical medicine, the herb enjoys a long history as an appetite stimulant, digestive aid, and mild sedative. Its flowers, dried leaves, and seeds are used medicinally; it also has an essential oil that is used in aromatherapy.

Common Uses

- Stimulate appetite, aid in digestion, and reduce intestinal gas.
- Alleviate stomach cramps and vomiting.
- Relieve constipation and increase flow of urine.
- Promote healing of minor cuts, wounds, and insect bites and stings.
- Ease nasal congestion when inhaled in steam.

How It Works

As a member of the mint family, basil has many of the same compounds and therapeutic properties. It also has concentrated amounts of beta-carotene, the plant precursor of vitamin A, as well as vitamin C and various flavonoids. These are powerful antioxidants that bolster immunity and protect cells from genetic damage caused by free radicals, the unstable molecules released when the body burns oxygen.

Basil seeds contain mild antibiotic substances that, when used as a poultice, help prevent skin infections and promote healing of minor skin wounds. Basil is also in some skin ointments, and it has been promoted as a treatment for acne.

Basil tea is said to be relaxing; a cup in the evening can help calm jittery nerves and promote drowsiness. Chewing a couple of basil leaves before a meal is said to stimulate the appetite. Basil tea after a meal promotes digestion by increasing the flow of gastric juices and also reduces gas and bloating.

The essential oil in basil is distilled and used in aromatherapy to reduce sinus and nasal congestion, promote relaxation, and improve mood.

◉ A LITTLE HISTORY

Basil has long been considered an herb of love and romance. In some parts of the world, women once placed a pot of basil on their windowsill as a sign they were ready to receive their suitors. It was said that a man could win a woman's affection by giving her a sprig of basil—she would fall in love with him and never leave him. But not all the references to basil are laudatory. Some ancient healers regarded basil as a poison, and some references suggest that its common name is derived from the legendary basilisk, a reptile that could kill with a glance. Another more likely derivation, however, is from the Greek word *basileus,* meaning king and signifying its place as a royal herb. It was a sacred herb to people in India, who put it on the chests of the dead to protect them on their journey to the next world. It is still used in parts of India as an air freshener and also to protect the family's spirit.

Evidence of Efficacy

Basil has not been studied extensively as a therapeutic agent, and the studies that have been done involve mostly animals or laboratory cultures. Results of one small study suggested that basil's essential oil may be helpful in controlling mild acne. Researchers have also found that basil can kill some intestinal parasites, and that the seeds and oil have mild antibiotic properties that may be useful in preventing skin infections and controlling the oral bacteria responsible for dental plaque.

Forms and Usual Dosages

Basil is available for external use as an extract, gargle, medicinal-strength oil, and ointment. It is available for internal use as an extract, fresh or dried leaves, tea, and tincture. To brew basil tea, use 1 to 2 teaspoons of the chopped herb (or dried leaves) per cup of hot water, and drink it after meals. A few drops of diluted basil oil may be massaged into the skin, added to bathwater, or inhaled in steamy vapors as part of aromatherapy.

Potential Problems

Basil is used worldwide as a culinary herb without reports of any adverse reactions. Even its essential oil is considered safe by American health authorities. At one time, there were fears that a chemical in basil called estragole caused liver tumors in mice, but those fears have been dispelled. Another component in basil, safrole, is also thought to promote cancer, but again, proof of this is lacking. However, German health authorities are more cautious, and warn that medicinal dosages of the essential oil should not be given to young children or pregnant or breast-feeding women.

BILBERRY (*VACCINIUM MYRTILLUS*)

◉ A LITTLE HISTORY
During World War II, British Royal Air Force pilots reported that they had better night vision during bombing raids when they ate bilberry jam beforehand. Medical scientists paid attention, leading to supportive research for this and other bilberry vision benefits.

A close relative of cranberries and American blueberries, bilberry is native to northern Europe and now also cultivated in Asia, Canada, and the United States. This perennial is a thickly branched shrub with oval leaves and pink-tinged greenish flowers. Its fruit is a blue-black wrinkled berry, darkly purple inside with multiple brownish-red seeds. The dried leaves and dried berries are used medicinally.

Common Uses

- Ease sore throats and mouth inflammation when used as a mouth-wash and gargle.
- Treat or prevent night blindness, retinopathy, and other vision disorders.
- Treat diarrhea.
- Treat or prevent circulatory disorders including decreased blood flow to the legs and atherosclerosis.
- Alleviate gastrointestinal, kidney, and urinary tract problems.
- Relieve arthritis, gout, and dermatitis symptoms.

How It Works

The primary active ingredients in bilberries are anthocyanosides, a bio-flavonoid complex with potent antioxidant effects. They are believed to strengthen capillaries and improve blood circulation, which may account for their wide use in Europe to treat diabetic retinopathy. Anthocyanosides also appear to have a positive effect on certain enzymes important in vision, especially the eye's ability to adapt to the dark.

The fruit also contains tannins, known for their astringency, and fruit pectins, both of which account for the benefits of bilberries in controlling simple diarrhea. Drying of the fruit enhances tannin content. In Europe, herbal teas containing bilberry powder are prescribed for infants with infectious diarrhea and indigestion. Its astringent quality also supports bilberry's use as a palliative for sore throats and mouth inflammation.

Evidence of Efficacy

Small, short-term studies suggest that bilberry may offer a number of eye-related benefits, including improved night vision and reduced eye fatigue for those who do visually demanding tasks, such as working at a computer terminal. Scientists believe that the anthocyanosides enhance blood supply to the eye, which also may protect against other eye diseases, such as cataracts, glaucoma, retinopathy, and macular degeneration. In a study of fifty people, progression of senile cataracts was halted in nearly all of those who supplemented their diets with vitamin E and bilberry extract.

The ability of bilberry to strengthen capillaries has led to its use in Europe for treating varicose veins, venous insufficiency of the legs, and atherosclerosis, but strong clinical research has not yet supported such benefits. Animal studies have shown that an extract of dried bilberry leaves lowers levels of blood sugar and triglyceride levels in rats, although the mechanisms remain unknown. A reduction in symptoms of diabetes and heart disease also have been observed in patients taking bilberry. Similarly, only laboratory and animal studies, and very small human trials, support its use to prevent or treat such diverse conditions as edema, liver damage, inflammation, angina, blood clots, high cholesterol levels, atherosclerosis, and painful menstruation.

Forms and Usual Dosages

A tea can be made by pouring boiling water over 2 or 3 tablespoons of dried berries and then straining them after ten to fifteen minutes of steeping. This is best used as a mouth rinse or gargle. Or 1 to 2 teaspoonful of dried bilberries can be chewed, along with some water or juice.

For internal use, practitioners recommend 240 to 480 mg of bilberry extract capsules or tablets that are standardized to provide 25 percent anthocyanosides.

Potential Problems

No side effects have been reported when bilberry extract is taken in the recommended doses. However, German health authorities warn that prolonged use of high doses have proven toxic in animal studies, causing wasting, anemia, and even death. In treating diarrhea, only dried bilberries should be used; fresh berries may actually worsen the condition.

See Also

Cataracts
Diarrhea
Irritable Bowel Syndrome
Macular Degeneration

BLACKBERRY (*RUBUS FRUTICOSUS, R. VILLOSUS*)

⊙ A LITTLE HISTORY

Blackberry was first used medicinally by ancient Greek physicians for gout. Subsequently, herbal practitioners prescribed the leaves, roots, and berries for conditions similar to those recommended for raspberries and blueberries, including diarrhea, sore throats, and wounds.

Also known as bramble, goutberry, and thimbleberry, various species of the blackberry plant grow in wet areas across North America and Europe. *Rubus fruticosus* is the most common European type, while *Rubus villosus* (also known as dewberry) is more common in the United States. It is a prickly flowering bush with palm-shaped leaves and white or pale pink flowers. Although the roots and berries are also used medicinally, the leaves are the part most highly praised for health benefits. They are gathered during the flowering period and dried.

Common Uses

- External applications are used to heal wounds and treat hemorrhoids.
- Treating diarrhea.
- Relieve a sore throat and mouth inflammations and sores.

How It Works

Large amounts of tannins, known for their astringent effects, give blackberry roots and leaves their effects. Tannins are believed to calm intestinal inflammation and therefore help control or stop diarrhea. Tannins also tighten tissue and control minor bleeding, so the same constituents are also helpful for soothing sore throats. In addition, blackberry contains fruit acids, including citric acid, and flavonoids, with their antioxidant benefits.

Evidence of Efficacy

Although the benefits have not been well studied, German health authorities recommend blackberry leaf or root bark tea for use in acute, simple diarrhea that is not caused by bacterial infection or an underlying medical disease. A tea made from blackberry leaves has been found to ease symptoms when used as a mouthwash or gargle to treat sore throats, oral sores, and other forms of mild inflammation or infection in the mouth and throat. The astringent benefits of blackberry explain why generations have used cool compresses of an infusion or decoction to soothe hemorrhoids and wounds. The latest area of research has begun exploring potential anticancer benefits of the blackberry plant.

Forms and Usual Dosages

Although the berries may be eaten whole, the plant is used medicinally primarily as a tea or a tincture. The tea infusion can be made by adding 1 to 2 teaspoons of chopped leaves to a cup of boiling water and allowing it to steep for ten to fifteen minutes. Three to six cups should be drunk daily. A root bark tea may be taken up to three times a day for diarrhea, but it should be made by the decoction rather than the infusion method to extract an adequate amount of tannins. (To make a decoction, simmer

2 tablespoons of bark per cup of water for one hour, or until one volume of water is reduced by one-third. Strain and store in a cool place.) For acute problems, up to 2 teaspoons of tincture can be taken daily in divided doses.

Potential Problems

In general, recommended doses of blackberry seem to pose no health hazards, according to German health authorities. However, as tea drinkers have long known, tannins can cause nausea and even vomiting in those with sensitive stomachs. So they should particularly be avoided by people who have chronic gastrointestinal problems, as well as those who are allergic to the berries. When used for diarrhea, a physician should be consulted if blackberry does not provide relief within three to four days.

BLACK COHOSH (*CIMICIFUGA RACEMOSA*)

Black cohosh, which is also called black snakeroot and cimicifuga, is a shrublike plant native to North America. Gardeners prize black cohosh for its tall spires of fluffy yellow flowers, but medicinally, it's the parts of the plant you can't readily see that matter most. The dark, tough, and knotty rhizomes—rootlike stems that grow under or along the ground—and the roots that emanate from the rhizomes contain the plant's medicinal compounds. These include triterpene glycosides, along with small amounts of a substance called formononetine, a flavonoid that has mild hormonal activity similar to estrogen. It also contains tannins and fatty acids.

For centuries, black cohosh has been used to treat disorders related to menstruation, menopause, and other "female complaints." In the 1980s, German researchers started studying the hormonal effects of formononetine, and results of these studies have spurred similar studies in the United States.

Common Uses

- Lessen symptoms of premenstrual syndrome (PMS).
- Alleviate menstrual cramps (dysmenorrhea).
- Reduce menopausal symptoms, including hot flashes.

In the past, black cohosh was also used to:

- Treat diarrhea.
- Loosen lung congestion and suppress coughs.
- Rid the body of excess fluid.
- Reduce inflammation and treat arthritis pain.
- Treat eczema and the irritation of insect bites.

How It Works

The formononetine in black cohosh acts as a plant (phyto) estrogen. It is weaker than the natural estrogen produced by the body, but by binding to estrogen receptor sites, it can mimic the effects of human estrogen. When menopause begins, estrogen production starts to drop off, causing numerous symptoms. In addition, menopause causes luteinizing hormone levels to rise, and a high concentration of LH fosters fluctuations in body temperature, resulting in hot flashes and night sweats. In addition to its estrogenlike properties, black cohosh's active ingredients, which include triterpene glycosides, counteract hot flashes by suppressing the secretion of luteinizing hormone (LH).

As for painful periods, black cohosh lessens discomfort by increasing blood flow to the uterus and decreasing severe contractions that cause the discomfort. When it comes to lessening the irritation of premenstrual syndrome, black cohosh may be able to stand in for estrogen to provide better hormone balance.

The tannins in black cohosh may help in treating diarrhea; when applied to the skin, they have an astringent action that can ease the irritation of insect bites and may also reduce the inflammation and itching of eczema and other types of dermatitis.

Evidence of Efficacy

The effects of black cohosh have been studied in the lab using both cells and animal models. Black cohosh studies involving women have also been conducted. In considering its effectiveness and safety, Germany's Commission E—the official body that has studied hundreds of botanical medicines and supplements—has found that black cohosh works to reduce the discomforts of PMS; reduces painful periods; and decrease the "nervous" conditions associated with menopause. No scientific studies have been conducted to validate other claims that black cohosh cures diarrhea, eases lung congestion, eases arthritis pain, and clears up skin inflammation, although some practitioners feel that the herb's components may have these effects.

Forms and Usual Dosage

Black cohosh is typically taken in the form of a 40 to 60 percent alcoholic extract that corresponds to 40 mg of crude drug daily. Black cohosh is available in capsule, tablet, tincture, and a dried form. You probably won't get instantaneous effects from black cohosh. It can take up to four weeks to establish a blood level that's adequate to ward off the discomforts associated with PMS and menopause.

Potential Problems

Some participants in controlled studies on black cohosh have suffered minor side effects, including weight gain, intestinal upset, dizziness, and headaches. Very high intakes of black cohosh can lead to vomiting, headache, dizziness, limb pains, and decreased blood pressure. Because so little is known about the ramifications of taking black cohosh for extended periods of time, experts recommend limiting its consumption to no more than four months at a time. (German health authorities recommended a six-month limit.) Experts also advise against taking black cohosh during pregnancy and when breast-feeding.

See Also

Endometriosis
Menopause
Premenstrual Syndrome

BLACK CURRANT (*RIBES NIGRUM*)

The black currant is a thornless shrub that grows wild in Yorkshire and the Lake District of England. Its buds and leaves have a distinctive perfume, and its berries are gathered to make jelly, brandy, and wine; the leaves are dried and used to make tea. The leaves, berries, and seeds are all used medicinally, especially to treat diarrhea and soothe a sore throat.

Common Uses

- Control diarrhea.
- Increase urine output when taken as a diuretic.

- Reduce arthritis pain and inflammation.
- Ease premenstrual swelling and other symptoms.
- Soothe a sore throat.
- Treat eczema and other inflammatory skin conditions.

How It Works

Black currant leaves and berries contain bioflavonoids and tannins; the seeds are rich in gamma-linolenic acid (GLA), a fatty acid similar to that found in evening primrose oil and borage seed oil. Black currant juice is a concentrated source of vitamin C, an important antioxidant; the berry skins are high in anthocyanin, a bioflavonoid that is also a potent antioxidant. These substances protect cells against the damage of unstable molecules called free radicals; they may also bolster immunity and inhibit cancer growth.

Black currant leaves and berries contain substances that have antifungal and antibacterial properties; the latter may explain its usefulness in treating diarrhea caused by the *E. coli* bacterium. The tannins in black currant leaves help counter diarrhea by reducing intestinal inflammation; they also soothe an inflamed sore throat. Black currant tea has mild diuretic properties, which helps rid the body of excess fluids and may help lower high blood pressure. The tea and black currant juice are rich in potassium, an essential electrolyte mineral that many pharmaceutical diuretics wash out of the body.

The GLA found in black currant seeds is thought to reduce the inflammation of arthritis, lupus, and other inflammatory diseases by increasing the body's production of prostaglandin E-1, a hormonelike substance that reduces inflammation. It also inhibits blood clotting and thus may protect against heart attacks and strokes. (See Essential Fatty Acids, p. 295.)

Evidence of Efficacy

Most of the evidence supporting the therapeutic uses of black currant is either anecdotal and based on a long tradition in herbal medicine or inferred from studies done on the plant's individual components. For example, numerous studies have documented the value of GLA in treating PMS. The mild diuretic action of black currant tea may help reduce swelling by ridding the body of excess fluid.

Forms and Usual Dosages

Black currant oil is available in a capsule form; the dried leaves are sold as a tea. The fresh fruit is sometimes available, but the juice is easier to find. The berries and juice tend to be quite tart; the juice is usually diluted and sweetened or it may be mixed with other berry juices. In Scandinavia, a powder made from black currant skins is used to treat diarrhea. Black currant lozenges are also available and used to treat sore throats.

To treat diarrhea, herbalists typically recommend drinking three or four cups of black currant tea or an equivalent amount of black currant juice. To reduce symptoms of arthritis, eczema, and other inflammatory conditions, take up to 1,000 mg of black currant oil, standardized to provide 14 to 19 percent GLA, two or three times a day. The daily dosage may be increased to 6,000 mg a day.

Potential Problems

Black currant tea, juice, and seeds have been used for many years with no reports of toxicity or other problems.

BLACK HAW (*VIBURNUM PRUNIFOLIUM*)

Also called sweet viburnum, black haw is a native shrub that grows in many parts of central and southern North America. It is distinguished by winter buds that produce clusters of small, white flowers in the spring and dark, edible berries in the fall. However, the plant's medicinal properties are concentrated in its distinctive bark, which is gray-brown on the outside and a reddish brown on the inside.

Traditionally, black haw has been used as a "uterine tonic" to treat disorders related to menstruation, pregnancy, and childbirth. Black haw is closely related to cramp bark (*Viburnum opulus*) and has many of the same antispasmodic and sedative effects.

Common Uses

- Ease menstrual cramps and uterine contractions after childbirth.
- Prevent miscarriage.
- May lower high blood pressure and calm bronchial spasms related to asthma.
- Reduce inflammation in arthritis and other conditions.

How It Works

The active ingredients in black haw are scopoletin, a coumarin compound that appears to help relax smooth muscles and may also inhibit blood clotting; tannins, which have a drying, or astringent action; salicin, a chemical relative of the active ingredient in aspirin; other substances that are muscle relaxants; and various plant acids and a volatile oil. Taken together, these ingredients appear to relax smooth muscles, including the uterus, to reduce cramping and uterine contractions. This action may also lower blood pressure by widening (dilating) the small blood vessels (arterioles) and also relieve asthma symptoms due to spasms of the muscles controlling the airways. Herbalists sometimes recommend black haw to stop the uterine contractions that may lead to premature birth or a miscarriage; however, this should be tried only under a doctor's close supervision. It has also been used to control heavy bleeding following childbirth (postpartum hemorrhage), but again, this is a serious situation that demands a doctor's attention.

Evidence of Efficacy

Researchers at both the University of Illinois and the Tufts University School of Medicine have confirmed that black haw extract appears to help relax contractions of smooth muscles, easing not only uterine contractions but also other types of muscle spasms.

Forms and Usual Dosages

Black haw is available as dried bark, an extract, a tincture, pills, and capsules. Herbalists typically recommend a tea made from 2 teaspoonfuls of dried bark to a cup of freshly boiled distilled water. Steep for ten to fifteen minutes and strain. Drink one cup two to three times a day to relieve cramps. As an alternative, 5 to 10 ml of the tincture may be taken three times a day.

Potential Problems

Black haw appears to be safe when used as directed to treat menstrual cramps, but it should not be taken during pregnancy except under the close supervision of a doctor or other health care professional who is experienced at using it to treat pregnancy complications. Even then, many experts advise against using black haw and, instead, recommend other, more reliable medications.

BLOODROOT (*SANGUINARIA CANADENSIS*)

◉ **A LITTLE HISTORY**
Not only did Native Americans use bloodroot to treat skin infections and cancers and as a skin and clothing dye, but bachelors of the Ponca tribe in North Carolina also used it as a love charm. A man would apply the red juice to his palms, then shake hands with the woman he wanted to marry. This ritual was repeated over the course of five or six days, or until the object of his affection got the message.

As an herbal remedy, bloodroot can be used externally or as a toothpaste or mouthwash, but it can be highly toxic if more than a tiny amount is swallowed. Named for the red extract made from its root, bloodroot is a perennial with beautiful white flowers that bloom in early spring. The leaves first appear wrapped around the flower bud and are grayish green and covered with a downy fuzz. After flowering, the leaves increase in size and have prominent veins on their underside. The roots are thick, round, and fleshy, slightly curved at the ends, and contain an orange-red juice.

The dried roots have a very bitter taste, and they release a powder that irritates the nose and causes sneezing. Native Americans used bloodroot to make dyes and body paint. Its medicinal use evolved when Indian medicine men noted that, when the extract was applied to the skin, it cleared up ulcers, ringworm, and other infections. Today it is used mostly to prevent or treat gingivitis, although some of its components are being studied as a potential treatment for skin cancer.

Common Uses

- Inhibit oral bacteria that cause gum disease and gingivitis.
- Treat various skin disorders and infections, including athlete's foot, eczema, ringworm, and warts.
- Soothe sore throat and coughs when used in small amounts mixed with other herbs.

How It Works

Bloodroot contains several alkaloids, the most important of which are sanguinarine and chelerythrine. When ingested—which is not recommended—sanguinarine stimulates saliva flow and raises blood pressure, among other effects. In small doses, it acts as an expectorant to clear mucus from the airways. In larger amounts, it induces vomiting. Both sanguinarine and cheleythrine inhibit the growth of the oral bacteria that form dental plaque and can lead to gum disease. It is used in natural toothpastes and mouthwashes, which should be used with caution to avoid swallowing. In addition, bloodroot has been proved effective in treating fungal infections, such as ringworm. There is also some evidence that the alkaloids in bloodroot can inhibit the growth of skin cancers, and sanguinanine may inhibit the growth of solid tumors.

Evidence of Efficacy

The toxic effects of bloodroot have been studied in animal experiments and reported anecdotally in humans. Although research results have been mixed, some laboratory studies indicate that sanguinarine and chelerythrine may inhibit the growth of oral bacteria and also reduce bad breath and numb local mouth pain. Researchers are also studying sanguinarine and chelerythrine as potential anticancer agents.

Bloodroot contains protopine, a substance that is also found in opium. In the 1800s, bloodroot extracts were sometimes used as narcotic painkillers. Fortunately, there are now many safer alternatives.

Forms and Usual Dosage

Bloodroot should only be used externally on skin conditions or in a mixture of alkaloids called sanguinaria extract found in mouthwashes and toothpastes that are not swallowed. For external use, bloodroot can be found as a decoction, in ointments, as a powder, and as a tincture. To make a decoction to use as a compress soak or mouthwash, boil 1 teaspoon of dried root in a cup of water, and let it sleep ten minutes. Bloodroot is also blended with red sage and cayenne to make a gargle to treat throat irritations.

Potential Problems

Bloodroot is safe only when used externally, and even then it can cause problems, including a rash similar to that of poison ivy in people who are allergic to it. Ingestion can cause nausea, vomiting, numbness, low blood pressure, shock, fainting, coma, and death. Since 1977, bloodroot has appeared on the U.S. Department of Agriculture (USDA) list of unsafe herbs. Fortunately, bloodroot has a very unpleasant, bitter taste that makes overdosing unlikely. Pregnant women should be especially careful to avoid any products containing bloodroot.

See Also

Tooth Decay and Gum Diseases

BONESET (*EUPATORIUM PERFOLIATUM*)

Before aspirin came on the scene, boneset was one of the remedies of choice to treat the aches and fever of flu and bad colds. In fact, the high fever and deep achiness of a bad case of flu probably gave rise to the herb's common names of boneset and feverwort; it is also called white snakeroot. The perennial grows wild in damp areas throughout the eastern part of North America and into the West Indies and South America and it is gathered after it flowers in the late summer and early autumn. The leaves and the heads of small, white flowers are dried and used medicinally to treat complications of the common cold and flu. Boneset has a bitter, astringent taste; the fresh herb is toxic, but the poisonous compound dissipates when the plant is dried.

Common Uses

- Reduces fevers, especially those associated with colds and flu.
- Alleviate achiness associated with arthritis, colds, and flu.
- Treat indigestion and stimulate appetite loss.
- In small amounts, may promote urination and exert a mild laxative effect.
- May have antibacterial and cancer-fighting components.

How It Works

The active ingredients in boneset include compounds called sesquiterpene lactones, especially eupatorin, a bitter-tasting substance that may be effective against minor infections. Other components include bioflavonoids, such as quercetin, astragalin, and rutin, which are antioxidants; polysaccharides, which help bolster immunity; sterols, which may have hormonelike activity; and a volatile oil.

To treat influenza, herbalists usually combine boneset with other herbs, such as yarrow, elder flowers, cayenne, or ginger. It may also be combined with pleurisy root and elecampane to treat bronchial conditions.

Evidence of Efficacy

Compounds in boneset have been studied in the laboratory, but it is unclear whether the herb itself has any real medicinal effects and there is little scientific evidence to substantiate many of its traditional uses. Even so, laboratory studies of some of the herb's active ingredients indicate they may have anti-infective and cancer-fighting properties, but it is not clear whether the herb carries these benefits, especially when consumed by humans.

Although a person may start to sweat after drinking a cup of boneset tea, it is unclear whether this effect is a sign that the decoction is working to lower a fever or is simply a reaction to its bitter taste. A concentrated boneset extract has been shown to have mild anti-inflammatory properties, which may help ease muscle aches and arthritis pain.

Forms and Usual Dosages

Only the dried herb should be used, as fresh leaves and flowers contain a toxic substance. Boneset is usually taken as a tea made with 1 to 2 teaspoons of the dried leaves and flowers per cup of water; the typical dosage recommended to relieve cold and flu symptoms calls for drinking a cup of the hot tea every thirty to sixty minutes until sweating begins or until three cups have been consumed. The commercially available tincture is taken in dosages of ½ to 1 teaspoon three times a day. Check labels on extracts for dosage information.

Potential Problems

When used as recommended, boneset is considered safe although high doses may cause vomiting and severe diarrhea. Even at the recommended dosages, however, it should not be used for longer than two weeks, especially if the condition does not improve. Other more effective remedies are available.

There is some concern that long-term use of boneset may result in liver damage. Researchers have found that many members of the genus *Eupatorium* contain dangerous chemicals—pyrrolizidine alkaloids (PAs)—that can cause liver damage and promote liver cancer. German health authorities recommend that PA ingestion be limited to less than 1 mcg a day. Because there is no way to determine how much PA is in any dosage of boneset, this warning is problematic to herbalists. However, there are no known cases of boneset actually causing liver damage. Certainly anyone with a liver disorder should avoid boneset. In addition, some people may develop a rash when handling the fresh plant.

BORAGE (*BORAGO OFFICINALIS*)

⊙ A LITTLE HISTORY
Centuries ago, Europeans made a "tea" of borage leaves, by soaking them in wine, to allay boredom and melancholy. It continues to be used as a kitchen herb in parts of Europe. However, GLA is widely used in Europe to treat diabetic neuropathy and eczema and, in both the United States and Europe, to treat fibrocystic breasts and PMS. Recent research has increasingly supported the use of GLA for rheumatic disorders.

Borage is also known as burrage, bugloss, ox's tong, cooltankard, starflower, and, because its pungent flower attracts bees, beebread and bee plant. Originally indigenous to the Mediterranean region, it is now grown all across Europe and the United States. This succulent herb grows on bristly stems to three feet in both height and width. Borage blooms with lavender-to-blue star-shaped flowers in the spring and summer. Both the leaves and flowers, which have a cucumber flavor, have been used in salads and to flavor punches and other beverages. The flowers can also be used to make a flavorful vinegar.

Dried leaves and the fatty oil of borage seeds have long been used for medicinal purposes. The active ingredient that makes borage a healthful supplement is gamma-linolenic acid (GLA), an omega-6 essential fatty acid. (GLA is also found in evening primrose oil and black currant seed oil.)

Common Uses

- Ease discomfort of fibrocystic breast disease.
- Relieve inflammation and pain of diabetic neuropathy, eczema, rheumatoid arthritis, and lupus.
- Alleviate PMS symptoms.

In folk medicine, borage also has been used for coughs, kidney and bladder disorders, as an astringent and diuretic, and as a heart tonic and sedative, but no scientific evidence supports these benefits.

How It Works

The body uses essential fatty acids (see p. 295) to make prostaglandins, hormonelike substances that influence inflammation and the pain it causes. Some prostaglandins increase inflammation, while others decrease them. GLA is one of the two main types of essential fatty acids. It is a "good" fat that can help the body manufacture prostaglandins that create a less inflammatory environment, thus easing the symptoms of diseases involving inflammation.

Very little GLA is found in the typical Western diet. However, the body normally makes all the GLA it needs from linoleic acid, an omega-6 essential fatty acid found in many foods. However, some conditions may impair the body's ability to convert linoleic acid to GLA efficiently. These include aging, alcoholism, diabetes, eczema, high intake of saturated fat, high cholesterol levels, mastitis, viral infections, and deficiencies of vitamin B_6, zinc, magnesium, biotin, or calcium.

Evidence of Efficacy

Multiple studies of people with rheumatoid arthritis have demonstrated a reduction in the number of tender and swollen joints when borage seed oil capsules are taken for long periods, usually several months. In one double-blind, controlled study of one hundred patients, about half took 2.8 g of borage daily while the other half took a placebo. The GLA group had significantly fewer symptoms, with benefits slowly growing over the course of the six-month study. Similar results have been seen in studies of systemic lupus erythematosus, a "cousin" disease of rheumatoid arthritis.

Both animal and human studies have demonstrated the ability of GLA taken orally to reduce skin inflammation in eczema (atopic dermatitis). Although some studies found notable relief of itching and the size and severity of skin lesions, others found no benefit.

GLA has become a standard treatment for fibrocystic breast disease in which breast pain occurs in association with the menstrual period and is even recognized in the AMA's official *Drug Evaluations* textbook. In one study, GLA was compared to three prescription drugs (danazol, bromocriptine, and progestins), and 56 percent of the GLA group found the therapy effective in reducing pain.

Although it is also widely used to ease other PMS symptoms, research evidence in support of such therapy is not strong. However, GLA is widely used in Europe to treat diabetic neuropathy and eczema and, in both the United States and Europe, to treat fibrocystic breasts and PMS. Recent research has increasingly supported the use of GLA for rheumatic disorders.

Studies have supported the benefits of GLA for treating diabetic neuropathy, if it is given enough time to work. In one double-blind placebo-controlled study of 111 people, those receiving 480 mg daily of GLA had a significant improvement in symptoms after twelve months.

GLA also has been proposed as a treatment for: asthma, allergies, bursitis, chronic fatigue syndrome, endometriosis, heart disease, irritable bowel syndrome, prostate cancer, and prostate enlargement (benign prostatic hyperplasia), among others. However, none of these potential uses has as yet any strong evidence behind it.

Forms and Usual Dosages

The oil is commercially sold in softgel capsules. Most commonly each 300-mg softgel contains 20 to 26 percent of GLA. It is the amount of GLA in each capsule that should affect dosing choice, so it's important to read labels carefully.

For fibrocystic breast disease, 200 to 400 mg of GLA daily is usually recommended. For diabetic neuropathy, treatment is typically 400 to 600 mg daily. Studies in rheumatoid arthritis have used 1.1 to 3 g a day of GLA, which may require taking more than a dozen softgels.

Borage also is available as a liquid leaf extract and a tea; follow label instructions for dosages.

Potential Problems

GLA benefits take time to develop. Thus you may have to take it for at least two months—or as long as six months—to experience an improvement. In large measure, no hazards or side effects have been proved when borage is used in appropriate dosages. However, some reports in the 1980s identified the presence of low levels of toxic unsaturated pyrrolizidine alkaloids (PAs) in borage plants. PAs have been implicated in liver damage and liver cancer, although it is not known whether the levels found in borage can cause such damage. Nonetheless, concerns about toxicity prompted the German government to refuse approval of borage for any medicinal use. Thus, to err on the side of caution, it may be wiser to obtain GLA from other plant sources, such as evening primrose or black currant oil.

BOSWELLIA
(*BOSWELLIA SERRATA*)

The boswellia is a medium to large branching tree native to the dry hilly areas of India. When its trunk is tapped, a gummy resin called boswellin or salai guggul is exuded. It is also known as Indian frankincense and Indian olibanum. The purified extract of this resin is used for medicinal purposes.

Common Uses

- Musculoskeletal pain, especially due to arthritis (external applications).
- Inflammatory musculoskeletal problems, such as rheumatoid and osteoarthritis, ankylosing spondylitis, and bursitis (ingested forms).
- Ulcerative colitis.

In addition, the salai guggul resin itself has been used for centuries for such diverse problems as:

◙ A LITTLE HISTORY
The history of boswellia—a close cousin of the biblical frankincense plant—stretches back some four thousand years to ancient Egypt. The classic Ayurvedic texts of India, dating from 700 B.C., praise boswellin as an antirheumatic medicine. It is grouped with other gum resins, collectively referred to as gugguls, which were recommended for a variety of conditions including arthritis, diarrhea, dysentery, pulmonary disease, and ringworm.

- Diarrhea and dysentery.
- Lung disease.
- Parasitic worms.

How It Works

Just as salicylic acid from the bark of the willow tree led to the development of aspirin, the resin of the boswellia tree also seems to have nonsteroidal anti-inflammatory benefits. Boswellin consists of essential oils, gum, and terpenoids. Recent research suggests that it is the terpenoids, which contain boswellic acids, that are responsible for its benefits. They appear to act in three ways:

- They inhibit leukotrienes, pro-inflammatory mediators in the body, by interfering with the inflammatory cascade reaction produced by the 5-lipoxygenase enzyme.
- They reduce the migration of inflammatory immune cells to inflamed tissues.
- They disrupt even earlier stages of the inflammatory autoimmune response, specifically primary antibody production and complement (immune protein) activity. However, because they do not block the COX enzymes, as traditional NSAIDs do, boswellia acids do not appear to have such toxic side effects as stomach ulcers, bleeding, or changes in blood chemistry.

Evidence of Efficacy

India's council for Scientific and Industrial Research has sponsored a series of studies of potentially anti-inflammatory herbal products, including the boswellic acids. In several studies in both rats and humans, boswellia's benefits have been compared to other NSAIDs. For example, 175 people with rheumatoid arthritis were given either 450 to 750 mg of boswellic acids daily or standard doses of ketoprofen or phenylbutazone. All were effective in reducing pain, swollen joints, and morning stiffness, and improving grip strength and physical performance.

In another study, 175 patients with either rheumatoid arthritis or ankylosing spondylitis received 600 mg daily of boswellia extract for at least four weeks; two out of three had good to excellent results on a standard measure of clinical improvement (the Mean Arthritic Score). One of the best studies to date was a double-blind, placebo-controlled crossover study of thirty patients who first received either a placebo or 600 mg of boswellic acids, and then were switched over to the opposite regimen; Mean Arthritic Scores dropped by 60 percent during the boswellia phase and rose again when placebo was introduced.

Because of its anti-inflammatory activity, boswellia is also being investigated for benefits in ulcerative colitis, but positive findings have not been reported.

Forms and Usual Dosages

For topical application, boswellia is available in pain-relieving creams, some of which also contain capsaicin, a simple analgesic made from the oils of hot chilies. For systemic benefits, capsules or tablets should be taken. Products are usually standardized to contain 37.5 to 65 percent boswellic acids and contain 150 to 250 mg of boswellic acids. For arthritis, practitioners recommend 400 mg three times per day of a 37.5 percent extract or 200 mg three times a day of a 65 percent extract.

Potential Problems

Boswellia is generally considered safe when used as directed. Rare side effects can include diarrhea, skin rash, and nausea.

See Also

Arthritis

BROOM
(*CYTISUS SCOPARIUS*)

◉ A LITTLE HISTORY

Broom was adopted at a very early period as the badge of Brittany and has a long and colorful history. Geoffrey of Anjou was said to have thrust it into his helmet before going into battle so that his troops could see him. Henry II of England adapted broom's medieval name, *Planta genista,* as his family name (Plantagenet). The shrub was seen on the great seal of Richard I and adorns the Westminster Abbey tombstone of Richard II.

Broom's medicinal uses were mentioned in fifteenth-century herbal texts, and it was listed in the *Pharmacopoeia* published in London in 1618. It was listed in the U.S. *Pharmacopoeia* until 1978, when it was withdrawn by the FDA because of its potential for dangerous side effects.

Also known as Scotch or Irish broom and broomtops, this shrub is native to western Europe but now grows in many parts of the world. In the United States, as well as Australia and New Zealand, it has overrun large areas of land once used for recreation and farming. It grows up to six feet in height and its stiff, angled branches were once used in Scotland and other parts of Europe to make brooms, giving rise to its popular name. The leaves and pods are mildly poisonous to farm animals if ingested in large amounts. The flowering tops are the parts of the plants used by herbalists.

Common Uses

- Rid the body of excess fluid, especially in congestive heart failure in which the heart is unable to pump adequately.

- Treat cardiac arrhythmias.
- Stimulate uterine contractions and help control heavy menstrual bleeding.
- Reduces varicose vein symptoms.

How It Works

Broom contains various alkaloids, including sparteine, which raises blood pressure by constricting peripheral blood vessels; isoflavone glycosides, which have estrogenlike effects; scoparoside, a glycoside that is believed to have diuretic and laxative effects; various flavonoids, which are antioxidants; tannins, which have astringent actions; coumarin compounds, which hinder blood clotting; and essential oils, among other ingredients. Sparteine has been shown to slow the heartbeat and may be useful in treating some types of cardiac arrhythmias. In Germany, broom is considered gentler and less toxic than the drug quinidine for treating heart arrhythmias.

In the presence of mild congestive heart failure, compounds in broom may strengthen the heartbeat and, along with the herb's diuretic effects, help rid the body of excess fluid. By constricting small arteries, broom is said to help control heavy menstrual bleeding, but this effect had not been proved.

Evidence of Efficacy

The effectiveness of some of the ingredients in broom has been demonstrated in laboratory studies. For example, the diuretic and laxative effects of scoparoside are well established. Sparteine is a potent alkaloid with actions similar to those of nicotine. Studies show that it can slow the heartbeat by suppressing certain nerve impulses. Other alkaloids in broom have been shown to raise blood pressure and stimulate uterine contractions. In some countries, broom is used to induce labor, although it is not approved for that use in the United States; there are other much safer methods.

Forms and Usual Dosages

Broom is available as an infusion, using its flower tops, and as a tincture. A tea is made by steeping 1 teaspoon of the dried herb in a cup of boiling water for ten to fifteen minutes. Do not exceed three cups of tea a day. As a tincture, 1 to 2 ml three times a day is the usual dosage.

Potential Problems

The toxic effects of broom limit its usefulness in treating humans. The Food and Drug Administration (FDA) lists broom as a dangerous herb with a high risk of harmful side effects, and German health authorities caution that it should be used only under the supervision of a health professional. The active ingredients in broom are potent and can cause toxic side effects, such as impaired vision, vomiting, diarrhea, and profuse sweating. It should never be used during pregnancy or by anyone with high blood pressure. When taken with a monoamine oxidase (MAO) inhibitor, it can cause a dangerous sudden rise in blood pressure. Farm animals that ingest large amounts, especially along with alfalfa, may suffer fatal internal bleeding.

BUGLEWEED
(*LYCOPUS VIRGINICUS*)

Bugleweed, a member of the mint family and a common weed throughout North America, favors damp, shady areas; it is also known as water bugle, sweet bugle, Virginian water horehound, and gypsyweed. Its leaves are paired and, from July until September, it produces clusters of small white and purple flowers. The whole herb, which has a minty odor and flavor, is used medicinally. In the past, it was used mostly to treat coughs, anxiety, fevers, and palpitations; today, it is an adjunctive treatment for mild overactive thyroid (hyperthyroidism or Graves' disease).

Common Uses

- As an adjunct to medical treatment of an overactive thyroid.
- Ease breast enlargement and tenderness in men.

In the past, bugleweed was also used as:

- A sedative to calm nerves and induce sleep.
- Calm coughs.
- Control nosebleeds and heavy menstrual bleeding (menorrhagia).

How It Works

In Graves' disease, the thyroid gland produces excessive hormones, resulting in accelerated metabolism and such symptoms as a rapid pulse, weight loss, sensitivity to heat and excessive sweating, fatigue, and physical changes, including development of an enlarged thyroid (a goiter) and bulging eyes. It is not clear how bugleweed works in treating hyperthyroidism, but some studies indicate that it may influence metabolism of iodine, which the thyroid uses to make its hormones. The lithospermic acid and other organic acids in bugleweed may work to lower levels of thyroid-stimulating hormone (TSH) or it may block the TSH receptors and prevent the hormone from entering the thyroid gland to stimulate production of other hormones. Substances in bugleweed also appear to decrease the pituitary gland's production of prolactin, a hormone that can stimulate breast growth and tenderness in men.

Evidence of Efficacy

German researchers have reported that bugleweed has some effect in regulating production of thyroid hormones in mild hyperthyroidism. There are also anecdotal accounts of bugleweed reducing symptoms of hyperthyroidism in some patients. German health authorities recommend that it be used in very mild Graves' disease, or as an adjunct to pharmaceutical prescription drugs, especially in controlling more severe hyperthyroidism.

Forms and Usual Dosages

Only a small amount of bugleweed is needed to decrease thyroid function, however, the amount needed is different for each individual. The German Commission E recommends a daily dosage of 1 to 2 g of the whole herb. Ingestion of the tincture should be limited to 1 to 2 ml three times a day. Modern herbalists recommend a tea made from 1 ounce of the dried herb to a pint of freshly boiled distilled water, taken several times a day. As a fluid extract, bugleweed can be taken in doses of ten to thirty drops. It is sometimes used in combination with lemon balm (*Melissa officinalis*), another herb that suppresses the thyroid.

Potential Problems

Thyroid disease is serious and should only be treated under the supervision of a health care professional. Bugleweed should not be taken by people with underactive thyroids. Sudden withdrawal from ingestion of bugleweed may lead to an abrupt increase in prolactin secretion and should be avoided. The herb should not be taken by pregnant or nursing women.

BURDOCK
(ARCTIUM LAPPA)

The carrotlike burdock root grows in the hedges and ditches of Europe and in parts of Asia and North America, and it is cultivated in Japan, where it is consumed as a vegetable called gobo. Also known as beggar's buttons, burdock is a biennial that produces pretty purple flowers that evolve into the dreaded burrs that get entangled in pets' fur and cling relentlessly to clothing and anything else that brushes against them.

All parts of the plant can be eaten while it is young, after which it grows bitter. Most of the burdock's medicinal properties are contained in the roots or rhizome, although the seeds are also crushed and used therapeutically. Burdock is used medicinally worldwide: in China it is believed to be an effective aphrodisiac and is used to treat impotence and infertility; in Russia and India, it is a popular cancer treatment. Closer to home, burdock is used as a diuretic and general blood "purifier."

Common Uses

- Treat indigestion and appetite loss.
- Rid the body of excess fluid and relieve mild constipation.
- Treat inflammatory skin conditions, such as acne, eczema, and psoriasis.
- Reduce symptoms of gout, arthritis, and rheumatism.
- May have antibacterial and cancer-fighting components.

How It Works

When consumed as food, burdock provides fair amounts of several vitamins and is also a good source of minerals, especially iron, chromium, cobalt, magnesium, phosphorus, silicon, zinc, and potassium. The root is high in mucilage, a gummy (demulcent) material that has a soothing effect when applied to inflammatory skin conditions, such as patches of psoriasis. It contains tannins, resins, and bitter compounds that stimulate appetite, aid digestion, and treat mild intestinal upsets; it also has a mild laxative effect that can alleviate constipation. It is reputed to have a diuretic effect that can reduce fluid buildup (edema), but the evidence for this is sketchy at best. The root is a good source of inulin, which is said to help regulate blood sugar, although it should not be confused with insulin, the hormone that is essential to metabolize sugar and other carbohydrates. The root also contains chemicals called polyacetylenes, which have antibacterial and antifungal properties; however, these sub-

◉ A LITTLE HISTORY
Shakespeare mentions burdock in quite a few of his plays, including *Troilus and Cressida, King Lear,* and *As You Like It.* Native Americans used the entire plant as food, and even made candy from it by boiling the stem in maple syrup, then storing it for the winter.

stances dissipate when the root is dried—the form that is most often used medicinally.

Evidence of Efficacy

There is little or no scientific evidence to back up the many claims for burdock. After extensive study, the German health authorities have declined to recommend burdock to treat any ailment. The idea that blood needs to be "purified" to maintain health has been discounted by modern medical science. The mucilage in burdock root may have a soothing effect, but it has not been shown to actually heal skin and other conditions.

There is some evidence—based on laboratory rather than human studies—that burdock root can stimulate the liver to produce bile and that inulin can help control blood sugar levels. Root infusions may also help dissolve kidney or bladder stones. Researchers are investigating whether the chemicals in burdock root or its seeds can protect against cancer and inhibit tumor growth, but much more study is needed to determine whether it has any potential for humans in these areas. There was some speculation that burdock extract can kill HIV, the virus that causes AIDS, but this has been disproved in test tube studies.

Forms and Usual Dosages

For internal use, burdock root is available in capsules and as a decoction, an extract, powdered root, tea, and tincture; it is also added to many herbal blends. The seeds are sometimes crushed and their oil and other components are available as capsules and extracts.

Dosages vary according to usage. A decoction is made using 1¼ teaspoons of the chopped root per cup of water. A tincture is taken in dosages of ½ to 1 teaspoon three times a day. Capsules generally contain 475 mg of burdock extract and may be taken several times a day. Burdock root tea, made from the plant's young leaves, is said to aid digestion. The leaves may also be used to make a poultice, which is said to reduce pain and swelling of arthritis, rheumatism, and gout; burdock poultices are also used to hasten the healing of bruises and minor skin wounds.

Potential Problems

Although burdock is safe to consume as food, when it comes to medicinal uses, the FDA classifies this herb as one of "undefined safety." It should be used with caution, if at all, and certainly avoided during pregnancy or if you have a serious chronic disease. Some people also develop allergic skin reactions from external applications of burdock.

BUTCHER'S BROOM
(*RUSCUS ACULEATUS*)

Butcher's broom is an evergreen bush native that grows all across Europe, western Asia, and northern Africa. It is also known as kneeholm,
knee holly, box holly, pettigree, sweet broom, and Jew's myrtle. The
shrub is spiny and heavily branched, with small triangular leaves and
short shoots with sharp tips. Its small greenish white flowers often grow
in clusters from the middle of the leaves. They develop into berries the
size and color of cherries, ripening in September and remaining on the
bush all winter.

A member of the lily family, butcher's broom is also similar to asparagus, and the young shoots have sometimes been eaten as a vegetable.
However, it is the roots and young stems of the bush that are used
medicinally.

Common Uses

- Hemorrhoids (external application).
- Varicose veins and reduced venous circulation in the legs.
- Atherosclerosis.

In addition, ancient physicians used the roots as a diuretic and a laxative,
but no recent research supports this application. Nonetheless, some
herbal practitioners continue to recommend butcher's broom to reduce
fluid retention and swelling in the feet and hands and to alleviate
arthritis-reed inflammation.

How It Works

Butcher's broom's active ingredients are believed to be steroidal molecules called ruscogenin and neoruscogenin. Ruscogenin is similar to
diosgenin, a substance found in wild yams. The substances appear to
decrease vascular permeability, thus yielding anti-inflammatory activity
and causing small veins to constrict.

Evidence of Efficacy

Animal studies in the 1950s demonstrated an increase in venous tone
and electrolytelike reactions on the cell walls of capillaries, thus narrowing these small blood vessels. Subsequent clinical trials also have supported such benefits in humans. In one study involving forty patients

with chronic venous insufficiency of the legs, half took a combination of butcher's broom, hesperidin, and vitamin C (ascorbic acid) for two months. After two months, those receiving the active substance reported a decrease in swelling, numbness, tingling, itching, heaviness, and cramping, compared to no such benefits in the placebo group. Similar, albeit not as dramatic, improvements were reported in a two-week double-blind study of fifty people with varicose vein problems.

The evidence in support of hemorrhoid benefits are not as clear. Laboratory studies show that the active ingredients in butcher's broom can inhibit inflammation and constrict blood vessels, both benefits likely to be useful in treating the swollen (dilated) veins of hemorrhoids. Although at least one animal study has indicated value, no clinical studies in humans have been done. Nonetheless, German health authorities have approved butcher's broom as a supportive therapy for the itching and burning of hemorrhoids and for venous problems, such as those that cause pain, heaviness, cramps, itching, and swelling of the legs.

Forms and Usual Dosages

Ointments and suppositories containing butcher's broom may be inserted before bedtime for hemorrhoids. For vein-related problems, German health authorities recommend raw extract equivalent to 7 to 11 mg ruscogenin. Some practitioners recommend 1,000-mg capsules of butcher's broom extract, combined with vitamin C or flavonoids, taken three times a day.

Potential Problems

No significant side effects or health hazards have been reported for the use of butcher's broom in recommended doses. However, there have been a few reports of stomach upset attributed to butcher's broom.

See Also

Circulatory Problems
Varicose Veins

CALENDULA (*CALENDULA OFFICINALIS*)

More commonly known as the garden or pot marigold, calendula is ubiquitous in flower gardens throughout the world. Gardeners prize this ornamental plant not only for its ease in growing and cheerful, nonstop yellow blossoms, but also for the fact that it appears to repel aphids and other common garden pests. For centuries, cooks have turned to calendula to add color and flavor to everything from porridge and puddings to salads and vegetable dishes. As if all this weren't enough, this humble little flowering plant has numerous medicinal properties and herbalists recommend it as an overall tonic and to speed healing of cuts and other skin wounds, aid digestion, and treat numerous disorders.

◙ A LITTLE HISTORY

Calendula was named by the ancient Romans, who observed that the plant was in bloom on the first day (*calends*) of every month. They looked upon calendula's nonstop blooming as a symbol of joy, and cultivated it in their gardens to spread the happiness. Calendula's emergence as a botanical medicine came later, and was led by Nicholas Culpepper, the seventeenth-century herbalist, who advocated it to strengthen the heart. During the American Civil War, calendula was used—with mixed success—in field hospitals to stop bleeding, prevent infection, and heal wounds.

Common Uses

- Hasten healing of minor skin wounds and irritations, including boils, cuts, burns, ulcers, rashes, and bruises.
- Treat ringworm and other fungal skin infections.
- Soothe inflammation of the mucous membranes of the mouth and throat.
- Help heal stomach ulcers and intestinal inflammation.
- Lower blood levels of cholesterol and other lipids.
- Bolster the immune system.

How It Works

When used as a mouthwash or gargle, diluted calendula extracts are soothing and appear to hasten healing of mouth ulcers and a sore throat. Herbalists maintain that the calendula blossoms and leaves have antiseptic qualities and promote the healing of skin wounds. When applied as a lotion or ointment, or applied as a poultice or compress, calendula does appear to relieve skin inflammation and enhance healing. Triterpenes may be responsible for the anti-inflammatory action, but to date, no specific compound has been discovered in calendula that would account for the many other benefits attributed to the plant. However, it is high in lutein and other carotenoids, the antioxidant flavonoids found in carrots and many other brightly colored vegetables and fruits. These substances may bolster immunity and help prevent the cellular damage that is thought to increase the risk of cancer.

When taken internally as a tea, calendula appears to reduce intestinal inflammation and symptoms, and it may be beneficial in healing small ulcers. It may also aid digestion by stimulating the flow of bile, the substance made by the liver that is instrumental in digesting fats. Animal studies indicate that it can lower blood levels of cholesterol and other fatty substances (lipids), but the mechanism for this is unknown.

Evidence of Efficacy

German health authorities have approved the use of calendula to heal minor skin wounds and inflammation. However, most of the evidence regarding calendula is either anecdotal or based on animal studies; there are no reports of controlled studies involving humans. Several animal studies indicate that calendula soothes inflammation and speeds wound healing in animals. There have also been reports that calendula may reduce the risk of cancer, but again, these are based on animal or test-tube studies.

Forms and Usual Dosage

Myriad products—lotions, creams, ointments, shampoos, and cosmetics—include calendula as a main ingredient. It is available as a dried herb, an essential oil, an extract, and a tincture. The tincture or dried flowers and leaves can also be used to make a tea—use 1 to 2 teaspoons of the dried plant per cup of water. In addition to being drunk as a tea, the infusion can be used as a gargle or mouthwash or to soak a compress. The flowers and leaves can also be used to make a poultice to apply directly to a skin ulcer, bruise, or other wounds.

Potential Problems

Calendula has been consumed for centuries as both a food and a botanical medicine without reports of toxicity. However, some people are allergic to calendula, and should not use it.

CAMPHOR (*CINNAMOMUM CAMPHORA*)

The camphor tree is native to Asia and now grown in many parts of the world. When its roots or bark is steamed, it produces a volatile, white,

The Chinese have used camphor, both medicinally and for many other uses, for centuries.
After his trip to China, Marco Polo described
its many uses there. It was virtually unknown
elsewhere at that time, but the trees that grow
naturally in China have since been cultivated
in subtropical countries such as India and Cey-
lon, and they now thrive in Egypt, Formosa,
Madagascar, the Canary Islands, Argentina,
and Brazil, as well as southern parts of Europe
and the United States.

crystalline compound with a characteristic pungent aromatic odor; this
is usually referred to as camphor. The aromatic oils in certain other
plants, such as tansy and feverfew, may also be referred to as camphor.

Trees that produce camphor are slow-growing—the Chinese believe
the camphor cannot be extracted from trees under fifty years old—so
camphor production is a long-term investment. In the United States,
camphor is extracted from leaves and twigs of the oldest trees, which
does less damage than the more invasive Chinese method. Even so, most
camphor now used in this country is produced synthetically.

Camphor is used in the manufacture of many products, including
celluloid, explosives, moth repellents, and soaps. Better known, however, are its medicinal uses in topical ointments, linaments, and creams.

Common Uses

- Soothe the pain of arthritis, sprains, bruises, and sore muscles.
- Soften chapped lips.
- Ease itchiness of minor skin irritations.
- Promote healing of minor burns and skin wounds.
- Relieve upper respiratory congestion due to colds and flu.
- Repel moths and other insects.

How It Works

Camphor has a strong, penetrating odor, a bitter, pungent taste, and,
like menthol, is slightly cool to the touch; it also has mild antibacterial
properties. When camphor is applied to the skin as a salve or linament,
it acts as a counterirritant that stimulates nerve endings and helps reduce
the number of pain messages that reach the brain. Thus, it is useful in
treating the discomfort of minor arthritis and muscle aches and strains;
it can also ease itchiness of eczema, insect bites, and external hemorrhoids.

Camphor has mild antibacterial properties, which may aid in the
healing of minor burns and skin wounds. As an ingredient in lip balms,
it softens and soothes chapped or blistered lips.

Used in steam vaporizers to produce an aromatic vapor, camphor is
thought to control coughs by producing a local anesthetic action to the
throat, and to loosen congestion due to colds. When a cream or ointment
containing camphor is rubbed onto the chest, throat, or back, body heat
helps release camphor vapors that, when inhaled, help loosen mucus and
relieve airway congestion.

Evidence of Efficacy

Camphor has been studied extensively, analyzed chemically, and produced synthetically. Commercially prepared forms, such as Ben-Gay,

Aurum Gold Analgesic, Vicks VapoRub and Vicks VapoSteam, are safe when they are used as directed. Studies have found that when camphor is used in concentrations of 3 to 11 percent it is an effective counterirritant that can relieve minor arthritis and muscle pain and may also be effective in easing nerve pain (neuralgia). Animal studies confirm that camphor vapors can control coughing, presumably by acting as a mild local anesthetic.

While the external uses and benefits of camphor have been subjected to considerable research, there is controversy over its internal use. German health authorities have approved the use of camphor as a tonic for circulation disorders, but the U.S. Food and Drug Administration cautions against any internal use of the substance.

Forms and Usual Dosage

For external use, camphor is found diluted in concentrations from 3 to 11 percent in gels, drops, oil, ointments, and other formulations for topical application to the skin. It is also available in hot steam vaporizer solutions. It can be applied to limited areas of the skin—for example, an aching shoulder or part of the upper chest—up to three or four times a day, but because camphor can be absorbed through the skin, it should not be used more often or applied to very large areas.

Potential Problems

Camphor is highly toxic to the liver, and should not be ingested, even in small amounts. In recommended concentrations, camphor is safe and not likely to produce any adverse reactions. In rare cases, it can produce a skin rash. Do not apply to skin more often than recommended, because it can irritate or damage the skin and there is a risk of absorption into the body with serious consequences. Camphor preparations should not be applied to skin that is badly burned or to open wounds. It also should not be used on babies and young children. Finally, caution is needed when using camphor mothballs because of its effects on the environment. For example, some gardeners scatter mothballs around plants to repel insects—a practice that should be discouraged because it can accumulate in the soil and also enter the water table.

CARAWAY
(*CARUM CARVI*)

A member of the carrot family, caraway is grown more for its culinary uses than for its medicinal purposes. Still, its seeds (technically, they are the plant's fruit) produce a medicinal oil, and for centuries people have chewed caraway seeds to promote digestion, perk up appetite, and treat a variety of intestinal problems.

Caraway, thought to have originated in ancient Asia Minor, was used to flavor bread in the time of Julius Caesar—a practice that continues today. The seeds are also used to flavor everything from cheese and soup to alcohol. In ancient times, superstition held that caraway possessed the gift of retention, preventing the theft of any object which contained it by holding the thief in custody within the invaded house. Likewise, it was used in love potions to keep lovers from straying, and in bird food to keep barnyard fowl from wandering away.

Throughout history, writers have referred to caraway—Dioscorides, for example, advised pale-faced girls to eat its oil (perhaps in recognition of caraway as an ancient remedy for anemia) and in Shakespeare's *Henry IV*, Squire Shallow invites Falstaff to a "pippin and a dish of caraways."

Common Uses

Traditionally, caraway is promoted to help regulate menstrual periods or prompt the return of menstruation in women whose periods have stopped (amenorrhea). The phytoestrogens may also help reduce menstrual cramps, but the mechanism for this is not known.

How It Works

Caraway seeds yield an essential oil that contains carvole and D-limonene (carvene), substances that soothe the digestive tract and reduce bloating and gas. A diluted caraway infusion is sometimes added to an infant's bottle to reduce gastric upset. The oil also promotes the flow of saliva and the secretion of gastric juices—actions that stimulate appetite and promote digestion.

Caraway seeds are thought to contain phytoestrogens, plant substances that mimic the effect of estrogen, which would explain how they may work against menstrual and other "female" problems.

Evidence of Efficacy

Most of the evidence regarding the effectiveness of caraway is either anecdotal or based on laboratory and animal studies. For example, substances found in caraway oil—carvole and carvene—have been shown to reduce muscle spasms in the digestive organs of lab animals. There is also some evidence carvole and carvene have antihistamine, antibacterial, and antifungal properties, but these effects have been demonstrated only in laboratory animals.

Other studies suggest that carvene may have cancer-fighting properties. When applied to the skin of laboratory mice, small tumors disappeared and new ones grew more slowly than the original ones. This has not been tested on humans, however.

Tea made from caraway seeds may prevent or treat iron-deficiency anemia. Laboratory studies have found that iron absorption is increased when research animals are fed caraway tea.

Forms and Usual Dosage

Caraway is available as a liquid extract, tincture, and essential oil, and the seeds themselves can be chewed whole or crushed to make infusions and teas. To make an infusion, use 1 to 2 teaspoons of freshly crushed seeds per cup of hot water. Let the infusion steep for ten to fifteen minutes, strain, and drink either before a meal (to stimulate appetite) or after eating (to aid digestion). Alternatively, three to four drops of liquid extract can be added to a cup of water. Or chew a teaspoon of the seeds three or four times per day. The tincture may be taken in doses of ½ to 1 teaspoon three times a day.

Potential Problems

Caraway seeds have been ingested by humans for centuries with no problem. However, people who are allergic to other members of the carrot family may also react to caraway.

CARDAMOM (*ELETTARIA CARDAMOMUM*)

Cardamom, a perennial that is native to India, is a tropical shrub that grows to some ten feet and has large leaves and white flowers with blue stripes and yellow borders. Its fruit is a small capsule that contains eight to sixteen seeds; the seeds are a distinctive spice that has been adopted by several different cuisines. They taste like a mild ginger and are often blended with cumin and coriander to season curries. Cardamom also combines well with orange, cinnamon, cloves, and caraway. The Scandinavians use cardamom to flavor pastries; it also enhances the flavor of squash, sweet potatoes, duck, pork, pickling brines, sweet and sour sauces, and coffee.

Medicinally, the seeds have been used by traditional Ayurvedic physicians in India to treat a number of disorders, ranging from digestive problems to asthma. In the West, cardamom is used mostly as a digestive aid.

A LITTLE HISTORY
Cardamom is one of the oldest spices used in India and the Middle East, as exemplified by the many references to it in *The Arabian Nights*. Sometimes called grains of paradise, cardamom was first used around the eighth century in India and was exported to Europe in the early thirteenth century. Today Bombay ships 250,000 pounds of seeds annually to London markets. The French use cardamom oil to make perfumes, and in many countries, it is a popular cooking spice.

Common Uses

- Aid digestion and relieve flatulence and constipation.
- Soothe a spastic colon.
- Sweeten bad breath.

How It Works

Cardamom seeds contain a volatile oil rich in mucilage and various resins, which are thought to aid digestion by stimulating the flow of various gastric juices. The resins also have antispasmodic properties that can help calm intestinal spasms and reduce bloating and gas.

Evidence of Efficacy

Most of the research on cardamom has been done in the laboratory and involves animals rather than humans. For example, researchers have shown that cardamom oil has strong antispasmodic effects on animal intestines, which would appear to support the traditional use in treating spastic colon, colic, and gas. German health authorities have approved the use of cardamom to treat indigestion.

Some preliminary studies cite cardamom as a potentially effective oil for fighting growth of cancer cells. As for its breath-sweetening powers, you can follow the Indian practice of chewing a few seeds after a meal and judge for yourself if it makes a difference.

Forms and Usual Dosage

Cardamom is available in many forms, including a tea or infusion made with crushed seeds, a tincture, and an essential oil, which is used in aromatherapy. Cardamom is also an ingredient in many commercial laxatives, digestive aids, and gas products. Most often, however, it is taken as seeds, which are chewed or crushed to make a tea. Use about fifteen to twenty seeds for every one-half cup of water. It can be used full-strength or diluted and sipped several times a day. Chewing on the seeds after a meal not only freshens breath but may also aid digestion.

Potential Problems

As with other essential oils, full-strength cardamom oil should not be ingested or applied to the skin; instead, it should be diluted with a neutral oil, such as vegetable oil. When used as a spice or as directed, cardamom poses no risk of toxicity; it has been used safely for centuries. However, when consumed in large amounts, it can cause watery diarrhea because of its laxative properties. Allergic skin reactions have been reported among some people exposed to large amounts of cardamom, such as workers in spice factories.

CASCARA SAGRADA (*RHAMNUS PURSHIANA*)

Cascara sagrada, also known as sacred or chittem bark, is a small tree that is valued for its medicinal bark, as is that of its European counterpart, the buckthorn tree. Once plentiful in mountainous areas of the Northwest, the number of cascara trees have been greatly reduced as a consequence of clear-cut logging. Although the tree still grows in the wild, it is also cultivated to provide the bark extract that is used in a number of commercial laxatives and herbal products.

Common Uses

Cascara sagrada bark is stripped from the tree in the spring and summer months and allowed to age for at least a year (ingesting extracts made from green bark can cause nausea and severe intestinal cramps). Extracts of the dried bark are then used mostly as a laxative although some herbalists also recommend it as a tonic for the digestive system and to treat liver and gallbladder disorders.

How It Works

Cascara sagrada is high in compounds called anthraquinone glycosides, which are rapidly broken down by intestinal bacteria. This action stimulates peristalsis, the rhythmic muscle contractions that move material through the digestive tract. In addition, another cascara glycoside derivative is absorbed into the circulation and stimulates the nerves that control the urge to defecate.

Evidence of Efficacy

The effectiveness of cascara sagrada as a laxative is well documented, both by a long history of successful use and by clinical studies. In fact, cascara sagrada is one of the most commonly used laxatives worldwide.

◉ **A LITTLE HISTORY**

For centuries, Native Americans have used cascara sagrada bark as a laxative and remedy for an upset stomach. The tree was dubbed "sacred bark" by early Spanish explorers who ventured into the Pacific Northwest and observed how the native peoples used the bark. Settlers in the area adopted the Native Americans' practice of soaking a piece of the cured bark overnight and drinking the "tea" in the morning as a general tonic.

It has been approved by the U.S. Food and Drug Administration and is also recommended by the German Commission E, the body that reviews and sets standards for natural products in that country.

Forms and Usual Dosage

Cascara sagrada is available in many forms—pill, capsule, liquid extract, powdered bark, and tincture. One popular method of taking cascara sagrada is to dissolve ½ teaspoon of the powdered bark or tincture in a glass of water or juice and drink it before going to bed, although some people prefer to take it in the early morning. Drink several glasses of water throughout the day.

Cascara sagrada has a very bitter taste, which can be masked by adding a little honey or drops of anise to the mixture. As noted, it is an ingredient in a number of commercial laxatives, and it is also included in many herbal combinations that are used as general tonics. Check the labels for ingredients and follow the product's dosage instructions.

Potential Problems

Cascara sagrada is considered one of the safest of the stimulant laxatives. Still, as with other stimulant laxatives, it should be taken for only a short time, certainly no more than a few days. Long-term use can result in a laxative habit, in which the colon becomes sluggish and unable to function normally. If chronic constipation is a problem, dietary changes (e.g., increasing intake of fluids and high-fiber foods) and increased exercise is usually all that is needed. Also, doctors usually recommend using a bulk-forming laxative, such as psyllium, before resorting to a stimulant laxative like cascara sagrada.

High doses of cascara sagrada can cause cramping and diarrhea. It should not be taken during pregnancy or by persons who have any type of intestinal obstruction or inflammatory bowel disease.

See Also

Constipation

CATNIP
(*NEPETA CATARIA*)

Catnip is a perennial and a member of the mint family; in fact, it is often called catmint. Like its botanical cousins, its leaves give off a pleasant, minty aroma when they are crushed. It is native to Europe and Asia, but has spread throughout North America and the rest of the world. Anyone who has ever grown even a single catnip plant can attest to its hardiness and tendency to spread to every part of a garden or yard.

The herb grows to a height of up to three feet and its leaves and flowers can be used fresh in salads or dried for their medicinal properties. While it is best known for inducing active euphoria in even the most docile of cats, it has the opposite effect on humans, who use it to calm jittery nerves and induce sleep, among other uses.

Common Uses

- Calm feelings of nervousness and help induce sleep.
- Ease coughs and other cold symptoms.
- Settle an upset stomach, promote digestion, and treat minor diarrhea.
- Alleviate menstrual and muscle cramps.
- Promote healing of minor cuts.
- Attract cats and repel cockroaches.

How It Works

The leaves contain a number of chemicals, including various acidic compounds, antioxidants, tannins, and volatile oils. Some of these compounds are known to have antispasmodic and astringent effects, which relax constricted muscles, reduce cramps, soothe intestinal passages, and calm coughs. Substances in catnip have a mild hormonal effect similar to that of estrogen, which may also help ease menstrual cramps. The aromatic oils stimulate the flow of gastric fluids and aid digestion; other ingredients appear to have calming effects on the central nervous system and also induce drowsiness.

Catnip leaves contain generous amounts of vitamins C and E and flavonoids, antioxidants that protect cells against the damage of unstable molecules (free radicals) that are released when the body burns oxygen. Antioxidants help lower the risk of cancer and slow the effects of aging. However, one would have to consume a lot of catnip to get enough of these nutrients to make an appreciable difference. Still, every little bit

◉ A LITTLE HISTORY

Catnip has been used for some two thousand years as a mild relaxant, a treatment for colds, stomachaches, and digestive ailments. Colonists brought it to the New World and it is mentioned in the writings of Washington Irving, Nathaniel Hawthorne, and Harriet Beecher Stowe.

Its effects on cats are well known, but for about 10 to 20 percent of cats, it has no effect. Those that do respond love to roll in it, chew the leaves, and play with toys stuffed with catnip. The effect is by no means limited to housecats—tigers, lions, leopards, and other "big cats" have similar responses, which last for about twenty minutes.

helps, and having a cup of catnip tea before retiring may produce benefits beyond simply falling asleep faster.

Catnip leaves have a mild antibiotic effect. Crushed leaves pressed against minor cuts and scrapes before bandaging them may protect against skin infection and promote healing. They may also be used to make a poultice.

Evidence of Efficacy

Most studies on the effects of catnip have been done on animals rather than humans. It is known that lactone, nepetalactone, and the alkaloid actinidine produce the so-called catnip response in cats. These compounds are also found in other herbs, such as valerian, and cats have a similar euphoric response to these plants. However, these substances are not stimultants and mood-elevators for humans. Instead, something in catnip has the opposite effect in humans—calming rather than stimulating or intoxicating.

Forms and Usual Dosage

Catnip is available in bulk as dried leaves and flowers, in capsules, liquid extracts, tinctures, and as an essential oil. Catnip is usually consumed as a tea by steeping an ounce of dried leaves in a pint of hot water for ten to fifteen minutes. This tea is said to soothe upset stomachs and have an overall calming effect on the digestive and nervous systems. Catnip is sometimes mixed with boneset, elder, yarrow, or cayenne as a treatment for colds. A very weak form of the tea may be given to babies to relieve gas and symptoms of colic, although this should be done only after consulting your child's doctor.

The essential oil of catnip is used in aromatherapy. Adding a few drops to bathwater or massaging the diluted oil into the skin has a calming effect. The dried leaves may be used to make a catnip pillow that can be slipped into a pillowcase to help promote sleep.

Potential Problems

Catnip is considered safe and nontoxic in humans when taken in the recommended dosages. In very high doses, however, it may depress the central nervous system. It should not be taken with alcohol or medications, such as sleeping pills, that have a similar effect. Because of its possible hormonal effects, catnip should not be taken during pregnancy. Long-term use of catnip may interfere with the absorption of iron and other minerals.

CAT'S CLAW (*UNCARIA TOMENTOSA*)

Cat's claw, a twining woody vine, is a native of South America. Its Spanish name, *uña de gato,* is derived from the fact that its hook has a curvature resembling a cat's claw. It is also called samento and life-giving vine of Peru. Although there are other varieties of cat's claw, only *Uncaria tomentosa,* the species native to Peru, has been shown to have medicinal qualities. However, the *U. tomentosa* species is now cultivated elsewhere, especially in Austria, where it has been extensively studied for more than twenty-five years. The inner bark and root of the plant are used medicinally.

Common Uses

- Boosting the immune system to fight infections, cancer, HIV infection, and allergies.
- Alleviating gastrointestinal symptoms, such as those arising from ulcers, gastritis, and hemorrhoids.
- Healing skin wounds.

In addition, cat's claw has been used in traditional Peruvian medicine for such disorders as:

- Asthma.
- Cancer.
- Inflammatory disorders such as arthritis.
- Bacterial, viral, and yeast infections.

How It Works

The biochemical activity of cat's claw depends on the environment, and soil conditions where it is grown. The preparations believed to boost immune-system activity are high in pentacyclic alkaloids and low in tetracyclic alkaloids. Indeed, the pentacyclic alkaloids seem to be responsible for its medicinal effects, and they are blocked by the tetracyclic alkaloids.

In laboratory research, the pentacyclic alkaloids appear to have a powerful effect on the process by which certain white blood cells engulf and destroy foreign particles (phagocytosis). This effect would, in theory, support the use of cat's claw to treat bacterial and viral infections as well as prevent or slow the progression of cancer. Researchers are also ex-

amining the potential anti-inflammatory and antiviral properties of qui-
novic acid glycoside, a nonalkaloid compound in cat's claw that has
never been found in nature before.

Evidence of Efficacy

Despite a wide range of anecdotal reports of cat's claw's benefits in
diverse conditions, little actual clinical testing has been done to support
such claims. In infectious disease, some reports suggest that it decreases
the risk of colds and flu in people who tend to have recurrent infections,
such as the elderly. There have also been reports that some patients
infected with HIV, the virus that causes AIDS, had increases in levels
of helper T cells and reduced viral loads, as well as increased vitality, a
better tolerance of anti-HIV drug therapy, and fewer opportunistic infections. Austrian physicians have reported that some cancer patients
have an improved ability to tolerate radiation and chemotherapy, including less nausea and a reduced susceptibility to infection.

Forms and Usual Dosage

Capsules, tablets, and liquid extracts and decoctions are available. Practitioners usually recommend one or two 500-mg capsules three times a
day.

Potential Problems

Cat's claw is generally regarded as safe, but an absence of toxicity has
only been well-documented in animals. However, because its effects
during pregnancy and breast-feeding have not been well studied, it
should not be taken by women who are planning a pregnancy, who are
pregnant, or who are breast-feeding. One researcher recommends avoidance by those taking ulcer medications.

Further, it should be avoided in people having organ transplants
because it may enhance immune function and lead to serious organ
rejection disease. For the same reason, its use may be risky in autoimmune diseases, possibly leading to flare-up, and in those with allergies,
which are disorders involving overactive immune reactions. Thus contradictory evidence that it has offered some benefit to people with
asthma, hay fever, and rheumatoid arthritis raises serious questions.
Nonetheless, for example, in a twenty-four-week study, seventeen of
eighteen rheumatoid arthritis patients who were given one Austrian
product made from cat's claw had a decrease in joint pain, compared to
ten of seventeen who received placebo.

In addition, in view of the seriousness of some of the diseases for which cat's claw claims are made, such as cancer and AIDS, it should only be considered as a supportive—not a primary—therapy for these illnesses. So far, cat's claw does not appear to interfere with the action of chemotherapy agents or radiation.

CAYENNE
(*CAPSICUM ANNUUM*)

Depending upon where it's grown, *Capsicum annuum* is called African, bird, chili, Hungarian, sweet, or zanzibar pepper. These various varieties are closely related to bell peppers, jalapeños, paprika, and other familiar peppers.

Cayenne plants originally grew only in Mexico and Central America, where they are perennials, but they are now grown as annuals in warm areas all over the world. The plants grow to three feet or more, with woody stems and green leaves. They have droopy white to yellow flowers. The fruits (also known as the berries) of these plants are peppers, used as food and medicine around the world. Peppers are a many-seeded pod with a leathery outside. They grow in various shades of red and yellow.

Capsaicin is the resinous, pungent substance in hot peppers that make them hot, yielding a burning sensation in the mouth when eaten. It stimulates the oral nerve endings, fooling your brain into thinking you're in pain. The brain responds by releasing substances called endorphins, which are similar in structure to morphine. A mild euphoria results, and chilies can be mildly addictive because of this hot pepper "high."

Common Uses

External preparations containing capsaicin are used to:

- Reduce arthritis pain and inflammation and relieve symptoms of bursitis, fibromyalgia, diabetic neuropathy, and the nerve pain that often follows shingles (post-herpetic neuralgia).
- Treat the skin rash and pain of psoriasis.
- Treat other nerve pain syndromes, including the severe facial pain of trigeminal neuralgia.

In addition, ingested capsaicin may be used to ease the pain and speed healing of ulcers. Cayenne and other peppers have a long history of folk medicine use as digestive aids in many parts of the world. It was considered helpful for various conditions of the gastrointestinal tract, in-

◉ A LITTLE HISTORY
In the early 1900s, a pharmacist named Wilbur Scoville developed a system for scoring the capsaicinoid content of hot peppers. Although Scoville units are still a recognized measurement of capsaicin level, many food writers use a new system called the Official Chili Heat Scale, with a rating of 1 to 10. Although peppers vary plant to plant, in general, following is an approximate scale for common varieties.

Chili Heat Scale	Scoville Units	Type
0	<100	Mild bells, pimento
1	100–500	Mexi-bells
2	500–1,000	Anaheim, big Jim
3	1,000–1,500	Ancho
4	1,500–2,500	Cascabel
5	2,500–5,000	Jalapeno, mirasol
6	5,000–15,000	Serrano
7	15,000–30,000	Chile de arbol
8	30,000–50,000	Aji, cayenne, tabasco
9	50,000–100,000	Santaka, chiltepin, Thai
10	100,000–350,000	Habanero, Scotch bonnet
	16,000,000	Pure capsaicin (only found in a laboratory)

cluding stomachaches, cramping pains, and gas. However, cayenne has entered conventional medical practice in recent years due to its external benefits as a topical remedy for arthritis pain.

How It Works

Initially, it was thought the pain-relieving benefits of cayenne arose solely from a counterirritant effect. A counterirritant is something that causes irritation to a tissue to which it is applied, thus distracting from the original irritation (such as joint pain). They send high levels of messages out, overwhelming the nerves' ability to communicate pain to the brain. They temporarily stimulate release of various neurotransmitters from local nerves, leading to neurotransmitter depletion. Without the neurotransmitters, pain signals can no longer be sent. Indeed, this is the way most topical creams used for arthritis work.

But capsaicin does more; it also neutralizes substance P, an inflammatory chemical involved in inflammation in the fluid that bathes the joints. Substance P is believed to be the primary chemical mediator of pain impulses from the periphery to the brain. The substance also has been shown to activate inflammatory mediators in psoriasis.

Evidence of Efficacy

Numerous studies support the pain-relieving benefits of capsaicin when applied externally. One double-blind, controlled study found that a capsaicin cream reduced osteoarthritis pain and tenderness by 40 percent. A study of diabetic neuropathy patients demonstrated a reduction of nerve pain, tingling, or numbness in 70 percent of patients. A study of patients with fibromyalgia reported less tenderness in trigger points and improved grip strength. A study of people with severe post-herpetic neuralgia—the painful condition that can follow shingles—yielded good to excellent relief in more than half of the patients who completed the study.

Research also supports benefits in psoriasis. In one study, ninety-eight patients applied a 0.025 percent capsaicin cream to psoriatic lesions four times a day for six weeks, while ninety-nine patients used a placebo cream. Those using the active ingredient had a significantly greater relief of itching as well as a reduction in psoriasis scaling, redness, and the thickness of the lesions.

There is no scientific evidence that cayenne pepper taken internally can help heart disease, as has been promoted by some people, but some research suggests that it can help heal ulcers and may protect the stomach against damage caused by anti-inflammatory drugs. Its local anesthetic effect has already been well demonstrated. It also brings blood to the surface of the tissue, which may ease healing.

Forms and Usual Dosages

Capsaicin creams are approved over-the-counter drugs and should be used as directed on the tube. Creams containing 0.025 to 0.075 percent capsaicin are generally available. Depending on the concentration, you must apply it two to four times a day and you should use it for at least a week to obtain pain relief. If you don't notice an improvement within a few weeks—or if you feel worse at any time, as happens to some people with rheumatoid arthritis—stop using it.

For internal use, a red pepper tea can be made by steeping ¼ teaspoon of cayenne pepper in a cup of hot water; sip it several times a day. Or one to two standard cayenne gelatin capsules can be taken one to three times daily, or a cayenne tincture can be used in the amount of 0.3 to 1 ml three times daily.

Potential Problems

Capsaicin should be handled carefully because some people are very sensitive to it. So test it on a small area of skin for a few days before using it on a large area. If you develop skin irritation, stop using it.

However, it's normal to experience a local burning sensation when you apply it to the skin. If you use it regularly, this usually disappears within a week.

After you rub it on, you should wash your hands carefully and thoroughly, or use gloves to apply it. If you don't, and then touch your eyes, genital tissue, or other delicate mucous membranes, you get that same burning pain that hits if you cut up hot peppers (the source of capsaicin) and then touch tender spots. So be sure to prevent the cream from accidentally reaching the eyes, nose, or mouth. (Another option is to purchase a brand that comes in an applicator bottle, which permits application of a thin layer—without your hands ever touching the medication.)

Do not apply the cream to areas of broken skin or to any rash other than diagnosed psoriasis. Also, do not use a heating pad on skin that has recently had an application of capsaicin cream. If you are taking the asthma drug theophylline, talk with your doctor before using cayenne because it might increase the amount you absorb, possibly leading to toxic levels.

See Also

Arthritis
Psoriasis

CHAMOMILE (*MATRICARIA CHAMOMILLA, M. RECUTITA, CHAMOMILLA RECUTITA*)

■ A LITTLE HISTORY

Women have used chamomile cosmetically for at least two thousand years. Hieroglyphic records show that Egyptian noblewomen used preparations of crushed petals on their skin. In more modern times, women who would like to lighten their hair without using harsh hair bleaches and dyes often turn to chamomile hair rinses as a gentler alternative. To give your hair blond highlights or to lighten it one or two shades, try this: Brew a strong cup of chamomile tea, and use it as a final rinse after shampooing. Do not rinse out the tea; instead, towel dry and then expose the hair to the sun for a few minutes.

The type of chamomile most widely available and used for medicinal purposes is the German or Hungarian variety, which is also known as genuine or true chamomile and pinheads. (It is biochemically distinct from Roman or English chamomile, chemically known as *Chamaemelum nobile.*)

Chamomile is a flowering plant with a branched stem and white flowers with yellow centers, similar in appearance to its cousin the daisy. Although native to Europe and northwest Asia, it has been cultivated in North America and other areas. True chamomile is differentiated from other types by the fact that the receptacle under the head of the flower is hollow. It is primarily the dried flower that is used medicinally.

Common Uses

- Speed healing of burns, cuts, scrapes, and other skin wounds.
- Reduce rashes and other skin inflammations.
- Promote relaxation and reduce anxiety.
- Treat insomnia, especially in children.
- Ease coughs and fevers due to colds and bronchitis.

How It Works

Chamomile has long been a folk remedy for such diverse problems as digestive disorders, colds, fever, menstrual discomfort, insomnia, and anxiety. However, it is most widely recognized for its cosmetic and healing benefits when used topically on the skin. The active ingredients in chamomile appear to be flavonoids, such as apigenin, and essential oils, such as levomenol (also known as bisabolol) and azulene (chamazulene). Both flavonoids and the essential oils have been shown to reduce inflammation and encourage wound healing. The antioxidant benefits of flavonoids also may protect the skin from UV radiation.

Apigenin may also be responsible for chamomile's anti-anxiety and

414   NUTRACEUTICALS

sedative effects, via action on receptors in the brain that are also affected by benzodiazepines such as Valium. Further, the anti-inflammatory effects of the flavonoids and the anti-inflammatory and anti-spasmodic benefits of the essential oils may contribute to chamomile's reputation for easing gastrointestinal inflammation and spasms. Levomenol can improve the texture of the skin, reducing fine lines caused by pollution, stress, and the sun.

Evidence of Efficacy

Numerous laboratory and animal studies have documented the anti-inflammatory and anti-spasmodic effects of chamomile, as well as its ability to reduce fever and prevent and heal gastric ulcers. German health authorities recommend chamomile tea and other preparations for peptic ulcers, gastrointestinal spasm, and inflammatory diseases such as arthritis. Although such antispasmodic activity may account for its reputation as a calmative, no clinical support for this benefit can be found.

Studies also suggest that chamomile may fight such infectious organisms as *Staphylococcus aureus* bacteria and *Candida albicans* fungi which, together with the anti-inflammatory properties, may play a role in wound healing. Again, although most studies have been in animals, a small double-blind study in humans found that chamomile significantly decreased the surface areas of wounds and helped them to dry, and another supported benefits for healing eczema. These studies and related research encouraged German health authorities to approve of chamomile for bacterial skin diseases and as a mouthwash for inflammatory mouth and gum problems.

Forms and Usual Dosages

A variety of creams and ointments containing 3 to 10 percent chamomile can be used on the skin, and bath salts and powders are also available. Or a poultice can be made by pouring one and a half cups of hot water over 2 teaspoons of dried chamomile flowers and allowing them to steep for fifteen minutes before draining. For a gargle, ten drops of fluid extract can be dissolved in a glass of water. For internal use, chamomile is available as a tea, as a liquid tincture or infusion, and in tablets or capsules. However, because the essential oil that is believed to be the active ingredient is not very water-soluble, only a small amount of it is released into the liquid when teas are prepared. Thus formulations containing whole flower heads (avoiding powdered formulations or those containing stems and other plant parts) should be purchased from reputable sources to help assure the highest potency. A tea can be made using 2 to 3 teaspoons of dried flowers per cup of water. Generally, 1 teaspoon of dried flowers equals 1 g of drug. For internal use, practitioners generally recommend 10 to 15 g of chamomile.

Potential Problems

With their long history of use, chamomile products are considered so safe that they can be used in children as well as by women who are pregnant or breast-feeding. Only a few cautions are known. First, chamomile-based skin creams should not come in contact with the eyes. Second, because it is possible that people who have allergies to other herbs in the daisy and aster family also might be allergic to chamomile, those with hay fever, ragweed, and other pollen allergies should use them with caution. Allergic sensitivity problems may not appear initially but build with continued use over extended periods. Finally, eating large amounts of the dried flowers may cause vomiting.

See Also

Heartburn
Mouth Sores
Psoriasis
Tooth Decay and Gum Disease

CHASTE BERRY (*VITEX AGNUS-CASTUS*)

The chaste tree, also called vitex, Agnus-castus, and monk's pepper, is a shrub that grows in Central Asia and the Mediterranean countries. Its reddish-black berries, which are about the size of peppercorns, have been used since ancient Greek times to the present for a variety of "female complaints." Ancient physicians used it to stop hemorrhages following childbirth. In the 1930s, Agnolyt, a patented medicine made from chaste berries, was widely used to treat a purported "imbalance of the female hormones." From the 1950s to the present, European physicians have recommended dried chaste berries for irregular menstrual periods, heavy periods (menorrhagia), and especially to ease symptoms of premenstrual syndrome.

◙ A LITTLE HISTORY

The chaste tree derives its name from the belief that its fruit fostered chastity by suppressing sexual desire. Medieval monks chewed on chaste berries to temper their libidos and make maintaining their vows of chastity easier. Likewise, in ancient Rome, wives whose husbands were off fighting wars used the herb to keep their sexual desires in line. But, chaste berry was also considered an aphrodisiac. The true effect may not be at these extremes but as a "normalizer" of sexual drive.

Common Uses

- Menstrual problems, including irregular periods, heavy bleeding, and cramps.
- PMS symptoms, including breast tenderness and sensitivity, irritability, bloating, depression, and mood swings.

- Regulation of ovulation after stopping the mini (progesterone-only) oral contraceptive.
- Endometriosis.
- Uterine fibroid growths.
- Menopausal symptoms such as hot flashes and night sweats.
- Acne related to hormonal imbalances

How It Works

Although its actions are largely hormonal, the chaste tree berry contains no hormones. But its active ingredients, including agnuside, are thought to work on the pituitary gland to stimulate production of luteinizing hormone (LH), which in turn increases production of progesterone and helps regulate the menstrual cycle. It also inhibits excessive production of prolactin, the hormone that regulates breast milk production.

Women with PMS usually get some relief within two or three menstrual cycles after beginning daily use of the herb, and more improvement may occur over subsequent months. It may take as long as six months of daily use for absent menstrual periods to return, and even longer to have an impact on infertility.

Evidence of Efficacy

European studies support the effectiveness of the chaste berry preparation used to make Agnolyt in treating PMS symptoms. There have been reports of up to 90 percent of women obtaining at least some relief of symptoms. It appears to be most effective in women with mild to moderately low progesterone levels.

Forms and Usual Dosages

Dried berries may be used to make a tea—1 teaspoon per cup—that can be taken three times a day. Forty drops of the tincture or 225 mg in a powder, tablet, or capsule, twice a day is commonly recommended to treat PMS and menstrual irregularity.

Potential Problems

Since chaste berry affects female hormones, it should not be taken along with other endocrine therapies or hormonal medication, such as birth control pills or estrogen replacement therapy. It should not be taken during pregnancy or breast-feeding. It is also contraindicated for women who are also taking dopamine-receptor antagonists, since the herb may interfere with the drug's effects.

There have been reports of chaste berry causing mild intestinal upset and an itchy skin rash. If stomach irritation is a problem, avoid taking it on an empty stomach and divide the dosage in half, taking some after breakfast and again after lunch. Stop the herb if a rash or other signs of an allergic reaction develop.

See Also

Breast Disorders (Benign)
Endometriosis
Infertility
Menopause
Premenstrual Syndrome

CHINESE CUCUMBER (*TRICHOSANTHES KIRILOWII*)

◉ A LITTLE HISTORY

Although virtually unknown in Western botanical medicine until recently, Chinese cucumber has a long history in traditional Chinese medicine. It is used for its cooling properties and used to treat "hot" diseases, such as those that produce fevers, to restore a healthy balance of the opposing life forces, yin and yang. It is also said to unbind qi, the essential life energy, in the chest and loosen sputum to make it easier to cough up. It also is said to moisten the intestinal tract and relieve dry constipation.

Chinese cucumber, also known as snakegourd, is a perennial and a member of the gourd family that grows only in China, hence its common name. While many of the seven hundred or so species of gourds found worldwide produce fleshy, seed-filled fruits (e.g., pumpkins, squashes, and melons), Chinese cucumber is a tropical species that has a larger, hard-shelled fruit. Although it is inedible, the Chinese cucumber is one of a group of gourds thought to have important medicinal properties. In fact, recent studies indicate that Chinese cucumber may be useful in fighting HIV, the virus that causes AIDS.

Common Uses

In traditional Chinese medicine, it is used to:

- Remove pus from boils and abscesses.
- Relieve dryness by stimulating production of body fluids.
- Reduce airway congestion.

How It Works

Western herbalists have only limited experience with Chinese cucumber, so not much is known about how it works. Chinese medical texts recommend it for its antibiotic, expectorant, laxative, and anti-inflammatory properties, and as a general tonic. It contains various sterols, saponins, fatty acids, and other compounds that may have medicinal properties. However, researchers in the United States and elsewhere have been studying a refined protein called trichonanthine, which is derived from Chinese cucumber and closely related members of the *Trichosanthes* genus. This protein appears to destroy an HIV-infected cell without affecting the surrounding healthy tissue.

Evidence of Efficacy

A group of New York University researchers have isolated a protein (trichonanthine) from Chinese cucumber that appears to inhibit HIV-1, the virus that causes most AIDS cases in the United States and other Western countries. This protein is the basis of an experimental HIV drug known as TAP29 or Compound Q. More research is needed, however, before it can be determined whether Compound Q will be an effective treatment for HIV.

Forms and Usual Dosage

Chinese cucumber is available as an extract in some Asian herbal outlets; it is also included in some Chinese herbal combinations. Follow label instructions for dosages.

Potential Problems

Some gourds are considered poisonous and should be avoided. Chinese cucumber appears to be safe, but should not be taken if it causes diarrhea or other intestinal problems. Japanese researchers have discovered a substance in Chinese cucumber that appears to cause spontaneous abortions (an abortifacient), so it should never be taken during pregnancy.

CINNAMON (CINNAMOMUM ZEYLANICUM/CASSIA)

Mentioned in the Bible and in Sanskrit writings, cinnamon is one of the world's oldest known spices. The spice itself is in the bark of an

Described in Chinese herbal texts as early as
2700 B.C., cinnamon was also an ingredient in
ancient Egyptian embalming mixtures and was
used by Moses as an anointing oil. It was so
highly prized that even after the fall of Rome,
when trade between Europe and Asia was difficult, cinnamon still found its way to the West.

evergreen laurel tree native to Sri Lanka; the tree bark is rolled into
sticks or ground into powder. "True cinnamon" comes from the *Cin-
namomum zeylanicum* tree; common cinnamon, the kind used in the
United States, comes from the *C. cassia* tree. There are many other varieties of cinnamon. Regardless of the specific variety, the tree's bark,
along with the leaves and roots, produces essential oils, extracted
through steam distillation, that are used not only to scent and flavor
incense and perfumes, but also in tonics, antiseptics, and remedies for
intestinal gas, nausea, colds, and high blood pressure.

Common Uses

- Relieve upset stomach and gas, diarrhea, and various other ail-
  ments.
- Stimulate appetite and enhance digestion.
- Reduce pain of minor cuts and abrasions.

How It Works

All types of cinnamon aid digestion in several ways. Cinnamon's entic-
ing aroma stimulates salivation; its volatile oils break down fats in the
digestive tract. The essential oils have been found to stimulate movement in the gastrointestinal tract. The bark of both cinnamon and cassia
has carminative (gas-reducing) and astringent properties. Cinnamon is
often used as a flavoring in toothpaste, not only because of its refreshing
taste but also because its antiseptic properties helps kill the bacteria that
cause tooth decay and gum disease.

Evidence of Efficacy

Research in lab rats has shown that the cassia variety may stimulate bile
production and it has demonstrated antidiarrheal properties in the test
tube. One study showed that cassia tea helped protect against ulcers in
rats and mice. It is not clear whether these findings relate to humans.
The essential oils have been shown to contain a substance that fights
and kills disease-causing microbes and fungi. According to one German
study, cinnamon suppresses the bacteria (*Escherichia coli*) that commonly
cause urinary tract infections and the fungus responsible for vaginal yeast
infections (*Candida albicans*). Researchers at Kent State University
showed that adding one part cinnamon to one thousand parts apple cider
can kill 90 percent or more of the *E. coli* bacteria, a potentially deadly
organism that is sometimes found in unpasteurized apple juice.

Cinnamon may also be beneficial to people with type 2 (adult-onset
or non-insulin-dependent) diabetes by reducing the amount of insulin

necessary to metabolize glucose. Researchers have found that ⅛ of a teaspoon of cinnamon can triple insulin efficiency.

A chemical called eugenol, found in the oils of cloves, allspice, and cinnamon bark (but not cassia bark), has topical anesthetic properties, probably the reason that cinnamon was once used as a painkiller for skin wounds. One Japanese study using animals shows cinnamon may help prevent ulcers.

Forms and Usual Dosage

Cinnamon is available as an essential oil, a powder, a tincture, and a dried herb from which to make tea. The essential oil is very strong (6 g of the oil is enough to kill a medium-sized dog in five hours) and it must be diluted in a neutral oil before it is used. Topically; it should not be ingested. Cassia, whether in oil or powder form, is half the strength of cinnamon (1 to 2 percent volatile oil compared to 4 percent), much more abundant and less expensive, and is the only form of the herb used in the United States. Again, the volatile oil should be diluted and used topically. A tea can be made by stirring ½ to ¾ teaspoon of powdered cinnamon in a cup of boiling water; up to three cups a day may be consumed to treat menstrual cramps and intestinal upsets, such as indigestion, gas, bloating, and other digestive problems.

Potential Problems

Powdered forms of cinnamon are nontoxic, but may cause allergic reactions in susceptible people. Cinnamon oil, however, may burn and cause redness on contact with skin. Taken internally, it can cause nausea, vomiting, and kidney damage.

See Also

Nausea

CLEAVERS (*GALIUM APARINE*)

Many of the popular names for this trailing weed—grip grass, catchweed, everlasting friendship, goosegrass, and, of course, cleavers—refers

Although farmers generally consider cleavers a noxious weed that crowds out crops, people in times past found many ways to use cleavers. Greek shepherds fashioned sieves from its vinelike stems, and in some areas of Sweden, some dairy farmers still strain milk through cleaver sieves. English poultry growers actually encouraged its growth because it was such a favorite food of geese. In fact, cleavers is still called goosegrass in England.

to its tendency to cling to anything that brushes against it with its Velcro-like bristles. Although livestock and birds relish its bitter flavor, cleavers are considered invasive weeds throughout North America because they have taken over farmers' fields, with each plant producing some 3,500 seeds and often getting a jump on planting season because of its ability to withstand cold winters.

Herbalists and homeopaths value all parts of the plant, from its roots to its seeds (which, when dried and roasted, make a passable coffee substitute). The plant can also be cooked and eaten as a vegetable.

Common Uses

- Rid the body of excess fluids.
- Treat mild constipation.
- Soothe inflammatory skin disorders, including sunburn, blisters, psoriasis, and eczema.
- May reduce discomfort associated with fibrocystic breasts.
- Help induce sleep.

How It Works

Cleavers has mild diuretic properties, probably from substances called iridoid glycosides. It helps reduce swelling from a buildup of body fluids and may reduce the discomfort of fibrocystic breasts and bloating during a woman's premenstrual phase. Because it promotes the flow of urine, it may be helpful in the treatment of cystitis, and other mild urinary tract conditions, but it should be avoided by anyone with chronic renal failure and other serious kidney disorders.

The plant's tannins give it astringent properties that may aid in the treatment of sunburn, psoriasis, eczema, and other skin inflammations. Cleavers powder or a poultice applied to the skin has been found to promote healing of minor skin wounds.

Evidence of Efficacy

There is very little actual data to support the traditional uses of cleavers. Tannins, with their astringent properties, are present in the plant in concentrations of 2.5 to 4 percent, and may explain why herbalists have traditionally relied on them to treat skin inflammation. Glycosides are present, explaining its diuretic and laxative action. Studies have shown that cleavers can kill the staph bacteria that sometimes cause skin infections, indicating that the plant also has antibacterial properties.

Forms and Usual Dosages

For internal use, cleavers is available as an infusion, a juice, or a tincture. For external use, the dried herb can be made into a compress or poultice, a powder, or used in a cream form.

To make a tea or infusion, steep 1 ounce, or about 1 tablespoon, of dried leaves in a pint of hot water and sip it during the day. The recommended dosage for cleavers juice calls for drinking up to 3 ounces twice a day. The tincture is taken in 5- to 10-ml doses three times a day.

Potential Problems

Cleavers should not be used by anyone with serious kidney problems, as its ability to increase urine output might irritate the renal system. Other than that caution, there are no known problems using cleavers at the recommended dosages.

CLOVES (*SYZGIUM AROMATICUM*)

The strong, pleasant aroma and the hot, pungent taste of cloves are distinctive features of this highly valued spice—they have set the mood at holiday parties and flavored everything from curry, pumpkin pie, and gingerbread to mulled wine for centuries. Cloves are the flower buds of a tropical evergreen tree believed to be indigenous to the Moluccas (Spice Islands) and now also grown on the island of Zanzibar as well as Madagascar and Indonesia. Cloves get their name from the French word *clou,* meaning nail; anyone who has ever stuck cloves into lemons or oranges to make pomander balls during the holiday season will know why. The buds contain essential oils (as do, to a lesser extent, the stems and leaves) that are as highly valued for their medicinal properties as they are for their flavor and distinctive aroma.

A LITTLE HISTORY

As early as 266 B.C., Chinese officials chewed cloves to sweeten their breath before audiences with the emperor. In the Middle Ages, Europeans wore necklaces made with cloves to ward off the plague. In the eighteenth century, the Dutch had a monopoly on the clove trade and the French smuggled it from the East Indies to islands they ruled in the Indian Ocean and the New World.

Common Uses

- Ease pain of a toothache and minor mouth irritations.
- Soothe a sore throat.
- Sweeten bad breath.
- Calm upset stomach.

- Treat mild skin infections, such as athlete's foot.
- Repel insects.

How It Works

The essential oil of cloves is rich in eugenol, which gives the spice its pungency and aroma. It is extracted by steam distillation and has numerous uses, as everything from a preservative on microscope slides, a topical anesthetic, a gargle and mouthwash, and a mild germicide to an ingredient in perfumes and aftershave lotions. When added to mouthwash and toothpaste, it not only gives them a refreshing flavor, but it also acts as a mild germicide to kill the oral bacteria that cause gum disease. As a gargle, diluted oil of cloves soothes inflamed tissue and may help overcome infection.

Dentists once relieved the pain of toothache by putting cotton saturated with clove oil directly on the tooth. Today they use it to prepare dental cements, fillings, and dry sockets. Sucking on cloves is said to reduce temporarily the craving for alcohol; smoking them likewise is said to aid tobacco smokers in kicking the nicotine habit; however, this can be a risky practice (see Potential Problems, below.)

Tea made from a few drops of clove oil is widely regarded as effective in relieving nausea. It is also a time-honored remedy for traveler's diarrhea. Clove oil is also used in aromatherapy to calm digestive tract upsets, including stomachache and flatulence. It also helps repel biting insects by masking the aroma of human flesh, which attracts mosquitoes and other pests.

Evidence of Efficacy

In the test tube, scientists have proved that eugenol kills certain bacteria that cause skin infections, as well as fungi that cause skin and vaginal yeast infections, viruses, larvae, and parasites. They have noted eugenol's ability to block sensory receptors that are instrumental in perceiving pain. No controlled trials have been performed on humans to test these properties, although the oil has withstood the test of time when put to these uses, with no ill effect.

Researchers are delving into other properties of cloves, such as their cancer-fighting potential, because they contain antioxidants, known to prevent the formation of free radicals, or chemicals in the body that have the potential to damage cells. The oil also seems to reduce blood clotting in laboratory animals by boosting the blood's antiplatelet properties.

Forms and Usual Dosage

Cloves are available as a potent oil, as a food spice either whole or powdered, in mouthwash and toothpaste, in teabags, and as cigarettes.

To make tea, a few drops of oil can be added to a cup of boiling water. In mouthwashes, the oil is used in concentrations of between 10 and 15 percent. For toothache, the oil can be applied directly to the tooth with a clean cloth, but care is needed because full-strength oil can damage delicate mucous membranes (see below). The full-strength oil should not be swallowed.

Potential Problems

Pure clove oil can burn tender skin tissue and mucous membranes. When applying it directly to a painful tooth, do not allow it to come into contact with surrounding mouth tissue. Although cloves have been used for centuries with no serious illnesses reported, too much of the oil in too concentrated a form can cause serious stomach upset. Teething infants and children are particularly vulnerable to the effects of excessive cloves, which may cause nervous and blood problems. Some people may be allergic to clove oil; sensitivity tests on a patch of skin are recommended. Health organizations, notably the American Lung Association, warn of the danger of smoking cloves to kick the nicotine habit. The smoke from cloves contains more cancer-causing substances than unadulterated tobacco smoke, but fewer than commercial cigarettes. It also numbs the smokers' throats, causing them to inhale more deeply than they would with tobacco cigarettes. Toxic lung reactions, such as coughing up sputum tainted with blood, have been reported by those who smoked clove cigarettes.

COMFREY (*SYMPHYTUM OFFICINALE*)

Comfrey is a hardy, leafy perennial that grows to about three to five feet. Native to Europe and Asia, it is now cultivated worldwide. Its rhizomes contain a gummy substance that gives the herb its nickname: slippery root. Traditionally, comfrey has been used by herbalists as a great healer until recent studies showed that, when taken internally, it can cause severe liver damage and may even induce cancer. Even so, when used externally, comfrey leaves are useful in healing stubborn skin ulcers, bedsores, and other lesions.

Common Uses

Note: Comfrey is for external use only, and should not be ingested in any form.

- Promote healing of minor burns and skin wounds or lesions, including bedsores, bruises, eczema, and psoriasis.
- Soothe bee stings and help heal spider bites, including those of the brown recluse spider.
- Treat skin infections, including those caused by staph bacteria.
- May have antifungal properties that are effective against athlete's foot.

How It Works

The active ingredients in comfrey are allantoin, a substance that fosters the growth of new cells; rosmarinic acid, which is an anti-inflammatory; and mucilage, a gummy substance that can soothe inflamed tissue. Unfortunately, comfrey also contains toxic substances called pyrrolizidine alkaloids (PAs), which can damage the liver and may promote cancer development.

Comfrey roots contain about twice as much allantoin as the dried leaves. Comfrey compounds are often added to creams or salves, sometimes in combination with arnica, witch hazel, calendula, and other herbs, and applied topically to promote healing of skin wounds and infections. Fresh leaves crushed in a blender and applied directly to the skin also promote regeneration of abraded tissue, help control infection, and promote healing. A soothing solution can be made from leaves that are steeped in hot water, although allantoin's effectiveness is lessened by heat.

Evidence of Efficacy

The healing properties of comfrey have been known to herbalists and farmers for centuries. Salves made from comfrey leaves applied to the skin abrasions of humans and farm animals reduced infection and allowed the skin to regenerate much more quickly than if left untreated. The thick sticky substance found in the roots was once thought to knit broken bones back together and heal open wounds. Although no longer used to heal broken bones, comfrey is still used to disinfect and heal skin wounds and to treat stubborn cases of eczema, psoriasis, and bedsores.

Forms and Usual Dosage

Comfrey leaves are dried, then ground up (their healing compounds are stable) and mixed with water, a moisturizing oil, or aloe vera to form

◉ A LITTLE HISTORY

Comfrey has been used as a healing herb at least since 400 B.C. Early Greek physicians used it to stop bleeding, treat bronchial problems, heal wounds, and mend broken bones. During the Irish potato famine of the 1840s, an Englishman named Henry Doubleday became convinced that the world could be saved from hunger and suffering by using comfrey. He established a charitable organization to research the cultivation and use of comfrey that exists to this day and continues to publish pamphlets and books on the uses of comfrey. Recent history has suggested, based on well-documented studies, that internal use of comfrey may be carcinogenic, although its benefits when used topically are well documented.

salves or pastes that are applied externally to the skin to promote healing and reduce inflammation and infection. A poultice can be made from fresh chopped leaves, applied directly to the wound and covered lightly with a bandage. It should be changed every day, the wound cleansed with water and a mild soap, and hydrogen peroxide applied if any infection is present. Pharmacists may add allantoin, the active ingredient in comfrey, to ointments and creams to enhance skin-healing properties. Extract of comfrey has many of the same properties. A lotion or solution of comfrey leaves, made from soaking them in hot (not boiling) water, may be applied to skin abrasions to soothe the irritation. Dried roots may be ground up and dissolved in hot water to form a mucilage that can bind together open skin ulcers, such as bedsores, that have resisted healing. It also smoothes the skin and is used in cosmetics for that purpose.

Potential Problems

There have been several reports of humans suffering severe liver damage attributed to ingesting comfrey. A number of animal studies also show that comfrey causes liver tumors. In one study, all of the animals fed comfrey leaves developed liver tumors within six months. Some herbalists note that comfrey comprised 8 percent of the laboratory animals' diet and argue that a person would have to eat much more comfrey than normal to suffer adverse effects. Still, the Food and Drug Administration has banned internal use of comfrey because of its toxic PAs.

Two species of comfrey, *S. asperum* (prickly comfrey) and *S. uplandicum* (Russian comfrey), contain very high levels of echimidine, one of the most potent of the PAs. Adding to the problem is the fact that these forms of comfrey are sometimes labeled "common comfrey." This is an additional reason why comfrey should never be taken internally.

CORIANDER (*CORIANDRUM SATIVUM*)

Coriander—the seeds of a plant that is also called cilantro or Chinese parsley—is native to southern Europe, even though its leaves are most closely identified with Mexican and Asian cuisine. It is an annual herb that grows twelve to eighteen inches high and produces white or pink-tinged flowers. The leaves are used to flavor spicy dishes; the fruit produces seeds with a distinctive, rather unpleasant odor reminiscent of burned rubber until they are dried. They then have a pleasant aromatic blend of sage and lemon.

Coriander seeds are used medicinally; they are also used to flavor gin, curry, and medicines. They are also one component of American cigarettes.

Common Uses

- Stimulate appetite, aid digestion, and treat mild intestinal upsets, including gas, bloating, diarrhea, and nausea.
- Calm jittery nerves and help induce sleep.
- May help control blood glucose levels.
- Sweeten bad breath.
- Lessen joint and muscle pain.

How It Works

While the major active ingredient in coriander seeds is an aromatic volatile oil, they also contain malic acid and tannins. These components have been shown to have soothing effects on the muscles of the digestive tract as well as antiseptic properties when applied to skin abrasions. The seeds are also made into poultices or salves for external use to prevent infection of wounds and to ease muscle and joint aches.

Evidence of Efficacy

Although there is a lot of research on the effects of coriander in laboratory settings, it is unclear how much of it applies to humans. German health authorities have approved the use of coriander seed preparations for digestive tract complaints, including loss of appetite. Researchers at Cairo University have shown coriander oil lowers glucose levels by normalizing insulin levels and supporting pancreatic function. Human studies indicate that coriander has a mild diuretic effect, but there are many other herbs that are more effective in ridding the body of excess fluids.

Forms and Usual Dosages

Coriander is available as a decoction, an infusion, a liquid extract, and as crushed, powdered, or whole seeds. The decoction is made by infusing 1 to 2 teaspoons of crushed seeds per cup of water; it should be consumed between meals. The liquid extract is taken in doses of 0.5 to 2 ml and the powder in doses of 0.3 to 1.

Potential Problems

The FDA considers coriander to be a safe herb when used in recommended amounts. Some people may experience allergic reactions. It may increase sun sensitivity, so caution is needed to protect the skin from sunburn.

CRAMP BARK
(*VIBURNUM OPULUS*)

Also known as Guelder rose and highbush cranberry, cramp bark is a shrub or tree that grows in North America and parts of Europe. In the spring, it is covered with white flowers that produce drooping clusters of bright red berries that ripen quickly and eventually turn purple. Birds relish the bitter berries, and in Canada, they are sometimes substituted for cranberries to make a piquant relish. When dried, the berries turn black and were once used to make ink. It is the shrub's bark, however, that is valued by herbalists for its sedative and antispasmodic properties.

Common Uses

- Calm colicky muscle spasms, especially those associated with menstrual cramps and endometriosis.
- Reduce the risk of miscarriage due to uterine contractions.
- Relieve anxiety and nervous conditions.
- Act as a diuretic to relieve bloating, especially that linked to premenstrual syndrome (PMS).
- Reduce palpitations and lower blood pressure.

How It Works

The active ingredient in cramp bark is thought to be bitter glucoside, which is similar to that of black haw (see p. 380), but milder. It also contains tannins, resin, valerianic acid, viopudial, and scopoletin; some of these substances have been shown to have antispasmodic properties. But precisely how cramp bark works is unknown.

◉ **A LITTLE HISTORY**
There are numerous literary references to Guelder rose and its berries. Chaucer, for example, described the berries as good for the health and advised eating them right from the bush. It is unlikely that many people did this, however, because the berries are very bitter and must be sweetened to be palatable. In Siberia, the berries were fermented and distilled into a type of spirits. They have also been used in Norway and Sweden to flavor a paste of honey and flour. Native American tribes in the Northeast were said to have used the bark and leaves from the cramp bark shrub as a diuretic and to treat swollen glands, mumps, and eye problems.

Evidence of Efficacy

Most of the evidence regarding cramp bark is based on a long tradition of its use as a botanical medicine and on animal studies. It was once listed in the U.S. *Pharmacopoeia* and in Britain's *National Formulary* as fluid extract, tincture, and compound elixir forms to treat nervous conditions and muscle spasms. However, there are no reported scientific studies that prove the efficacy of this herb. A team of American researchers reported that cramp bark had an antispasmodic effect on rat uterine tissue, but it is not known whether this holds true for humans. Animal studies also indicate that substances in cramp bark can slow a rapid heartbeat and lower high blood pressure. Again, more research is needed to demonstrate whether these findings also apply to humans.

Forms and Usual Dosage

The bark is collected in very thin strips, dried, and used to make teas, decoctions, lotions, and tinctures; it is also included in a number of herbal combinations, especially those used to treat menstrual problems. Dosages vary according to the problem under treatment. To relieve PMS and other symptoms related to menstruation, it is often combined with other so-called female herbs, such as vitex, pau d'arco, and dong quai, and taken for two weeks before the onset of menstruation.

Potential Problems

Given the lack of scientific data associated with cramp bark, there is no way to determine what if any health risks its use might have. There are no reports of any adverse effects but, because of its possible effects on the uterus and heart, pregnant women and people with heart disease should either avoid the herb or check with a doctor before taking it.

CRANBERRY (*VACCINIUM MACROCARPON*)

The cranberry is a native American plant that grows in bogs. Although the bright red berries are associated more with Thanksgiving than medicine, alternative practitioners and physicians alike recommend cranberry juice or pills as a preventive measure for people who suffer from frequent bladder infections.

Common Uses

- Prevent and treat urinary tract infections, especially those caused by the *E. coli* bacterium.

In the past, cranberries were also used to:

- Promote healing of skin wounds.
- Treat scurvy, a vitamin C–deficiency disease.

How It Works

Cranberries fight urinary tract infections in several ways: When consumed in large amounts, cranberries acidify the urine and raise its level of hippuric acid, a substance that creates an inhospitable environment for *E. coli* and other bacteria. Cranberries, along with their blueberry cousins, contain a substance that prevents invading bacteria from adhering to the bladder wall where they would normally reproduce. The high vitamin C content of cranberries may also bolster the body's immune system to fight off the infection. By making the urine more acidic, cranberries increase the effectiveness of nitrofurantoin, an antibiotic commonly prescribed to treat urinary tract infections.

Evidence of Efficacy

A number of controlled studies in the United States and Europe have confirmed that consuming large amounts of cranberry juice, or taking the fruit in concentrated pill form, reduces the incidence of urinary tract infections among susceptible people. It also appears to shorten the duration of symptoms.

Forms and Usual Dosage

The typical dosage used in clinical studies to treat a urinary tract infection calls for taking 800 mg of cranberry extract a day. This is equivalent to drinking two 8-ounce glasses of undiluted cranberry juice. (The commercial juice sold in supermarkets is too diluted to be of much therapeutic value; either make your own with a juicer or buy full-strength juice at a health food store.) However, many people find the unsweetened and undiluted juice too sour. This can be remedied by combining it with plain blueberry juice, which contains similar beneficial ingredients.

◉ A LITTLE HISTORY

While it's doubtful that the Native Americans and Pilgrims who celebrated the first Thanksgiving sat down to roast turkey with cranberry relish, the early settlers did observe how the Indians used the bog berries and followed suit. The dried berries helped prevent scurvy by providing a good source of vitamin C during the long New England winters. Native Americans also applied poultices of crushed cranberries to heal skin wounds.

So instead of 16 ounces of cranberry juice, try mixing 8 ounces of each. Or the 16 ounces of cranberry juice can be diluted with an equal amount of apple juice, which is naturally sweet.

To prevent a recurrence, cut the dosage in half. Be sure to drink at least eight to ten glasses of water or other nonalcoholic fluids during the course of the day to promote the flow of urine, which also helps wash bacteria out of the urinary tract and bladder.

Potential Problems

Cranberries, even in large amounts, are safe. While they interact favorably with some prescription antibiotics by acidifying the urine, they should not be used with another popular botanical remedy—uva ursi—which works best in an alkaline environment.

DANDELION (*TARAXACUM OFFICINALE*)

Dandelion, which is closely related to chicory, is a common weed found worldwide. The plant grows to a height of twelve inches and produces bright yellow flowers that, when they mature, become white, globular seed heads. Each seed has a tiny parachute that even the gentlest breeze can carry far and wide. The plant gets its name from the Old French term *dent de lion,* which means lion's tooth and refers to its lance-shaped leaves. Herbalists have used dandelion roots and leaves for centuries to treat numerous disorders; the leaves are also highly nutritious and a plentiful, inexpensive source of many vitamins, minerals, and other nutrients.

Common Uses

The bitter, milky sap is used externally to:

- Heal wounds.
- Remove warts, moles, pimples, calluses, and sores.
- Soothe bee stings and blisters.

The sap, leaves, and root extracts are ingested to:

- Increase urine output and help rid the body of excess fluid.
- Stimulate stomach secretions and aid in digestion.
- Relieve constipation and control diarrhea.
- Stimulate bile production and treat liver disorders.
- Prevent formation of gallstones.
- Prevent or lower high blood pressure.
- Stimulate milk flow in nursing mothers and relieve pain of endometriosis.
- Inhibit plaque buildup on teeth.

Aside from dandelion's many medicinal uses, it is also highly nutritious. The greens are rich in antioxidants, including beta-carotene (the precursor of vitamin A), vitamin C, and flavonoids; minerals, including calcium, iron, silicon, boron, magnesium, and zinc; and many of the B-complex vitamins. The leaves can be steamed or boiled and served as a green vegetable; very young leaves are also tasty in salads. The roots are sometimes used as a coffee substitute, in much the same manner as those of its cousin chicory. They may also be boiled and eaten as a root vegetable.

How It Works

Dandelion leaves and roots have been used for hundreds of years to treat liver, gallbladder, kidney, digestive, and joint problems. Dandelions contain certain unique bitter compounds that help stimulate digestion and may increase bile production and its flow; these properties lower the risk of gallstones and may also help lower blood cholesterol levels. The bitter compounds may also have an antifungal effect.

Dandelion tea and extracts have a diuretic effect that reduces the body's fluid volume. This can help lower high blood pressure, and also prevent the uncomfortable bloating and swelling that many women experience during their premenstrual phase. Dandelions are high in potassium, an electrolyte that many pharmaceutical diuretics wash out of the body; thus, dandelion tonics may be doubly useful in treating mild high blood pressure.

Dandelions contain several other chemical compounds, which may have a theraputic effect on the body:

- *Inulin,* which converts to fructose in the body. The liver can convert fructose into glycogen without requiring insulin. Thus, inulin may be beneficial to people with diabetes.
- *Pectin,* a soluble fiber that is helpful in preventing constipation, controlling diarrhea, and lowering blood cholesterol.
- *Coumestrol,* a plant (phyto) estrogen that may promote milk production in nursing mothers and balance the body's hormones by reducing the effects of natural estrogen.

Evidence of Efficacy

Although scientists have studied the compounds contained in the dandelion, there have been few formal studies of the plant's effects on the human body. Much of our knowledge of dandelion is based on traditional folk medicine. The few studies that have been reported confirm dandelion's high vitamin and mineral content, from which benefits to the body can be attributed. A patent was filed in Japan in 1979 for a freeze-dried extract of dandelion root for antitumor use, after it was shown to inhibit the growth of some tumors. (Some anecdotal evidence exists of dandelion's cancer-fighting properties—the Chinese are using it to treat breast cancer—but these results may be due to other factors and have not been scientifically proved.) Dental researchers at the University of Indiana reported on dandelion's role in anti-plaque-formation preparations. From 1941 to 1952, a French scientist named Henri Leclerc demonstrated that the bitter white milky latex that dandelions produce in late summer aided chronic liver problems related to gallstones. In the late 1950s, some studies were able to confirm antibacterial effects of dandelion pollen, which has been used for centuries by Koreans to prevent infections and edema, and to promote blood circulation.

Forms and Usual Dosage

Dandelion leaves are steamed or boiled and eaten in salads or made into tonics. The leaves may also be dried and drunk as a tea to stimulate digestion and treat constipation. Use 4 to 10 g of dried leaves added to one cup of boiling water, or 5 to 10 ml of fresh juice from the leaves, or 2 to 4 ml of tincture made from the leaves. These mixtures can be ingested three times a day.

Dandelion roots are boiled and the cooking water is used as a tonic. Either 3 to 5 g (1 or 2 tablespoons) of dried root, boiled in one cup of water, or 5 to 10 ml of a tincture made from the root, can be taken three times per day. Some experts recommend an alcohol-based tincture because the medicinal bitter compounds are more soluble in alcohol. The roots may also be dried and roasted and added to coffee, much as chicory is, or used as a coffee substitute.

Potential Problems

Because dandelion is known to increase bile flow, persons suffering from gallstones or other bile duct obstructions should not take this herbal in any form. Dandelion also increases production of gastric juices, and so is not recommended for anyone with stomach ulcers or gastritis. Do not use dandelion as a diuretic without the advice of a nutritionist, and, if taken for that purpose, potassium levels should be monitored. Because of the herb's effect on hormonal balance, pregnant women or those who wish to become pregnant should consult their doctor before taking this substance. The plant's milky latex, found in the stem, may cause an allergic skin rash in some individuals. Certain medications may become less effective if dandelion is ingested, so be sure to check with a doctor about possible drug interactions when taking dandelion.

See Also

Anemia

DEVIL'S CLAW (*HARPAGOPHYTUM PROCUMBENS*)

Devil's claw—also known as wood spider and grapple plant—is native to the Kalahari Desert and other arid areas of southwestern Africa. Its various names are derived from the appearance of its fruit, which looks like it is covered with tiny hooks, claws, or spider legs. The plant also has underground tubers in which it stores the water it needs to survive the harsh desert climate, and it is these tubers that African healers have used for centuries to treat everything from cancer, intestinal disorders, and fevers to menstrual and pregnancy problems. Devil's claw is now cultivated in other parts of the world and has become a popular botanical medicine in Europe, where it is taken as a painkiller, diuretic, and sedative. It is also gaining popularity in the United States.

Common Uses

- Reduce arthritis pain and inflammation.
- Calm jittery nerves and ease anxiety.
- Help rid the body of excess fluid.
- Treat mild digestive problems and stimulate appetite.

How It Works

Active ingredients of devil's claw include harpagoside, a member of the ididoid glycoside family. It has been shown to reduce inflammation, especially that associated with rheumatoid arthritis. Unlike many non-steroidal anti-inflammatory drugs (NSAIDs), which relieve arthritis pain

⊙ A LITTLE HISTORY

Used in traditional medicine of Africa for centuries, devil's claw was unknown in Europe until the beginning of the twentieth century. At that time, a German farmer heard stories about the medicinal properties of devil's claw while traveling in South Africa. He decided to try cultivating the plant in Germany, and it soon became very popular as a botanical medicine in his homeland. Over the next few decades, it gained a wide following in Europe and, more recently, in the United States. It is also being cultivated in China and has been added to the list of traditional Chinese botanical medicines.

but may also increase cartilage damage, devil's claw appears to protect cartilage while relieving pain and increasing joint flexibility.

Devil's claw is high in bitters, compounds that stimulate the flow of saliva and digestive juices. These effects help perk up appetite and may also improve digestion and reduce gas. Other active ingredients include beta-sitosterol (which may lower cholesterol), stigmasterol and other fatty acids (which may act as natural estrogen to relieve menstrual and menopausal symptoms), various acidic compounds, triterpenes, resins, and flavonoids.

Evidence of Efficacy

Devil's claw has been studied extensively in Europe and China, but so far, results have been somewhat disappointing. A few studies show that it may reduce arthritis inflammation and pain, but those that have compared devil's claw with standard NSAIDs and a placebo have produced very mixed results. Some have found that devil's claw is not much more effective than placebo, while others—most notably a small study done by a team of French researchers—deemed it more effective than the pharmaceutical products. A study in China involving patients with rheumatoid and osteoarthritis reported that more than 50 percent experienced improvement in their symptoms.

Some studies have shown a reduction of blood cholesterol and uric acid levels, but more recent research was unable to substantiate those findings. Researchers have also shown in lab animals that devil's claw can help correct an irregular heartbeat, but this has not been demonstrated in humans.

Despite these mixed or conflicting studies, European herbalists continue to recommend devil's claw tea to treat arthritis and other inflammatory disorders. German health authorities have also approved devil's claw tea for appetite loss, stomach disorders, and other disorders.

Although devil's claw has been prescribed in Africa for many years for such ailments as skin cancer, fever, and malaria, none of these uses have been studied scientifically.

Forms and Usual Dosages

Devil's claw is available as a capsule, liquid extract, and chopped or powdered root. The decoction is made with 1 teaspoon of powdered or finely chopped root dissolved in two cups of water; this is sipped through the day. If taking the herb in capsule form, the usual daily dosage is 4.5 g.

Potential Problems

Devil's claw is generally considered safe when used in the recommended dosages, but there are reports of adverse reactions, including appetite loss, ringing in the ears, and headache. It is not known whether the herb interferes with the actions of other drugs. Some have cautioned that devil's claw should not be used by anyone with ulcers, gallstones, or heart problems, because the herb's actions on these conditions isn't known. It also should not be taken during pregnancy because its effects on the uterus and fetus are unknown.

DILL (ANETHUM GRAVELONS)

Dill is a popular garden herb that is native to the Mediterranean and southern Russia, but is now grown widely throughout Europe, Asia, and North America. It is in the same plant family as fennel; in fact, its feathery leaves are similar to those of fennel. But dill has a much tangier taste, and is most familiar as a pickling herb and to season fish. Although dill is no longer used extensively as a medicinal herb in the United States, many European herbalists rely on it as a digestive aid and to treat intestinal gas and flatulence.

Common Uses

- Stimulate appetite, aid digestion, and settle an upset stomach.
- Reduce intestinal gas and flatulence.
- Freshen bad breath.
- Increase the flow of breast milk.

In the past, dill was also used to:

- Alleviate infant colic.
- Induce sleep.
- Treat kidney disorders.

How it works

Dill seeds contain an oil that has mild antibacterial properties, which may help destroy intestinal micro-organisms that cause ulcers and intestinal problems. Dill may also quell intestinal spasms. Chewing a few dill seeds stimulates the flow of saliva, which can help freshen breath; in addition, the dill itself has a fresh, pleasant odor.

Evidence of Efficacy

Most of the studies into dill's medicinal properties have been done on laboratory animals and cell cultures rather than human subjects. German researchers have documented antibacterial activity of ingredients in dill oil, and German health authorities have approved dill as a treatment for intestinal complaints related to bacteria. Experiments using laboratory animals have also found that dill oil can relax the smooth muscles that control intestinal motility, and thus may reduce colicky abdominal pain. Other studies indicate that dillweed (the leaves and stems) contain substances that lower blood pressure and slow the heartbeat in laboratory animals. It is not known, however, whether these effects apply to humans.

Forms and Usual Dosages

Medicinal dill is available in pill, tincture, and powder forms. The dried dillweed and seeds can be used to make a tea or infusion. As a digestive aid, experts recommend making a tea using up to 1 to 2 teaspoons of crushed seeds per cup of hot water; let it stand for ten to fifteen minutes and drink a cup following each meal. To treat gas or a stomachache in a young child, use ½ teaspoon of dill seeds per cup of water, and give the child one-fourth cup at a time. Experts disagree, however, on the safety of this for very young children. Some say that cooled diluted dill tea is safe for colicky infants, and others, caution against giving it to babies under twelve months. To be safe, check with your doctor before giving dill—or any other herbal remedy—to a young child.

Potential Problems

Dill is safe when used in the recommended dosages.

DONG QUAI (*ANGELICA POLYMORPHIA, A. SINENSIS, A. ACUTILOBA*)

This traditional and respected Asian herbal medicine comes from the thick, yellowish brown root of *Angelica sinensis,* a plant found in China and Korea, and *A. acutiloba* of Japan. (European and American varieties do not seem to have the same powerful attributes as the Asian ones.)

Dong quai—or dang gui, as it is usually written in Chinese medicine texts—is one of the most popular of the Asian herbal remedies. It is often taken in combination with other herbs as a "female tonic" for various menstrual problems, ranging from premenstrual syndrome to irregular and/or painful periods, as well as symptoms of menopause. Because it's so often recommended for menstrual disorders and for restoring or improving a woman's sexual desire, dong quai is often referred to as "women's ginseng."

Blood dominates women's health, according to the principles of Chinese medicine, and dong quai is said to nourish and invigorate the blood, and it's sometimes prescribed as a blood builder or blood tonic. It also acts as an antispasmodic and a mild sedative. Despite its reputation as a remedy for "female problems," herbalists sometimes recommend it for men, too, especially if they are suffering from blood-related or circulatory problems, such as fatigue or high blood pressure.

Common Uses

- Menstrual problems, including absent or irregular periods, cramps, and premenstrual syndrome.
- Lack of sexual desire and fertility problems.
- Liver disorders.
- Inflammation.
- Sciatica and rheumatism.
- Digestive problems, including upset stomach, ulcers, and constipation.
- High blood pressure.
- Fibrocystic breasts.

How It Works

The root is a rich source of vitamin B_{12}, folic acid, and niacin, which may explain its blood-building attributes because these B vitamins are

◉ A LITTLE HISTORY

Dong quai, also known as Chinese angelica, is a botanical cousin of European angelica (*Angelica archangelica*), which was used in medieval times to ward off the plague and witches. Legend has it that in the mid-1600s, an angel appeared to a monk during a dream with a message that the wild celery plant could protect against the plague. The monk renamed the plant angelica, and the British Royal College of Physicians used it to formulate the "King's Excellent Plague Recipe." Sadly, it didn't stop the plague, and it soon fell out of favor.

instrumental in making blood cells. It also contains coumarins, substances that increase blood flow, relieve inflammation, stimulate the central nervous system, and have antispasmodic effects. Experts disagree as to whether dong quai contains plant (phyto) estrogens or has any direct hormonal action.

Evidence of Efficacy

Most of the studies that attest to the wide variety of actions of dong quai have been done in China and involve laboratory animals rather than humans. This animal research indicates, however, that dong quai directly affects the uterus, causing both contracting and relaxing effects. In addition, the herb's active ingredients appear to affect nearly every part of the body, including the central nervous and immune systems, muscles, the digestive tract, kidneys, and the blood vessels and blood cells.

Despite the fact that Chinese studies have substantiated many of the claims for dong quai, some American herbalists remain skeptical of the root's benefits. It also should be noted that, in Asia, dong quai is frequently used in combination with other herbs such as chaste tree berry (vitex), licorice, and ginseng, and so it's difficult to isolate the effectiveness of dong quai alone.

Forms and Usual Dosages

The powdered root is available alone or in combination with other herbs in the forms of capsules, tablets, tinctures, and tea. An injectable form is available in the Far East, but is rarely used elsewhere. Recommended dosages range from 600 mg to 3 or 4 g a day. A tea can be made from a teaspoon of the crushed root.

For PMS symptoms, dong quai is typically used on the days before menstruation begins. For cramps, it is advised to begin using it on the day the menstrual period should begin and continue until bleeding stops. For relief of menopausal symptoms, dong quai can be taken daily. Two months or so of daily use may be necessary before problems such as hot flashes subside, although one study by Stanford University researchers found the herb no more effective than placebo in reducing hot flashes.

Potential Problems

Because the root contains chemicals call psoralens, serious sun sensitivity can occur, so unprotected sun exposure should be avoided while taking it. In Asia, women may take it every day, and sometimes drink the tea three times a day; however, this overuse can cause diarrhea. Stop taking dong quai if diarrhea develops. Dong quai should never be taken during pregnancy or lactation and it is contraindicated in women with breast cancer.

See Also

Bladder Control Problems
Menopause

ECHINACEA (*ECHINACEA PURPUREA, E. ANGUSTIFOLIA, E. PALLIDA*)

Also known as purple coneflower, echinacea is a daisylike wildflower native to North America. There are nine species, four of which (*Echinacea angustifolia, E. pallida, E. purpurea*, and the endangered *E. tennensiensis*) are used medicinally; most scientific studies, however, have used *E. purpurea.* Their stems, roots, flowers, and leaves are part of hundreds of commercial preparations that claim to boost the immune system and ward off cold and flu symptoms. Over the decades, the popularity of echinacea has ebbed and flowed: Once used by Native Americans, pioneers, and earlier generations of doctors, the herb fell out of favor with the discovery and then widespread use of antibiotics in the 1930s and only recently has been rediscovered by herbalists everywhere.

Common Uses

- Speed healing of various skin problems, including minor wounds, inflammation, boils, abscesses, eczema, burns, and cold sores.
- Reduce intensity and duration of cold and flu symptoms.
- Help the body fight recurrent infections, such as those of the respiratory system, middle ear, and urinary tract, as well as vaginal yeast infections.
- Bolster immunity and relieve symptoms of chronic fatigue syndrome and reduce opportunistic infections in people who are HIV-positive.

◉ A LITTLE HISTORY

Long before colonists arrived, Native Americans on the Great Plains were using echinacea for its antiseptic properties, placing it on insect bites, skin wounds, and rattlesnake bites. They used it to calm toothaches and sore gums, and drank it as tea to treat colds, mumps, arthritis, and other conditions. American Eclectics, a group of doctors prominent from 1830 to 1930 who used botanicals in their practices, were a major force in bringing echinacea to the forefront of herbal medicine. They promoted it as a "blood purifier" (venereal disease remedy) as well as an agent for treating migraine headaches, rheumatism, tumors, malaria, and hemorrhoids. After falling out of favor in the 1930s, the herb regained its stature when interest in herbal medicine revived in the 1970s and 1980s.

How It Works

The precise disease-fighting substances in echinacea have not been identified. However, when echinacea preparations are taken internally, injected into the bloodstream, or inhaled, they appear to stimulate immune system responses: The body steps up production of defensive white blood cells to fight off infecting organisms. The herb also appears to boost production of interferon, a natural compound that fights viruses. When taken at the first sign of cold or flu symptoms, echinacea may prevent the infection from taking hold or shorten the duration of full-blown symptoms.

Echinacea also appears to stimulate the immune system to respond to internal threats; for example, seeking out and destroying mutant precancerous cells. When applied to the skin in the form of a poultice or lotion, echinacea appears to speed the healing of boils, abscesses, cold sores, and other minor infections. Gargling with echinacea tea can soothe a sore throat and may speed healing of canker sores.

Evidence of Efficacy

Echinacea has been studied extensively in Europe, especially in Germany. At least three double-blind, placebo-controlled studies have been published showing that echinacea either prevents a full-blown cold or flu from developing or shortens its duration. Some studies, however, have produced mixed or conflicting results, so more study is needed to determine that echinacea does, indeed, live up to the many claims made for it. In the meantime, German health authorities have approved it as a supportive treatment for colds and flu.

Forms and Usual Dosage

Because echinacea's effects are relatively short-lived, it is most effective if taken every two or three hours initially until symptoms are relieved and then three times a day for a week to ensure complete recovery and optimal immune function. One dose is two tablets or capsules containing between 500 and 1,000 mg of the ground herb; forty drops of the extract; or 4 to 8 ounces of a strong tea made from the ground root. Potency varies among manufacturers, so be sure to follow instructions on the label of commercial preparations. Echinacea also comes in various manufactured forms, such as capsules, tablets, softgels, lozenges, tincture, liquid, or dried herb (tea). Look for a liquid that is either fresh-pressed juice (standardized to contain 2.4 percent of beta-1,2-fructofuranosides) or an alcohol-based tincture (in a 5:1 concentration of the herb). Pills should contain at least 3.5 percent echinacosides. Echinacea is often blended with other immune-enhancing herbs such as goldenseal, astragalus, and pau d'arco, but these additions raise the price and many experts feel they are not needed. Many herbalists and premier E. researcher Rudy Bauer of Germany suggest that the herb be hyperdosed at onset of symptoms, then used as indicated above.

Potential Problems

Echinacea is safe and effective when used in recommended dosages. No known side effects have been reported. However, it should not be taken longer than eight weeks, because its immune-enhancing effects decrease. It is most effective if stopped for a week and then resumed. If you have an allergy to daisies or other wildflowers, this herb may cause a similar reaction. Contact a doctor if you develop a skin rash or shortness of breath when taking echinacea. Persons with autoimmune disorders such as lupus, rheumatoid arthritis, and MS, as well as those with TB or HIV disease, are generally advised not to take echinacea until its immune-stimulating effects are better studied.

See Also

Bronchitis
Common Cold and Flu

ELDER (*SAMBUCUS CANADENSIS*)

Known commonly as American elder, elderberry, and sweet elder, *Sambucus canadensis* is one of more than a dozen varieties that are native to North America. It grows up to ten feet tall, and in the spring it produces masses of whitish flowers that evolve into small clusters of berries that range in color from amber and red to deep purple and black. Since ancient times, elder flowers, berries, and the inner bark have been used medicinally; elderberries are also used to make dyes, wine, liquors, jellies, perfumes, and cosmetic creams and lotions. Caution is needed when gathering and consuming elder, however, because the leaves and stems contain the deadly poison cyanide.

Common Uses

- Induce sweating to help "break" the fever of a bad cold or flu and reduce nasal and airway congestion.

- Increase the flow of urine to rid the body of excess fluid.
- Induce vomiting.
- Reduce swelling of sprains and bruises and lessen skin inflammation; may also relieve joint and muscle pain.

How It Works

Elder flowers contain triterpenes, which may have anti-inflammatory action similar to steroids; oils, including linoleic and linolenic fatty acids; various flavonoids, including rutin and quercetin; pectin, a soluble fiber; and sugars. The bark, inner bark, and berries contain various resins, tannins, acidic compounds, vitamin C, volatile oils, and wax. It is believed that elder's most common medicinal use—inducing perspiration associated with the fever of cold and flu symptoms—is caused by flavonoids and viburnic acid, since these substances have produced similar effects when isolated from other plants. When consumed as a hot tea, elder bark and berries loosen the mucus that causes airway and nasal congestion, making it easier to expectorate. The hot tea can also cause profuse sweating, which naturopaths and other practitioners associate with reducing a fever and other flu symptoms.

Elder may also produce a diuretic effect by increasing the flow of urine. Tea made from the elder root is very bitter and has a purgative effect and can induce vomiting and diarrhea. Purgatives were once thought to be useful in "cleansing the system," but people now recognize their danger and they are no longer recommended.

As noted, elder leaves and stems contain cyanide and should never be ingested. However, they contain other ingredients that may be used externally as a salve, emollient, or to reduce swelling and inflammation of sprains, bruises, and arthritis. An oil extracted from the seeds may also be massaged onto painful joints to relieve arthritis pain.

Evidence of Efficacy

There is very little medical research to back the various claims for elder; most of the evidence is either anecdotal or based on a long tradition of botanical medicine. German health authorities have approved the use of elder-flower preparations to treat fever and cold and flu symptoms. There is also ample research into some of the components of elder, such as flavonoids and phenolic acids, to substantiate their use as a diuretic and to promote sweating.

One small study, conducted in Skokie, Illinois, and reported by a company that sells nutraceuticals, found that elderberry capsules shortened the duration of flu symptoms in a large majority of patients. The capsules were taken at the first sign of flu symptoms; those who took the elderberry recovered in an average of two to four days, compared to an average of six days for those who received a placebo. The active

◉ A LITTLE HISTORY

Throughout history, elder shrubs have been thought to have great powers of healing as well as offer protection against evil spirits. The cross on which Jesus was crucified was said to have been made of elder wood. In the Middle Ages, it was thought that a baby who slept in an elder cradle was destined to fall ill and die. Similarly, the appearance of elder in a dream was considered a bad omen. In contrast, the seventeenth-century diarist John Evelyn called elder a remedy against all infirmities. In Tyrol—the alpine parts of Austria and northern Italy—green elder branches were buried in graves to protect the dead from evil spirits. At one time, winemakers in Portugal added elderberry juice to cheap wine to make it taste like expensive port. Indeed, this practice gave rise to a popular medicinal use of elderberries after sailors reported that drinking large amounts of adulterated port cured their rheumatism.

ingredients in elderberry were thought to inactivate an enzyme that normally allows the flu virus to penetrate cell walls. An Israeli study using a different elder product produced similar results. More study is needed, however, to duplicate these findings.

Forms and Usual Dosage

The dried flowers can be made into emollient creams, infusions, flower water, tablets, teas, and a tincture. To make an elder-flower tea or infusion, use 2 teaspoons of dried flowers per cup of hot water. Dried elderberries are available in capsules, decoctions, liquid extracts, lozenges, ointments, and tea bags. Follow dosages recommended on the labels. Topical elder preparations are available as skin lotions, creams, ointments, and emollients. A compress soaked in elder-flower tea can be applied directly to the skin; fresh or dried leaves may be used to make a poultice.

Potential Problems

Elder stems, leaves, and outer bark are extremely toxic, containing enough cyanide to quickly kill small children after ingesting only a handful of leaves. The leaves are safe when used externally as a skin preparation to relieve inflammation and swelling. Elder flowers and berries are safe if used as directed.

EUCALYPTUS (*EUCALYPTUS GLOBULUS*)

Eucalyptus is a tall evergreen tree that is native to Australia and Tasmania, and now grown in subtropical climates worldwide. Both eucalyptus oil, which is distilled from the leaves, bark, and roots, and the leaves themselves, are used medicinally. The oil has a strong, pleasant fragrance that not only has medicinal properties, but also is used in bathwater, as an air freshener, and as an insecticide and insect repellent.

Eucalyptus stores a lot of water in its roots, making it a useful tree to plant in areas that suffer periodic droughts. Traditionally, eucalyptus trees have been planted near mosquito-infested swamps to drain them and help reduce the spread of malaria.

Common Uses

- Ease stress when the oil is massaged into the skin or added to bathwater.
- Promote healing of minor skin infections, cuts, and abrasions.
- Relieve upper respiratory and nasal congestion to ease cold symptoms.
- Soothe a sore throat.
- Sweeten bad breath.

How It Works

Eucalyptus oil contains a substance called eucalyptol, which has been shown to have many therapeutic properties; it also contains tannins, ketones, flavonoids, and other substances. Eucalyptol (also called cineole) helps thin and loosen sputum and make it easier to cough up. It stimulates the flow of saliva, which helps reduce the cough reflex caused by a dry throat. Eucalyptus also contains tannins, which have an astringent effect and reduce inflammation.

The odor of eucalyptus oil, like that of camphor and menthol, elicits a two-phase nasal response. In the initial phase, which lasts about thirty minutes, the nasal passages actually constrict and feel even more obstructed. This is followed by an opening of the passages, which allows more air to flow through them and results in a distinct feeling of being able to breathe more easily. It is not known precisely how eucalyptol achieves this benefit, but some researchers theorize that it stimulates the tiny hairs in the nasal passages to help clear them of mucus. The essential oil can be put in boiling water so that it rises in the steam to the nasal passages. Another effective way to inhale the vapors is to sprinkle a few drops of the oil on a handkerchief and hold it under the nose on a pillow at night.

Eucalyptus tea is used as a gargle to soothe mouth ulcers and an inflamed sore throat. The oil's antibacterial and astringent properties make it useful in treating minor skin infections. Before applying the oil to the skin, however, be sure to dilute it with alcohol, water, or a neutral oil, such as vegetable or olive oil; the full-strength oil can damage the skin. Use 1 teaspoon of eucalyptus oil per cup of the diluting substance. A poultice made from the dried leaves can also be made and applied directly to the skin.

Evidence of Efficacy

Numerous studies in both animals and humans have documented the therapeutic benefits of eucalyptus oil. It is an approved ingredient in many prescription and over-the-counter cough and cold preparations.

◉ A LITTLE HISTORY

The eucalyptus has played an important role in its native Australia. In addition to its many medicinal properties, eucalyptus was an important food. Aborigines and early settlers ground and ate the roots of smaller plants in the eucalyptus family and mixed "lerp," a sugary substance secreted by parasites that live in the plant, into their foods and beverages. The aborigines also discovered that the roots of eucalyptus trees stored much-needed water that was easily accessible if they dug up the roots. As a source of hardwood, eucalyptus trees became important to the economies of many countries. The trees were also planted near mosquito-infested marshes because of their ability to absorb great quantities of water and dry the swamps, killing the mosquitoes and reducing the spread of infection. The blue gum tree (*E. globulus*) thus earned the nickname of the Australian fever tree.

German health authorities have approved eucalyptus as a treatment for upper respiratory congestion, bronchitis, and throat inflammation.

Forms and Usual Dosages

Eucalyptus is available as dried leaves that can be used to make teas and poultices, tinctures, and oil. To be effective, dried eucalyptus leaf must contain at least 2 percent volatile oil. Eucalyptus oil is an ingredient in many commercial lozenges, cough syrups, skin salves and creams, balms, linaments, ointments, lotions, nasal inhalants, air fresheners, and other products. A few drops of eucalyptus oil can be added to a room vaporizer. Or add a half cup of leaves to a quart of oil, bring to a boil, and then inhale the steamy vapors. Eucalyptus tea can be made by steeping 1 to 2 teaspoons of leaves in a cup of water for ten minutes, strain, and drink two or three cups a day.

Potential Problems

Eucalyptus is generally safe, although it should not be used by individuals with inflammation of the gastrointestinal tract and the bile ducts, or those with serious liver disease. It should never be applied directly to the face, as the fumes from the oils can irritate the nasal passages. In some cases, the person who ingests eucalyptus preparations may experience nausea, vomiting, or diarrhea.

EVENING PRIMROSE (OENOTHERA BIENNIS)

The evening primrose, a native of North America, is a biennial herb that produces only leaves the first year and bright yellow flowers and seeds the second. It is the oil from its small, reddish seeds that is responsible for evening primrose's medicinal effects. Evening primrose oil (EPO) is 60 to 80 percent linoleic acid and 8 to 15 percent gamma-linolenic acid (GLA), one of the omega-6 fatty acids. While there is little or no proof that EPO lives up to some of the claims of its advocates, some scientific studies do support its use in treating eczema.

Common Uses

- Reduce the skin itchiness, flaking, and inflammation of eczema.
- Ease symptoms of premenstrual syndrome (PMS).
- Ease the pain and inflammation of rheumatoid arthritis.

How It Works

It is the GLA that is the active ingredient in evening primrose oil. The body uses GLA to manufacture a certain prostaglandin that fights inflammation. The body can convert linoleic acid into GLA but some people with neurodermatitis—an itchy skin condition—lack the enzyme necessary to do this. Thus, GLA supplements can compensate for the missing enzyme and allow the body to make anti-inflammatory prostaglandins. In that role, gamma-linolenic acid may also reduce the inflammation and pain of rheumatoid arthritis and the swelling that causes the pain and discomfort of premenstrual syndrome. (See Essential Fatty Acids p. 295.)

Evidence of Efficacy

In one year-long study, people with active rheumatoid arthritis aged eighteen to ninety took 2.8 g of GLA daily. During the first six months, the study subjects reported marked decreases in tenderness, pain, and stiffness, and doctors' assessment of their conditions revealed improvement in the disease as well. Fewer strides were made in the following six months of the study, but improvements continued.

A team of British researchers analyzed results of several studies in which patients with severe eczema were treated with evening primrose oil. The researchers rated the extent of the skin disorder and improvement in such symptoms as inflammation, dryness, itchiness, and scaliness. Both the treating physicians and the patients reported improvement among those receiving the GLA when compared to the placebo-treated group. Although other studies have produced mixed results, many experts suggest trying evening primrose oil for at least four weeks to treat skin inflammation rather than starting treatment with prednisone or another steroid medication.

Form and Usual Dosages

Evening primrose oil is available in capsule form. Look for products that provide at least 40 mg of GLA per 500 mg of EPO. The usual daily dosage is 2 to 3 g of EPO, or enough to provide 160 to 240 mg of GLA, divided into two or three doses. Higher amounts, up to 360 mg of GLA, may be needed to treat arthritis and severe eczema.

◉ A LITTLE HISTORY

Although evening primrose is a native plant of North America, it has found its way around the world. Seeds from the plants hitched rides in the ballasts of ships traveling from North America to Europe in the seventeenth century, effectively allowing evening primrose a chance to take root in the Old World. From Europe, the plant spread to Asia. It is now cultivated widely for its medicinal oils. However, the early European settlers in the New World copied the Native American practice of using the entire evening primrose plant to treat coughs and intestinal upsets. Of course, they would have done better to use just the seeds, which are the most therapeutic part.

Possible Problems

There is no evidence of side effects or health hazards when you take evening primrose oil at the recommended therapeutic dosages. Very high doses may produce nausea, stomach upset, and headaches.

FENNEL (*FOENICULUM VULGARE*)

Fennel is a perennial plant that is often planted as an ornamental in flower gardens. Fennel's bulb and tall stalk, which look like celery, are consumed as a vegetable; the leaves and seeds are used to flavor soups and other dishes. The taste and aroma of fennel are sometimes mistaken for anise and licorice—two other herbs that have important medicinal uses—but the plant is actually related to caraway. It's fennel seed oil, however, that has medicinal properties.

Common Uses

- Stimulate appetite, aid digestion, prevent nausea, and reduce gas and flatulence.
- Relieve heartburn and indigestion.
- May ease symptoms of premenstrual syndrome (PMS) and menstrual cramps.
- Freshen bad breath.
- Reduce upper respiratory congestion.
- May help soothe infant colic.

How It Works

Fennel seeds contain an oil that is 50 to 60 percent anethol, which is also the chief component of anise oil, and 18 to 22 percent fenchone, a pungent gas. They also contain 2 to 6 percent volatile oil that appears to relax smooth muscles and calm intestinal spasms. Diluted fennel water is a time-honored treatment for infant colic and gas; fennel also helps relieve bloating and intestinal gas in adults.

Fennel oil also contains a substance, estragole, that is a plant (phyto) estrogen, which appears to mimic some of the actions of this female sex hormone. In fact, estragole was once used to produce a synthetic version, and this component may be useful in treating bloating, breast tenderness, and other PMS symptoms as well as menstrual cramps.

⊙ **A LITTLE HISTORY**
Some ancient people believed that fennel restored the vision of snakes after they shed their skins, and they often used fennel for vision problems—a use that has long since been disproved. During the Middle Ages, fennel was placed on doors and windows to prevent the entry of witches. In Colonial times, Puritans were said to carry fennel seeds to church to keep their stomachs from rumbling during the long services; it also masked the odor of alcohol on the breath.

Evidence of Efficacy

A number of studies appear to document at least some of the benefits attributed to fennel. Laboratory studies show that fennel seed extract calms muscle spasms by reducing smooth muscle contractions. German health authorities approve of using fennel for a variety of purposes: treating mild stomach upset, indigestion, bloating, gas, and abdominal cramps. They recommend giving fennel seed to hyperactive children to calm them down, as the seeds may have mild sedative effects. They also approve of various uses of fennel, such as in syrup or honey, to clear upper respiratory congestion.

Studies indicate that substances in fennel can reduce airway congestion by thinning and loosening phlegm; these findings tend to support the addition of fennel in numerous European cough remedies.

In laboratory studies using rats, estragole has been shown to promote lactation as well as menstruation, increase the female sex drive, and decrease the male's. Studies to document these effects in humans, however, have not been done.

Forms and Usual Dosages

Fennel is available in capsules, tea, oil, powder, seeds, and a tincture. It is used to make poultices and as a compress soak. A tea can be made using 1 to 2 teaspoons of bruised seeds per cup of water; double the amount of water or reduce the seeds to ½ teaspoon or less if the tea is intended for a young child.

The tincture is taken in dosages of ½ to 1 teaspoon up to three times a day. Fennel capsules typically provide 455 mg of fennel, and can be taken up to three times per day. Follow package instructions for commercial preparations of this herb.

Potential Problems

Fennel is considered safe when taken in recommended dosages and there is no evidence that it interacts with other botanical or pharmaceutical products. However, some people may experience an allergic reaction to fennel; it has also been reported to increase sun sensitivity in some people. Full-strength fennel oil must be diluted, either in water or a neutral oil, such as olive or vegetable oil. Ingesting even small amounts (1 to 5 ml) of undiluted fennel oil can cause nausea, vomiting, seizures, and respiratory problems, particularly in children. When fed to rats, the oil worsened any existing liver disease, and people with hepatitis, cirrhosis, and other liver disorders are advised not to take fennel. Because of fennel's estrogenlike properties, any woman who has had breast cancer or has been told not to take birth control pills should probably not consume medicinal amounts of fennel.

The Food and Drug Administration (FDA) classifies fennel as GRAS (generally recognized as safe) when used as food. However, the FDA has found that some samples of imported fennel are contaminated with disease-causing bacteria, such as streptococci and salmonella.

FENUGREEK (*TRIGONELLA FOENUM-GRAECUM*)

Fenugreek is an annual herb with leaves that look like those of clover and small, white flowers similar to those of peas. It is a native plant of western Asia and the Mediterranean, but is now grown in northern Africa, India, and parts of the United States.

Through history, fenugreek has been prized not only as a spice but also for its medicinal powers and as cattle feed. In the past, fenugreek was considered a cure for many ailments—indigestion, respiratory infections, skin wounds and inflammation, arthritis, and kidney disorders, among others. Today, fenugreek seeds are used mostly for digestive and skin problems, although some herbalists also recommend it to treat or prevent atherosclerosis and to help control diabetes.

Common Uses

- Treat or prevent digestive problems, including ulcers, bowel inflammation, and constipation.
- Relieve bronchial congestion, calm coughs, and soothe a sore throat.
- Soothe and promote healing of minor skin wounds and infections.
- Lower high blood levels of cholesterol and triglycerides.
- Help manage diabetes.
- Ease menstrual cramps, stimulate uterine contractions during labor, and perhaps relieve menopausal symptoms.

How It Works

The active ingredients in fenugreek are saponins, specifically substances called diosgenin and tigogenin, which are chemically similar to estrogen and steroidal hormones. These may help balance female hormone levels, and perhaps compensate for the lack of estrogen after menopause.

Fenugreek seeds are also rich in mucilage, a soluble fiber that absorbs

⬤ **A LITTLE HISTORY**
Although fenugreek does not have a wide following among many American consumers, our great-grandmothers may well have taken the herb without realizing it—fenugreek was the major ingredient in Lydia Pinkham's Vegetable Compound, a popular nineteenth-century patent medicine used for menstrual problems. Today, fenugreek is used as a flavoring for artificial maple syrup and the bitter seeds are added to curry powder and other flavorings.

large amounts of water and swells to form a soft mass in the intestinal tract, thereby preventing constipation. Mucilage also has a soothing effect on inflamed mucous membranes; when used as a gargle or mouthwash, it can relieve a sore throat and mouth ulcers. Soluble fiber helps control blood sugar (glucose) levels, making fenugreek a beneficial adjunct in treating diabetes. In addition, fenugreek may reduce cholesterol absorption and synthesis, which would explain fenugreek's apparent lipid-lowering effects. A fenugreek ointment or poultice can soothe and promote healing of a boil or other minor skin infections. The oil in fenugreek seeds is also used as a skin softener and emollient.

Evidence of Efficacy

Studies conducted in Europe and Asia have found that fenugreek seeds can help lower blood sugar levels in diabetic animals as well as patients with type 2 (adult-onset) diabetes. Controlled studies in India and elsewhere have also found that fenugreek can reduce total cholesterol levels without lowering the beneficial HDL cholesterol.

A group of French researchers reported studies showing that fenugreek seeds contain substances that stimulate the pancreas to release digestive enzymes and thereby aid digestion.

Animal studies have found that fenugreek extracts can stimulate contractions of the uterine muscles, but this has not been documented in human research. However, herbalists in Asia and the Mediterranean countries often recommend fenugreek to stimulate contractions in delayed or sluggish labor. Some Asian herbal texts claim that fenugreek is also an effective treatment for both male and female infertility, but these claims have not been proved. The estrogenic compounds in fenugreek may help relieve menstrual problems, but this is also unproved.

Forms and Usual Dosages

Fenugreek is available as capsules and tinctures and as whole, crushed, or powdered seeds. It is also an ingredient in some skin ointments and moisturizers. The seeds can be used to make an infusion for a gargle or compress soak. Plain fenugreek seeds have a very bitter taste; however, debittered seeds are available.

The dosage recommended to lower cholesterol or help control blood sugar calls for taking capsules containing 5 to 30 g of fenugreek with each meal. Alternatively, 3 to 4 ml of fenugreek tincture can be taken three times a day.

Potential Problems

Fenugreek appears to be safe, but high doses can cause nausea and an upset stomach; there have also been reports of skin irritation among some people who have used fenugreek ointments or poultices. Because fenugreek contains hormonelike substances, it should not be taken during pregnancy unless specifically recommended by a doctor. The herb also contains ingredients that may interact with blood-thinning drugs, MAO inhibitors (used to treat depression and lower blood pressure), and some diabetes medications. If you are taking these or other medications, check with your doctor before trying fenugreek.

FEVERFEW (*TANACETUM PARTHENIUM*)

This member of the chrysanthemum family is one of the few botanical medicines whose common name is based on an ancient health claim. The name feverfew is derived from the Latin term *febrifugia,* which translates to "driver out of fevers." Also known as the midsummer daisy, feverfew is a perennial that has feathery leaves and numerous small yellow and white blossoms. The plant is often confused with chamomile, but unlike this distant cousin whose flowers contain medicinal oils, it's the feverfew leaves that contain therapeutic ingredients. In the past, feverfew was considered an effective remedy for fevers and a number of other ailments, including menstrual cramps, digestive problems, and intestinal parasites. Feverfew is no longer used for these conditions, but it has gained recognition among both alternative practitioners and traditional physicians as an effective treatment for migraine headaches. This effect is attributed to a compound called parthenolide that is found in feverfew leaves.

Common Uses

- Prevent and perhaps abort a migraine headache if taken during the warning (prodromal) stage.
- Alleviate pain and inflammation from arthritis and other rheumatic diseases.
- Cleanse and disinfect minor skin wounds.
- Relieve skin irritation and inflammation.
- Repel insects.

◉ A LITTLE HISTORY

Throughout history, healers have turned to feverfew for a variety of ailments. Dioscorides, the ancient Greek physician, gave it to women during childbirth to increase uterine contractions and speed the birth process. For centuries, it was thought to lower a fever and treat such diverse ailments as infant colic, depression, vertigo, kidney stones, and constipation. Cotton Mather, the famed American clergyman and writer of the early 1700s, recommended chewing feverfew to ease a toothache. In 1633, the British herbalist Gerard wrote that feverfew was an effective headache remedy, but it wasn't until the 1980s that a team of British researchers discovered that feverfew did, indeed, contain compounds that can prevent or lessen migraine symptoms.

How It Works

Parthenolide—the principle active ingredient in feverfew—appears to work against migraine headaches by reducing blood platelet activity and the release of histamines and prostaglandins, body chemicals that are instrumental in the inflammation and sudden widening of the blood vessels in the head. It also helps prevent the fluctuations in levels of serotonin, another chemical that is instrumental in migraine symptoms.

Feverfew's action in inhibiting production of certain prostaglandins may also explain the herb's apparent effectiveness in reducing menstrual cramps and relieving arthritis and other inflammatory conditions.

Evidence of Efficacy

A number of scientific studies have found that feverfew reduces the frequency and intensity of migraine headaches. However, feverfew is more effective as a preventive measure; it has little effect in relieving symptoms of a full-blown migraine. A two-year British study involving fifty-nine patients who normally suffered at least one migraine headache a month found a significant drop in headache frequency among those who took the feverfew. When headaches did occur, vomiting and other symptoms were milder, but there was no change in the duration of the headaches.

Animal studies have found that feverfew reduces joint and skin inflammation by preventing white blood cells from releasing certain inflammation-causing compounds. However, clinical studies involving patients with rheumatoid arthritis have failed to document any benefit of feverfew on pain, inflammation, and other symptoms. Similarly, there is no scientific evidence that feverfew is effective in treating inflammatory skin conditions.

Forms and Usual Dosages

Feverfew is sold in many forms—pills, capsules of freeze-dried powdered leaves, and liquid leaf extracts. It is also available in combination with magnesium and riboflavin—nutrients that have been shown to reduce the incidence of migraines.

The recommended daily dosage to prevent migraines calls for taking the equivalent of 250 mcg of parthenolide a day. This would require taking about two 400-mg tablets that are standardized to contain 0.4 percent parthenolide. Unfortunately, the quality of many commercial feverfew products is very uneven. Laboratory analyses of products often find little or none of the active ingredient, parthenolide. As an alternative to pills, some experts recommend chewing two or three dried or fresh feverfew leaves a day. The plants are very easy to grow, even in window containers. Some health food outlets also sell the whole dried leaves, which can be chewed or brewed to make a tea. Infuse 2 teaspoons of dried leaves in 8 ounces of hot water; let the brew steep for fifteen minutes before straining. Up to three cups a day can be consumed. A stronger brew is used to treat skin inflammation and minor wounds: Infuse about one-fourth of a cup of the leaves and allow it to steep for about thirty minutes. Soak a compress in the liquid and apply to the skin. (It should be noted, however, that there are no clinical studies to document the efficacy of this use.)

Potential Problems

Chewing fresh or dried feverfew leaves can cause mouth ulcers and a sore tongue. Switch to tea, pills, or liquid extract if sores develop, although similar symptoms may occur. Otherwise, feverfew is quite safe. An exception might be among people who are allergic to other members of the chrysanthemum plant family, which includes ragweed and daisies. They may develop a skin rash and other allergic symptoms when taking feverfew. When used externally, feverfew may cause skin irritation, especially among people with related allergies.

Some experts advise against taking feverfew along with blood-thinning drugs, such as aspirin and warfarin (Coumadin), high-dose vitamin E, and ginkgo biloba extract. It should be avoided by people taking calcium channel blockers or ticlopidine (Ticlid). Feverfew also has mild anticoagulant properties, and combining it with other anti-clotting products may result in bleeding problems. Similarly, feverfew should not be taken with prescription antimigraine drugs. Because feverfew can cause uterine contractions, it should not be used during pregnancy.

See Also

Migraine Headaches

FLAX (*LINUM USITATISSIMUM*)

Also known as flaxseed, linseed, lint bells, linum, and winterlien, this slender-stemmed plant is grown throughout the world in temperate and tropical areas, including North America. It grows eight to sixty inches

The flax plant originated in central Asia, and it has been cultivated for at least five thousand years. Egyptians, Hebrews, Greeks, and Romans used the seeds as food, the oil as medicine, and the fibers to weave clothes, sails, and other items. The Roman legions were renowned for its ability to march long distances and then do battle. Interestingly, their bread was made with flaxseed flour. In more modern times, Roman meal bread also used flaxseed flour. Today, the linseed oil extracted from flax is mainly used in the manufacture of varnish, paint, linoleum, and soap.

tall, producing gray-green leaves and five-petaled, light-blue flowers that open only in the morning. The fruit is a 2½-to-3-inch almost round capsule, containing flat, brown, glossy seeds.

Flax is one of the best plant sources of alpha-linolenic acid, which the body converts to the same heart-protective omega-3 fatty acids found in salmon, sardines, and other cold-water fish. The seeds (but not the seed oil) also contain both soluble and insoluble fiber, which promotes intestinal health, and lignans, a form of phytoestrogens believed to help protect against colon, prostate, and breast cancers. Flaxseeds must be ground into meal before ingestion, because whole seeds will pass through the body undigested. Flax meal has a sweet, nutty flavor.

Common Uses

- Reduce skin irritation.
- Prevent and treat constipation.
- Soothe an irritable colon.
- Treat various intestinal disorders, including diverticulitis, gastritis, and enteritis.
- Reduce high blood cholesterol levels.
- Relieve symptoms of inflammatory arthritis, including rheumatoid arthritis and lupus.

How It Works

When mixed with liquid, flaxseeds swell and form a gelatinous substance that is soothing to the gastrointestinal tract when ingested or to irritated skin and mucous membranes when applied externally. Flax is also a good source of dietary fiber. The seeds absorb fluid in the intestines, forming a soft mass that moves easily through the intestinal tract, thereby preventing or alleviating constipation.

Flax is a good source of lignans, a type of phytoestrogen, which are believed to offer health benefits related to cardiovascular diseases and other disorders. The body uses essential fatty acids to make prostaglandins, hormonelike substances that influence inflammation and the pain it causes. They are classified as omega-3 and omega-6 fatty acids. Sources of omega-3 fatty acids are limited, but include flaxseed and cold-water northern fish, such as salmon, tuna, sardines, mackerel, and herring. Omega-3s are a "good" fat that can help the body manufacture prostaglandins that create a less inflammatory environment, thus easing the symptoms of diseases involving inflammation. The anti-inflammatory impact of flax also may play a role in its cardiovascular benefits. (See Essential Fatty Acids, p. 295.)

Evidence of Efficacy

Research in cardiovascular disease has shown that daily flax can help reduce total serum cholesterol, as well as LDL—the "bad" cholesterol—while leaving intact HDL—the "good" cholesterol. Flax in the diet also may reduce the risk of blood clots, which can cause heart attacks and stroke. Studies have included one in which participants took 15 g of flaxseed daily, as well as ate a bread containing flaxseeds, for three months; another involved a daily supplement of 50 g of ground flaxseed.

Studies of the benefit of flax oil supplements for inflammatory diseases have not had uniform results. Animal and human studies of lupus showed reductions in inflammation and other symptoms and improvements in kidney function. The patients took doses ranging from 15 to 45 g of flaxseed oil a day. But research involving people with rheumatoid arthritis has not been as promising. Extensive research is examining the impact of flax on hormone function, which may have implications for the prevention of breast and colon cancer.

Forms and Usual Dosages

As a good overall health tonic; 1 or 2 tablespoons of ground flaxseed daily is often recommended. As a laxative or therapy for gastritis or enteritis, 1 tablespoon of the whole or crushed seeds should be taken with 5 to 8 ounces of water two or three times a day. Be sure to drink extra water between doses—several glasses throughout the day—because the fiber absorbs fluid as it moves through the digestive tract.

To lower high cholesterol and reduce inflammation, one softgel of 1,300 mg of flax oil (or an equivalent amount of bottled flax oil), is taken once a day to obtain 740 mg of linoleic acid for its anti-inflammatory benefits.

For external use, 30 to 50 g of ground seeds are mixed with warm water to form a poultice or compress.

Potential Problems

Flaxseed oil and ground flax meal should be kept refrigerated in a dark, airtight container to prevent it from turning rancid. It will generally keep for up to a month. Flax that has an oily or "off" odor has spoiled and should be discarded.

Flax is safe for almost everyone (including women who are pregnant or breast-feeding), although its mild laxative effect at recommended doses may trouble people with inflammatory bowel disease. Further, it should not be used by those who have strictures or any other obstruction of the esophagus or bowel or acute inflammatory diseases of the gastrointestinal system.

Flax should not be taken simultaneously with other drugs, because it may delay their absorption.

A word of caution: Only flax preparations designed for human consumption should be used because linseed oil intended for carpentry or cleaning use can be toxic. The medical literature contains at least one report of a woman who had a life-threatening allergic reaction after using linseed oil as a laxative.

See Also

Constipation
Endometriosis

GARLIC
(*ALLIUM SATIVUM*)

◉ A LITTLE HISTORY
Cultivated for more than five thousand years, garlic is mentioned in the Old Testament and has been handed down through the centuries as a preventive medicine and folk remedy. The ancient world recorded its uses: Hippocrates and Artistotle recommended garlic therapies; the Roman naturalist Pliny listed more than sixty uses for the herb, including driving away scorpions and curing asthma and epilepsy. Its antibiotic properties were first studied by Louis Pasteur in the mid-nineteenth century. In the twentieth century, Albert Schweitzer used it to treat amebic dysentery in Africa. It has been prescribed for tuberculosis and was used as an antiseptic during World War II when penicillin and sulfa drugs were in short supply.

Garlic is the bulb of a tall flowering plant in the lily family, which includes onions, leeks, chives, shallots, and scallions. The bulb is made up of individual garlic cloves surrounded by layers of thin papery skin that are usually peeled away to prepare the garlic for consumption. Garlic may be consumed raw, cooked, or in any number of prepared forms, such as oils, pills, extracts, and juices.

It has been cultivated for thousands of years and used to flavor food and for its medicinal qualities. For centuries, garlic has been an accepted treatment for numerous disorders—colds and flu, coughs, ringworm, intestinal worms, fever, and digestive disorders. Recent studies indicate that garlic may be an effective treatment for hardening of the arteries (atherosclerosis), high blood pressure, elevated blood cholesterol, and a tendency to form blood clots. In dosages high enough to be therapeutic (usually the equivalent of one or two cloves a day), bad breath and intestinal upsets are common complications.

Common Uses

- Help lower mild high blood pressure.
- Reduce blood cholesterol levels.
- Hinder blood clotting, thereby lowering the risk of heart attack and stroke.
- Alleviate cold symptoms.
- Promote healing of minor skin infections and wounds.

- Treat or prevent common fungal infections, including ringworm, swimmer's ear, and athlete's foot.
- May aid in digestive and intestinal disorders.

How It Works

Although garlic has traditionally been prescribed for everything from warding off witches' spells to treating leprosy and intestinal worms, researchers today are concentrating on its ability to reduce the risk factors associated with heart disease. Studies suggest that it can lower several cardiovascular risk factors, including lowering high blood pressure and cholesterol levels, reducing clot formation, and helping prevent atherosclerosis. It may also be helpful in preventing certain cancers.

The key therapeutic ingredient in garlic is alliin, which is converted to allicin and other compounds when the bulb is crushed or ingested. Allicin contains sulfur and sulfur compounds that are responsible not only for garlic's characteristic odor but also for derivative compounds such as ajoene, methyl ajoene, and dithiins.

Garlic appears to lower the risk of heart attack and stroke by inhibiting the ability of blood platelets to clump together to form clots. Garlic contains polyphenol—a substance also found in red wine and certain vegetables—which helps prevent the formation of plaque, the fatty substance that leads to atherosclerosis when it collects in the artery walls. It is thought to help lower blood pressure by relaxing the smooth muscles that control artery walls, thereby allowing the vessels to open wider and carry more blood with less pressure. It is not known how garlic lowers cholesterol levels, but medical scientists theorize that allicin somehow interferes with the liver's ability to make cholesterol.

Researchers are also investigating whether garlic may prevent certain cancers. So far, the evidence is mixed, although population studies indicate that people who eat a lot of garlic have a reduced risk of certain cancers. Garlic's antiviral, antibacterial, and antifungal properties may derive from allicin's ability to block the enzymes that normally allow these organisms to invade body tissues.

Evidence of Efficacy

Researchers have been studying the effects of garlic on the body for years, and hundreds of studies have been published suggesting how garlic works and trying to pinpoint the specific properties of the herb that are responsible for its metabolic and disease-fighting effects. Many positive results have been found in animal studies, but the findings have not been duplicated in controlled clinical studies in humans. For example, garlic has been fed to hypertensive rats and dogs, with statistically significant reductions in blood pressure. Other animal studies suggest that garlic's sulfur-containing compounds inhibit the stiffening of the aorta in an aging population. But human studies have not been so conclusive. Although many researchers believe that garlic has definite health benefits, it is not known how much must be consumed to be effective. Nonetheless, population studies in Italy and Spain, where large amounts of garlic are consumed, have found that atherosclerosis is uncommon, despite a high-fat diet, although it's becoming more common in large cities even there.

Compounds in garlic have been shown to have anticlotting properties when mixed with blood platelets in a test tube. In one laboratory study, ajoene prevented the formation of blood clots in dogs undergoing open-heart surgery. Other studies have found that ajoenes and dithiins may possess antitumor and antifungal activities, and thus may help prevent cancer and various yeast infections.

Researchers are also investigating the antioxidant properties of compounds in garlic, which may also help prevent cancer. Sixteen separate studies in animals suggest that garlic inhibits the development of tumors, even in those exposed to carcinogenic materials such as carbon tetrachloride, isoproterenol, and heavy metal poisoning. But other studies found that, in rats, garlic does not inhibit tumor growth once cancer has developed.

Forms and Usual Dosages

Garlic is available in many forms—fresh bulbs that can be bought in any produce market as well as pills and extracts. Many experts believe that the most benefits are obtained from the whole garlic, preferably raw or very lightly cooked. When pills are taken, the recommended daily dosage is 300 mg of powder a day, the equivalent of the allicin in one or two whole cloves.

Potential Problems

Garlic is notorious for causing an unpleasant breath and body odor. This problem can be lessened by taking deodorized garlic pills, but even in pill form, large dosages of 900 to 1,200 mg a day can cause a garlicky body odor. Some people also experience an upset stomach, heartburn, and other intestinal problems, even when they eat only a small amount of garlic. Because of its anticlotting properties, high doses of garlic should not be used by anyone taking blood-thinning medications or who have bleeding problems.

See Also

Cancer
Cholesterol Disorders and Atherosclerosis

Common Cold and Flu
High Blood Pressure
Leg Cramps and Restless Legs

GINGER (*ZINGIBER OFFICINALE*)

Ginger, a perennial that is native to India and parts of China, is now cultivated in most tropical parts of the world and in containers or greenhouses in temperate climates. Fresh or dried, the rhizome of the underground ginger stem has a distinctive spicy taste and lemony scent that has been used both to flavor foods and to ease nausea and promote digestion in nearly every culture since ancient times. In addition, practitioners of Chinese medicine and Ayurvedic physicians in India have relied on it for centuries for its anti-inflammatory properties and have used it as a "carrier" herb, one that enables other herbs to be more effective in the body. Jamaicans as well as early American settlers made beer from it, and today, natural ginger ales made with fresh ginger are available as a digestive tonic. These should not be confused with most commercial brands of ginger ale, however; these contain so little ginger that they are simply sweet soft drinks with no medicinal value.

Modern herbalists use ginger root for the same purpose, and often suggest it for nausea regardless of cause, from motion sickness to morning sickness, and other gastrointestinal upsets from heartburn to stomach cramps. Ginger has been approved by German health authorities for medicinal uses.

⊙ A LITTLE HISTORY

Medieval theologians believed that ginger came from the Garden of Eden. While this claim remains unproved, there's no doubt that ginger enjoys a long and colorful history. Indeed, an ancient Indian proverb holds that "everything good is found in ginger," perhaps a reflection of the fact that ginger has played a central role in Asian cuisine and medicine for thousands of years. Greek bakers used the spice to flavor bread more than four thousand years ago, and perhaps even made the first gingerbread man. Spanish explorers brought it to the New World via Jamaica; where ginger beer remains a favorite drink.

Common Uses

- Nausea due to motion sickness, early pregnancy, chemotherapy and other cancer treatments, and miscellaneous other causes.
- Numerous digestive problems, including indigestion, upset stomach, gas, and abdominal cramps.
- Loss of appetite.
- Cold and flu symptoms.
- Menstrual irregularities and problems.
- Impotence.
- Depression.
- Mild pain such as that of inflammatory arthritis.
- Migraine headaches.
- High blood cholesterol.

- Dandruff, skin inflammation, and minor burns.
- Sore throat.

How It Works

Ginger is believed to stimulate appetite, soothe the intestinal tract, and promote digestion by increasing the flow of saliva and gastric juices. In addition to quelling nausea, its antispasmodic action may relieve the uterine contractions of menstrual cramps. It also contains zingibain, an enzyme that has anti-inflammatory properties, and many antioxidants that also counter inflammation. Other natural anti-inflammatory components reduce production of certain prostaglandins, thereby easing the pain of arthritis, headaches, and muscle pain. The components that give ginger its pungency—substances called gingerols—are thought to be responsible for its usefulness in treating fever and pain. Its volatile oils may be natural killers of cold and flu viruses.

When used externally in a poultice or as an ointment, ginger soothes inflammation and promotes healing. Some herbalists recommend mixing fresh ginger juice with a neutral oil, such as sesame or olive oil, and applying it to the scalp to control dandruff. Mixed with lemon juice, vinegar, and honey, ginger makes a soothing gargle for a sore throat.

Evidence of Efficacy

In a Danish study involving naval cadets who were prone to developing seasickness, subjects in the group receiving ginger were less likely to develop symptoms than those in the placebo group. Another study found that ginger was about as effective as Dramamine—a drug commonly used to prevent motion sickness. However, other placebo-controlled studies have produced mixed results, with some showing that ginger reduces nausea, vomiting, and other symptoms, while others have found that a placebo works just as well.

Some migraine sufferers report that ginger can abort a headache when taken during its early stages. Researchers theorize that this benefit may come from substances called shogaols, as well as gingerols, which reduce platelet clumping and may prevent the blood-vessel inflammation that causes migraine pain. The evidence that ginger root improves arthritis conditions is mostly anecdotal, although one small study involving women with rheumatoid arthritis found that most obtained relief of joint pain and inflammation when taking 1 g of powdered ginger a day. More clinical studies are needed, however, to verify ginger's effectiveness against arthritis. Still, because ginger is quite safe, many practitioners suggest there is no harm in trying ginger to see if it alleviates arthritis pain and inflammation.

Forms and Usual Dosages

Typically ginger is taken in powdered form in a capsule, but it's also available fresh or dried, as a liquid or tincture, tea, honey syrup, or covered in sugar and eaten as a candy. Tea can be made from the dried powder or by boiling slices of the root in water. The usual daily recommended dose is 3 to 10 g of fresh ginger or 2 to 4 g of dried ginger. For motion sickness, 1,000 to 1,500 mg in a capsule is suggested a half hour before traveling, as is nibbling on crystallized ginger candy during travel. A square inch of candy is equal to about 500 mg. For digestion, take 2 teaspoons of powdered ginger or a teaspoon of grated ginger root in a cup of water. For pregnant women, a cup of ginger tea or real ginger ale may help relieve nausea. However, a pregnant woman should check with her doctor before taking ginger, or any herbal preparation.

Potential Problems

Some people develop heartburn from ginger, but this is an uncommon side effect. However, it should not be taken by people with a history of gallbladder disease because it may provoke a flare-up. People with mouth sores may find fresh or candied ginger is too irritating; powdered ginger and tea are unlikely to cause problems.

There have been reports that large amounts of ginger root may affect hormone levels in the fetus. This has led some doctors to advise against its use during pregnancy, although small amounts taken to ease morning sickness are probably safe.

See Also

Arthritis
Migraine Headaches
Nausea

GINKGO
(*GINKGO BILOBA*)

Originally native to China, the ginkgo tree is now cultivated around the world. It is also known as bai guo, kew tree, and maidenhair tree. It grows up to 120 feet in height and can live for hundreds of years. The rough-grooved bark is light to dark brown; in the male trees the grooves are broad and in the females they are pointed. Both have green, leathery, fan-shaped leaves that turn yellow to golden in the fall. The trees start to flower only when they are more than twenty years old. The female develops apricot-sized seeds, sometimes called fruit, that have a foul smell.

Both the leaves and the seeds have been used for medicinal purposes. In the 1930s, flavonoids in the leaves were first identified. In the 1970s, an extract of the leaves was developed. In the United States, plantations grow ginkgo and process the dried leaves to create a concentrated extract standardized to a potency of 24 percent flavone glycosides (primarily quercetin, kaempferol, and isorhamnetin) and 6 percent terpene lactones (about equal parts of bilobalide and ginkgolides A, B, and C). This extract, called GBE for ginkgo biloba extract, is the form of ginkgo now used medicinally and under study for its active ingredients and effects.

Common Uses

- Preserve memory.
- Treat mild depression and reduce symptoms of early Alzheimer's disease and other cognitive problems.
- Improve circulation and treat leg pains due to reduced blood flow (intermittent claudication).
- Treat erectile dysfunction.
- Reduce risk of blood clots.
- Treat inner ear disorders such as tinnitus and vertigo.
- Possible treatment for allergies, asthma, and inflammatory disorders.

How It Works

The primary benefits of ginkgo seem to derive from its ability to promote the widening (dilation) of blood vessels, which improves blood flow in tiny vessels throughout the body. For example, this can reduce the buildup of fluids (edema) throughout the body and reduce symptoms of a wide range of disorders affecting the legs, brain, eyes, ears, and other organs. It also seems to inhibit the formation of blood clots and functions as an antioxidant, reducing the cellular damage caused by free radicals, unstable molecules that are a by-product of oxygen metabolism and that form as a response to inflammation and exposure to the sun and certain pollutants. It also may affect brain chemicals (neurotransmitters), such as norpinephrine, serotonin, monoamine oxidase, acetylcholine, and nitric oxide, as well as inhibit the synthesis of corticosteroids.

Evidence of Efficacy

In addition to hundreds of years of medicinal use in China and other parts of Asia, numerous studies from around the world document the benefits of ginkgo. For example, studies in Europe and more recently in the United States indicate that GBE may improve circulation to the brain, especially among older people with atherosclerosis, the clotting of arteries with fatty plaque. In one clinical study, people with uncomplicated dementia had a 25 percent improvement in cognitive function after four to six weeks of ginkgo. Other dementia studies have reported benefits on cognitive and social function for six months to a year. A study of 112 people, their average age seventy, showed improvements in short-term memory and an easing of such symptoms as headache, vertigo, tinnitus (ringing in the ears), and mood disturbance after a year of ginkgo therapy.

Research on disorders directly related to circulatory problems includes a study on impotence related to impaired blood supply to the penis, in which half of sixty participants regained erectile function after twelve to eighteen months of ginkgo. A study of patients with intermittent claudication, caused by arteriosclerosis, demonstrated significant improvement in the distance people could walk before experiencing pain. Other research has shown improvements in visual acuity in people with macular degeneration.

In a study of people with asthma, dosing with ginkgo seemed to help prevent bronchospasm in response to a challenge with dust or pollen. Other research has supported the benefits of ginkgo in hearing problems related to poor blood flow to nerves critical to hearing, and in vertigo associated with inner-ear problems.

Although the theoretical basis of ginkgo's benefits would support its use in many other conditions, clinical research has not yet confirmed its value in the treatment of asthma, inflammatory conditions, heart attack, ischemic stroke, shock, abnormal heart rhythms, hemorrhoids, leg ulcers, phlebitis, Raynaud's syndrome, anaphylaxis, kidney disease, or graft rejection. Only laboratory—not human—studies support its potential antioxidant benefits for inflammatory conditions.

Forms and Usual Dosages

GBE, the standardized extract, is available as a liquid or powder in capsules and tablets, as well as in an injectable form used for intravenous dosing in Europe and the Far East. The typical dose recommended is 40 mg of a standardized extract taken three times a day with meals, although 60 mg may be taken by those fifty and over to help prevent age-related circulatory problems. However, studies have reported doses as high as 120 to 240 mg three times a day in people with cerebral insufficiency and dementia. Further, doses as high as 6 g of leaves as an infusion are prescribed in traditional Chinese medicine.

Benefits may begin as early as three weeks after initiating ginkgo, although at least six weeks is usually necessary. Improvement often is not evident for several months. Its benefits appear to increase over time.

Potential Problems

Because of its antithrombotic activity, ginkgo can present problems for people taking blood thinners, such as warfarin (Coumadin) or aspirin, by increasing their risk of severe bleeding. Anyone with ulcers or heavy menstrual periods should not take ginkgo. For the same reason, doctors advise that ginkgo should be discontinued at least two weeks before elective surgery. In the event of emergency surgery, be sure to tell your surgeon about all supplements you have been taking, especially ginkgo. Further, ginkgo should be avoided by people with bleeding disorders, such as hemophilia, and those at risk for hemorrhagic stroke, especially those who smoke or use amphetamines or cocaine. Practitioners advise discontinuing ginkgo use during pregnancy and breast-feeding.

Other than this risk, ginkgo use is generally known for its safety when taken in the recommended doses. About 4 percent of users have minor gastrointestinal problems. Only rarely have other problems occurred, such as headache or dizziness, even in people who have taken much higher than recommended dosages. Serious allergic and hypersensitivity reactions are extremely rare, but there have been a few reports of skin rashes and other allergic responses.

See Also

Alzheimer's Disease and Memory Loss
Circulatory Problems
Depression
Dermatitis/Eczema
Leg Cramps and Restless Legs
Migraine Headaches
Sexual Dysfunction

GINSENG (*PANAX QUINQUEFOLIUS*—AMERICAN; *PANAX GINSENG*—ASIAN)

Ginseng is perhaps the best known and most widely used of the panacea botanical medicines—substances that foster good health and are effective against a wide variety of ailments. Indeed, *panax,* the scientific name for American and Asian ginseng, means "all healing," although there is little scientific evidence to back the myriad claims for the herb.

The roots of the ginseng plant have been highly valued in Asian medicine for thousands of years as a general tonic to boost energy, relieve stress, and bring various body functions into balance. The plant grows in wooded areas and has yellow-green flowers and red berries, with roots that are said to grow in the shape of the human form. Since it's a slow-growing plant—it takes six years to mature—it is difficult and expensive to grow.

The American version (*P. quinquefolius*) is virtually identical to the Asian variety (*P. ginseng*), although some herbalists believe it is more sedative and relaxing, producing yin energy to balance the Asian variety's yang. Until recently, most of the ginseng grown in this country was exported to China and other Asian countries, but this is changing because a growing number of Americans are taking ginseng. The Siberian variety (*Eleutherococcus senticosus*) is considered more adaptogenic than the other varieties. However, the plant matures more quickly than the Asian and American varieties, and is therefore less expensive to cultivate. Its active ingredients are lignans and coumarin derivatives, with effects that are considered to be milder than those of the American and Asian varieties.

Common Uses

- Increase physical stamina and mental alertness, as a general health tonic.
- Counter stress (*E. senticosus* only).
- Relieve symptoms associated with fatigue, such as insomnia, poor appetite, nervousness, and restlessness.
- Balance female sex hormones and relieve symptoms of premenstrual syndrome, menstrual problems, and menopause (*P. quinquefolius* only).

How It Works

The major active ingredients in the Asian and American ginsengs are ginsenosides, which are composed of more than twenty saponin triterpenoid glycosides. In the body, these substances are thought to function like steroid hormones, but herbalists value them for what they call adaptogenic (body-balancing) properties. Ginseng also contains polysaccharides and other compounds that may have medicinal effects, such as bolstering immunity and helping control blood sugar (glucose) levels.

Although American herbalists do not make distinctions between the varieties, Asian herbalists do and find that American ginseng is rich in the Rb1 group of ginsenosides, which are said to have a more sedative,

◉ A LITTLE HISTORY
Ancient Chinese medical texts advocate ginseng to "quiet the spirit and increase wisdom." At one time, ginseng was so valued in China that only those designated by the emperor were allowed to gather it. But ginseng was also prized in the New World. Long before the arrival of European explorers and settlers, Native Americans gathered the ginseng root to use as a general tonic to help restore health to the weak and wounded and to "help the mind."

Jesuit settlers in Canada began exporting American ginseng to China in the early 1700s, and China continues to import large amounts of ginseng from the United States and Canada. However, wild ginseng has been harvested so heavily that it has disappeared in many places where it was once abundant. To compensate, the Canadian government now restricts the gathering of wild ginseng and, to meet consumer demands, the plant is now being cultivated in North America, Europe, and many Asian countries.

or "cooling," effect on the central nervous system. In contrast, Asian ginseng has a somewhat different Rg1 group of ginsenosides that are more arousing and stimulating, or "warming" to the body. Both forms are said to improve circulation, including increasing blood flow to the brain and producing a sense of mental alertness; the increased blood flow may also slow the progression of Alzheimer's disease. Siberian ginseng, which is used by the Russian cosmonauts and many athletes, is said to improve stamina and resistance to stress.

Asian herbalists recommend ginseng to enhance male sexual performance although there is marginal evidence to support this belief. It is also said to balance the female sex hormones and lessen symptoms associated with menstruation and menopause (although it can cause heavy bleeding), much in the same way that the closely related dong quai, also known as the female ginseng, works.

Evidence of Efficacy

Most of the published research on the effects of ginseng have been done in Asia and Russia, although a number of European and American researchers are also studying its properties. Human studies have produced mixed results, with some showing benefits in improved endurance and others finding no measurable effects. This could be because different types of ginseng were used or because of differing chemical makeup of the extracts used.

A number of animal studies have found that those receiving ginseng are more resistant to infection and stress-related problems. Some studies have focused on the animals' mental function—for example, the ability to learn and remember tasks. Others have looked at physiological effects, such as metabolism, control of blood sugar, and increased immune-system activity. Many have produced positive results, but it is not known whether these findings apply to humans. However, a large-scale population study in Korea found that people who took ginseng had a much lower incidence of cancer when compared to a similar group that did not take the substance.

Of course, there are many anecdotal accounts of ginseng's benefits. Many athletes and bodybuilders insist that it improves stamina, mental alertness, and ability to compete. Efforts to isolate compounds in ginseng that may account for these benefits have so far been fruitless and studies aimed at documenting physical changes, such as more efficient use of oxygen, have produced conflicting results.

Forms and Usual Dosages

Fresh or dried ginseng root may be added to soup or can be taken as infusions or in capsules. To make ginseng tea, pour boiling water over 3 g of the chopped root and steep for five to ten minutes. The average daily dose is 1 to 2 g of the root. The tea may be taken three to four times a day. Various commercial ginseng root preparations are also available. Such standardized extracts are often taken at the rate of 100 to 200 mg daily, although commercial strengths can vary, so follow manufacturer's recommended dosages. The quality of products also varies widely; one well-publicized study analyzed fifty-four ginseng products and found that one-fourth of them contained no ginseng at all, and others provided less than the stated amount. Some even contained dirt, filler, and other substances.

Potential Problems

Ginseng is safe when used in recommended dosages, but the best advice is to start with a low dose, give it some time to work (usually a few weeks), and then, if necessary, increase the dosage slowly. It should not be taken for several weeks without a break. Very high doses can cause nausea, vomiting, sleeplessness, muscle tension, and fluid retention. Anyone with high blood pressure should check with a doctor before taking ginseng. Its safety during pregnancy and breast-feeding has not been established so it's wise not to take it during these times. Avoid taking ginseng in extremely hot weather. Individuals with ischemic or vascular heart disease, thyroid disease, diabetes, or migraine should not take ginseng.

See Also

Chronic Fatigue Syndrome
Menopause
Sexual Dysfunction

GOLDENSEAL (*HYDRASTIS CANADENSIS*)

Goldenseal, a perennial, has a flowering stem that appears in the spring and yields small three-petaled, greenish white flowers. Its inedible fruit looks like oblong raspberries. Goldenseal is native to the eastern coast of North America but is becoming rare in the wild because of over-harvesting. However, herb growers have begun to domesticate and cultivate it, so supplies are increasing.

Many of the alternate names for goldenseal refer to the color of its pulp and root, such as yellow root, yellow puccoon, wild curcuma, jaundice root, and turmeric root. Others are derived from its history as a remedy among Native Americans, such as Indian dye, Indian paint, and Indian plant. Others include ground raspberry, hydrastine, eye root, and eye balm. The medicinal parts are the root and the long yellow rhizome, an underground stem out of which the root fibers grow. These parts are dug up in the autumn and dried; the powdered root is then made into various botanical medicines. One of its key compounds, an alkaloid called hydrastine, is sometimes used alone.

Medically, goldenseal is used to bolster the immune system and to treat diverse infections. Modern herbalists prize it for its antiseptic, anti-inflammatory, astringent, and tonic benefits; in fact, it is often called the "poor man's ginseng." It is often taken in combination with echinacea to treat colds and flu since it has a reputation for boosting the effectiveness of other herbs.

Common Uses

- Treat upper respiratory infections, including the common cold, flu, and sore throats.
- Heal minor eye infections such as conjunctivitis and blepharitis.
- Soothe intestinal problems, including indigestion, ulcers, constipation, diverticulitis, and Crohn's disease.
- Relieve the pain of sciatica and muscle and joint disorders.
- Treat gynecological disorders, including vaginitis, menstrual disorders, and postpartum bleeding.
- Treat urinary tract infections.
- Treat or prevent various skin problems, including herpes cold sores, chapped lips, eczema, acne, dandruff, and ringworm.

How It Works

The two primary alkaloids in goldenseal are hydrastine and berberine; it also has lower levels of canadine. Berberine is the most extensively researched of these components and seems to have some antibiotic properties. Further, the alkaloids have mild laxative, astringent, antiseptic, and anti-inflammatory effects. On the negative side, they can cause constriction of small blood vessels, which can raise blood pressure. Also, prolonged use depletes intestinal flora; supplement with acidophilus.

Evidence of Efficacy

Evidence of goldenseal's benefits come mostly from anecdotal accounts and folklore; there are no recent clinical studies of the herb or its active ingredients. However, hydrastine and berberine are recognized as drugs in a number of countries. Based on documented studies, the most justifiable uses for goldenseal are likely as a mouthwash for canker sores and other minor sores involving mucous membranes; it may also be helpful in treating minor infections.

Although goldenseal causes blood-vessel constriction, which may help stop bleeding, there is no evidence that it reduces postpartum bleeding or heavy menstrual flow. Animal studies have yielded contradictory results, sometimes calming uterine spasm but also stimulating uterine contractions.

Human studies done nearly fifty years ago showed some benefits for berberine as a digestive aid because it stimulates bile secretion. It may also kill some of the intestinal bacteria that can cause ulcers and diarrhea.

Although the alkaloids may have some tumor-fighting potential, no human studies have been done. Similarly, although they may help lower blood sugar levels, much more research is needed before goldenseal can be considered an effective treatment for diabetes.

Forms and Usual Dosages

For external use, goldenseal is available as a tea and hydrastine is an ingredient in many eyewashes. For internal use, in addition to the tea, health food stores carry capsules, extracts, gargles, powders, and tinctures, as well as the raw or dried goldenseal rhizomes and roots. Practitioners recommend varying doses, from 500 to 6,000 mg a day of the dried root powder, 4 to 6 ml of liquid herbal extracts, or one dropperful of tincture two to three times a day. A gargle or mouthwash can be made by adding a teaspoon of the powder to one cup of water.

Long-term use is not recommended. Some practitioners suggest discontinuation after a week, while others recommend not using it for more than three weeks without a break of at least two weeks.

Potential Problems

Compared to similar infection-fighting herbs, such as echinacea and astragalus, goldenseal is more expensive and probably less effective. As a result, some manufacturers adulterate it with less costly herbs, such as yellow dock, bloodroot, barberry, and wild Oregon grape. Some of these can cause unpleasant side effects. Goldenseal has a potent, bitter taste. Because of this, its use as a tea or mouth rinse can be very unpleasant unless you mask the taste with honey, lemon, or sugar.

Taken as recommended, goldenseal is generally safe. However, high doses or long-term use can lead to vomiting and other intestinal symptoms, a slowed heartbeat, and possible nervous system effects, including anxiety, hallucinations, delirium, and muscle spasms.

Topical formulations can cause skin sores. Goldenseal douches can cause vaginal irritation and should not be used. Although goldenseal is sometimes recommended as an eyewash, doctors strongly advise against this use as possible contamination can cause a serious eye infection.

Goldenseal should not be used by women who are pregnant or breast-feeding or by anyone who is allergic to plants in the daisy family, such as chamomile and marigold. Finally, it should not be taken by people who have high blood pressure, diabetes, glaucoma, a history of stroke or heart disease, or any autoimmune disease such as multiple sclerosis, rheumatoid arthritis, or lupus.

See Also

Bronchitis
Common Cold and Flu
Mouth Sores
Nausea

GOTU KOLA (CENTELLA ASIATICA)

Gotu kola is a perennial herb that thrives in the swampy areas of the tropics. It has clusters of red flowers and bears fruit, but the small, fan-shaped leaves are where its medicinal value lies. It enjoys a long history as a healing herb in the Ayurveda medicine of India and herbalists in other tropical areas prize it for its wound-healing properties. Since the late 1800s, gotu kola has been used in France and other European countries to promote healing of burns and other skin wounds. It is relatively new in the United States, but interest in its healing properties has increased in the last few decades.

Gotu kola appears to be most useful in building healthy connective tissue, thereby reducing formation of scar tissue. It may also improve circulation, probably by strengthening the walls of veins and other blood vessels.

Common Uses

- Promote healing of skin wounds and disorders, including psoriasis and leprosy.
- Reduce scarring of surgical incisions and other wounds.
- Treat varicose veins and improve circulation, especially to the lower legs.

- Help build connective tissue.
- Improve memory and slow the aging process.

How It Works

Gotu kola contains two important glucosides: asiaticoside prompts wound healing and madecasosside is an anti-inflammatory. These actions are believed to account for the herb's wound-healing properties. In addition, these substances appear to reduce the risk of scarring.

Gotu kola strengthens the wall of veins, thereby helping to prevent varicose veins. It contains substances that are used to build brain chemicals (neurotransmitters) that are instrumental in memory and learning. In this regard, it shows promise in slowing progression of Alzheimer's disease; it may also improve learning among children with developmental disorders.

In Sri Lanka and other tropical areas, gotu kola has a long tradition of use in treating leprosy. Studies attribute its apparent effectiveness to asiaticoside, a substance that destroys the protective cell walls of the bacterium that causes leprosy.

Evidence of Efficacy

Numerous clinical studies have documented the value of gotu kola in treating skin ulcers, wounds, and chronic disorders such as psoriasis. A standardized gotu kola extract, called TECA, has been shown to speed healing of burns, skin ulcers, skin grafts, and surgical incisions. It has also been used to heal skin tuberculosis and bladder ulcers. These various studies showed that TECA not only promoted healing, but it also reduced the formation of scar tissue. In a small study involving patients with severe psoriasis, five of the seven participants had their skin lesions disappear within seven weeks. More clinical study is needed, however, to prove that gotu kola is an effective psoriasis treatment.

A well-controlled double-blind study involving patients with reduced circulation in their legs (intermittent claudication) compared gotu kola and a placebo. After eight weeks of treatment, patients receiving a standardized extract of the herb showed marked improvement in symptoms, including reduced pain, swelling, and sensation of heaviness.

In a study of thirty children with learning disabilities, researchers found that the youngsters who received gotu kola for twelve weeks showed improvement in their concentration and attention span. Laboratory studies have also found that the herb improves the ability of animals to remember how to perform certain tasks.

In 1995, researchers reported that gotu kola extract killed cancer cells in a laboratory culture. Much more study is needed, however, to establish that the herb can help prevent cancer.

Forms and Usual Dosages

Gotu kola is available in capsule, tablet, powder, and tincture forms, and as dried leaves that can be brewed as a tea. The recommended dosage for varicose veins and poor leg circulation calls for taking one 200-mg pill of standardized gotu kola extract three times a day. Instead of pills, a tea can be made using ½ to 1 teaspoon of dried leaves per cup; drink two cups a day. To heal burns and other skin wounds, take 200 mg twice a day. Compresses soaked in gotu kola tea also promote healing.

Potential Problems

Gotu kola is safe in the recommended dosages, although there have been reports of some people developing skin irritation from external applications. Very large doses may cause drowsiness.

See Also

Varicose Veins

GUARANA (*PAULLINIA CUPANA, P. SORBILIS*)

Guarana, a perennial climbing shrub that grows in the Amazon, produces brightly colored red and orange fruits that have black seeds. These seeds are dried and crushed to make a thick paste, which is one of our richest sources of caffeine.

Common Uses

- Promote mental alertness, stave off drowsiness, and improve memory.
- Suppress appetite.
- Enhance athletic performance.

In addition, native tribes in the Amazon use guarana as a general tonic and as a:

◉ A LITTLE HISTORY

The Maues-Sateres Indians of the Amazon are credited with discovering the medicinal properties of guarana seeds. For thousands of years, the native peoples of the Amazon have made a paste of crushed guarana seeds and used it as a general tonic and to treat dysentery. To stave off hunger during periods of fasting, they consumed guarana paste; they also considered it an aphrodisiac. French traders and explorers took guarana to their homeland, where it became a popular stimulant during the nineteenth century; this continues to be the major use of guarana. In fact, a carbonated soft drink called simply Guarana is touted as the national drink of Brazil.

- Diuretic to prevent swelling from excessive body fluid.
- Painkiller for headaches, arthritis, muscle aches, and menstrual cramps.
- Fever and malaria medication.

How It Works

Most of guarana's effects are attributed to its high caffeine content. The seed paste contains 3 to 8 percent caffeine, compared to coffee beans' 1 to 2 percent. The tannins in guarana are thought to slow the body's absorption and metabolism of the plant's caffeine, so that its effects are not experienced as quickly as those of coffee but they last longer. In addition to promoting mental alertness and wakefulness, caffeine enhances athletic endurance, perhaps by reducing a buildup of lactic acid in the muscles. Because caffeine helps suppress appetite, guarana may be a useful weight-loss aid. There is also some evidence that caffeine has a positive effect on memory; it also has a diuretic effect, but there are other more effective botanicals to treat fluid retention.

Evidence of Efficacy

Guarana itself has not been studied extensively, but caffeine—its major active ingredient—has been widely researched in both animals and humans (see Caffeine, p. 277). Animals studies have found that guarana may improve physical performance and memory, but human studies have produced mixed or negative results.

Forms and Usual Dosages

Guarana is available as dried seeds and in powdered form, which can be used to make a stimulating tea. It also may be taken in capsule, pill, and syrup forms, and it is an ingredient in some herbal weight-loss products. Dosages range from 250 to 1,200 mg, with the caffeine content varying from 10 to 15 percent, or about 20 to 200 mg.

Potential Problems

Guarana appears to be safe for adults when consumed in moderate amounts, but like other sources of caffeine, it can cause insomnia, jittery nerves, palpitations, and an upset stomach. It may also interact with a number of medications, including cimetidine, a histamine blocker that is used to treat heartburn; antianxiety drugs such as diazepam (Valium); MAO inhibitors, drugs used to treat anxiety and depression; antihypertensives, and some antibiotics and decongestants. It should not be taken during pregnancy and breast-feeding or by patients with cardiac arrhythmias, anxiety, high blood pressure, and other disorders in which caffeine should be avoided.

GUGGUL (*COMMIPHORA MUKUL*)

⊙ **A LITTLE HISTORY**

The earliest known reference to the medicinal properties of guggul is in one of the Vedas, or holy scriptures of the Hindus. Freely translated, it states that "consumption does not afflict and the curse never affects he who is penetrated with the delicious odor of the healing Guggul. The disease flees from him in all directions, like horses and deer." The classic Ayurvedic medical text, the Sushrutasamhita, describes the usefulness of guggul in treating obesity and other disorders of fat metabolism including "coating and obstruction of channels"—an apt description of atherosclerosis.

Guggul grows throughout the arid areas of northwest India and in Pakistan and Bangladesh. Also known as the Indian myrrh tree, it has been used in Ayurvedic medicine for centuries. (Guggul should not be confused with its close relative of the same family, *Commiphora molmol,* which is simply called myrrh; see p. 508.)

Guggul is a bushy shrub with thorny branches and ovoid fruits that ripen to a red color. Of interest medicinally is its ash-colored bark, which peels into thin rolls. Like most members of the Burseracea family, guggul has ducts in the bark that hold a liquid called a gum resin. The trees are tapped from November through June by shaving a thin band of bark from the base. The resin soon begins to ooze and up to a kilogram can be harvested from each tree. The gummy drops vary in color from pale yellow, to brown or dull green. It has a bitter, aromatic taste and balsamic odor.

The resin contains a combination of steroids, diterpenoids, alipathic esters, and carbohydrates. The steroids, called guggulsterones, differentiate guggul from the nearly two hundred other *Commiphora* species and are believed to be the source of the resin's benefits in lowering cholesterol levels and promoting weight loss. When the resin is distilled, it yields an aromatic essential oil that is believed to have anti-inflammatory and antibacterial benefits. The flowers are rich in flavonoids, especially quercetin, which also help control blood cholesterol levels.

Common Uses

- Lower high cholesterol and triglyceride levels.
- Treat obesity.
- Relieve arthritis pain and other symptoms.

How It Works

Guggulsterones are believed to help lower cholesterol and triglyceride levels by various mechanisms, including:

- Hindering the formation of lipoproteins by inhibiting the liver's manufacture of cholesterol and thereby increasing the liver's uptake of the harmful LDL cholesterol.
- Increasing the excretion of bile acids and cholesterol in the feces.
- Stimulating the thyroid gland to increase its hormone production and increase metabolism, which promotes weight loss and may reduce the amount of fats (lipids) circulating in the blood.

Guggul also may promote cardiovascular health through its antioxidant activity, thus reducing free radicals and potential cell damage, and its ability to inhibit platelet aggregation, thus reducing the risk of blood clots.

Evidence of Efficacy

A derivative of guggul, called gugulipid, gained approval as a lipid-lowering drug in India in 1986, although the herbal use dates back centuries. Numerous studies in animals and humans over the past thirty-five years, conducted by researchers in India and elsewhere, have demonstrated the ability of guggul to lower cholesterol and triglycerides. Research was prompted by exploration of the association between obesity and atherosclerosis in ancient Ayurvedic texts. This led to animal studies showing that it lowered both weight and cholesterol levels in rabbits, and further studies in humans. In one study involving 50 patients with coronary artery disease, those who took 10 to 15 g of guggul daily for three months showed an average 25 percent drop in total cholesterol and a 30 percent reduction in triglyceride levels. In another study, 22 patients with high blood cholesterol and other lipids were given 1,500 mg of gugulipid daily. Cholesterol levels began to drop within two weeks and were significantly reduced in 59 percent of the patients at the end of six weeks. Among responders, serum cholesterol and triglyceride levels were lowered 24.5 percent and 27.3 percent respectively. In a multicenter trial involving 205 patients, 1,500 mg of gugulipid daily for three months resulted in a 23.6 percent lowering of total cholesterol and a 22.6 percent decline in serum triglycerides in 70 percent of patients treated. In yet another study, the effects of gugulipid on cholesterol and triglyceride levels were found to be similar to those of clofibrate, a popular cholesterol-lowering drug.

Preliminary studies also support guggul's antioxidant properties and ability to inhibit blood clots, although more research is needed to prove this effect. Similarly, although the oldest uses of guggul was as an anti-inflammatory agent for such conditions as arthritis, less research has been done in this area as scientists have focused on its potential cardiac benefits. Thus, only a few animal studies have been done demonstrating its anti-inflammatory value and it is not known whether this will translate into clinical benefits in humans.

Forms and Usual Dosages

Although guggul is available in its crude resin form, clinical studies have involved capsules and tablets that are purified to remove the insoluble components and standardized for gugulipid or guggulsterone. Indeed, the gugulipid dosage is usually based on the guggulsterone concentration. Most commonly prescribed in clinical trials has been 25 mg of guggulsterones (or 500 mg of a product standardized for 5 percent guggulsterone content), to be taken three times a day. A comparable dose of the crude gum guggul powder would be 4 to 16 g per day, divided into three doses.

Potential Problems

The only side effects associated with guggul are transient and minor gastrointestinal problems such as nausea and diarrhea and, less commonly, restlessness, headache, and hiccups. Such problems are less likely when purified gugulipids are given, rather than the crude resin. However, because Ayurvedic doctors consider it an agent that stimulates the uterus and promotes menstrual discharge, it is not recommended during pregnancy. Further, it should be used cautiously in those already taking other medications for heart disease, especially antihypertensive drugs. In one study, for example, guggul reduced the peak plasma concentration of propranolol and diltiazem—drugs commonly used to treat high blood pressure and heart disease.

See Also

Cholesterol Disorders and Atherosclerosis
Heart Disease
Weight Problems

HAWTHORN (*CRATAEGUS* SPECIES)

Although hawthorn can grow to a thirty-foot spiny tree, it is more often grown as a low, bushy shrub or hedge plant. Indeed, its name is a corruption of "hedgethorn." It is also known as haw, may, mayblossom, maybush, mayflower, and whitethorn. Originally native to Europe, it now also grows in the temperate zones of North America and Asia. Its thorns indicate it is a member of the rose family; the plant has yellowish green, glossy leaves and white flowers that have an unpleasant smell. It yields bitter-tasting red to blue berries.

The berries, flowers, and dried leaves of the *Crataegus* species that have white flowers (*C. oxyacantha, C. laevigata, C. monogyna*) all share similar properties that benefit the heart; the garden hawthorn that has red flowers has no medicinal value. Although its medicinal use dates to ancient times, hawthorn's heart benefits were only recognized in the late nineteenth century. Since then, it has become a widely prescribed heart tonic, available in both prescription and over-the-counter preparations.

Common Uses

- Ease symptoms of congestive heart failure.
- Lower high blood pressure.
- Rid the body of excessive fluid (edema).
- Correct irregular heartbeat.

How It Works

The active ingredients of hawthorn are flavonoids and compounds called procyanidins oligomers (PCOs), along with a number of other compounds that are thought to benefit the heart and circulation. Flavonoids are potent antioxidants that help increase the amount of vitamin C inside cells, and stabilize vitamin C by protecting it from oxidative damage. Vitamin C also strengthens capillary walls.

Hawthorn seems to help the heart by multiple routes. It improves the blood supply to the heart by relaxing vascular smooth muscle and dilating blood vessels, particularly the coronary vessels. Such dilation can reduce blood pressure. Hawthorn also contains substances that inhibit angiotensin-converting enzyme (ACE), an approach used by some of the most widely prescribed medications to lower blood pressure. Furthermore, increasing blood and oxygen to the heart muscle lowers the risk of angina and strengthens the heart's muscle, allowing it to pump more effectively.

The improvements in circulation account for its ability to reduce swelling in the legs and feet. Hawthorn also may eliminate some types of abnormal heart rhythms. Its antioxidant properties are believed to reduce cholesterol levels and reduce the buildup of fatty plaque in the arteries—the hallmark of atherosclerosis.

Evidence of Efficacy

Considerable research, both in animal and human studies, supports the claims about hawthorn's heart benefits. For example, double-blind studies of hawthorn versus placebo have shown improvements in people with

◙ A LITTLE HISTORY

Hawthorn was long used in Germany as a hedge to divide plots of land, its sharp thorns serving to ward off intruders. One of its botanical names, *Crataegus oxyacantha*, comes from the Greek words *kratos*, meaning hardness, *oxus*, meaning sharp, and *akantha*, meaning a thorn. To the ancient Greeks and Romans hawthorn was a symbol of happiness and hope; it was often woven into bridal bouquets. In ancient Rome, sprigs of hawthorn were placed in babies' cradles to ward off evil spirits. But people of the Middle Ages had a much different view of hawthorn; to them, it was a symbol of evil, and bringing its branches into a house was a sign of impending death.

heart failure, demonstrating better heart function, less shortness of breath, and fewer palpitations. In a study of thirty patients with congestive heart failure, half were given placebo and the other half given twice daily capsules of hawthorn extract standardized to contain 15 mg procyanidin oligomers per 80-mg capsule. After eight weeks, the hawthorn group had statistically significant improvements in heart function and lower blood pressure, with no adverse reactions observed. In a study of seventy-eight patients with the same level of heart failure, those given 600 mg of standardized hawthorn extract were able to exercise much longer than those who received the placebo. Based on numerous studies, German health authorities have approved of hawthorn for treating mild heart failure, stable angina, and the slow heart rhythms known as bradycardia.

Lesser evidence, in animals only, is available to support hawthorn's potential benefits in lowering cholesterol, triglyceride, and blood sugar levels. Similarly, no human research supports its use in treating insomnia, although it is known that high doses can markedly slow down the central nervous system.

Forms and Usual Dosages

Hawthorn is available in many forms, including dried leaves, berries, and flowers, and in elixirs, extracts, infusions, capsules, and tinctures. Usually taken two or three times a day, the dosage depends on the type of preparation and source material. An infusion dose can be made with a teaspoon of chopped leaves and flowers. Tinctures may be recommended at 4 to 5 ml per dose. Flower extracts, standardized to contain 1.8 percent vitexin-4'-rhamnoside, may be prescribed at 100 to 250 mg per dose. It may take up to three months to note improvement; hawthorn may be taken indefinitely to treat chronic heart failure and other disorders.

Potential Problems

Toxic problems with hawthorn are not common and usually seen only when it is overdosed. In such cases, dangerously low blood pressure and sedation may occur. However, because of its potent effects, it should be used with care and only under the supervision of physicians experienced in its impact. In particular, it should be used very cautiously in conjunction with other heart medications. For example, because beta-blockers lower blood pressure by reducing cardiac output, simultaneous use of hawthorn may produce a mild rise in blood pressure. In contrast, hawthorn can markedly increase the effects of digitalis and other herbs containing cardiac glycosides to enhance their effects. When used with prescription heart drugs, the dosage of the latter can often be lowered. It should be noted that hawthorn will not stop an angina attack.

See Also

Heart Disease
High Blood Pressure
Leg Cramps and Restless Legs

HOREHOUND (*MARRUBIUM VULGARE*)

Horehound, a member of the mint family, is a perennial that is native to Europe and Asia and has been naturalized in North America. It grows to a height of about twelve inches and has hairy grayish leaves and a long woody stem that bears rings of white flowers that evolves into a burr containing a few brown or black seeds.

When in flower, the entire plant is used medicinally, especially to treat the airway congestion and cough of the common cold. It is also used to flavor candies and some beverages. Also known as white horehound and houndsbane, the *Marrubium vulgare* variety should not be confused with black horehound (*Ballota nigra*), which has a bitter, unpleasant taste.

Common Uses

- Relieve cold symptoms and congestion; ease coughing spasms associated with asthma and bronchitis.
- Soothe a sore throat.
- Stimulate appetite and aid digestion.

How It Works

Horehound has several active ingredients, including alkaloids, flavonoids, and trace amounts of volatile oils, but it is a substance called marrubiin that is believed to be responsible for its expectorant action in thinning and loosening airway mucus, making it easier to cough up. Horehounds volatile oils, tannins, and saponins may also have expectorant actions. Tannins and other substances soothe inflamed mucous membranes, relieving a sore throat. Bitters in horehound stimulate appetite and aid digestion by increasing the flow of saliva and gastric juices.

◉ A LITTLE HISTORY

The Latin name for horehound, *Marrubium,* is thought to have been named by the Romans after the ancient town of Maria urbs. Its name may also have been derived from the Hebrew *marrob,* meaning bitter herb; it is still eaten at the Passover seder.

The Romans and other ancient populations relied on horehound to treat numerous ailments, including whooping cough, tuberculosis, jaundice, menstrual cramps, and constipation. The Europeans believed that horehound helped ward off witches' spells. The Egyptians called it the seed of Horus and used it as an antidote for certain poisons and to repel flies.

Evidence of Efficacy

Traditional herbalists have been recommending horehound for coughs and other cold symptoms for centuries. In addition, German health authorities have approved the use of horehound juice or tea as an appetite stimulant and digestive aid. But the U.S. Food and Drug Administration removed horehound from its list of approved nonprescription cough remedies in 1989, saying there was not enough evidence that it had any medicinal properties. Naturopaths, herbalists, and other practitioners continue to recommend it, however, based on its long history as a botanical medicine.

Forms and Usual Dosages

Horehound is available in many forms: tea, tincture, liquid extract, lozenges, powder, syrup, and dried leaves. To make horehound tea, use 1 teaspoon of dried leaves per cup of boiling water; let it steep for ten minutes, and drink three or four cups a day to relieve congestion and a cough. Alternatively, horehound lozenges or candies can be used to still a cough.

The usual recommended dosage for the other forms calls for taking 2 to 4 tablespoons of the pressed juice per day; 1 to 2 of the dried herb three times a day; or ½ teaspoon of the liquid extract three times a day.

Potential Problems

Horehound is considered quite safe and poses no known risks when used in the recommended amounts. However, it should be avoided by people who have heartburn from gastroesophageal reflux disease (GERD) or peptic ulcers; the increased flow of digestive juices may worsen symptoms. In addition, like other members of the mint family, horehound may relax the sphincter between the esophagus and stomach, allowing a backflow (reflux) of stomach contents into the esophagus. As with other herbs and, indeed, all medications, it should not be taken during pregnancy without consulting a doctor first. Finally, long-term use of horehound may interfere with the absorption of iron and other minerals, so persons with anemia should take horehound in small amounts, if at all.

HORSERADISH (*ARMORACIA RUSTICANA*)

Horseradish is a perennial herb that probably originated in Russia and now grows worldwide. Best known today for its pungent taste (it is one of the five "bitter herbs" consumed at a Passover seder), horseradish is a member of the mustard family whose root is used for both its culinary and its medicinal properties. Its huge leaves (sometimes two feet long and six inches wide) are sometimes eaten in salads.

In the past, horseradish was a common folk remedy for digestive problems, gout, rheumatism, and liver and gallbladder diseases. Today, it is valued mostly as a condiment, although it is also effective in clearing sinus congestion.

Common Uses

- Ease minor muscle aches and arthritis pain.
- Reduce sinus congestion and symptoms of bronchitis and other upper respiratory disorders.
- Stimulate appetite and aid digestion.

How It Works

The active ingredients in horseradish are essential oils and mustard glycosides. When served as a condiment, horseradish stimulates appetite and aids digestion by increasing the flow of saliva and gastric juices.

The pungent mustard glycosides, oils, and possibly other components are said to help loosen mucus and relieve sinus and bronchial congestion. Certainly, anyone who has taken a deep whiff of horseradish knows that it can bring tears to the eyes and seem to clear the sinuses. Whether these effects are of any medical value in easing cold symptoms is unknown, but many people maintain that horseradish is an effective cold remedy.

Applied to the skin as a poultice, horseradish may relieve joint and muscle pain by creating warmth and stimulating circulation to the area. It also acts as a counterirritant to interfere with the transmission of pain messages from peripheral nerves to the brain.

Evidence of Efficacy

The glycosides in horseradish are responsible for its reddening effect on the skin, an indication, along with a sensation of warmth, of increased

◉ A LITTLE HISTORY

Horseradish derives its popular name from its similarity to oversized radishes, and sometimes it is used as a substitute for radishes. But for centuries, it was valued for its medicinal properties rather than as a food. Pliny, the first-century Roman scholar, recommended it for respiratory problems and many other ailments, but did not advise eating it. By the Middle Ages, some Europeans—most notably the Germans—had adopted it as a condiment to eat with fish and meat. But it wasn't until the 1600s that the English considered horseradish fit to eat, and then, according to John Parkinson, a popular herbalist of the time, only for "country people and strong laboring men."

circulation to the area. Volatile oil and isothiocyanates contained in the root may have mild antibiotic properties, and thus may be beneficial in treating throat and upper respiratory infections.

Forms and Usual Dosages

Horseradish is readily available as the fresh root in many produce markets; grated horseradish is sold in many forms as a condiment. The medicinal forms include the grated root and juice; horseradish pills are also available.

For external use, ointments containing up to 2 percent horseradish oils are available; this can be applied directly to the skin. To make a poultice, mix grated horseradish with cornstarch, spread it on cheesecloth or thin cotton, and apply to the skin.

As a digestive aid, consume ½ to 1 teaspoon juice three times a day, just before meals. Horseradish tincture, made from pressing the juice from the root, is also available and can be used in the amount of 2 to 3 ml three times per day. Ground fresh horseradish mixed with a little honey and added to a cup of hot water is a time-honored cough remedy.

Potential Problems

Some people cannot tolerate the pungent bitterness of horseradish. Even among those who can tolerate it, large amounts can cause vomiting or excessive sweating; it may also irritate the stomach lining and other mucous membranes, and may worsen symptoms in people who have ulcers. Care should be taken when applying directly to the skin, as irritation and burning can result. Be careful to keep horseradish away from the eyes and other delicate tissues.

HYSSOP (*HYSSOPUS OFFICINALIS*)

Hyssop is a bushy perennial herb that grows up to two feet in height and produces spires of fragrant blue or purple flowers. The plant originated in southern Europe and parts of Asia and now thrives in many parts of the United States, especially in the South and Southwest; it is also cultivated as a showy ornamental in flower and rock gardens.

Medicinally, hyssop is used both internally and externally to treat a variety of ailments. Its essential oils are used in perfumes and aromatherapy and as a food and beverage flavoring. Young hyssop leaves have a minty flavor and may be used to flavor tea, salads, fruit soups, and as a substitute for sage in poultry stuffing.

Common Uses

- Relieve coughs, airway congestion, and other cold and flu symptoms.
- Reduce intestinal gas and help settle an upset stomach.
- Promote sweating during a fever.
- Promote healing of minor burns, bruises, and skin sores.
- Repel insects.

How It Works

Hyssop contains a number of active ingredients, including terpenines, camphones, and other volatile oils; glycosides (hyssopin); a bitter substance called marrubiin; and tannins, flavonoids, and resins. Marrubiin is an expectorant that helps thin phlegm and make it easier to cough up. When used as a gargle, hyssop soothes a sore throat. It is often combined with other expectorant herbs, such as licorice and anise, which increases effectiveness and helps mask the herb's bitter taste.

Externally, diluted hyssop oil may be used as a chest rub to help reduce congestion. Hyssop compresses are said to help prevent skin infection and promote healing of bruises, minor burns, and injuries.

The odor of dried hyssop leaves is reminiscent of camphor and is sometimes used to repel moths and other insects.

Evidence of Efficacy

Hyssop has not undergone many scientific studies, thus most of the evidence regarding the herb is either anecdotal or based on traditional uses. It does appear to have expectorant qualities and hyssop tea is a soothing gargle. So far, no antibiotic substances have been isolated from hyssop, so claims that it prevents or treats skin infections are questionable, although the plant's volatile oils may be soothing and promote healing.

Forms and Usual Dosage

Hyssop is available in many forms; in addition to the dried flowers and leaves, these include liquid extract, tincture, essential oil, and tea. To make a tea or gargle, pour one cup of boiling water over 1 to 2 teaspoons of dried hyssop leaves and flowers, steep for ten minutes, and strain. The tea has a bitter taste; add a little honey to make it more palatable. The

◉ A LITTLE HISTORY

There are references to hyssop in the Bible, but it is unknown whether they are to the *Hyssopus officinalis* herb or to similar plants. However, hyssop's name is derived from the Greek *hussopos* and Hebrew *esob*, which both mean holy herb.

At one time, hyssop leaves were strewn on kitchen floors to mask unpleasant odors and repel insects. Today, hyssop is the major flavoring in such liqueurs as Chartreuse and Benedictine.

tea can also be used as a compress soak and moistened leaves and flowers can be placed directly on skin or between layers of cheesecloth to make a poultice.

Potential Problems

Hyssop is considered safe, although high doses may cause an upset stomach. The essential oil should be diluted with water or a neutral oil; taken full-strength, it can cause convulsions and vomiting.

KAVA
(PIPER METHYSTICUM)

◉ **USE IN ATTENTION DEFICIT DISORDER**

Over-the-counter products sold in health food stores for attention-deficit/hyperactivity disorder (ADHD) often contain herbs with sedative properties such as kava. Be careful when using such products in conjunction with standard sedative drugs because their impact may be increased. Kava has not been studied in rigorous clinical trials for effectiveness in ADHD. However, there seem to be no contraindications for its use as a mild sleep aid in the form of tea.

◉ **A LITTLE HISTORY**

Although kava has been used by Pacific Island natives for thousands of years, it first gained world attention after Capt. James Cook's explorations in the mid-eighteenth century. J. G. A. Forster, a botanist on Cook's ship, gave the plant its name, which means "intoxicating pepper." Cook's journals describe the plant's central role in the cultural, economic, political, and religious lives of South Pacific societies as a social relaxant and ceremonial means to achieve an altered level of consciousness.

Kava, a member of the pepper family Piperaceae, is also known as ava, ava pepper, kava kava, and kawa. The plant is a bushy perennial shrub that does best in sunny, humid conditions. It can grow taller than six feet, but it is usually harvested at about two feet. It has a knotty, underground root, large, green, heart-shaped and pointed leaves, and numerous small flowers, with an odor reminiscent of lilacs.

Kava is native to the Pacific Islands, but today it is cultivated on many islands in the South Pacific, including New Guinea, Vanuatu, Fiji, Polynesia, and Hawaii. The plant's active ingredients are a group of substances known as kavalactones, four of which have been found to have significant analgesic and anesthetic effects: kavain, methysticin, dihydrokavain (DHK), and dihydromethysticin (DHM). Modern medicinal extracts are usually prepared from the plant's root and rootstock, but abovegroumd portions of the plant have the highest concentration of DHK and DHM, which may have the strongest relaxant properties. However, these compounds must be taken in a particular ratio with the other active kavalactones (as occurs naturally in the root), to avoid adverse affects such as headaches. It has complex psychoactive effects that have variously been described as hypnotic and sedative; it differs from many narcotics in that it does not appear to work through the body's opiate pathways.

Common Uses

- Reduce anxiety and nervousness.
- Ease insomnia.
- Relax muscle tension.

How It Works

In South Pacific societies, where kava is used socially much as Western societies use alcohol, a type of tea is prepared by steeping the root. Drinking it induces mild euphoria, lively speech, and an increased sensitivity to sound. Medically, kava has been used for more than a century as a treatment for colds, migraine headaches, gonorrhea, vaginitis, menstrual problems, nocturnal incontinence and other urinary problems, gout, bronchial congestion, and rheumatism. However, research has only documented its benefits in easing anxiety, insomnia, and restlessness.

The anti-anxiety benefits of kava seem to be explained by the impact of kavalactones on slowing down the nervous system. It does this by several mechanisms, including blocking the uptake of norepinephrine. A study published in the journal *Neuropharmacology* described a study of kavain's chemical actions, which may contribute to kava's anticonvulsive, analgesic, and muscle-relaxing effects. The researchers found that kavain has a fast and specific inhibition action on pain pathways in the brain. Another study reported that kavalactones may mediate sedative effects through effects on the receptors of GABA, a brain chemical (neurotransmitter). In addition, the *Journal of Medicinal Plant Research* published a study demonstrating its positive impact on contraction activity in smooth muscle tissues in guinea pigs.

Evidence of Efficacy

Kava is more effective than placebo in relieving symptoms of anxiety. Further, multiple studies support the use of kava as an effective and safe alternative to tranquilizers and antidepressants in the treatment of anxiety disorders because patients do not develop tolerance, with a consequent need for increasing doses, as is seen with benzodiazepine drugs. In a recent German study, 52 patients with nonpsychotic anxiety were given kava; at the end of the study, 80 percent rated its benefits as "good" or "very good." Research has focused on how it reduces psychological stress and muscle tension. A study reported in the journal *Pharmacopsychiatry* described a clinical trial involving 101 patients suffering from anxiety in which the researchers concluded that kava is a viable alternative to tricyclic antidepressants and benzodiazepines in treating anxiety disorders. In animal studies, kava was also shown to slow hyperactive behavior, but not as effectively as some prescription medications.

Forms and Usual Dosages

Kava is available in capsule, powder, liquid extract, and decoction forms; it is also an ingredient in many herbal drinks and teas. A traditional bowl of kava drink or tea contains about 250 mg of kavalactones and, in South Pacific cultures, several such bowls may be sipped in one sitting.

For anxiety, the recommended dose is kava extract standardized to 60 to 75 mg of kavalactones per capsule taken two or three times daily. For insomnia related to anxiety or muscle tension, two or three capsules of such a standardized extract should be taken an hour before bedtime

Potential Problems

Although kava is generally considered a safe herb when taken in recommended dosages, serious problems can occur if it is not used carefully. These may include allergic reactions, gastrointestinal complaints, visual disturbances, and slowed reaction times. It has also been known to increase the effects of barbiturates, alcohol, and other psychopharmacological drugs, leading to overdose situations. Even recommended doses may impair reflexes, judgment, and other skills needed for driving and operating heavy machinery safely. Confusion and depression may accompany kava abuse syndrome.

However, the most common side effect, usually seen only with long-term, heavy usage of kava, is a scaly skin rash called kava dermopathy, which is accompanied by reddened eyes and yellowing of the skin, hair, and nails.

There is only modest evidence that kava is addictive, but German authorities advise that it should not be taken for more than three months without a doctor's supervision. It should not be used during pregnancy or breast-feeding.

See Also

Anxiety
Insomnia

LAVENDER (*LAVENDULA ANGUSTIFOLIA* AND OTHER SPECIES)

Lavender is a perennial shrub known for its refreshing aroma and spikes of purple or light blue flowers. It grows wild in mountainous areas in many parts of the world and is a favorite in herb and flower gardens. For centuries, lavender has been used to repel moths and other insects. The English and French varieties are especially prized for their essential oils, which are used in perfumes, cosmetics, skin-care products, and air fresheners. Lavender flowers are generally picked by the end of July to obtain maximum-strength essential oils, with sixty pounds of flowers yielding some 16 fluid ounces of oil.

Medicinally, lavender has found many uses, especially in aromatherapy; it is also used by midwives, massage therapists, and some hospitals for its relaxing properties and pleasant odor. It is also brewed as a tea and digestive aid.

Common Uses

- Calm an upset stomach, promote digestion, and relieve abdominal cramps and intestinal gas.
- Relieve tension-type headaches.
- Calm anxiety and lift mood.
- Promote deep, restful sleep.
- Prevent infection and hasten healing of minor cuts, wounds, and burns.
- Treat eczema, psoriasis, and other skin inflammations.
- Reduce itching of insect stings and bites.

How It Works

Lavender's essential oil is made up of complex and highly aromatic esters, including linalyl ester, which is also a major component of bergamot. Other components include tannins, pinene, limonene, geraniol, and borneol. Linalyl esters are responsible for the oil's fragrance as well as its medicinal properties, which include antispasmodic, antiseptic, sedative, and gas-reducing properties. Tannins in the oil also have antibacterial properties that are useful in treating minor skin wounds.

Lavender oil is often mixed with other oils and creams or with water for internal and external uses, and the dried flowers themselves are often hung in rooms to perfume the air and repel moths and other insects. When placed near or inside the pillow, dried lavender is said to help induce restful sleep.

Although lavender tea and other ingested preparations are still used, external applications are more popular and probably more effective. Diluted lavender oil is used in therapeutic massage and aromatherapy to help relax tensed muscles and relieve stress. When massaged into the temples, it can relieve tension headaches. A few drops added to hot bathwater can relieve tension and mild depression and promote sleep; added to cool bathwater, it becomes an energizing stimulant. Drops of

⊙ A LITTLE HISTORY

Lavender originated in the Mediterranean area, where ancient Romans used it as a bath perfume. In fact, its name is derived from the Latin *lavare,* meaning to wash. Shakespeare makes several references to lavender, but it probably wasn't widely cultivated in England until the late sixteenth century. It quickly became a favorite among gardeners, however, and English settlers brought it to the New World. The oil has also been used to kill lice and fleas and as an embalming fluid.

lavender oil are sometimes added to water and used as an astringent for cleaning the face and treating acne.

Evidence of Efficacy

The medicinal properties of lavender have been noted in the earliest English herbals and in the British *Pharmacopoeia* for some 250 years. A small British study found that lavender was more effective than a pharmaceutical sleep drug in helping nursing home patients get more restful sleep. German health authorities have approved lavender tea or tincture as a sleep aid and a treatment of minor digestive problems, including an upset stomach and intestinal gas. They also recommend it to promote healing of skin wounds and calm feelings of anxiety.

Animal studies appear to confirm that lavender calms the central nervous system, relaxes smooth muscles, and reduces muscle spasms. Other studies indicate that it has mild analgesic properties, but there are other more effective painkillers. Lavender has been shown to lower blood sugar levels in rats, but it has not been studied for this purpose in humans.

Forms and Usual Dosages

Lavender is available as dried flowers, teas, tinctures, and as a diluted or full-strength essential oil. Only a few drops of essential oil are needed to scent a bath and release its relaxing properties. Full-strength lavender oil should not be applied to the skin; instead, it should be diluted with alcohol or a neutral (carrier) oil. Lavender oil is a common ingredient in many skin creams, lotions, and other cosmetic or body-care products.

Lavender tea is made by pouring a cup of boiling water over 1 to 2 teaspoons of the dried flowers; steep for five to ten minutes, strain, and drink after meals or, as a sleep aid, just before going to bed.

Potential Problems

In recommended dosages, lavender is considered safe. Ingesting more than a few drops of full-strength oil, however, can cause convulsions and even death. Some people develop an allergic skin reaction to lavender oil; discontinue use if itching, hives, or a rash develop.

See Also

Insomnia

LEMON BALM
(*MELISSA OFFICINALIS*)

Also known as balm, Melissa, and sweet Mary, lemon balm is a perennial plant that originated in southern Europe, the Mediterranean region, and North Africa and is now cultivated worldwide. It is highly valued for its lemon-scented leaves and white or light yellow flowers that have been used medicinally for some two thousand years to treat such diverse conditions as digestive upsets, sleep problems, depression, and various skin sores. It is also used as a substitute for lemon or mint to flavor tea and as an ingredient in skin creams and lotions.

Common Uses

- Treat digestive problems, including indigestion, gas, and "nervous stomach."
- Relieve stress, anxiety, and depression, and promote sleep during bouts of insomnia.
- Hasten healing of cold sores, fever blisters, and minor skin infections.
- Repel mosquitoes and ease itching of insect bites.
- Ease muscle spasms and menstrual cramps.

How It Works

The active ingredients in lemon balm include various bioflavonoids, such as quercetin, luteolin, and apigenin. It is rich in tannins and various terpenes, including citronellal, the pleasant-smelling oil that has become a popular mosquito repellent. Lemon balm also relieves the itchiness of mosquito and other insect bites when applied topically. Similarly, application of lemon balm cream to a cold sore or other herpes sore when the warning tingling sensations are felt appears to reduce the size and hasten healing of the sore, probably because its tannins act as an astringent and kill surface viruses.

Terpenes account for the herb's antianxiety properties and also act as a digestive aid to stimulate the flow of bile, which is needed to digest fats, and to reduce gasiness. It is sometimes combined with other herbs to treat digestive upsets; for example, with peppermint to relieve an upset stomach. It may also be taken with valerian to relieve insomnia and tension. The rosmarinic acid in lemon balm has been shown to reduce smooth muscle spasms, and thus may be responsible for easing intestinal and menstrual cramps. There is some evidence that lemon

◎ A LITTLE HISTORY
Some of our earliest writings cite the medicinal use of lemon balm. The Roman scholar Pliny and the Greek physician Dioscorides both recommended it, as did Nicholas Culpeper, the famous English herbalist, in 1653 in his *Complete Herbal*. Charlemagne ordered that it be planted in every monastery garden, a testament to the plant's beauty and importance. American colonists brought it to the New World, and Thomas Jefferson grew it at Monticello.

balm inhibits the production of thyroid hormones; indeed, it is a traditional treatment for hyperthyroidism (Graves' disease).

Evidence of Efficacy

Lemon balm has been used for centuries by herbalists, and a number of recent studies appear to support at least some of the many medicinal claims made for this herb. For example, laboratory studies in Germany have demonstrated that balm leaves contain compounds with sedative, digestive, and antispasmodic properties. German health authorities have approved it for nervous sleeping disorders and indigestion.

A cream containing highly concentrated balm compounds, available in Europe but not in the United States, has been shown to speed the healing of herpes sores and reduce the number of recurrences.

Forms and Usual Dosage

Lemon balm is available as fresh or dried leaves, extract, tincture, and essential oil that can be diluted and used in aromatherapy. Lemon balm is also very easy to grow. Herbalists typically recommend a balm tea made from fresh (preferably) or dried leaves to calm nerves, aid sleep, ease menstrual cramps, and promote digestion. Use 2 teaspoons of chopped leaves to one cup of boiling water, let the brew steep for ten to twenty minutes, and drink it after meals and before going to bed. A popular aromatherapy remedy for insomnia involves adding a few drops of lemon balm oil to a warm bath and sprinkling a few drops on an herbal pillow. A poultice of crushed leaves can be made to soothe insect bites and stings and promote healing of cold sores and minor skin wounds.

Potential Problems

Lemon balm is generally recognized as safe when used for mild nervousness, insomnia, and indigestion. Because of its sedating qualities, lemon balm should not be taken by anyone who is operating machinery or driving a vehicle, or who must remain mentally alert. It may affect the actions of tranquilizers and sedatives, and so should not be used by anyone taking those medications. Lemon balm should not be used by pregnant or nursing women or any woman who plans to become pregnant, because of its possible effects on the uterus and the body's hormonal balance. Likewise, it should not be used by anyone with thyroid disease unless prescribed by a doctor.

LICORICE
(*GLYCYRRHIZA GLABRA*)

Licorice gets its common name from a Greek word meaning "sweet root," an apt description for this herb, which is native to southern Europe and central Asia. Now widely cultivated for commercial use, licorice is used to make candies and food flavorings. The licorice plant grows up to seven feet in height, and it produces spikes of blue-violet flowers. It is the licorice root, however, that gives the plant its medicinal properties. The Chinese have used it for more than five thousand years to treat a variety of ailments, including coughs, sore throats, food poisoning, and liver and stomach disorders. Modern herbalists value licorice root for its anti-inflammatory and antibiotic properties.

Common Uses

- Relieve eczema and other inflammatory skin disorders and treat minor skin infections.
- Soothe a sore throat and mouth ulcers, treat gum disease, and help prevent tooth decay.
- Relieve congestion, coughing, and other symptoms of bronchitis and common cold.
- Treat indigestion, heartburn, peptic ulcers, and intestinal inflammation.
- Alleviate symptoms of chronic fatigue syndrome, premenstrual syndrome (PMS), fibromyalgia, and arthritis.

How It Works

Licorice's most important uses are as a demulcent to coat and soothe inflamed tissues of the mouth, throat, and digestive and urinary tracts. Licorice's major active ingredients are glycyrrhizin, which has anti-inflammatory properties and suppresses coughs, and various flavonoids, which are potent antioxidants. Glycyrrhizin also acts as an expectorant by thinning and loosening sputum, making it easier to cough up. It is thought to stimulate the production of two of the body's steroid hormones: cortisone, which fights inflammation, and aldosterone, which raises blood pressure, among other functions.

Licorice may aid digestion by stimulating the liver's production of bile, a substance needed to digest fats. Recent studies indicate that licorice also contains substances that kill certain bacteria, viruses, and yeast

◉ A LITTLE HISTORY

Licorice is one of the world's oldest botanical medicines. It was used by the ancient Assyrians and Egyptians to treat various respiratory disorders. Hippocrates and other early physicians prescribed it, and Chinese physicians have used it even longer. Today, licorice root is the second-most-prescribed herb in China, exceeded only by ginseng.

organisms, which would support its traditional uses in treating herpes cold sores, candida vaginitis and other yeast infections, and some bacterial sore throats and respiratory infections. Some of the licorice flavonoids have been found to help heal peptic ulcers and canker sores. Their antioxidant properties may also protect against cancer.

The steroidlike properties of glycyrrhizin may be helpful in controlling PMS symptoms, such as achiness, as well as those of fibromyalgia and chronic fatigue syndrome.

Evidence of Efficacy

There is mounting scientific evidence that supports the traditional uses of licorice to treat many diverse disorders and more may be in the offing. For example, the National Cancer Institute is investigating compounds derived from licorice root for their ability to inhibit the growth of cancer, and other researchers are studying the potential of licorice in preventing tooth decay. Glycyrrhizin has been shown to posses antiviral properties and may be effective against herpes simplex and HIV in the test tube. No studies on humans have been completed, although clinical studies in Japan are being conducted to see how glycyrrhizin might prevent the progression of the HIV virus by inhibiting cell infection and boosting the body's own production of interferon. Researchers in Great Britain are studying the effectiveness of glycyrrhizin in treating chronic hepatitis C. More research is needed, however, to determine if it is effective against this common liver disorder.

As for some of the older uses of licorice, medical researchers have isolated several active substances in licorice root, including glycosides, flavonoids, asparagine, isoflavonoids, chalcomes, and coumarins that act as anti-inflammatory agents and are included in drugs used to treat intestinal and mouth ulcers.

Forms and Usual Dosages

Licorice is available as capsules, extracts, tinctures, teas, lozenges, ointments, and as the whole root (rhizome) or its juice. Many of these products are available in a deglycyrrhizinated licorice (DGL), in which the glycyrrhizin has been removed. (See below.)

Licorice is also an ingredient in many cough syrups and drops, tobacco flavoring, and occasionally, as imported licorice candy. (The licorice candy made in the United States is actually flavored with anise, an herb with a similar taste).

Dosages vary according to the form used and the condition that is being treated. The typical dosage for digestive problems, for example, calls for chewing two or three 380-mg tablets of the DGL form before meals. A cough and chest congestion is treated with up to 5 to 6 g of licorice root capsules taken three times a day, or by drinking two or three cups of licorice tea during the course of a day. To make the tea, put ½ ounce of the crushed root in one pint of water, bring to a boil, let it steep for fifteen minutes, and strain. This dosage is also recommended for PMS, chronic fatigue syndrome, and fibromyalgia.

Licorice ointment can be applied to painful joints as needed. For mouth ulcers, make a mouthwash by dissolving 200 mg of DGL powder in warm water; the mixture can be gargled to soothe a sore throat. Licorice cream or gel can be applied directly to a cold sore or fever blister three or four times to relieve pain and hasten healing.

Potential Problems

Long-term (more than a month) use of licorice containing glycyrrhizin can raise blood pressure and cause water retention. Anyone who has high blood pressure or disorders that cause fluid retention should not take regular licorice; it is also contraindicated during pregnancy. It may increase the effects of steroid medications, such as prednisone; if you are taking any medication, check with your doctor before trying medicinal licorice. The DGL form does not raise blood pressure, and has no known adverse side effects.

See Also

Allergies
Bronchitis
Chronic Fatigue Syndrome
Dermatitis/Eczema
Heartburn
Inflammatory Bowel Disease
Liver Diseases
Mouth Sores
Psoriasis
Ulcers

MARIJUANA
(CANNABIS SATIVA)

In the public mind, marijuana is an illegal street drug with many names—hemp, pot, Mary Jane, grass, hash, and reefer, among others. In some parts of the world, however, cannabis is cultivated legally for its fibers, which are used to make rope, and its seeds and leaves, which

Since ancient times, many cultures have used marijuana as a psychoactive drug, and today, smoking marijuana is an accepted social custom in many parts of Asia and Africa.

Until the 1950s, hemp seeds were fed to canaries and other pet birds in the United States because it seemed to induce them to sing more than other types of birdfeed did. Hemp birdseed was banned, however, when illegal pot smoking became so popular during the 1960s and authorities discovered that the seeds were being used to grow marijuana. The plant also thrived in landfill areas like the New Jersey Meadowlands, where undigested hemp birdseeds that had been discarded in trash sprouted into fields of hemp and were gathered by savvy drug users and dealers.

are used medicinally and for their oil. Today, the medical uses of marijuana are hotly debated, especially in Congress and other legislative bodies.

Common Uses

In the United States and other developed countries, marijuana is used mostly as an illegal street, or recreational, drug. But it also has medicinal uses, which include:

- Relieving mild to moderate pain and reducing inflammation.
- Stimulating appetite.
- Quelling nausea, especially that caused by cancer chemotherapy.
- Controlling glaucoma.

How It Works

Marijuana contains many compounds, but most of its actions are attributed to substances called cannabinoids. The most active of these is THC, short for tetrahydrocannabinol. THC is thought to be responsible for the euphoria and other psychological effects of marijuana; researchers think that it also accounts for many of the plant's medicinal properties. For example, THC is thought to help quell nausea and vomiting, relieve muscle spasms, reduce seizures in epilepsy, and control eye pressure in some types of glaucoma. It may also perk up a flagging appetite and help prevent the severe weight loss of AIDS and some types of cancer.

Evidence of Efficacy

Because marijuana is a mind-altering, illegal substance—at least in the United States—legal and political problems surrounding its use have limited research into its medicinal properties. This is beginning to change, however, following recommendations by a National Institutes of Health panel urging increased study of marijuana as medicine. Studies here and abroad document the effectiveness of THC in treating nausea and vomiting, and an artificial form of THC, which does not have any psychoactive effects, is available for this purpose. However, proponents of legalizing medical uses of marijuana contend that the artificial THC is not as effective as the natural form; it is also much more expensive and it is available only by prescription. More research is needed to establish the value of THC in treating glaucoma; in the meantime, there are numerous anecdotal accounts of its effectiveness.

Forms and Usual Dosage

In most parts of the United States, growing, possessing, and using marijuana in any form is illegal. A few states have legalized its medical use in treating some of the symptoms associated with AIDS, cancer, and other serious diseases. An artificial form of THC is available by prescription only in capsule or pill form; the prescribing doctor determines the appropriate dosage.

Potential Problems

Aside from the legal and political issues surrounding the use of marijuana, opponents of its use maintain that it is a gateway drug that can lead to addiction to more dangerous substances, including heroin and cocaine. Smoking marijuana can cause lung damage similar to that of smoking tobacco. Its psychological effects can impair judgment and coordination, and it has been linked to numerous car accidents. It speeds up the heartbeat, which can be dangerous for persons with cardiac arrhythmias and other forms of heart disease.

MARSHMALLOW (*ALTHAEA OFFICINALIS*)

Marshmallow is a perennial herb that grows near salt marshes worldwide; despite its name, it is totally unrelated to the soft, sugary confection that today is a favorite for toasting over a campfire. The entire plant can be used medicinally, but it's the roots that are the most valuable because of their high content of mucilages, compounds that are used to soothe inflamed tissues and calm coughs. The roots and leaves can also be boiled and eaten as a vegetable, although it has a somewhat gummy consistency.

Common Uses

- Promote healing of chapped skin, minor burns, cuts and scrapes, and inflammatory skin disorders, such as eczema.
- Soothe mouth ulcers, sore throats, and coughs; relieve other symptoms of colds and bronchitis.

⊙ A LITTLE HISTORY
Marshmallow has a long history as both a food and a botanical medicine. The ancient Romans considered cooked marshmallow a delicacy, and it is credited with sustaining some populations during famines. The plant's sweet, mucilaginous properties were once used to make a type of candy, and the modern marshmallow confection derives its name from this early sweet.

- Alleviate inflammatory intestinal disorders and ease symptoms of urinary tract infections.
- Help control blood sugar in diabetes.
- Treat and prevent constipation.

How It Works

The gummy mucilages in marshmallow have demulcent properties that soothe inflammation and promote healing of ulcers, skin sores, and burns. They may enhance immunity by stimulating macrophages, the white blood cells that engulf and destroy bacteria. The other active ingredients in marshmallow include asparagine, an amino acid; tannins, which have astringent and soothing properties; and pectin, a water-soluble fiber that helps control blood sugar levels and prevent constipation.

Mucilage and tannins help soothe a sore throat, calm coughs, and reduce bronchial congestion. Ointments, creams, and other skin products containing marshmallow help moisturize chapped skin and counter the inflammation and itchiness of eczema.

Evidence of Efficacy

The soothing and healing effects of mucilage on inflamed tissue are well known. Otherwise, most of the evidence of marshmallow's effectiveness is based on laboratory studies. For example, animal studies have demonstrated the effectiveness of marshmallow extracts in treating coughs. Other laboratory studies show that marshmallow lowers blood sugar levels in diabetic mice.

Marshmallow's value in treating various skin disorders is supported mostly by anecdotal accounts and a long tradition in botanical medicine.

Forms and Usual Dosages

Marshmallow is available in many forms: capsules, tablets, liquid extracts and tinctures, powdered root, and dried leaves. It is also an ingredient in some cough medications, skin ointments and gels, and gargles. An infusion can be made from the crushed roots or dried leaves, and consumed as a tea or used as a gargle or compress soak. The potency of commercial preparations varies widely, so check the labels for content and instructions. The typical daily dosage calls for taking 5 to 6 g of powdered marshmallow or 15 to 30 ml of tincture.

Marshmallow tea, used to treat coughs, ulcers, urinary tract disorders, and digestive tract irritations, is made by cold infusion. Cover 4 to 5 teaspoonfuls of crushed leaves and stems with one cup cold water and allow the mixture to stand for about two hours before straining. Dilute with an additional three cups of water and drink three or four cups a day until symptoms abate.

Potential Problems

Marshmallow is generally considered safe, and allergic reactions or other adverse effects are rare. However, the syrup that is made from the mucilage extracted by boiling the plant's roots, stems, and leaves has high sugar content and should be used with caution, if at all, by people with diabetes. Because of its high mucilage and pectin content, marshmallow may delay the absorption of some medications. Check with your doctor or pharmacist if you are taking prescription medications and want to try marshmallow.

MILK THISTLE (*SILYBUM MARIANUM*)

Milk thistle, a prickly annual or biennial herb that grows worldwide, has tall, furrowed, branched stems that sport a spiny, violet flower at the end of each. Its common name is derived from its rather bitter milky sap. At one time, it was thought that the sap increased milk flow of nursing mothers, but there is only anecdotal evidence to support this. But the plant has other medicinal uses that have been well documented. Young thistle leaves, shoots, stems, and roots are all edible, and good sources of flavonoids, vitamin C, iron, and other minerals. It is the seeds, however, that are used medicinally.

Common Uses

- Treat liver and gallbladder diseases.
- Help prevent liver damage due to alcoholism.
- Anecdote for death-cap (*Amanita*) mushroom poisoning.

How It Works

The ripe fruits and seeds of the milk thistle plant contain fatty oil, proteins, an essential oil, and bitter compounds. But the most important medicinal compounds are silybin and silymarin, flavones that have been shown to protect against liver damage and stimulate regeneration of damaged liver cells. Silymarin speeds recovery from hepatitis, liver in-

◉ A LITTLE HISTORY

Milk thistle is also known as Mary's or Our Lady's thistle, a reference to the legend that the thistle got its milky sap when the Virgin Mary sprinkled some of her milk on it. The plant was revered by early healers, but more recently, it has been considered a noxious weed that takes over farm and pasture land. In England, allowing thistles to grow on your land can bring a heavy fine. But some farm animals, especially hogs, love thistles, and finches relish its seeds. They also use soft thistle down to line their nests.

flammation that may be caused by viruses, medications, and toxic substances. Silymarin is also a powerful antioxidant, a substance that protects cells against damage from unstable molecules (free radicals) that are released when the body burns oxygen. Silymarin may also prevent formation of gallstones by reducing cholesterol levels in the bile.

Evidence of Efficacy

Scientific studies in many centers in the United States and abroad tend to confirm the time-honored use of milk thistle to treat liver and gallbladder diseases. Animal studies indicate that silymarin protects against liver damage. A series of animal studies found that silymarin fostered regeneration of liver cells when part of the organ was surgically removed. Human studies show that hepatitis patients recover more quickly when given silymarin, compared to those who receive a placebo.

Studies have also found that silymarin is an effective antidote for the toxins in death-cap mushrooms. This particular toxin kills by destroying the liver, a consequence that silymarin appears to prevent.

Forms and Usual Dosage

Silymarin and milk thistle extracts are available as tinctures, drops, tablets, powders, and tea. A standardized silymarin extract used in Europe to treat liver disease is available in the United States (see Appendix A, p 635). The recommended dosage for people with impaired liver function is 420 mg of silymarin. Look for milk thistle extracts that are standardized to provide 70 to 80 percent silymarin, and calculate the dosage accordingly. After improvement is noted—usually two or three months—the dosage may be reduced to 280 mg of silymarin. This dosage is also recommended as a preventive measure for alcoholics and others who are at high risk of developing liver disease. The herbal treatment of gallbladder disease calls for taking 600 mg of milk thistle extract, standardized to 70 to 80 percent silymarin, daily.

Potential Problems

Liver disease is always a serious medical condition, and should not be self-treated. Although studies support the use of milk thistle, it should be taken only with your doctor's knowledge and guidance. When silymarin is used, frequent liver-function blood tests should be done to make sure that it is helping.

See Also

Cancer
Liver Diseases

MINT/PEPPERMINT (*MENTHA* SPECIES)

Mints are aromatic perennial plants that will quickly take over a garden by sending up new offshoots from their rapidly spreading roots in addition to scattering seeds far and wide. Various species of mint grow naturally worldwide, but the most familiar originated in Europe and Asia. Their leaves grow in pairs along branching stems that end in clusters of small flowers that may be pink, white, or lilac. Many of the mint family members—peppermint, spearmint, cat mint, pennyroyal, and Japanese mint, among others—interbreed readily and are sometimes difficult to tell apart. But all have a distinctive minty odor and a fresh, pleasant taste.

Peppermint (*Mentha piperita*) is the one that is most often used medicinally. Menthol, which is found in peppermint and its close cousin, Japanese mint, is a potent herbal remedy for a variety of ailments. First commercially cultivated in England in the eighteenth century, peppermint was soon brought to the Americas. Today, the United States is the world leader in peppermint production. The leaves and flowering tops of the plant are used fresh or dried, though some experts recommend harvesting the leaves before the plant flowers.

The menthol is distilled from peppermint oil. Peppermint is best known for its stomach-soothing qualities, but it has a variety of nonmedicinal uses as well. For instance, it's a popular flavoring for candy and products such as antacids, toothpaste, and mouthwash, and as a soothing, cooling ingredient in lotions, cosmetics, aromatherapy and bath products, and even cigarettes.

Common Uses

- Counter common digestive problems including indigestion, gas, and flatulence; help quell nausea and treat irritable bowel syndrome.
- Stimulate appetite.
- Treat headaches and other stress-related disorders (aromatherapy).
- Ease congestion of common cold, flu, or sinusitis (inhaled vapors).

⊙ A LITTLE HISTORY

The mint derives its genus name from the Greek legend involving their jealous gods. As the story goes, the goddess Persephone turned Minthe, a beautiful nymph and her rival for Pluto's love, into a plant. Pluto was unable to undo the spell, but could lessen its impact a bit by ensuring that whenever Minthe was trod upon, her leaves would release a sweet odor. While few today take the legend seriously, the fact is that throughout history, *Mentha* plants have been valued for their pleasant odor and sweet taste. The Romans and Greeks used mint in temple rites and for its medicinal qualities. In medieval times, Europeans strewed their homes and beds with dried mint leaves to ward off fleas and other insect pests and to mask less pleasant smells. Even today, dried mint leaves are an alternative to camphor mothballs, and commercial room fresheners often give off a minty odor.

- Soothe muscle aches, hives, itchiness from insect bites (poultice or ointment).
- Suppress a dry, hacking cough.
- Freshen breath and treat gingivitis and help counter a dry mouth.
- Ease menstrual cramps.
- Overcome insomnia.

How It Works

The volatile oils in peppermint—primarily menthol—relieve spasms of the smooth muscle of the digestive tract, making the herb especially helpful for a variety of stomach ailments and digestive complaints. The antispasmodic action may alleviate menstrual cramps. Peppermint also contains flavonoids, which may explain why it stimulates the flow of bile. The herb also helps relieve intestinal gas by causing belching.

The potent mint flavor masks unpleasant scents, making it a useful ingredient in lozenges, breath fresheners, toothpastes, and mouthwashes. It also increases the flow of saliva; a dry mouth is a common cause of bad breath, tooth decay, and gum disease. Peppermint oil is said to have mild antiseptic qualities, too, which may be beneficial in treating a mild sore throat when used as a gargle. Inhaling menthol vapors helps thin mucus and ease congestion. By increasing the flow of saliva, peppermint causes you to swallow more often; this may help suppress a cough reflex.

The volatile oils in peppermint and other members of the mint family have cooling, anti-inflammatory properties. Applying a poultice or ointment containing menthol and other mint oils can soothe minor muscle aches and the itching of insect bites and hives. Applying a few crushed fresh peppermint leaves to a cold sore or fever blister is said to ease its pain and hasten healing.

Evidence of Efficacy

Despite the long history of peppermint oil's use as an herbal digestive aid, the Food and Drug Administration (FDA) has concluded that it is ineffective for digestive problems and does not allow its sale for that purpose. In contrast, German health authorities have found peppermint useful for these complaints—particularly when the upper gastrointestinal tract is affected. In several European countries, peppermint oil is also marketed as an antibacterial agent and to promote gastric secretions.

The FDA does feel it is helpful for relieving cold symptoms and allows peppermint in cough and throat lozenges, nasal decongestants and inhalers, and other products.

Laboratory experiments have shown peppermint oil kills bacteria and viruses, such as those that cause cold sores. Thus, the herbal remedy of applying fresh mint leaves to a cold sore may well have a scientific basis.

German researchers have also found that a mixture of eucalyptus and peppermint oils and ethanol rubbed on the forehead and temples relieves headache. Some German studies also indicate that peppermint may ease the colic-like pain and bloating of irritable bowel syndrome.

Forms and Usual Dosages

Peppermint is available in every form imaginable for internal and external use: Tea can be made from peppermint leaves, though there is not enough of the active ingredients to have a strong medicinal effect. Nevertheless, a tea made from 1 tablespoon of leaves, taken three to four times a day between meals, may stimulate a flagging appetite and help ease mild intestinal complaints. Some experts suggest 2 teaspoons in a cup of water for relief of gas. (Covering the steeping brew will prevent the oil from evaporating.) A cup of peppermint, spearmint, or bergamot mint tea in the late evening may help overcome insomnia problems. A gargle made of strong peppermint tea can ease a sore throat. To sweeten the breath and stimulate the flow of saliva, experts advise placing a drop or two of peppermint tincture on the tongue; chewing a couple of fresh mint leaves may have the same effect.

Digestive problems are usually treated by taking enteric-coated capsules containing 0.2 ml of peppermint oil an hour or so before a meal. The coating prevents the pill from dissolving before it reaches the small intestine, where it helps stimulate the flow of bile to break down fats. By acting directly in the intestines, the peppermint oil may also reduce bloating, gas, and flatulence.

A few drops of peppermint oil can be used in boiling water for steam inhalations. It can also be added to ointments and oils and rubbed on painful muscles for pain relief up to four times a day. Crushed leaves can be applied directly to the skin. Or make a poultice by dipping crushed leaves in hot water, draining immediately, and spreading the leaves between two layers of cheesecloth. Place the warm poultice on the aching muscles and cover with a towel to retain the heat.

To treat a cold sore, crush a few fresh leaves and apply them directly to the sore. Do not put them in hot water, however; heat can worsen a cold sore or fever blister.

Potential Problems

Pure menthol can be fatal if ingested; it must always be diluted. In addition, even diluted mint oils can provoke an allergic reaction in some people when they are applied to the skin or mucous membranes. Stop using immediately if symptoms such as a headache, rash, or flushing develop.

Since menthol can stimulate the gallbladder, do not take any form of peppermint if you have gallstones. Peppermint is also contraindicated in those who have a hiatal hernia or heartburn due to gastroesophageal reflux disease (GERD). Menthol can worsen GERD by relaxing the sphincter between the esophagus and stomach, allowing the stomach acids to flow upward into the esophagus.

Very young children should not be given strong peppermint tea or rubbed with ointments containing menthol, since it may cause them to gag and choke. As with other herbal and pharmaceutical medications, a pregnant or breast-feeding woman should consult her doctor before using peppermint.

See Also

Irritable Bowel Syndrome
Nausea

MULLEIN (*VERBASCUM THAPSUS*)

Mullein is a hearty biennial that grows almost everywhere. It is easily distinguished by its long, rodlike stem, velvety leaves, and long column of bright yellow flowers.

Mullein leaves, flowers, and seeds are all used medicinally. The plant is high in mucilage, a slippery substance that coats and soothes inflamed mucous membranes, making it especially valuable in treating sore throats and other inflammatory conditions. The herb also has astringent properties, and the seeds are sometimes used as a mild sedative.

Common Uses

- Soothe minor skin abrasions, burns, and insect bites, and help prevent infection.
- Relieve hemorrhoid pain and itching.
- Soothe sore throats and other throat irritations.
- Reduce coughs and help clear the airways of sputum.
- Control diarrhea.
- Promote healing of ulcers.
- May counter insomnia.

How It Works

Mullein acts as a demulcent to coat irritated throat tissues to relieve a sore throat and calm a cough. It also has expectorant actions that thin and loosen mucus in the upper airways. Mullein's saponins, tannins, and mucilage have anti-inflammatory properties, and the volatile oils and other mullein components may act as a mild antibiotic and promote healing of minor skin infections.

The mucilage, tannins, and perhaps other components of mullein help control diarrhea. In addition, these substances soothe inflamed and irritated intestines and, when applied as a poultice or ointment, mullein relieves hemorrhoids. The tannins also reduce swelling, not only of hemorrhoids but also of inflamed airways. Mullein tea has been reported to help induce sleep, but the mechanism for this is not known.

Evidence of Efficacy

Mullein has not been studied scientifically, although some of its components, especially mucilage, have. Most of the evidence for mullein's effectiveness is either anecdotal or based on observation of results. German health authorities have approved its use for coughs and bronchitis.

Forms and Usual Dosages

Mullein is available as a tincture and dried flowers and leaves, and the fresh herb can be gathered in the wild. To make a tea, use 1 teaspoon of finely cut leaves, flowers, and stems per cup of boiling water. Steep for ten to fifteen minutes, strain, and drink up to three cups a day. Some people dislike the flavor of mullein; adding honey to the brew improves its taste. Alternatively, a soothing cough remedy can be made by simmering an ounce of dried leaves, or 1 to 2 tablespoons of fresh leaves, for ten minutes in a pint of milk. Strain and drink it while warm. This can also be used to settle an upset stomach or as a bedtime drink.

The leaves and flowers can be used to make a poultice to apply to hemorrhoids or skin sores and inflammations. Mullein tea can also be used as a compress soak for external use, or as a soothing gargle to treat a sore throat.

Potential Problems

There are no reports of adverse effects caused by mullein in any form.

MUSTARD
(BRASSICA SPECIES)

Mustard belongs to the same plant family (Cruciferae) as broccoli, cabbage, and other cruciferous vegetables, so named because their flowers have four petals arranged in tiny crosses. Mustard is thought to have originated in Europe and Asia, but there are now dozens of different varieties that grow worldwide. All are characterized by their pungent seeds, which almost every culture uses to make condiments. The seeds are also pressed to produce oil, which is used for cooking in some parts of the world and as a food and beverage flavoring. Mustard greens can be added to salads or steamed to make a highly nutritious vegetable dish.

Both the mustard seeds and oils have many medicinal uses. The most familiar are external applications, such as mustard poultices, plasters, and liniments. There are also mustard preparations that are taken orally to treat various systemic disorders.

Common Uses

- Reduce chest congestion.
- Relieve muscle aches, inflammation, and joint pain.
- Stimulate appetite.
- Induce vomiting.

How It Works

The active ingredients in mustard seeds are two chemical compounds, called myrosin and sinigrin, glycosides that give mustard its strong odor and pungent flavor. When added to water, they form the volatile oil of mustard, which can cause severe burning when applied directly to the skin or mucous membranes. In a diluted form, however, the oil can be used as a liniment to soothe painful, inflamed arthritis joints. Athletes also use it to ease aching muscles. The diluted volatile oil acts as a counterirritant to reduce the number of pain messages transmitted to the brain by peripheral nerves. It may also interfere with substance P, a body chemical (neurotransmitter) that carries pain messages.

Although not as popular in the United States as in the past, mustard plasters are still used in many parts of the world to treat chest congestion from colds, flu, and bronchitis. The plaster is made by mixing crushed seeds or powdered mustard with flour and adding a little water to make a paste. The paste is spread between two pieces of cotton and then

Mustard is mentioned in the Old and New Testaments of the Bible, and in India, it is a symbol of fertility. It is also one of the world's oldest botanical medicines. Some two thousand years ago, the Greek physician Dioscorides described making mustard plasters to treat chest congestion, a usage that continues to the present. Roman soldiers took mustard seeds to Great Britain, and by the tenth century, mustard was a popular cure-all throughout the British Isles. Even before Pasteur discovered that germs cause infection and disease, the antiseptic properties of mustard were recognized. For example, barber-surgeons were said to have used a mustard solution as a surgical scrub long before the development of antiseptic washes. Mustard gas was a lethal weapon in the early part of the twentieth century, but its use gave rise to the first successful anticancer drug, which is still used to treat leukemia.

wrapped in flannel. The plaster is placed on the patient's chest, and removed as soon as a burning sensation is felt.

The internal uses of mustard are not as well known. A small amount of mustard stimulates appetite by increasing the flow of saliva and digestive juices. Diluted mustard oil is said to have diuretic properties, although it is rarely used for this purpose because of its irritating qualities. At one time, it was also used as a purgative to induce vomiting. Some commercial products marketed to repel dogs, cats, and garden pests contain mustard oil. The irritating nature of mustard oil, combined with its pungent odor, makes it ideal for this purpose.

Evidence of Efficacy

The therapeutic uses of mustards have stood the test of time—they have been used successfully for thousands of years. Scientific studies have isolated the active ingredients in mustard oil, and have also established that they have antibiotic and antifungal properties. In some countries, a few drops of mustard oil added to a foot bath is used to treat athlete's foot.

Forms and Usual Dosage

In addition to the dozens of different condiments, mustard is also available as seeds, powder, liniments, and paste. Mustard oil is also available, typically in concentrations of 0.5 to 5 percent. Full-strength oil should be diluted in a ratio of 1 part mustard oil to 50 parts water, neutral oil, or another suitable dilutent. Dosage depends upon the usage and type. Typically, a small amount—a teaspoon or less—of prepared mustard is used to stimulate appetite.

Potential Problems

Mustard oil is highly irritating; a single drop on the skin can cause a severe burn. Taken internally, it can damage tissue and cause severe vomiting. Care must also be taken not to inhale concentrated mustard fumes; mustard gas is highly toxic to the lungs, and was one of the lethal forms of chemical warfare used in World War I. A mustard plaster should not be left on the skin too long; it can cause serious burning.

MYRRH (*COMMIPHORA MOLMOL*)

Myrrh is made from the sap of a tree that grows mostly in the arid regions of North Africa and parts of the Middle East. When the myrrh tree's bark is cut, it oozes an aromatic whitish sap that hardens into a type of gum. The sap is the source of an incense that has been used in religious ceremonies since ancient times. It also has a long history as a botanical medicine, and today it is a popular treatment for gum and mouth problems. It is also a topical antiseptic that is used to cleanse minor wounds and prevent or treat skin infections. Recent studies indicate that myrrh may help prevent some types of cancer.

Common Uses

- Sweeten bad breath.
- Promote healing of canker sores, gingivitis, and fever blisters or cold sores.
- Soothe a sore throat and intestinal inflammation.
- Shrink hemorrhoids.
- Treat vaginitis caused by bacterial or yeast infections.
- May bolster the immune system.
- Act as a topical antiseptic.

How It Works

The therapeutic ingredients in myrrh include volatile oils, such as limonene, eugenol, and pinene, and astringent resins and gums. The volatile oils reduce airway congestion by thinning phlegm and making it easier to cough up. The astringent properties help stop superficial bleeding and oozing by tightening the skin and constricting peripheral blood vessels. This action may also help reduce excessive menstrual bleeding as well as help shrink hemorrhoids and reduce itching and other symptoms.

When used as a gargle or mouthwash, myrrh soothes inflamed tissue and promotes healing of swollen and bleeding gums (gingivitis), canker sores, and fever blisters. Because myrrh helps control oral bacteria, it can counter bad breath caused by their overgrowth. This is why myrrh is a popular ingredient in mouthwashes, gargles, and some toothpastes.

Myrrh's antibacterial and antifungal properties may be helpful in treating vaginitis. They may also help prevent skin infection and promote healing of wounds. In this regard, it is used as an antiseptic wash to cleanse wounds, bed sores, and skin ulcers.

◉ A LITTLE HISTORY

Myrrh has a long and colorful history. In ancient Egypt, myrrh resin was used to preserve mummies, and it was one of the gifts that the three wise men brought to the Christ child. In biblical times, it was also used to treat leprosy and syphilis. Chinese physicians used it to treat bleeding disorders, including heavy menstrual periods, and to heal skin ulcers and other wounds.

Myrrh may bolster immunity by stimulating macrophages—white blood cells that engulf and destroy bacteria and other foreign invaders—to go into action. This may also help prevent cancer. When taken as a digestive aid, myrrh is thought to prevent or treat indigestion by increasing the flow of pepsin, a major digestive acid.

Evidence of Efficacy

Myrrh's long history as a botanical medicine attests to its effectiveness. In addition, scientific studies have documented its ability to kill certain bacteria and fungi. Animal studies indicate that myrrh may bolster immunity; it also appears to reduce pain and help lower high blood sugar levels. However, these effects have not been studied in humans.

German and British health authorities have approved the use of myrrh to treat canker sores, gingivitis, sore throat, and other oral problems and as a topical agent to treat minor skin inflammations and infections.

Forms and Usual Dosages

Myrrh is available in many forms, including capsules, pills, tinctures, powder, and tea. It is also an ingredient in many commercial mouthwashes, gargles, lip and skin balms, and toothpastes and powders. A gargle can be made by adding ten drops of myrrh tincture to a glass of water. To make myrrh tea, use 1 teaspoon of powdered myrrh per cup of hot water; two or three cups may be consumed a day to treat digestive problems. Myrrh tea can also be used as a compress soak to treat hemorrhoids, or as a wash to cleanse skin ulcers and sores. The typical oral dosage calls for two or three myrrh capsules or pills (usually about 650 mg each) a day.

Potential Problems

Myrrh is considered safe, although some people experience irritation when it is applied to the skin. Be sure to dilute the tincture before applying it.

See Also

Mouth Sores

NETTLE
(URTICA DIOICA)

Also known as common or stinging nettle, *Urtica dioica* is the most common of the five hundred or more species of the plant. It grows in temperate climates worldwide and is characterized by hairy leaves that, when touched, release formic acid—a substance that stings and can cause a painful skin rash. Despite its sting, the plant has been valued throughout history for its sturdy stem, which is similar to flax or hemp and can be used to make fabrics ranging from fine linen to burlap and rope. Its leaves, roots, and flowers, which are high in nutrients, are used in making tonics and beer. The flowers and leaves are also used medicinally to treat a variety of disorders, especially allergies and liver, respiratory, and urinary disorders.

Common Uses

- Increase urine output and perhaps prevent kidney stones.
- Reduce symptoms of an enlarged prostate due to benign prostatic hyperplasia (BPH).
- Help stop bleeding and promote healing of cuts, bruises, and other skin wounds.
- Reduce airway congestion.
- Control hay fever and other allergies, including allergic asthma.
- Alleviate skin itchiness caused by eczema, psoriasis, and other inflammatory skin disorders.
- May reduce excessive menstrual bleeding and the risk of postpartum hemorrhaging.
- Relieve arthritis, fibromyalgia, and other muscle and joint pain.

How It Works

Nettle is a source of 5-HTP, tannins, mucilage, various astringent and acidic compounds, and several important nutrients, including beta-carotene, vitamins C and K, iron and other minerals, and protein. The vitamin K is important in clotting function, and it may be responsible for nettle's reputed ability to reduce heavy menstrual bleeding and hemorrhaging following childbirth.

Tannins and other astringent compounds soothe inflamed skin and membranes, and another ingredient in nettles—5-HTP—has been found to reduce muscle and joint pain. Consuming a tea made of nettle leaves has been shown to increase the flow of urine, which may help prevent kidney stones and ease some of the symptoms of an enlarged prostate gland. It should be noted, however, that nettle tea and other compounds do not actually shrink the prostate.

It is not known how nettles reduce allergy symptoms. The plant does contain anti-inflammatory compounds, which may be helpful in managing asthma and also reducing airway congestion due to inflammation. Mucilage acts as a demulcent to coat irritated mucous membranes and quell coughs. Topical applications appear to reduce minor bleeding and ease the itchiness of eczema and other skin inflammations.

Nettle tea has long been promoted as a tonic to fight fatigue and a general run-down feeling. This benefit may be due to nettle's high iron and vitamin C content—the iron is used to build red blood cells and vitamin C increases its absorption.

Evidence of Efficacy

The scientific evidence on nettles is rather limited, but a few studies appear to document at least some of the medical claims. For example, studies have found that nettle tea and tincture have a mild diuretic effect that increases urine output. A small controlled study involving allergy sufferers found that, in this group at least, nettle preparations were more effective than a placebo, and many of the participants rated the herb higher than their regular allergy medications. No clinical studies have been done to test the herb's effectiveness in treating arthritis and rheumatism, but the German Commission E has approved its use for these conditions. The German health authorities have also approved nettle as a diuretic to treat lower urinary tract problems, including symptoms arising from an enlarged prostate, and to prevent and treat kidney stones.

Forms and Usual Dosages

Nettle is available in capsule, extract, tincture, powdered, and topical forms. A tea can be made from either fresh or dried nettle leaves and stems; use the equivalent of about 1 tablespoon per cup of boiling water. The infusion can be consumed as a tea or used as a gargle or compress soak. Nettle leaves and the powdered root can be used to make a poultice, although nettle lotions and tinctures are available to treat skin problems.

The typical daily dosage to treat urinary problems calls for 8 to 12 g (2 to 3 tablespoons) or 4 to 6 g of powdered root. Some herbal products for benign prostate hyperplasia (BPH) combine nettle root with saw palmetto or pygeum. To alleviate hay fever and other allergy symptoms, many herbalists recommend nettle capsules or tablets in dosages of two or three 300-mg capsules a day, or 2 to 4 ml of tincture three times a day.

Nettles grow wild in most places and are best collected in the late spring just before the plant flowers. Young nettle leaves can be steamed and served as a vegetable. The leaves can also be dried and stored in airtight containers.

Potential Problems

Nettles found in the wild or in gardens should always be handled with leather gloves to protect hands from contact with formic acid. In a meadow or open field, stinging nettles are usually found near plantains. The green juice extracted from the plantain by crushing its leaves against affected skin areas will ease the discomfort of the skin's reaction to the acid. The plantain juice will also relieve the itching of mosquito bites.

Very strong nettle tea can cause digestive problems and a burning sensation on the skin. If this occurs, either stop using the tea or dilute it. Be sure to drink plenty of other fluids—at least eight to ten glasses a day—when taking nettles for a diuretic effect. Because concentrated nettle products may cause uterine contractions, they should not be used during pregnancy. Some people are allergic to nettle; watch for reactions.

See Also

Allergies
Benign Prostate Enlargement

OAK (*QUERCUS ALBA*)

Oaks are among our most stately trees, long revered as a source of wood, shelter, food, and medicine. The white oak, which probably originated in England and grows throughout most of North America, can reach a height of one hundred feet and live up to one thousand years. White oak bark and sometimes the acorns are also used medicinally to treat both external and internal ailments.

Common Uses

- Reduce bleeding, inflammation, and oozing of skin wounds, ulcers, and disorders such as eczema.
- Soothe inflammation of oral tissue and throat membranes.
- Relieve hemorrhoids.
- Control diarrhea.

How It Works

White oak bark is harvested from young branches and saplings in the spring and dried. It is high in tannins, which give white bark preparations their bitter and astringent properties; triterpene glycosides, including saponins, which may lower blood cholesterol levels and bolster immunity; and resins, pectin, calcium, and starches. Oak bark's astringent action soothes inflamed skin and mucous membranes, making gargles and other preparations made from it useful in alleviating a sore throat, mouth ulcers, and gingivitis. The major tannin in oak bark, a substance called quercitannic acid, is also a mild antiseptic that can help prevent minor skin wounds from becoming infected.

The astringent action of tannins reduces bleeding and oozing from skin ulcers, eczema, and other skin disorders, and helps shrink hemorrhoids and stop their bleeding. Tannins and other ingredients in oak bark can help control diarrhea, although there are other botanical medicines that may be more effective.

Evidence of Efficacy

Oak bark itself has not been studied extensively, although some of its astringent ingredients have been researched and found effective in treating inflammation, diarrhea, and other conditions. Recent animal studies indicate that the saponins in white oak bark may help lower high cholesterol, but it is not known whether this finding applies to humans. Saponins also appear to bolster immunity in animals by increasing antibody production. Again, more study is needed to determine whether these benefits extend to humans.

Forms and Usual Dosage

Oak bark for internal use is available in capsule, liquid extract, and tea forms. Chopped and powdered bark is used to make decoctions, gargles, poultices, and compress soaks. Oak bark is an ingredient in some skin lotions, disinfectants, and bath products. To make an oak bark decoction or gargle, use about 2 tablespoons of chopped or powdered bark per pint of hot water; one cup of the decoction can be added to bathwater.

Potential Problems

Oak bark appears to be safe when used as directed. However, German health authorities caution against applying oak bark solutions to large areas of damaged skin and adding it to bathwater if you have extensive oozing eczema.

POPPY (*PAPAVER SOMNIFERUM*)

Poppies are annuals that produce showy, brightly colored flowers with black centers that evolve into round seedpods. Poppies grow wild in most parts of the world. They are also popular in flower gardens and one species—*Papaver somniferum*, which is cultivated in the Middle East and parts of Asia, gives rise to two major commercial products: poppyseeds that are crushed to make oil or used whole to flavor breads, cakes, and other baked goods; and opium, a highly addictive drug that is one of our most effective painkillers and has numerous other medicinal uses. Opium, which is derived from the milky sap of the green seedpods, is the basic substance needed to make heroin, one of our most notorious illegal substances that has ruined countless lives over the years.

Common Uses

- Control pain, especially that following surgery or other severe pain that cannot be alleviated by other means.
- Stop severe diarrhea.
- Calm a hacking dry cough.
- Reduce muscle spasms.
- Induce sleep.

How It Works

Opium contains several alkaloids, morphine being the most important. Its derivatives include codeine, laudenine, narcotine, and papaverine. Morphine is widely regarded as our most effective painkiller. It is often given during a heart attack to calm the patient and ease chest pain; it is also used to ease postoperative pain and that of cancer, broken bones, and many other causes of extreme, intractable pain. It works through the brain's opiate receptors, which block pain messages from reaching the areas of the brain where they are interpreted.

All the morphine derivatives have important painkilling and sedating qualities that make them highly effective in many situations. They also quell muscle spasms, which can stop diarrhea and a hacking cough. Papaverine is especially effective in relaxing smooth muscle contractions, making it an effective treatment for intestinal cramps, diarrhea, and the spasms that tighten the airways during an asthma attack. Codeine, while not as effective as morphine, is considered a safer drug because it is not as addictive. It is used to treat everything from menstrual cramps to back pain due to muscle spasms.

Morphine and its derivatives have other important properties—they ease anxiety, calm jittery nerves, and induce feelings of euphoria. On the surface, these would seem positive attributes; in fact, they are what make morphine a dangerous, double-edged sword because users quickly become addicted to the drug and suffer withdrawal symptoms when they try to stop taking it (see Potential Problems, below).

Evidence of Efficacy

There is no question that morphine is one of our most effective painkillers; it has been used for this purpose for thousands of years. In recent decades, neuroscientists have identified the brain receptors that allow opium to block out pain messages. Artificial forms have been developed; these, called opioids, include some of our most effective painkillers. Because they are still narcotic substances, they—like morphine and other natural opium derivatives—are addictive.

Forms and Usual Dosage

Medications derived from the opium poppies are classified as controlled substances and are available only with a doctor's prescription. They are given by injection or may be taken orally in pill, capsule, or liquid form. A new form of administration, using an automated morphine pump, allows patients to control their own dosage. Studies have found that this method of administration is more effective in controlling pain than giving the drugs according to a set schedule, which often means that pain is already intense when the morphine is administered. In addition, patients usually get relief with smaller dosages, perhaps because they can give themselves an injection at the first perception of pain rather than waiting for it to become so severe that a large dosage is needed.

Potential Problems

Addiction is the major problem with all the opium-based drugs. In fact, it is the fear of addiction that keeps many doctors and patients alike from using these narcotic substances even when they are indicated. Recent studies indicate, however, that people who are given opiates to control severe, temporary pain such as that associated with surgery or a broken bone are unlikely to become addicted unless they have a history of alcoholism or other addiction problems. In the case of pain caused by terminal cancer, the patient's comfort is certainly more important than concerns about possible addiction. Otherwise, use of these drugs for more than a few weeks poses a problem of becoming dependent on them. Of course, use of heroin and abuse of prescription opiates invariably lead to addiction.

Even short-term, medically supervised use of codeine and other morphine derivatives can cause severe constipation, especially if the person is bedridden. When taking any opiate, it's important to increase fluid and fiber intake, and a bulking laxative, such as psyllium seeds, may be needed.

RED CLOVER (*TRIFOLIUM PRATENSE*)

◉ A LITTLE HISTORY

In the past, red clover tea was often recommended as a spring tonic to "cleanse the blood" and was said to prevent cancer. It was also used to treat whooping cough, tuberculosis, and syphilis and other venereal diseases. These remedies have been replaced by more effective treatments, but many continue to believe that red clover contains important unknown compounds that protect against cancer and other diseases. Ongoing studies may justify some of these beliefs. For example, some research suggests that daidzein and genistein—two of the isoflavones found in red clover—may have anticancer properties.

Red clover is a perennial that is thought to have originated in the Mediterranean and now grows wild throughout much of Europe and North America. It is cultivated as a farm crop to make hay and silage.

Red clover, characterized by its pink flowers and leaves that grow in clusters of three, is a legume, and as such, related to soybeans, chickpeas, and other peas and beans. In addition to being a highly nutritious food for livestock, red clover is said to have important medicinal properties, especially in easing menopausal symptoms.

Common Uses

- Reduce hot flashes and night sweats associated with menopause.
- Prevent mood swings.
- Increase flagging libido.
- May help prevent osteoporosis and postmenopausal heart disease.
- Possibly treat eczema, psoriasis, and other skin disorders through anti-inflammatory actions.
- Treat coughs and chest congestion caused by colds and flu.

How It Works

Like soybeans and its other legume relatives, red clover is rich in isoflavone compounds—plant (phyto) estrogens that have effects similar to estrogen, the major female sex hormone. Phytoestrogens mimic some of the effects of estrogen because they have similar chemical structures and are able to interact with estrogen receptors. Consequently, they are thought to reduce hot flashes, night sweats, and other menopausal symptoms caused by the decline in production of natural estrogen.

Phytoestrogens may also help maintain vaginal tissue and lubrication—important factors in a woman's sexual function and pleasure. Phytoestrogens may also help prevent the accelerated loss of bone mass that is common following menopause. Unlike natural estrogen, phytoestrogens do not appear to stimulate breast tissue, so they are probably not linked to an increased risk of breast cancer.

Red clover also contains coumarins, substances that reduce blood clotting, and volatile oils, which are thought to have mild anti-inflammatory properties that are useful in treating eczema and other skin inflammations. It also contains compounds that may help calm a cough and reduce airway congestion.

Evidence of Efficacy

Most of the evidence for red clover is based on traditional uses rather than scientific studies. In recent years, medical researchers have identified four different isoflavones in red clover—genistein, daidzein, biochanin, and formononetin. Population studies have found that women who consume large amounts of soy products, which are high in genistein and daidzein, have fewer menopausal symptoms and a lower incidence of breast cancer compared to women whose diets are low in soy and other legumes. Promoters of red clover contend that it may be even more beneficial than soy because it contains two extra isoflavones, as indicated by studies conducted in Australia. There is little or no scientific proof, however, that red clover is effective in treating skin inflammation. Red clover tea does appear to reduce coughing and airway congestion, but similar effects can be obtained by drinking any number of other hot liquids.

Forms and Usual Dosages

Red clover is available in tablet and capsule forms; dried red clover flowers are marketed as tea. To treat menopausal symptoms, the typical recommended dosage entails taking red clover extracts standardized to provide 40 mg of isoflavones per day.

To make red clover tea, steep four to six dried blossoms in a cup of boiling water for fifteen minutes, then strain and sweeten if desired. Two or three cups a day are recommended to ease menopausal symptoms. A cough remedy can be made by adding honey and vegetable glycerin to the tea to make a syrup and then consuming 1 tablespoon four or five times a day and before going to bed. Compresses soaked in red clover tea may ease muscle and joint pain.

Potential Problems

Do not take red clover extracts if you are taking Coumadin or other blood-thinning medications. Red clover contains compounds similar to those in Coumadin and the combination may cause bleeding problems. When gathering clover in the wild, check the blossoms carefully to make sure they are not moldy, diseased, or sprayed with pesticides; dry them carefully, too, before storing them; if in doubt, use a reliable commercial product. Otherwise, red clover is considered safe when used as directed.

See Also

Menopause

RED RASPBERRY (*RUBUS IDAEUS, R. STRIGOSUS*)

Raspberries are members of the Rosaceae family, which also includes blackberries, another berry plant that is widely used in herbal medicine. Raspberries, both black and red, grow wild in wooded areas of Europe and the United States; they are also cultivated for home and commercial use.

While the tasty, sweet raspberries are a favorite summer fruit and flavoring for everything from soft drinks and ice cream to pharmaceutical products, it's this thorny shrub's leaves that are used medicinally. For centuries, Native American midwives and their Old World counterparts—from the British Isles to the woodlands of central Russia and into Asia Minor—have treated various pregnancy-related problems with raspberry leaf teas and extracts. Raspberry leaf is also used to treat menstrual and fertility problems. Although it is generally considered an herb for "female complaints," it may also be recommend for diarrhea, stomach upsets, edema, and lung congestion due to a common cold or flu. The leaves are also added to some blends of drinking tea to improve their flavor.

Common Uses

- Relieve morning sickness and prevent a threatened miscarriage.
- Maintain healthy pregnancy and ease labor pains during childbirth.
- Help restore the uterus to its normal size following childbirth.
- Ease menstrual cramps and reduce premenstrual breast tenderness, swelling, and other PMS symptoms.
- Help overcome female fertility problems.
- Treat intestinal problems, including diarrhea and upset stomach.

- Reduce nausea, especially motion sickness.
- Treat skin inflammation, fever blisters, hemorrhoids, and other irritations of the skin and mucous membranes (external use).
- Relieve mouth sores and a sore throat (as a gargle).

How It Works

Native American herbalists and midwives recommend drinking red raspberry leaf tea in the early months of pregnancy to "strengthen the uterus," prevent miscarriage, and relieve morning sickness. During the final month or so of pregnancy, the tea is again recommended to prepare the uterus for childbirth and reduce labor pains. There is no scientific evidence that raspberry leaves contain any substances that can effect these benefits (see Evidence of Efficacy, below).

In contrast, there is an explanation for some of the other recommended uses. Raspberry leaves are rich in tannins, which have astringent properties, and pectin, a soluble fiber. These substances may explain the beneficial effects of raspberry leaf teas in stopping simple diarrhea. The astringent action of tannins are also useful in treating mouth or throat inflammation. Raspberry leaves are also relatively high in vitamin C and flavonoids, which may promote healing of mouth sores and other skin irritations.

Evidence of Efficacy

There is little or no scientific evidence that raspberry leaf teas or extracts are of value during pregnancy. Animal studies have found that raspberry leaves contain substances that affect the uterus in ways that tend to cancel each other out. In a laboratory study using human uterine tissue, a raspberry leaf extract promoted muscle contractions when applied to strips of tissue from a pregnant uterus; no such effect was noted in tissue from a nonpregnant uterus. It is not known, however, whether similar effects take place in a pregnant woman's body.

Forms and Usual Dosage

Steeping 2 teaspoons of raspberry leaves in a cup of boiling water makes a soothing tea that may be taken three times a day. Some herbalists recommend combining raspberry leaf tea with ginger and dried mint leaves to relieve nausea and calm an upset stomach. An infusion can also be used as a mouth rinse, gargle, solution for compresses, and a soak.

Potential Problems

Commercial red raspberry leaf tea actually contains very little active ingredients, so drinking it in moderation—for example, two or three cups a day—is unlikely to cause problems. Stronger homemade brews from dried leaves can provoke nausea and diarrhea in some people.

Although eyewash made with a raspberry leaf infusion is said to help reduce inflammation, unless the liquid is sterile, it could cause an eye infection, so homemade eye solutions are never advisable.

The use of red raspberry leaf tea during pregnancy remains controversial. No long-term studies have been done to prove raspberry leaf is safe for a developing fetus, so many experts advise against it. In contrast, others note that traditional healers have recommended it during pregnancy for centuries with no reports of ill effects. Still, to be safe it's wise to check with a doctor before taking it—or any other herbal or pharmaceutical product—during pregnancy.

See Also

Diarrhea

ROSE (*ROSA CANINA* AND OTHER SPECIES)

Roses are cultivated worldwide and are prized for their beautiful flowers and fragrance. Rosehips are the bright red fruits that form on rosebushes after the flower petals have fallen off. The rosehips that are most often used medicinally come from the climbing varieties known variously as briar or dog rose and witches' briar.

Common Uses

- Prevent and treat the common cold.
- Treat urinary tract infections by increasing the flow of urine.
- Treat constipation.
- Relieve mouth ulcers, cold sores, and sore throat.

How It Works

Rosehips are one of our richest sources of vitamin C, an essential anti-oxidant that bolsters immunity and may well protect against the cold virus or shorten the duration of a cold. They also contain pectin (a soluble fiber) and various acidic compounds that have laxative effects. Rose oil, which is distilled from the petals, is used in aromatherapy. A tea made from the rosebush roots has soothing astringent properties that may relieve the pain of mouth ulcers (canker sores), fever blisters, and—when gargled—a sore throat. Similarly, drinking or gargling rosehip tea has a soothing effect.

Evidence of Efficacy

Whether vitamin C can actually prevent the common cold remains an issue of scientific debate. Numerous studies have been conducted trying to prove or refute the contention that high doses of vitamin C will prevent the common cold, and they have produced mixed results. Some show no difference, while others indicate that vitamin C may shorten the duration of a cold by a few days.

Drinking several cups of rosehip tea a day increases fluid intake, an important factor in treating cold symptoms and urinary tract infections. There is no doubt, however, that vitamin C—when taken in moderate amounts—possesses important antioxidant properties and helps boost immunity against common infections. It also promotes healing of minor skin sores.

Forms and Usual Dosage

Rosehips are available fresh or dried and in pill, capsule, and tincture forms. To make a tea, use about ½ teaspoon of powdered rosehips or a scant teaspoon of dried or chopped fresh hips per cup of hot water. Let it steep for ten to fifteen minutes, strain, and drink. Three or four cups a day are recommended, starting at the first hint of cold or flu symptoms. Otherwise, a cup a day made from high-quality rosehips more than meets the recommended dietary allowance (RDA) for vitamin C; in fact, some provide more than 1,000 mg of vitamin C per cup.

Potential Problems

Excessive intake of rosehip tea and other products can increase the risk of kidney stones in susceptible people. Some people are allergic to roses, and may react to rosehips as well. Recent studies indicate that when vitamin C is taken in very large amounts of more than 2,000 mg a day, it becomes a pro-oxidant and actually has the opposite effect of an antioxidant by increasing cellular damage of unstable free radicals. Some experts contend that this pro-oxidant activity begins at dosages as low as 1,000 mg (see Vitamin C, p. 210).

Consumers also should be aware of the fact that much of the natural vitamin C in some rosehip products is lost in the manufacturing process. To compensate, some manufacturers fortify the products with artificial vitamin C. For example, 100 g of high-quality rosehips may provide 1,000 mg or more of vitamin C; some commercial products contain only a fraction of this amount.

ROSEMARY (*ROSMARINUS OFFICINALIS*)

◉ A LITTLE HISTORY
Rosemary's reputation as a memory enhancer dates to ancient Greece. Instead of cramming all night to prepare for a big test, early Greek students were more likely to wear a garland of rosemary in the belief that the herb would help improve their memory.

In medieval times, the faithful placed sprigs of rosemary under their pillows to ward off evil spirits. Brides wove rosemary into their bridal bouquets as a symbol of love. And at funerals, mourners would toss fresh rosemary into a grave as an act of remembrance.

French medics in World War II burned a mixture of rosemary leaves and juniper berries in field hospitals to prevent infection—a practice that dates to the Middle Ages. Recent studies indicate that rosemary oils do have antibiotic properties, but they should not be used in place of standard antibiotics.

Rosemary is a perennial evergreen shrub that is native to the Mediterranean and now cultivated worldwide. Its needle-like leaves and tiny pale blue flowers have been used for centuries to preserve fish and meat, flavor food, and scent cosmetics, soaps, and shampoos. The list of rosemary's medicinal uses past and present is equally varied. Throughout history, herbalists and traditional healers have recommended rosemary to cure baldness and paralysis, improve memory, treat depression and headaches, and help heal bruises and skin wounds. Aromatherapists recommend it as a stimulating bath solution and massage therapists use the diluted oil to help increase peripheral circulation. Today, researchers are studying its cancer-prevention potential; it may also play a role in preserving memory. It may be ingested, inhaled, and applied externally as an ointment, in shampoo, or a soaking solution.

Rosemary oil contains tannins and a mix of cineol, camphor, monoterpene hydrocarbons, and borneol. Some of these chemicals are potent antioxidants that may play a role in preventing cancer and the effects of aging.

Common Uses

- Alleviate intestinal symptoms, including indigestion, upset stomach, and gas.
- Improve circulation.
- Repel insects.
- Speed healing of bruises and skin wounds.

- Relieve joint and muscle pain.
- Treat stress, mild depression, and mental fatigue.
- Slow hair loss of male-pattern balding.
- May slow or prevent memory loss.

How It Works

The potent oil in rosemary has multiple actions: it calms the intestinal tract, lessens muscle spasms, and relieves bloating and gas. Camphor in the oil has an irritating effect, so that when it is applied externally as an ointment or liniment it stimulates peripheral circulation that may help ease muscle and joint pain. When used on the scalp, the stimulating effects of rosemary may improve circulation to the scalp, which may have some effect in slowing premature baldness. Inhaling rosemary's aromatic vapors is said to help ease nervous tension and may lift a depressed mood.

Rosemary does contain antioxidants, which make it a good food preservative. In the body, antioxidants protect cells against oxidative damage caused by unstable molecules (free radicals), and thus may slow aging and help prevent cancer and numerous other diseases.

Evidence of Efficacy

There is little proof that rosemary accomplishes all the therapeutic and preventive claims made for it, but studies in Japan have documented rosemary's high content of antioxidants. They identified carnosol and carnosic acid in rosemary, both of which protect cells from oxidative damage. Animal studies have found that rosemary slows the growth of breast cancer in mice, and other studies have found that rosemary applied to the skin of laboratory animals halved their incidence of skin cancer. German health authorities have approved claims that rosemary ointments can alleviate muscle and joint pain.

Forms and Usual Dosages

A tea made using 1 teaspoon (2 g) of the leaves in a cup of water can be drunk three times a day. Doses of the tincture range from 0.3 to 1.2 ml, taken up to three times a day.

Diluted rosemary oil can be used externally in a variety of preparations, but the full-strength oil should never be taken internally or rubbed into the skin in large amounts, since it can cause kidney damage. A few drops under the nose may revive a person who has fainted. For a relaxing, pain-relieving bath, fill a cheesecloth bag with 2 ounces of dried or fresh rosemary and add it to the bathwater.

Potential Problems

Full-strength rosemary oil should never be ingested, and high doses can be fatal. Even diluted oil can irritate the stomach and intestines and damage the kidneys. Rosemary tea is safe when used as directed. Aromatic bath preparations, shampoos, and other external uses are generally safe.

SAGE (*SALVIA OFFICINALIS*)

This aromatic perennial is commonly used in food preparation; for centuries the Greeks have preserved meat with it, and today it's a popular food flavoring. But throughout history, many cultures have employed sage for uses that extend far beyond the kitchen. As with many kitchen herbs, women have relied on sage to ease their "female complaints"; for example, sage is said to bring on and/or slow menstruation and ease menstrual cramps.

The medicinal uses of sage run the gamut from antiseptic to antidepressant, but sage may be most famous for its ability to decrease perspiration. Sage tea was used to stop the night sweats of people suffering from tuberculosis, and today a German company markets a natural antiperspirant that contains sage. More recently, herbalists and other alternative practitioners have started to tout its antioxidant activity, which may help prevent cancer and diseases of aging.

Common Uses

- Soothe mouth or throat inflammations, canker sores, and gum disease.
- Relieve toothache.
- Soothe dry skin.
- Relieve insects bites.
- Reduce excessive perspiration.
- Treat fever.
- Ease dry cough.
- Calm digestive upsets, including stomach cramps, gas, and diarrhea.
- Treat menstrual problems, including cramps and irregular periods, and menopausal symptoms.
- Treat depression and other nervous disorders.
- Relieve rheumatic (joint and muscle) pain.

- Stop lactation.
- Boost appetite.

How It Works

The astringent quality of the tannins in sage are responsible for its use as a gargle and mouthwash to soothe sore throat inflammation in the mouth. Also, it contains phenolic acids, which help fight the bacteria that can cause gum inflammation and some sore throats.

The volatile oil in sage contains cimene, cineole, limonene, terpinene, camphor, and thujone, among many other constituents. The oil promotes blood flow to the area when the herb is used in a rinse or a poultice. And when taken internally, the diluted oil may help calm the digestive tract and relieve upset stomach. It's also said to stimulate bile production.

Sage is purported to have mild estrogenlike effects, which may explain its benefits in treating menstrual problems and menopausal symptoms, but the constituent responsible has not been identified.

Evidence of Efficacy

Proof of its principal use—as a natural antiperspirant—is lacking, and animal studies done decades ago failed to show the effect. While American medical textbooks no longer suggest sage gargles for sore throat, German health authorities continue to recommend it for this purpose. Animal studies have shown that it soothes the smooth muscle of the intestinal tract, and in Germany it is officially approved for relief of indigestion.

The strong antioxidant activity of the components of sage oil has been documented, but whether that actually helps prevent cancer and heart disease is not known. However, American researchers have found that it enhances the effects of insulin, so it may have some effect on diabetes.

Forms and Usual Dosages

A tea can be made with 2 teaspoons to a cup of hot water, steeped in a covered container. When the tea cools a bit, it can also be used as a gargle or mouthwash. The tea or mouthwash can be used three times a day, but prolonged use should be avoided.

Two to three drops of sage oil in about ¼ cup of water can be used as a gargle or rinse. The same solution can be used to soak compresses as well. Chewing on a leaf may remedy bad breath, especially if it is due to a food, such as onions.

Potential Problems

Pure sage oil—as with all essential oils—should not be ingested or applied to the skin in its full strength. Instead, the oil should be diluted in a neutral carrier, such as olive or another vegetable oil.

Thujone, a chemical in sage oil, can cause convulsions. (Thujone is the notorious ingredient in absinthe, which is said to have been the cause of Vincent Van Gogh's insanity.) It's unwise to use the tea for a prolonged period of time for similar reasons. (Mouthwashes and gargles appear to be safe since the liquid is not swallowed.) Pregnant women are cautioned to avoid sage tea because its estrogenlike effects are not clear.

See Also

Tooth Decay and Gum Disease
Menopause

ST. JOHN'S WORT (*HYPERICUM PERFORATUM*)

St. John's wort is a perennial shrub that produces bright yellow flowers with tiny black dots in their petals and sepals. When squeezed, these dots ooze a red pigment; according to legend, the pigment represents the blood of St. John the Baptist, and some think that this is the origin of the plant's popular name. Another theory holds that the plant got its name because it usually blooms by June 24, the day of the feast of St. John, and, according to tradition, this is the best day to gather the herb. Whatever the origin of its name, St. John's wort enjoys a long history as a medicinal herb, and today it is one of the most touted natural treatments for mild to moderate depression.

Common Uses

- Lift mood and help overcome mild or occasional bouts of depression.
- Promote sleep.
- Calm feelings of anxiety.
- Aid healing of minor skin wounds and infections.

How It Works

One of the active ingredients in St. John's wort is hypericin, a substance that if thought to increase circulating levels of serotonin, a brain chemical (neurotransmitter) that is instrumental in controlling mood, by selectively preventing its reuptake by cells. This mechanism of action is similar to that of Prozac, Zoloft, and other antidepressants known as SSRIs, or selective serotonin reuptake inhibitors. It may also inhibit monamine oxidase (MAO), a brain enzyme that destroys serotonin, epinephrine, and dopamine, the mood-elevating neurotransmitters.

Evidence of Efficacy

More than two dozen studies have found that St. John's wort is more effective than a placebo in treating mild to moderate depression. In addition, controlled studies in Germany have found that St. John's wort compares favorably with Prozac and other pharmaceutical SSRIs in relieving mild to moderate depression: other studies have found it is comparable with tricyclic antidepressants such as Elavil. It has the added advantage of not causing dry mouth and other side effects that sometimes occur with the pharmaceutical products; it is also more economical.

In Germany, St. John's wort is by far the most popular prescription drug to treat mild to moderate depression. In addition, other healing properties of St. John's wort are under study. Its flowers and leaves have mild antibiotic properties, a finding that tends to substantiate its ancient use to heal wounds. In addition to depression, German health authorities have approved external applications of an oil extract of the herb to treat minor burns, skin wounds, and inflammations and a diluted oral solution to treat heartburn. Researchers are studying the plant's apparent antiviral actions to determine whether hypericin may be effective against HIV, the virus that causes AIDS. So far, laboratory findings are promising, but it has not been studied for this purpose in humans.

Forms and Usual Dosage

St. John's wort is usually taken in pill or capsule form; it is also available as a tincture and tea, and as an ointment for external application. Most of the clinical studies to assess St. John's wort in the treatment of depression used 300-mg tablets or capsules, standardized to provide 0.3 percent of hypericin, taken three times a day. St. John's wort may also be taken in tea form, made with tincture, a liquid extract, or a capsule dissolved in a cup of hot water. It usually takes at least two to six weeks to notice improvement.

◉ A LITTLE HISTORY

Since ancient times, St. John's wort has been accorded medicinal and supernatural powers. A brew of St. John's tea was said to drive out demons—perhaps an early recognition of the herb's antidepressant properties. It was worn as a protection against witches, and placing a sprig of the herb under a pillow on St. John's Eve was said to induce the saint to appear in a dream and ensure another year of life.

St. John's wort was introduced into the United States by European settlers and, like many weeds, it quickly established itself and then went on to take over vast tracts of pasture and farmland in the Pacific Northwest, where it is called Klamath weed. Cattle love the weed, but those that eat large amounts of it become sun-sensitive and can develop severe sunburn. When herbicides applied in 1946 failed to control the plants' spread, an Australian beetle that loves St. John's wort was imported and within a decade the weed was declared under control. The beetle has continued to thrive and control the spread of St. John's wort. This is now something of a mixed blessing, however, because the beetle is thwarting recent efforts to cultivate St. John's wort for commercial purposes.

Potential Problems

St. John's wort is not effective against the more severe forms of clinical depression. Although the plant causes sun sensitivity in cattle that consume large amounts of the herb, this does not seem to occur in humans unless they take a synthetic form of hypericin. Still, experts caution that it is always prudent to protect the skin against exposure to direct sun, perhaps even more so if you are taking this herb.

Because St. John's wort may act as a mild MAO inhibitor, some experts caution against eating foods that are high in tyramine while taking the herb. These include red wine, aged cheeses, and beans and other legumes, among others. However, many other experts discount the danger and there have not been reports of MAO-like reactions, which include a dangerous rise in blood pressure.

St. John's wort should never be taken with prescription antidepressants (Prozac, Paxil, Zoloft) lithium, Demerol, or dextromethorphan, a common ingredient in cough syrups. The combination can result in a very dangerous reaction called serotonin syndrome, marked by a high fever, confusion, muscle rigidity, diarrhea, and possibly death.

There have been some reports of allergic reactions to St. John's wort, and a few people experience mild diarrhea and other intestinal problems. On the whole, however, St. John's wort is safe and most people do not experience adverse side effects.

See Also

Anxiety
Depression

SAW PALMETTO (*SERENOA REPENS, S. SERRULATA*)

Saw palmetto, a shrubby, bushy plant that grows in sandy soil in the southeastern United States, is also known as the American dwarf palm tree or cabbage palm. It also grows in the Caribbean and certain parts of the Mediterranean. It reaches a maximum height of about ten feet.

The plant is characterized by long, swordlike, yellow-green leaves, cream-colored flowers, and purplish to black fruits. These berries are similar to olives in their size and shape, each with one pale brown seed. But unlike the pleasant-tasting olive, saw palmetto seeds have an unpleasant soapy taste. However, it is the partially dried berries that are used medicinally. Active components of the berries include plant sterols, flavonoids, water-soluble polysaccharides, and free fatty acids.

Common Uses

- Relieve excessive urination and other symptoms of benign prostate enlargement (BPH).
- Reduce bladder irritation.

How It Works

Historically, Native Americans used saw palmetto for various urinary tract disorders, such as bladder inflammation and infection and as a diuretic to increase urinary output. It was also recommended for respiratory diseases and reproductive tract disorders, such as impotence and male fertility problems, and—in women—to increase sexual desire and promote breast growth. However, only its benefits against symptoms of prostate enlargement have been well documented.

The prostate is a small gland in men that wraps around the urethra. With increasing age, the prostate tends to enlarge—the phenomenon is called benign prostate hyperplasia, or BPH—and this may result in urinary problems. Saw palmetto has been shown to reduce symptoms resulting from BPH, but researchers do not fully understand how it works. Some theorize that it directly reduces swelling, others believe that it actually decreases the size of the gland, (although this has never been proved), and still others think it may increase the bladder's ability to contract and expel its contents. In fact, saw palmetto works faster than Proscor, a drug prescribed for this condition.

Newer theories hold that saw palmetto may inhibit the action of an important hormone-regulating enzyme that converts testosterone into dihydrotestosterone, a process believed to be important in the development of both BPH and prostate cancer. Preventing this conversion is also the way finasteride—the standard medication prescribed for BPH—works. However, saw palmetto does not produce the negative side effects that sometimes occur with finasteride.

Evidence of Efficacy

A number of clinical trials have shown that saw palmetto is more effective than a placebo and also works as well or better than finasteride, the most-used pharmaceutical drug prescribed to relieve BPH. In general, studies show about a 50 percent improvement in urinary flow rate and a decreased number of nighttime urinations. It also improved the maximum flow, increased the volume of urine per voiding, lengthened the interval between voidings, and reduced the sensation of incomplete voiding. Further, it does not impair male sexual function as finasteride may. In one study of quality-of-life scores after ninety days of treatment with saw palmetto, 37 percent of men were satisfied with the results, 29 percent were very happy or delighted, 21 percent reported that their symptoms were lessened, and only 13 percent were unsatisfied, unhappy, or hopeless about their situation. In further contrast, finasteride took up to a year to produce positive results.

Forms and Usual Dosage

Experts recommend a daily dose of 1 to 2 g saw palmetto, or 320 mg of its hexane extract. In a large double-blind, randomized clinical trial at eighty-seven urology centers in nine European countries, Permixon, a liquid/sterol extract of 320 mg per day of saw palmetto, was given to more than two thousand German men with BPH. In some studies, doses of 160 mg were prescribed twice a day.

Potential Problems

In contrast to finasteride, which decreases libido and causes impotence in some men, saw palmetto has minimal side effects. Stomach complaints are rare. An extract standardized to contain 85 to 95 percent fatty acids and sterols should be used because an equivalent dose using crude berries, fluid extracts, or tinctures would require very large doses and would not be reliable.

See Also

Benign Prostate Enlargement

SENECA ROOT (*POLYGALA SENEGA*)

Also known as snakeroot, milkwort, and senega, seneca root is a perennial that is native to North America, growing from Canada in the north to as far south as Georgia and Tennessee. Its popular names are derived from the fact that the Seneca Indians and other Native Americans used it to treat snakebites. There are now more effective snakebite treatments, and the popularity of seneca root as a botanical remedy for its other major medical indications—coughs and airway congestion—has waned. Still, some herbalists recommend it, and Native Americans in the Plains states and parts of Canada still gather and dry it.

Common Uses

- Loosen phlegm and make it easier to cough up (expectorant).
- Increase sweating with a goal of lowering the fever of colds and flu.

How It Works

Seneca root is high in saponin glycosides—specifically polygalic acid and senegin—which form a soapy froth when mixed with water. When ingested, these substances act as an expectorant to thin and loosen phlegm. These compounds also stimulate the sweat glands to increase perspiration, and when taken in large amounts, they increase the output of urine and act as purgatives to cause vomiting and diarrhea. These functions were once considered helpful in "cleansing the system," but this is no longer thought necessary or even beneficial.

Seneca root also contains mucilage, a slippery substance that coats and soothes inflamed and irritated mucous membranes, thus relieving a sore throat, as well as resins, a volatile oil, and methyl salicylate, which gives it a refreshing minty flavor and odor. An acidic compound in seneca root is thought to have anti-inflammatory properties.

Evidence of Efficacy

The expectorant properties of the type of saponin glycosides in seneca root are well established and German health authorities have approved seneca root as a cough and cold remedy. It is no longer listed in the *National Formulary* of the United States because other more effective treatments are available.

Forms and Usual Dosage

Seneca root is usually taken as a tea, extract, cough syrup, or tincture. In Europe, it is an ingredient in some throat lozenges. A tea is made by steeping about 0.5 to 1 g (just under ¼ to ⅓ teaspoon) of dried seneca root per cup of water. Up to three cups a day may be consumed.

Potential Problems

High doses (2.5 to 3 g a day) can cause vomiting, diarrhea, and profuse sweating. Stop taking seneca root immediately if vomiting or diarrhea develop and don't use it if you have ulcers, colitis, or other chronic intestinal disorders. It should never be taken during pregnancy; its effects on the uterus are unknown, but it was purportedly used to induce abortion by some tribes of Native Americans.

SENNA
(*CASSIA SENNA*)

Senna, the popular name for two varieties of cassia shrubs, is native to India, Pakistan, and parts of China. Asians and north Africans have used senna to treat constipation for centuries, and it is an ingredient in several over-the-counter laxatives sold in the United States. Taken plain, it has a very unpleasant taste; its use is also limited by its potential side effects.

A LITTLE HISTORY
Senna has been used as a laxative for hundreds of years. According to legend, during the ninth century, Mesue the Elder, a famed court physician to the court of Baghdad, treated the calif with senna as a gentler alternative to his usual laxatives. It's hard to imagine harsher laxatives, but as the story goes, the calif was delighted with the preparation.

Common Uses

• Treat occasional, severe constipation.

How It Works

Senna leaves are high in substances called anthraquinone glycosides, which are powerful stimulant laxatives. These compounds, which are also found in buckthorn and cascara sagrada (see p. 405), act on the muscles that encircle the colon and control peristalsis, the muscular contractions that move waste through the large intestine. Increased peristalsis shortens the transit time of material passing through the colon. Anthraquinones also increase the amount of fluid in the colon, resulting in a more fluid fecal mass that is easier to pass than a compacted, hard stool.

Evidence of Efficacy

The laxative effects of anthraquinones are well documented by long experience with botanical medicine and by well-controlled scientific studies.

Forms and Usual Dosage

Senna is available in capsule or tablets, usually in dosages providing 20 to 60 mg of sennosides. As noted, senna is included in many non-prescription pharmaceutical and herbal laxatives; check labels for ingredients—it may be listed as senna or sennosides. Many doctors advise that senna be used as a last-resort laxative. First try lifestyle changes, especially dietary changes (increased fiber and fluid intake) and regular exercise. If constipation persists, start with a gentle, bulk-producing laxative such as psyllium seeds. The next step would be a lubricant laxative, such as mineral oil suppositories. If a stimulant laxative is considered necessary, cascara sagrada is gentler than senna and may be preferable to start with first.

Potential Problems

Use of senna, or any stimulant laxative, should be limited to seven to ten days, and should be taken only after consulting a doctor. Long-term use can result in laxative dependency, a condition in which the colon becomes sluggish and ceases to function normally on its own.

Even a moderate senna overdose can cause severe cramping and diarrhea, and possible dehydration and excessive loss of potassium and other electrolytes. Thus, it's a good idea to stick with commercial products with fixed dosages. If you do decide to brew your own senna tea, start with a scant teaspoon of dried leaves per cup of boiling water and drink only one cup a day. It usually takes six to twelve hours to work. To reduce the risk of cramping and intestinal upsets, senna may be combined with licorice, anise, fennel, or other soothing herbs. Do not take senna if you have ulcers, diverticulosis, colitis, or another intestinal disorder, and avoid it—and all other laxatives—during pregnancy unless your doctor specifically recommends it.

See Also

Constipation

SLIPPERY ELM (*ULMUS RUBRA*)

Slippery elm is a botanical medicine that comes from the inner white bark of the American elm tree, which was once prolific throughout much of North America. The stately tree, also known as the Indian, moose, or sweet elm, grows to a height of some fifty feet and was a favorite shade tree throughout the United States until Dutch elm disease decimated the species in the 1960s. Fortunately, some hardy trees survived the blight, and elms are making a comeback in many parts of the country.

For centuries, Native Americans have used slippery elm to treat a wide range of ailments. Many of these practices were quickly adopted by the early colonists, and slippery elm soon became an indispensable botanical medicine. In recent years, it has enjoyed a resurgence of popularity, and it is now used to ease coughs, colds, and inflammatory disorders.

Common Uses

- Soothe skin abrasions, minor burns and wounds, and eczema and other inflammatory skin conditions.
- Relieve coughs, congestion, sore throat, and other symptoms of colds and bronchitis.
- Treat peptic ulcers and intestinal inflammation and relieve indigestion and heartburn.
- Prevent or treat constipation.
- Promote weight loss.

How It Works

The inner bark, or bast, of the slippery elm is noted for its soothing properties and is effective both internally and externally. The major healing compounds in the bark are polysacharides, a type of complex carbohydrate. Polysaccharides are rich in mucilage, a type of soluble fiber that swells when water is added to it. Powdered bark is used to make a soothing poultice that not only eases pain and itchiness but also promotes healing of cuts, bruises, insect stings and bites, minor burns, and skin inflammation. When the bark itself is moistened, it forms a flexible, spongy tissue that can be molded and applied to the anal area to ease the discomfort of hemorrhoids.

Powdered bark can be made into a type of gruel or a thick drink to relieve heartburn and indigestion and soothe ulcers and other intestinal inflammatory disorders. The mucilage acts as a demulcent to coat irritated or inflamed mucous membranes and promote their healing. Like other types of soluble fiber, it absorbs large amounts of water and softens the stool, thus preventing or treating constipation. When used as a cereal or high-fiber drink, slippery elm fosters a sense of fullness and helps prevent overeating.

Evidence of Efficacy

The Food and Drug Administration has approved the use of slippery elm as an ingredient in lozenges and cough syrups to treat sore throats and coughs. Otherwise, not much research has been done on slippery elm per se, but the effectiveness of mucilage in treating skin and intestinal inflammation is well established.

Forms and Usual Dosages

Powdered elm bark is sold in two forms: a coarse powder from which poultices are made and used externally, and a fine powder that is made into a mucilaginous drink or gruel. As noted, it is also used in throat lozenges, and may be taken in tablet or capsule form. A typical dosage to treat intestinal inflammation calls for two or three 500-mg capsules to be taken three or four times a day. As an alternative, take 5 ml of slippery elm tincture three times a day.

To make slippery elm tea; pour a cup of boiling water over ½ to 1 teaspoon of powdered bark and drink as soon as it cools enough. If it gets too thick, it can be diluted with more water. Three or four cups of this tea can be taken per day. Slippery elm can also be made into cereal by moistening 1 to 2 teaspoons of powdered bark in cold water; then, while stirring the mixture, pour 1½ cups of hot water or milk over it. Flavor with cinnamon, nutmeg, honey, or fresh fruit, and eat as you would oatmeal or other hot cereals.

Potential Problems

Slippery elm is quite safe when taken at recommended dosages. It has no known side effects and does not appear to interact with other medications.

See Also

Bronchitis
Diverticular Disease

TEA TREE (MELALEUCA ALTERNIFOLIA)

⊙ A LITTLE HISTORY

Native Australians have used tea tree oil for centuries, but it was unknown to the rest of the world until the late 1700s when Capt. James Cook led an expedition there and began experimenting with the leaves. The crew brewed a lemon-flavored tea from the leaves and added it to a beer made from spruce leaves. The tea reduced the astringency of the beer, and the crew grew to accept it; they also gave the shrub its popular name.

On later voyages, a botanist traveling with Captain Cook observed how the aborigines used the shrub to heal infected wounds. But word of the medicinal properties of tea tree oil did not spread until the 1920s, when a Syndey researcher, A. R. Penfold, started to study the oil and discovered its antiseptic properties.

During World War II, tea tree oil was included in soldiers' first aid kits for skin injuries in tropical areas. After the discovery of penicillin, tea tree oil was pretty much forgotten until recently. With the growing problem of antibiotic-resistant organisms, a number of researchers are investigating tea tree oil as a substitute for pharmaceutical products.

Despite its common name, this shrub or small tree, which is native to Australia, is not a source of tea. Instead, it produces an essential oil that has unique infection-fighting properties. Also known as Australian tea tree or cajeput, the shrub is related to the myrtle tree. It has needle-like leaves and produces heads of yellow or purplish flowers.

Scientists have identified eighty of the estimated one hundred compounds in tea tree oil, a few of which are unique to this plant. Some of these compounds are active against viruses, fungi, and bacteria, and in recent years, demand for tea tree oil has grown tremendously, rising from about ten tons in the early 1990s to more than two hundred tons a year today. Although tea trees are now grown on plantations in Asia and other parts of the world, the swampy areas of New South Wales and Queensland are the only places where the shrub grows naturally, and Australia remains the chief source of the prized medicinal oil.

Common Uses

Tea tree oil has scores of medicinal uses, most of them external.

- Kill bacteria associated with minor skin infections (as an antiseptic skin wash or application).
- Treat inflammatory skin conditions, including dermatitis, acne, and blackheads.
- Soothe chapped lips and hands.
- Relieve itching of insect bites, chicken pox, shingles, poison ivy, and other minor skin irritations.
- Control oral bacteria, sweeten bad breath, and reduce buildup of plaque and gum disease (gingivitis).
- Promote healing of canker sores and fever blisters (herpes cold sores).
- Treat various fungal infections including ringworm, athlete's foot, thrush, nail fungus, and jock itch.
- Soothe sore throat.
- Relieve nasal and sinus congestion when inhaled.
- Ease muscle and joint pain and inflammation.
- Help shrink hemorrhoids and relieve itching and other symptoms.
- Reduce dandruff and cradle cap.

How It Works

Most of the eighty known compounds in tea tree oil are chemicals classified as either terpene hydrocarbons, such as pinene, or oxygenated terpenes, especially terpinen-4-ol and cineole. Terpinen-4-ol makes up some 60 percent of the essential oil and is a powerful germicide and fungicide. Cineole, a prominent essential oil also found in eucalyptus, has expectorant and antiseptic properties.

The antiseptic properties of tea tree oil make it especially valuable in treating various skin infections. When used as an antiseptic wash, it helps prevent infection and promotes healing. When inhaled in steamy vapors, tea tree oil eases nasal and sinus congestion. A gargle or mouth rinse containing diluted tea tree oil soothes a sore throat and mouth ulcers and hastens their healing. Tea tree lotion, cream, or compress can ease the itchiness of insect bites, poison ivy rash, chicken pox or shingles blisters, and numerous other skin irritations. When used as a shampoo, tea tree oil is an effective treatment for dandruff and cradle cap, the thick, scaly rash that many babies develop.

Although expensive, tea tree is also an effective household and hospital disinfectant. It is used to soak soiled cloth diapers and to disinfect kitchen and bathroom surfaces. It is especially useful as a hospital disinfectant because it kills antibiotic-resistant strains of *Staphylococcus*.

Evidence of Efficacy

Tea tree oil has been studied extensively in many laboratories, especially in Australia, and found to be effective against a host of disease-causing organisms. For example, one study tested tea tree oil's ability to inhibit the growth of various yeast organisms in a test tube. It proved effective against all strains of candida except *Epidermophyton floccosum*, all sixty-four strains of *Malassezia furfur*, and eighty other types of disease-causing fungi. A 1995 laboratory study showed that tea tree oil kills certain antibiotic-resistant strains of bacteria, including a strain of *Staphylococcus aureus* found in hospitals.

In another study, Australian researchers compared a 5 percent solution of tea tree oil with a 5 percent solution of benzoyl peroxide to treat acne. They found the two substances equally effective, but tea tree oil produced fewer side effects. Researchers also tested a cream containing 5 percent tea tree oil and 2 percent butenafine hydrochloride in a randomized, double-blind, placebo-controlled study involving sixty persons with nail fungal infections. Eighty percent receiving the cream were cured after sixteen weeks, compared with no cures in the placebo group. Studies also indicate that tea tree applications are effective in treating vaginal yeast infections.

Form and Usual Dosages

Tea tree oil is used primarily externally and is available as an essential oil, usually in a diluted form. (Most experts advise against ingesting tea tree oil because it may provoke a toxic reaction.) Full-strength essential oil is sold primarily in dropper bottles of 1 and 2 ounces, but it should always be diluted before using it except when treating fungal nail infections.

Tea tree oil is often combined with vitamin E and other essential oils. It is used in virtually every type of body-care product, including toothpastes, mouthwashes, lip balms, shampoos, skin conditioners, hand creams, soaps, deodorants, body and foot powders, and face gels. It is used in lozenges to soothe sore throats and coughs.

As a steam inhalant for upper respiratory congestion, put two drops of oil in a bowl of steaming water, cover with a towel over the head, and inhale for five to ten minutes. To relieve muscle and joint pain, add three to five drops to 30 ml of a neutral base oil and massage twice daily to relieve muscle pain. As a disinfectant, add three to five drops to bathwater to help heal minor skin infections.

Potential Problems

The essential oil of tea tree is less toxic than most essential oils, but it should never be applied full-strength to any part of the skin, particularly broken skin, as it may cause irritation, burning, or a rash. As noted, the only exception is to treat fungal nail infections, in which applications of the full-strength oil are used.

See also

Acne

THYME
(*THYMUS VULGARIS*)

Thyme, an aromatic perennial that is native to southern Europe and the Mediterranean, is cultivated worldwide and is best known as a culinary herb. But thyme—a member of the mint family—is also valued as a medicinal herb. Both the leaves and flowering tops have medicinal properties, but it is thyme's essential oil that is especially prized. Although it takes about one hundred pounds of flowering tops to produce 8 to 16 ounces of essential oil, the plant is so abundant that the oil is relatively inexpensive. Thus, it is a popular ingredient in many over-the-counter cold remedies, mouthwashes, toothpastes, and similar products.

Common Uses

- Soothe sore throats, laryngitis, dry coughs, and other symptoms of colds, flu, and bronchitis.
- Relieve an upset stomach.
- Relieve minor muscle aches, joint pain, and inflammation.
- Aromatherapy remedy for premenstrual syndrome (PMS), stress, fatigue, and mild depression.
- Prevent skin infections and promote healing of minor wounds (as an antiseptic wash).

How It Works

Thyme contains many medicinal compounds, including tannins, flavonoids, bitters, resins, and saponins, but the most active are two phenols called thymol and carvacrol. Thymol has antiseptic properties that are effective against certain bacteria, fungi, and viruses. Thymol, carvacrol, and the saponins also act as expectorants to loosen and thin mucus, thus relieving upper respiratory and sinus congestion.

Thymol and carvacrol may help relax smooth muscles, thereby easing menstrual cramps and aiding in indigestion. Thyme's tannins have astringent properties that may relieve mild diarrhea. When applied to the skin, thymol causes blood to rush to the site, creating a sense of warmth and relief from pain and inflammation from arthritis, sprains, muscle aches, and possibly tension headaches.

Evidence of Efficacy

Japanese researchers isolated flavonoids and phenolic compounds in thyme that are well-known antioxidants, substances that protect cells against damage from unstable molecules (free radicals) that are released when the body burns oxygen. Researchers have also demonstrated that thyme's essential oils are effective in killing *E. coli* and certain other bacteria that cause food poisoning.

German health authorities have approved of the herb's use for treating mild upper respiratory infections and coughs.

Forms and Usual Dosages

Thyme is available as a liquid extract, essential oil, tea, syrup, elixir, and tincture, as well as the fresh and dried herb itself. It is also a key ingredient in cough drops, gas remedies, mouthwashes, antifungal medicines, dental products, and cosmetics. A tea brewed by steeping 1 teaspoon of the dried herb per cup of water can be consumed up to three times a day. Thyme syrup is taken by the teaspoon several times a day to relieve upper respiratory congestion. The liquid herb extract is taken in doses of 0.6 to 4 ml, and the elixir in doses of 4 to 8 ml. A few drops of the tincture may be applied to the skin as an antiseptic. The essential oil must be diluted in a neutral oil—for example, olive or salad oil—before it can be applied to the skin.

Potential Problems

Thyme is generally safe when used as directed. As with other botanical medicines and nutraceuticals, it should not be used during pregnancy without first consulting a doctor. The essential oil is more potent than the herb and should never be taken orally; it has been reported to cause many adverse reactions, including nausea, stomach pain, dizziness, headache, convulsions, coma, and cardiac and upper respiratory distress.

Some people have allergic reactions to thyme, so it should be used cautiously by people with allergies. Be especially careful with thyme bath preparations and oral products until you are sure you are not allergic to the herb's oils.

TURMERIC (CURCUMA LONGA)

Turmeric is a perennial, broad-leafed shrub that is grown in India and other tropical areas of Asia for its large underground stem (rhizome). Cooks recognize turmeric as the source of a hot, yellow spice that is used to flavor and color curries and other spicy dishes; it is also added to some mustards to give them extra "bite." The dried and powdered rhizome also has a long history of medicinal uses. In Ayurveda, the traditional healing system of India, turmeric is prescribed as a general body tonic, whereas Chinese physicians recommend it to treat intestinal problems, especially liver disease. Western herbalists use it mostly to treat inflammatory disorders, especially rheumatoid arthritis.

Common Uses

- Reduce joint pain and inflammation.
- Treat indigestion and heartburn.
- Improve liver function and stimulate flow of bile.

How It Works

The active medicinal ingredient in turmeric is curcumin, one of several curcuminoids in the rhizome and the substance that gives it its distinctive pungent flavor and its bright yellow color. Curcumin is thought to reduce inflammation by lowering histamine levels; it may also stimulate the adrenal glands to increase production of cortisone—a hormone that reduces inflammation. Curcumin is also said to protect against liver damage; this may be due to its potent antioxidant properties. Curcumin also has antiplatelet activity, which reduces the ability of the blood to form clots. This may improve circulation and also offer some protection against heart attacks and strokes.

Turmeric also contains a volatile oil, bitters, and other compounds that may also have therapeutic properties. Bitter principles, for example, stimulate the flow of bile and other digestive juices and may relieve indigestion, gas, and other intestinal problems.

Evidence of Efficacy

Most of the evidence supporting age-old claims for turmeric are based on either its long tradition in Indian and Asian medicine or recent animal studies. Researchers in India have found, for example, that curcumin has anti-inflammatory actions. Two clinical studies in which curcumin was compared to a powerful anti-inflammatory drug (phenylbutazone) produced mixed results: it was found to be less effective than the drug in relieving rheumatoid arthritis symptoms, but more effective in treating postsurgical inflammation. Of the two substances, curcumin carries a much lower risk of adverse side effects.

A small clinical study reported in a Thai medical journal found that turmeric was helpful in treating indigestion; other studies found it less effective than antacids in treating patients with peptic ulcers.

One interesting laboratory study demonstrated that curcumin inhibited HIV, the virus that causes AIDS, in a test tube. It has not been studied for this purpose in humans, however. Test-tube studies also indicate that curcumin destroys some types of cancer cells; this may be due to its antioxidant properties or some other antitumor activity. Obviously, more research is needed to determine whether turmeric is a potential anticancer agent.

◉ A LITTLE HISTORY

Turmeric has been grown for hundreds of years in India and other tropical places, not only for its pungent spice and medicinal properties, but also for various ceremonial purposes. For example, in some Pacific cultures the yellow powder is sprinkled on the shoulders during ceremonial dances to ward off evil spirits and for good luck. It was also thought to prevent skin disease. In parts of India, new mothers consumed turmeric to increase milk production.

Forms and Usual Dosages

Turmeric is widely available as a powdered spice; it is also sold in pill and capsule forms; look for standardized extracts that provide 400 to 600 mg of curcumin. The recommended dosage is three capsules a day. Turmeric is also sold as a tincture; the typical daily dosage is 0.5 to 1.5 ml a day. Of course, turmeric can be incorporated into the diet by using it to flavor foods. Some herbalists recommend dissolving 1 to 3 g of powdered turmeric in a glass of milk and drinking it after or between meals.

Potential Problems

Turmeric has been used as a spice for hundreds of years without reports of toxicity or other problems. Some people do not like its pungent flavor, but this is a matter of taste. Medicinal dosages may pose a problem for some people. German health authorities warn of possible problems in people with gallbladder disease because the increased flow of bile may provoke a flare-up of symptoms. People with bleeding problems or who are taking Coumadin or other blood-thinning medications should not take large amounts of turmeric. One animal study suggested that high doses of curcumin may affect fertility, but more study is needed to determine whether this is indeed so.

See Also

Gallstones

UVA URSI (*ARCTOSTAPHYLOS UVA-URSI*)

◉ A LITTLE HISTORY
After his return from China, Marco Polo described how Chinese doctors used the herb to treat urinary disorders. Before long, European healers were following suit, and herbalists continue to recommend it for kidney and bladder disorders.

Also known as bearberry, beargrape, mountain and upland cranberry, and hogberry, uva ursi is a low-growing perennial that some gardeners cultivate as an attractive ground cover. Bears feast on its red berries and bitter leaves; hence its common name of bearberry. The red fruits resemble cranberries, but have a bland taste. It is the bitter leaves—not the berries—of the uva ursi shrub that have been used medicinally from the Himalayas to North America for more than a thousand years. Recent chemical studies document that the leaves do contain antibacterial chemicals, which appear to validate the long-standing use of uva ursi to treat urinary tract and bladder infections.

Not all the uses are medicinal, however. In Russia, dried uva ursi leaves have been used to make a type of bitter tea. Native Americans smoked the leaves in combination with tobacco.

Common Uses

- Treat urinary tract infections, especially cystitis.
- Help dissolve kidney and bladder stones.
- Reduce premenstrual bloating and swelling.
- Heal minor cuts and abrasions.
- Ease muscle pain.

How It Works

Uva ursi leaves contain a number of active ingredients that have anti-inflammatory, diuretic, astringent (drying), and antibacterial properties. Arbutin, which becomes hydroquinone in the body, is an antiseptic that can kill bacteria and other micro-organisms. Ursolic acid and isoquercitrin have diuretic properties, but it is not known whether uva ursi can actually rid the body of excess water.

Evidence of Efficacy

Laboratory tests show that uva ursi has antibacterial effects on several organisms, such as *Escherichia coli* and *Staphylococcus aureus*, which are common causes of urinary tract infections. It also appears to destroy *Candida albicans*, a cause of yeast infections. Clinical trials in humans to determine just how effective uva ursi is in treating infections in humans have not yet been done. Even so, German health authorities have approved uva ursi for the treatment of mild urinary tract inflammation.

Although uva ursi is reputed to aid weight loss, probably because of its diuretic action, this effect is mild and brief—if it occurs at all. Still, when increased urination does occur, it may help urinary tract infections by helping to flush bacteria from the kidneys and bladder.

Forms and Usual Dosages

Uva ursi is available as capsules, tablets, and tincture, which are standardized to contain 20 percent arbutin. (It is also available as dried leaves that can be brewed into a tea, but the dosage of this form is difficult to control.) In Germany, the recommended dosage for cystitis and other mild urinary tract inflammations calls for up to 500 mg to be taken three times a day.

To make a tea low in tannic acid, use 1.5 to 2.5 g of dried leaves per cup. Use cold, not hot, water and allow the mixture to soak overnight (twelve to twenty-four hours). Drain and dilute the mixture if the tea is still too bitter. Uva ursi tea made with hot water will be very high in tannic acid, which can irritate the stomach.

In order for the antiseptic uva ursi to work, the urine must be alkaline. Therefore, while taking uva ursi, vitamin C and acid-rich foods such as oranges, cranberries, and many other fruits must be avoided. Eating alkaline foods, such as milk and vegetables, is advised. A quick way to ensure alkaline urine is to dilute a teaspoon of baking soda (bicarbonate of soda) in a glass of water and drink it when taking the uva ursi. People who have high blood pressure should not take bicarbonate of soda, however, and even healthy people should not use uva ursi or bicarbonate of soda for more than a week at a time.

To ease muscle pain and sprains, make a poultice of crushed leaves. Boil the leaves in a small amount of water and drain. Cover the aching muscle or sprain with cheesecloth and place the leaves over it; cover with a towel to retain the heat. The treatment can be repeated two or three times a day until healing takes place.

Potential Problems

The high tannin content of uva ursi can cause nausea and vomiting. It should not be taken during pregnancy or by children under the age of twelve. Consult a doctor for a diagnosis before taking uva ursi to treat cystitis or other urinary tract problems. High doses and long-term use can cause serious urinary tract irritation.

Hydroquinone, which is derived from arbutin, may be toxic to the liver. Perhaps for this reason, the Food and Drug Administration placed it on its list of "Herbs of Undefined Safety."

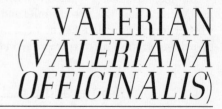

VALERIAN (*VALERIANA OFFICINALIS*)

Valerian is a perennial herb with a massive root system, short rhizome, and clusters of small white or pink flowers; it is also known as heliotrope, vandal root, and all-heal. Valerian grows as a weed in Europe and most parts of the British Isles, but it is also cultivated commercially for its medicinal roots and rhizomes. In cats, it acts as a stimulant and can be used as a substitute for catnip. In humans, however, it has the opposite effect and is a popular remedy for insomnia.

Common Uses

- Treat mild insomnia.
- Relieve muscle spasms and ease menstrual cramps and symptoms of irritable bowel syndrome (IBS).
- Calm jittery nerves and may lower blood pressure.

How It Works

Valerian roots contain valepotriates, which act as mild muscle relaxants, tannins, small amounts of alkaloids, and bitter compounds. Researchers once thought that each component produced the herb's sedative qualities, but it is now believed that it is the combination of ingredients that gives valerian its various medicinal properties. Some researchers theorize that the combination of compounds affects the brain receptors for a neurotransmitter called gamma-aminobutyric acid, or GABA; it also appears to affect the autonomic nervous system. In essence, valerian seems to work by calming the brain and relaxing tensed muscles so that sleep can occur naturally. Valerian also relaxes the smooth muscles of the digestive tract, thus reducing symptoms of irritable bowel syndrome. A similar action on the uterus may help relieve menstrual cramps. The calming effect of valerian may also help prevent stress-related disorders, including flare-ups of IBS and insomnia.

Unlike many common pharmaceutical tranquilizers, sedatives, and muscle relaxants, valerian is not habit-forming when used in moderation and does not cause a morning hangover. In Germany, valerian is used to treat childhood attention deficit hyperactivity disorder (ADHD) and behavior problems.

Evidence of Efficacy

Valerian has been studied extensively in both animals and humans, especially in Germany and other European countries, with generally positive results. Its calming and sedating properties have been demonstrated in a number of studies using a German drug (Valmane) that is standardized to contain concentrated valepotriates. For more than a decade, it has been the medication of choice to treat children with ADHD. Researchers have reported that it is as effective as pharmaceutical agents—or even more so—and has fewer adverse effects. Studies have also found that it may help lower high blood pressure.

◉ **A LITTLE HISTORY**

The plant was named valeriana in the ninth or tenth century; this is thought to be derived from the Latin verb *valere,* meaning "to be happy." Valium, the most widely prescribed antianxiety medication, is said to derive its name from the same source and from valerian itself.

According the legend, the Pied Piper of Hamelin used valerian to attract the rats that he led out of the town. Be that as it may, valerian is known to attract both rats and cats.

For centuries, valerian has been taken as a sedative and sleep aid, its major uses today. During the Middle Ages, it was also used to treat epilepsy and there is some evidence to support it as an anticonvulsant.

Forms and Usual Dosages

Valerian is available as capsules, tablets, tinctures, and softgels; look for a product that is standardized to 0.8 percent valeric or valerenic acid. However, the whole valerian root may provide other effective ingredients that are not in a standardized extract. Use dried valerian root to make a tea by combining 1 teaspoonful of crushed herb with ⅔ cup hot water; steep it for ten to fifteen minutes, strain, and drink before going to bed. The typical daily dose ranges from 250 to 500 mg in pill or capsule form or 1 teaspoon of tincture. Anxiety is treated with two or three cups of tea consumed during the day and another before going to bed, or a 250-mg dosage twice a day and 250 to 500 mg before retiring at night.

Valerian has a rather bitter taste and acrid odor; try adding honey or a little sugar to make it more palatable. It should not be taken with Valium or other pharmaceutical sedatives, but it is safe to take with the other calming herbs, such as lemon balm, chamomile, catnip, or kava, and with 5 HTP, GABA, and other calming supplement ingredients.

Potential Problems

Valerian is safe when used in recommended dosages at the appropriate time of day, but as with any herbal extract, be careful about using large amounts over an extended period. High doses of valerian have been reported to cause headaches, grogginess, and restlessness. Taking it during the day may induce drowsiness, so don't use it if you are going to drive or need to be wide awake and alert. If you are pregnant or breast-feeding, or are being treated for a psychiatric condition, do not take valerian without consulting a physician.

See Also

Anxiety
Insomnia

WHITE WILLOW (*SALIX ALBA*)

White willow trees, also known as European or weeping willows, are native to central and southern Europe. They were brought to the American colonies by the earliest settlers and now grow nationwide. Worldwide, there are hundreds of willow species and many are the sources of botanical medicines. But it is the bark of the white willow—a tree distinguished by its towering height and drooping branches with long, silvery green leaves—that is rich in salicin, a chemical that is very similar to modern aspirin. In fact, white willow is often referred to as Nature's aspirin. Although white willow bark has been largely supplanted by aspirin and other painkillers classified as nonsteroidal anti-inflammatory drugs (NSAIDs), a growing number of pain sufferers are returning to the botanical product in the hopes that it has a lower risk of side effects than its pharmaceutical cousins.

Common Uses

- Lower fever and reduce muscle aches associated with colds and flu.
- Reduce joint inflammation caused by arthritis, bursitis, and rheumatism.
- Relieve headaches, minor backaches, and other common pain syndromes.
- Provide temporary relief for such conditions as menstrual pain, toothache, gout, angina, and sore muscles.

How It Works

The salicin contained in willow bark is a glycoside that the body metabolizes into salicylic acid, whose chemical composition is similar to that of aspirin's acetylsalicylic acid. White willow is assumed to work in much the same manner as aspirin to relieve pain, reduce inflammation, and lower a fever. Unlike aspirin, salicin does not interfere with platelet function so it is not likely to help prevent a heart attack or stroke. By the same token, it does not pose aspirin's risk of causing bleeding ulcers and other bleeding problems.

In addition to salicin, white willow contains other phenolic glycosides, tannins, and quercetin, isorhamnetin, and other flavonoid compounds. The tannins have an astringent effect that tightens skin and inflamed tissue, thereby reducing swelling. Tannins and other ingredients in white willow are effective in treating mild diarrhea and intestinal upsets. When applied to the skin and scalp, the astringent effect can treat dandruff and may reduce the risk of infection.

Evidence of Efficacy

Numerous scientific studies, as well as hundreds of years of traditional use, have demonstrated the effectiveness of white willow in treating various pain syndromes. Researchers have also demonstrated that white willow has fewer adverse side effects than aspirin. However, because the potency of salicin is much less than that of aspirin, white willow is

◉ A LITTLE HISTORY

White willow has been used for thousands of years to treat fevers, pain, and inflammation. For example, Chinese medical texts dating from 500 B.C. recommend willow bark for these conditions, and the ancient Greeks and Romans also used it. Europeans discovered its medicinal properties almost by accident. In the mid-1700s, a British minister and physician named Edmund Stone was seeking an inexpensive substitute for South American cinchona bark—the source of quinine—to treat malaria. Cinchona was very bitter tasting; willow bark looked like cinchona bark and when brewed as a tea, it tasted bitter. So Stone gave it to his patients—and it worked!

It was not until the mid-1800s, however, that salicin, the bark's active ingredient, was isolated. At the dawn of the twentieth century the German drug company Bayer marketed the first aspirin, a purified and more potent form of the chemical, acetylsalicylic acid, as an arthritis remedy. To this day, aspirin—which is now synthesized artificially rather than derived from plant sources—remains one of the world's most popular and widely used drugs.

unlikely to be very effective against rheumatoid arthritis and other inflammatory disorders that require high doses of aspirin or other NSAIDs to control. Also, the potency of willow bark can vary from batch to batch and species to species, so consumers have no way of knowing how much salicin is being consumed.

In Germany, where the active ingredients in botanical medicines are standardized, health authorities have approved willow bark as a treatment for fever and headaches. Although sometimes promoted as a weight-loss aid, no studies have proved this use.

Forms and Usual Dosages

Willow bark is found in capsules, liquid extracts, and tea bags, as well as the dried and powdered bark itself. To make a tea, use 1 to 2 teaspoons of powdered bark per cup of boiling water. Let the mixture steep for eight hours and strain. The tea is quite bitter; this can be masked by adding a little honey or lemon, or mixing it with another herbal tea, such as mint or lemon balm. Three cups of tea may be consumed during the course of a day.

When taken in pill or tincture from, the usual dosage is 60 to 120 mg of salicin a day. The standardized extract, which is available in Europe but not in the United States, is standardized to provide 7.8 percent salicin.

Willow bark is sometimes included in weight-loss formulas, and there are claims that it works synergistically with caffeine and ephedrine to speed metabolism and burn calories; these effects have not been proved. It is also combined with other herbs, such as feverfew, meadowsweet, and garlic, to increase its effectiveness, and is a common ingredient in botanical combinations to treat anxiety, increase energy, boost immunity, and enhance mood.

Potential Problems

Because the potency cannot be assured, it is difficult to know how much willow bark is required to relieve pain, lower a fever, and achieve other benefits. Also, it is not recommended as an aspirin substitute in treating or preventing heart attacks and strokes. Experts advise against taking white willow if you are allergic to aspirin. Although salicin is gentler to the stomach than aspirin, it is wise to avoid it if you have ulcers or other intestinal problems. As with aspirin, white willow should not be given to children under age eighteen who have viral illness because of the possible risk of Reye's syndrome, a rare but potentially fatal disease that has been linked to aspirin.

WILD YAM
(DIOSCOREA VILLOSA)

The other names for this perennial vine—colic root, devil's bones, and rheumatism root—provide clues to some of its many medicinal qualities. However, they do not include what has become its most common use—the relief of symptoms related to menstruation and menopause. Modern herbalists, aware of wild yam's estrogenlike effects, suggest making a salve out of it to use vaginally for dryness that sometimes occurs after menopause. And some women going through menopause rub wild yam cream on their abdomen and thighs in the belief that enough active ingredient is absorbed to act as a natural alternative to hormone replacement therapy. Although proof that it aids menopausal symptoms is lacking, at one time wild yam was used in the commercial production of hormones, particularly contraceptives. Breast enlargement is a side effect, which prompts some women to use it in hopes of developing bigger breasts. In recent years, it has also become quite popular as a treatment for premenstrual syndrome (PMS).

Common Uses

- Treat menstrual cramps and premenstrual symptoms.
- Relieve vaginal dryness after menopause.
- Ease arthritis and muscle pain.
- Lower high cholesterol.
- Treat gallstones and other intestinal disorders, including diverticulosis and irritable bowel syndrome.

How It Works

The outer bark of the wild yam root is high in saponins (including dioscin or diosgenin) and alkaloids, including dioscorin, and these have anti-inflammatory and muscle relaxants that work on the muscles of the abdomen and pelvis. Saponins are the source of hormones such as cortisone, estrogen, and progesteronelike compounds, although the human body lacks the enzymes to convert wild yam into these substances. The anti-inflammatory action makes wild yam especially helpful when arthritis pain is due to inflammation. Wild yam root also contains compounds that can lower high blood cholesterol. In turn, this reduces the risk of gallstone formation and has a favorable effect on the liver.

Evidence of Efficacy

Although it's well established that wild yam contains several active constituents, there are few clinical studies to attest to its effectiveness.

Forms and Usual Dosages

Capsules or tablets containing the dried root (500 mg) can be taken three times a day with food. It's also available as a tincture, and 2 to 4 ml may be taken three or four times a day. A tea can be made with 1 to 2 teaspoons of powdered bark in a cup of water and taken three times a day. (The bitter taste may be made more palatable by adding honey and lemon.) To make a vaginal salve, some women shave the outer bark off the root and mix it with a vaginal cream, although this is not an advisable practice.

Potential Problems

Large amounts should not be taken because the dioscorin can be toxic. Nausea and diarrhea may occur when wild yam is taken in large doses.

See Also

Bladder Control Problems
Endometriosis

WITCH HAZEL (*HAMAMELIS VIRGINIANA*)

Also known as spotted alder, winterbloom, and snapping hazelnut, witch hazel is a shrub that is native to the northeastern United States and eastern Canada. When its leaves fall in late autumn, yellow flowers appear in clusters at its joints and then evolve into black nuts that look like hazelnuts and contain oily, edible seeds. The seeds are burst from the tree when they are ripe, hence the plant's alternate name, snapping hazelnut.

The leaves and the bark are used in extracting the herb's medicinal witch hazel. However, the product sold as an astringent in stores contains very little actual witch hazel; instead, its astringent properties come from the alcohol used in its commercial preparation. To get the full medicinal benefits of witch hazel, you should use the actual botanical product.

Common Uses

- Shrink hemorrhoids and ease pain and itching.
- Soothe minor burns including razor burn and skin abrasions and prevent infection.
- Ease pain of muscle aches.
- Reduce bleeding of minor cuts and oozing of certain skin conditions.
- Relieve itching of insect bites.
- Soothe sore throat and alleviate intestinal inflammation.

How It Works

The leaves contain tannic and gallic acids as well as some volatile oil. The bark is high in astringent tannins, resins, gallic acid, and sterols. These components all have astringent properties; some also have sedative and analgesic actions. When applied topically to inflamed skin or mucous membranes, these astringent substances tighten the superficial layers, resulting in constriction of small superficial blood vessels. This reduces bleeding and may also lessen inflammation. The ability to shrink swollen tissue and relieve itching makes witch hazel a good remedy for mild hemorrhoids.

Some compounds in witch hazel have mild antibiotic properties, which helps prevent infection and promote healing of minor burns and skin wounds. Tannins have a mild topical anesthetic action that eases pain and itching. When taken internally, witch hazel soothes a sore throat and inflamed intestinal membranes. Tannins help control diarrhea, although there are other botanical medicines that are more effective than witch hazel in treating diarrhea.

Evidence of Efficacy

The astringent and healing properties of witch hazel are well documented. Most commercial witch hazel preparations are based on a distilled extract (hamamelis water) that is made by soaking the crude drug in water for about twenty-four hours, then distilling it and adding ethanol to it. These distillates contain almost no active tannins; their astringent properties are due to the added ethanol. However, even these preparations were found to shorten bleeding time and constrict blood vessels when tested in rabbits. Other tests using hamamelis ointments applied topically produced improvement in skin conditions in 50 percent of patients within three weeks. The efficacy of a combination product of hamamelis bark extract (10 percent) in an ointment was tested in patients with mild hemorrhoids. Between 70 and 90 percent of patients experienced relief from their bleeding, soreness, itching, and burning symptoms.

Forms and Usual Dosages

Witch hazel is available as a distilled liquid product. Some botanical medicine outlets also sell witch hazel tincture and dried or powdered leaves and bark. These can be used to make a poultice, decoction, or tincture. Witch hazel is the active ingredient in some commercial hemorrhoidal products.

To make a witch hazel decoction, boil 5 to 10 g (1 to 2 tablespoons) of dried leaves in a pint of water; strain and use the liquid as a compress soak or gargle. For internal use, brew a weaker tea (1 teaspoon of leaves per cup of water) and drink two or three cups a day.

Potential Problems

Witch hazel is safe when used externally, although some people develop skin irritation. Discontinue use if this occurs. When taken internally, witch hazel can interfere with the body's absorption of iron, which precludes its long-term use, especially by people who have anemia. Internal use is also contraindicated for people who have certain digestive disorders, including gastroesophageal reflux disease (GERD), ulcerative colitis, and diverticulitis. Commercially prepared witch hazel contains isopropyl alcohol and should never be taken internally. It is for topical use only.

Other Useful Botanical Medicines

The following table lists miscellaneous botanical medicines that are often recommended, but are not as commonly used as those in the preceding section. Consult a practicing herbalist or health care provider for directions and cautions if you choose to use any of these botanicals. Also, some are hazardous, so pay special attention to the Cautions section.

NAME OF PLANT/FORMS	TRADITIONAL USES	EFFICACY	CAUTIONS
Black walnut *(Juglans nigra)* Capsule, tea, tincture, poultice.	Astringent for skin problems; laxative; relieve hemorrhoids.	Juglone in black walnut appears to be effective in treating some skin disorders; may have antifungal properties.	Appears to be safe, but few studies have been done; may provoke allergies in some people.
Boldo *(Peumus boldus)* Dried leaves, pills, tea.	Digestive problems; liver disease; diuretic.	Contains alkaloid (boldine) that appears to protect liver, stimulate gastric secretions to aid digestion, and ease muscle spasms. Also stimulates kidneys to increase flow of urine.	Use only in limited amounts; volatile oils in boldo may be toxic; overdoses can cause convulsions and death.
Chicory *(Cichorium intybus)* Fresh plant, dried root, poultice, tea.	Coffee substitute; strengthen heartbeat; digestive aid; diuretic; sedative; poultice to ease skin inflammation.	Bitter compounds may stimulate appetite and stimulate flow of bile; animal studies show mild anti-inflammatory effects. Contains substance similar to digitalis that may affect heart, but no human studies have been done.	Chicory is considered safe, but may provoke allergic reaction in persons allergic to ragweed and other plants in daisy family. Check with a doctor before using if you have gallbladder disease.
Cocoa *(Theobroma cacao)* Extract, powder, cocoa butter, syrup, liquor; main ingredient in chocolate.	Cocoa butter for chapped lips and skin, burns, sore breasts due to breast-feeding; cocoa for a soothing drink, to stimulate appetite.	Stimulant action comes from small amount of caffeine in cocoa; cocoa butter has softening and soothing properties when used externally. Claims for cocoa as an asthma treatment are unfounded because very large amount must be consumed to affect airways.	Cocoa is safe, but may provoke sleep problems, nervousness, and other symptoms in people who are very sensitive to caffeine.

Other Useful Botanical Medicines, continued

NAME OF PLANT/FORMS	TRADITIONAL USES	EFFICACY	CAUTIONS
Coltsfoot *(Tussilago farfara)* Extract, infusion, juice, ointment, powder, tincture, fresh or dried leaves.	Expectorant; cough remedy; soothe skin inflammation.	Mucilage in coltsfoot soothes inflamed mucous membranes to ease sore throat and calm a cough. Poultices of coltsfoot leaves have been shown to reduce skin inflammation and irritation.	Coltsfoot is generally considered safe when used in small amounts and as directed. However, the pyrrolizidine alkaloids (PAs) in coltsfoot have been found to cause liver tumors in research animals. Coltsfoot should not be taken by anyone with liver disease, and some experts believe it should not be ingested in any form. (Also see in table, Dangerous Botanicals, p. 560)
Gentian *(Gentiana lutea)* Tincture, fluid extract, tea, whole root; flavoring in bitter tonics.	Stimulate appetite; aid digestion.	Bitter glycosides (gentiopicrin and amarogentin) stimulate appetite and aid digestion by increasing flow of saliva, bile, and gastric juices.	Should not be used by people with ulcers, heartburn, or other acid disorders.
Goldenrod *(Solidago* species) Dried herb, tea, poultice.	Diuretic when taken internally; promote healing of minor cuts and skin inflammations.	Appears to stimulate kidneys and increase flow of urine; plant's astringent tannins may stop minor bleeding and oozing and reduce inflammation.	May provoke allergies in persons allergic to other members of daisy family, such as ragweed.
Hops *(Humulus lupulus)* Liquid drops, tea, bath additive.	Appetite stimulant; sleep aid; calm anxiety.	Bitter compounds stimulate appetite and aid digestion by increasing flow of gastric juices; use as a sedative based mostly on tradition rather than scientific evidence.	Generally safe; may contain mild plant (phyto) estrogens, so experts caution against use during pregnancy.
Horse chestnut *(Aesculus hippocastanum)* Capsule, pill, extract, skin lotion, gel, ointment, powder.	Calm cough; treat skin ulcers, inflammation, hemorrhoids, varicose veins, and other skin disorders.	Research supports use as a topical anti-inflammatory and to treat varicose veins and reduce leg and hemorrhoid swelling.	Horse chestnut seeds, leaves, and bark are poisonous; use only commercially prepared products.

Other Useful Botanical Medicines, continued

NAME OF PLANT/FORMS	TRADITIONAL USES	EFFICACY	CAUTIONS
Horsetail *(Equisetum arvense)* Capsule, pill, extract, tincture, dried herb, tea, compress, poultice, bath additive.	Stop bleeding, promote wound healing; mild diuretic.	Astringent compounds help stop bleeding from minor cuts and hasten healing; animal studies show mild diuretic properties.	
Iceland moss *(Cetraria islandica)* Powder to make tea; ingredient in European cough and cold remedies.	Soothe cough and ease airway congestion; soothe sore throat and mouth ulcers.	High mucilage content soothes inflamed mucous membranes and calms cough due to irritation; laboratory studies show mild antibiotic activity which may promote healing.	Generally safe but long-term use is discouraged because of possible contamination with lead and other industrial wastes.
Ipecac *(Cephaelis ipecacuanha)* Syrup, tincture, fluid extract.	Induce vomiting in case of accidental poisoning; expectorant when taken in very small doses.	Acts directly on brain's vomiting center; also irritates stomach lining to induce vomiting. Loosens phlegm to make it easier to expel.	Must be taken only in recommended amounts and with ample fluids; do not try to induce vomiting if person has ingested lye or other corrosive poisons. Use syrup rather than fluid extract, which is highly concentrated.
Jasmine *(Jasminum grandiflorum and other species)* Tea, oil.	In aromatherapy, to ease stress, elevate mood, increase sexual desire; tea to calm anxiety and help induce sleep.	There are no scientific studies to validate aromatherapy uses of jasmine; laboratory studies indicate tea may reduce risk of some cancers, but this has not been proved.	Appears safe although some people develop rashes and other skin allergy symptoms.
Jojoba *(Simmondsia chinensis)* Oil; ingredient in many hair and skin products.	Lubricate and condition skin and hair; possible acne treatment.	Oil is absorbed by skin and may help improve mild acne by loosening the sebum that can clog hair follicles and pores.	Generally safe when used externally; toxic if swallowed.
Lady's mantle *(Alchemilla xanthochlora, A. vulgaris)* Tincture, dried herb, tea, douche solution, gargle, bath solution, poultice, compress, bath products.	Reduce heavy menstrual bleeding and regulate periods; diuretic; treat mild diarrhea; stop bleeding of minor cuts and promote wound healing.	Tannins may reduce diarrhea, reduce bleeding, and promote wound healing; little or no scientific evidence to support use in treating menstrual problems.	Appears safe although toxicity has not been studied.

Other Useful Botanical Medicines, continued

NAME OF PLANT/FORMS	TRADITIONAL USES	EFFICACY	CAUTIONS
Lime/linden (*Tilia* species) Liquid extract, dried flowers, tea; an ingredient in many herbal combinations.	Reduce cold symptoms; promote sweating to help lower a fever.	Hot tea soothes a sore throat and helps calm a cough. Increased perspiration has been noted, but benefits of this are doubtful. Laboratory studies suggest it may also bolster immunity.	Appears safe but toxicity studies have not been done.
Lovage (*Levisticum officinale*) Capsule, pill, liquid extract, dried root, tea; an ingredient in many herbal combinations.	Diuretic; treat upset stomach; reduce gas.	Volatile oil in lovage tea is thought to reduce intestinal spasms and lower gas production; animal studies show increased urine production, perhaps by irritating the kidneys.	Appears safe but should not be used by people with kidney inflammation or other kidney problems.
Meadowsweet/spirea (*Filipendula ulmaria*) Liquid extract, tincture, dried flowers, tea.	Diuretic; anti-inflammatory; mild painkiller; lower a fever.	Meadowsweet contains salicin, which acts as a mild natural aspirin and is known to reduce inflammation and pain, lower a fever, and perhaps increase urine flow.	Is generally safe but should not be used by people who are allergic to aspirin or by children under 18 because it may increase the risk of Reye's syndrome. In general, however, it is not as likely as aspirin to cause stomach upset, and it does not cause bleeding problems.
Motherwort (*Leonurus cardiaca*) Liquid extract, tincture, dried herb, tea.	General heart tonic, especially to treat fast heartbeat; sedative; treat menstrual problems; help regulate thyroid function.	Approved in Germany as a heart tonic; contains alkaloids that may lower blood pressure and slow a rapid heartbeat. Has been shown to reduce symptoms of overactive thyroid when used as an adjuvant treatment to conventional therapy. Also contains alkaloids that may stimulate uterine contractions.	Generally considered safe but should not be used as a substitute for prescribed heart or thyroid medications; should not be taken during pregnancy because effects on uterus are unclear.

Other Useful Botanical Medicines, continued

NAME OF PLANT/FORMS	TRADITIONAL USES	EFFICACY	CAUTIONS
Oregano (*Origanum vulgare, Lippia graveolens*, and other species) Dried herb, tea, infusion, oil.	Stimulate appetite; aid digestion and reduce gas; relieve airway congestion and coughs.	Phenols in oregano are known expectorants that loosen phlegm and make it easier to cough up. Oregano extracts have been found to reduce muscle spasms, alleviate indigestion, and treat mild diarrhea. Diluted essential oil is used in aromatherapy to counter stress and calm jittery nerves.	Widely used as an herb with no reported adverse effects; full-strength oil should not be ingested or applied to the skin.
Parsley (*Petroselinum* species) Liquid extract, tincture, tea; fresh or dried leaves, roots, and seeds.	Freshen bad breath; settle upset stomach and aid digestion; reduce intestinal gas; diuretic; promote healing of minor skin infections and bruises.	Volatile oils contain apiole and myristicin, which are known to increase urine output; may also stimulate the uterus. Long tradition supports use as a breath freshener; tea made from crushed seeds contain more volatile oil than fresh or dried leaves. Leaves have mild antiseptic properties, which may promote wound healing.	When used as a food flavoring, parsley is very safe. Large amounts of the volatile oils may cause stomach and intestinal irritation and overdoses can cause convulsions and other serious toxic reactions. Should not be taken in therapeutic dosages during pregnancy or by people with kidney disease.
Passionflower (*Passiflora incarnata*) Extract, concentrated drops, tincture, dried flower, tea, poultice.	Calm anxiety and jittery nerves; help induce sleep; promote wound healing and help prevent skin infections.	Flower and fruits contain substances that calm the central nervous system and have a tranquilizing or sedating effect, although experts debate the usefulness of passionflower to treat anxiety, insomnia, and nervous disorders. Plant's leaves contain antibiotic substances that may promote wound healing.	Generally considered safe in recommended dosages.

Other Useful Botanical Medicines, continued

NAME OF PLANT/FORMS	TRADITIONAL USES	EFFICACY	CAUTIONS
Savory *(Satureja hortensis, S. montana)* Oil, tincture, fresh or dried herb, tea.	Treat stomach upset; cough and cold remedy.	Contains tannins that may calm an upset stomach, reduce diarrhea, and soothe inflamed throat membranes and help calm a cough.	Generally considered safe, although full-strength oil should not be ingested or applied to skin. Instead, dilute in water or a neutral (carrier) oil.
Soapwort *(Saponaria officinalis)* Tea; ingredient in some European cough remedies.	Treat constipation; calm a cough; acne treatment; soap substitute.	Saponins in soapwort produce a foamy lather that can be used to cleanse skin and hair. Soapwort saponins can reduce airway congestion and calm a cough; extracts have anti-inflammatory actions that may be useful in treating acne and other skin inflammations.	Should not be ingested by people with ulcers or other intestinal disorders. May be toxic if taken in large amounts.
Vervain *(Verbena officinalis)* Liquid extract, tincture, fresh or dried herb, tea, compress, poultice, tooth powder.	Elevate mood; promote healing of skin wounds; diuretic; general tonic during convalescence.	No recent studies have been done on vervain, so claims are supported mostly by traditional use.	Appears safe when used in recommended amounts, but toxicity has not been studied.
Wild (choke) cherry *(Prunus serotina)* Dried bark, syrup, tincture, tea; ingredient in some commercial cough remedies.	Cold and cough remedy and treatment for other respiratory ailments; calm anxiety; treat mild diarrhea.	Inner bark contains prunasin, which acts as an expectorant to reduce airway congestion. Tranquilizing properties are attributed to hydrocyanic acid. Tannins help reduce diarrhea and also soothe a sore throat.	Generally safe when consumed in small amounts. However, hydrocyanic acid in wild cherry bark, leaves, and fruit has properties similar to cyanide when consumed in large amounts. Never chew raw bark or leaves.
Wintergreen *(Gaultheria procumbens)* Gargle, liniment, ointment, oil; ingredient in lotions, gels, and other skin products.	Treat muscle and joint pain, inflammation, and swelling; soothe mouth ulcers, gingivitis, and sore throat.	Methyl salicylate in wintergreen reduces inflammation and pain when applied externally; methyl salicylate and tannins in wintergreen also soothe sore throat and oral lesions when used as a mouth rinse or gargle.	Full-strength wintergreen oil is highly toxic and should never be ingested; fatalities have been reported, especially among children. Methyl salicylate also should not be swallowed. Wintergreen used as flavoring in commercial products are safe when taken in moderation.

Other Useful Botanical Medicines, continued

NAME OF PLANT/FORMS	TRADITIONAL USES	EFFICACY	CAUTIONS
Yarrow *(Achillea millefolium)* Capsule, juice, liquid extract, tincture, tea, ointment, lotion, poultice.	Promote wound healing; reduce inflammation; treat minor digestive upsets.	Chemical components have antiseptic and astringent properties that reduce inflammation and promote wound healing; bitter compounds stimulate appetite and aid digestion; antispasmodic compounds reduce intestinal cramps and help counter diarrhea. Some animal studies have found mild blood-pressure lowering and diuretic properties, but these effects have not been studied in humans.	Appears safe when used in recommended amounts; high doses can cause drowsiness, diarrhea, and urinary urgency. People allergic to ragweed and other members of the daisy family may also react to yarrow.
Yellow dock *(Rumex crispus)* Capsule, liquid extract, powder, dried root, tea.	Stimulant laxative; promote wound healing; treat fungal skin infections and skin inflammation.	Yellow dock contains anthraquinones, the substances in senna and cascara sagrada that act as stimulant laxatives. Tannins and yellow dock extracts have astringent and antibiotic properties that help prevent infection and promote healing of minor skin wounds.	Yellow dock roots and rhizomes are considered safe when used as recommended. The leaves contain toxic substances that can damage mucous membranes, damage kidneys, and cause other adverse reactions; the leaves should not be ingested or applied to open wounds.

Dangerous Botanicals

The following herbs are sometimes listed in botanical medicine texts and recommended by herbalists. However, all have potentially dangerous components and should not be ingested in any form. Some are also hazardous when applied to the skin because the toxic substances may be absorbed into the body.

NAME OF PLANT/FORMS	TRADITIONAL USES	POTENTIAL DANGERS
Angelica (*Angelica archangelica*) Capsule, concentrated drops, extract, tincture, powdered root, infusion.	Promotes sweating; aid digestion; kill lice; treat skin irritations.	High levels of furocoumarins can cause severe sun sensitivity; animal studies indicate these substances increase cancer risk; fresh root is poisonous.
Bayberry (*Myrica cerifera*) Capsule, extract, infusion, tincture, powder.	Expectorant; induce vomiting; poultice to treat skin ulcers.	Animal studies have found substance causes cancer.
Blue cohosh (*Caulophyllum thalictroides*) Capsule, pill, liquid extract, tincture.	Uterine stimulant; treat irregular menstrual periods; treat muscle spasms and a variety of disorders.	Blue cohosh (not to be confused with black cohosh, see p. 376) can cause serious heart damage and increase blood pressure. Seeds are poisonous if ingested; berries and roots cause serious cell damage.
Calamus (*Acorus calamus*) Tincture, extract, infusion, powdered root, bath product.	Upset stomach, epilepsy, anxiety, arthritis, and miscellaneous ailments.	Isoasarone in calamus has been found to cause cancer in laboratory animals; has been banned by U.S. health authorities for human use.
Chaparral (*Larrea divaricata*) Extract, capsule, infusion; included in some herbal combinations.	Weight-loss aid; antioxidant to slow aging and prevent cancer; cough and cold remedy; treatment for numerous other ailments.	Has been reported to cause serious liver damage in people taking preparation; FDA has barred sale to consumers.
Clematis (*Clematis virginiana*) Infusion or tea made from leaves.	Treat skin disorders, nervousness, tics, sleep problems, and other disorders.	All parts of the plant are toxic; external applications can cause severe skin irritation and ingestion can cause severe bloody diarrhea, vomiting, kidney damage, and convulsions.
Coltsfoot (*Tussilago farfara*) Extract, infusion, tincture, powder, ointment.	Cough and cold remedy; soothe skin inflammation.	External uses may be safe, but ingestion can cause serious liver damage. (Also see in table, Other Useful Botanical Medicines, p. 553).

Dangerous Botanicals, continued

NAME OF PLANT/FORMS	TRADITIONAL USES	POTENTIAL DANGERS
Comfrey (*Symphytum officinale, S. asperum*) Infusion, tincture for internal use. Balm, ointment, salve, and other products for external use.	Digestive aid; treat internal bleeding; airway congestion; skin sores and irritations.	External use is safe, but ingestion can cause serious liver damage.
Deadly nightshade (*Atropa belladonna*) Tincture, ointment, injection.	Dilate pupils; antispasmodic to treat intestinal disorders; treatment for tremors and other Parkinson's symptoms.	All parts of plant are highly poisonous and should not be ingested. Medical uses, such as dilating pupils, should be done only by a doctor using commercial preparations.
Ephedra (*Ephedra sinica*) Capsule, pill, tincture, dried herb, tea, or decoction.	Treatment for asthma; reduce airway congestion; appetite suppressant to aid in weight loss.	Alkaloids in ephedra can raise blood pressure, speed the heartbeat, and cause nervousness, insomnia, urinary retention, and other adverse effects. A number of deaths have been attributed to its use, and the FDA has issued a warning on its potential dangers.
Foxglove (*Digitalis purpurea* and other species) Prescription digitalis preparations.	Treatment for heart disease.	Digitalis glycosides are highly toxic and an overdose can cause abnormal heart rhythms, dizziness, confusion, and convulsions. Use must be carefully monitored by a doctor.
Germander (*Teucrium chamaedrys*) Capsule, decoction, or tea.	Appetite suppressant to aid in weight loss.	Can cause severe liver damage.
Lobelia (*Lobelia inflata*) Capsule, pill, infusion, liquid extract, powder, lozenge, dried herb.	Expectorant; alleviate symptoms of nicotine withdrawal; alleviate skin irritations.	Lobeline in lobelia can cause vomiting, diarrhea, tremors, dizziness, and palpitations. Overdose can also cause drop in blood pressure, shock, coma, and death.
Mayapple (*Podophyllum peltatum*) Powder, tincture, prescription tinctures for external use.	Folk treatment for cancer; topical treatment for genital warts.	Mayapple is highly poisonous if ingestesd; external use should be supervised by a doctor.

Dangerous Botanicals, continued

NAME OF PLANT/FORMS	TRADITIONAL USES	POTENTIAL DANGERS
Mistletoe *(Phoradendron flavescens and other species)* Capsule, liquid extract, tincture, infusion, or tea.	European varieties: tranquilizer, antispasmodic; lower high blood pressure; possible anticancer agent. American varieties: raise blood pressure; stimulate uterine contractions.	All parts of both European and American varieties are considered toxic and should not be ingested. Can cause liver damage and there have been reports of fatal poisoning of children who ingested berries.
Pau d'arco *(Tabebuia impetiginosa)* Capsule, extract, bark, tea.	Natural or folk cancer treatment; general tonic and digestive aid.	Ingestion can cause nausea, vomiting, bleeding, anemia, and other adverse effects.
Pennyroyal *(Hedeoma pulegioides)* Extract, oil, tincture, decoction, dried herb, tea.	Cold and flu remedy; treatment for eczema and other inflammatory skin conditions; induce menstruation and cause an abortion.	Volatile oil contains pulegone, a toxic substance that can cause vomiting, diarrhea, fever, internal bleeding, palpitation, high blood pressure, liver damage, seizures, and shock leading to death.
Periwinkle *(Vinca minor)* Tincture.	Reduce heavy menstrual bleeding; slow effects of aging; increase mental alertness; reduce bleeding and promote healing of skin wounds.	Animal studies show periwinkle can reduce levels of white blood cells and impair immunity.
Pokeweed *(Phytolacca americana)* Capsule, tincture, dried root, poultice.	General tonic to "cleanse" system; promote healing of skin ulcers, infection, hemorrhoids; folk or natural cancer treatment.	All parts of mature pokeweed are toxic, although cooked berries are safe. Ingestion can cause vomiting, breathing problems, drop in blood pressure, confusion, and convulsions. Toxic substances can enter body through broken skin.
Rue *(Ruta graveolens)* Oil, tincture, infusion, dried herb.	Calm coughs; ease intestinal and menstrual cramps; induce menstruation or abortion.	Volatile oil in rue is highly toxic and can cause vomiting, convulsions, miscarriage, severe intestinal pain, and death.
Sassafras *(Sassafras albidum)* Tincture, tea, infusion, extract without safrole.	Ease rheumatism and arthritis; cold and flu remedy; reduce mastitis following childbirth; kill lice and repel other insects.	Sassafras volatile oil contains safrole, which can cause vomiting, paralysis, and death; also increases cancer risk.

Dangerous Botanicals, continued

NAME OF PLANT/FORMS	TRADITIONAL USES	POTENTIAL DANGERS
Tansy *(Tanacetum vulgare)* Oil, infusion, tea (sale is prohibited in the U.S.).	Treat migraines and nerve pain; kill intestinal worms; external application to reduce itching and repel insects.	Tansy contains thujone, a substance that is highly toxic in both external and ingested forms. There have been reports of deaths from consuming tansy tea or ingesting even a few drops of tansy oil.
Wormwood *(Artemisia absinthium)* Liquid extract, powder, tea, tincture, enema, infusion.	Kill intestinal worms; flavoring for vermouth, absinthe, and other beverages after toxic substances are removed.	Thujone in wormwood essential oil is highly toxic and can cause convulsion; is addictive in small doses and can cause personality changes.
Yohimbe *(Pausinystalia yohimbe)* Capsule, pill, concentrated drops, tincture, tea, bark; active ingredient (yohimbine) is available by prescription.	Male (and female) aphrodisiac; treatment for impotence.	Overdose of yohimbine (alkaloid in yohimbe) can cause anxiety, panic, tremor, rise in blood pressure, and hallucinations. Higher doses can cause dangerous drop in blood pressure, weakness, and possible paralysis.

PART 4

Nutraceuticals in Practice

CHAPTER 3

Nutraceuticals Just for Women

For thousands of years women have turned to herbal teas and extracts for relief of "female problems." In the first century A.D., Dioscorides, author of one of the first Western medical texts, listed herbal formulas to treat everything from menstrual irregularities to fertility problems. Traditional healers worldwide have depended on raspberry leaf tea as a "uterine tonic." On this continent, Native Americans prized black cohosh (or squaw root) for the relief of similar ailments and to stimulate the menstrual flow. Eventually black cohosh (not to be confused with blue cohosh, which can raise blood pressure dangerously) became one of the principal ingredients of Lydia Pinkham's Vegetable Compound, which had such a favorable reputation for boosting fertility that it made its way into song:

> Widow Brown she had no children,
> Though she loved them very dear;
> So she took some Vegetable Compound,
> Now she has them twice a year.

Today, scientific studies have revealed that black cohosh has estrogen-like activity, and it is widely used in Europe for relief of premenstrual syndrome, menstrual cramps, and symptoms of menopause.

Another ingredient in Lydia Pinkham's Vegetable Compound, life root—also known as ragwort, false valerian, and squaw weed—was touted for its ability to promote menstrual flow. According to a turn-of-the-century medical advice book:

> Life-root exerts a peculiar influence upon the female reproductive
> organs, and for this reason has received the name of Female Reg-

ulator. It is very efficacious in promoting the menstrual flow, and is a valuable agent in the treatment of uterine diseases.

For centuries women in Asia have turned to dong quai root, a mild laxative, to treat almost every gynecologic complaint, from menstrual irregularities to menopausal symptoms. Modern herbalists now understand that some benefits of dong quai result from the coumarin it contains, which dilates the blood vessels and stimulates the nervous system.

Folk medicine sources have often used the term *emmenagogue* to describe an herb that promotes menstrual flow, but in the era before legalized abortion, the term denoted any herb that could trigger a miscarriage. Pennyroyal, for example, when taken as a tea relieves menstrual problems; used in its more potent oil form, pennyroyal is said to cause miscarriage. Sadly, women who took the toxic oil for this reason risked severe liver damage, convulsions, and even death. In contrast, raspberry tea remains a popular folk remedy for relieving morning sickness and preventing miscarriage, and it's reported to relax the smooth muscles of the uterus.

In recent decades, scientists have been isolating some of the active ingredients of some of the foods, roots, and herbs that women have traditionally relied on for their health. Many traditionally trained physicians have been joining naturopaths and practitioners of Chinese and Ayurvedic medicine in incorporating these natural medicines into their treatment of specific conditions that affect the female reproductive system, urinary tract, and breasts.

As you look through the following pages, be sure to review the full entry for any nutraceuticals you consider taking.

BLADDER CONTROL PROBLEMS

SYMPTOMS
- Involuntary urination.
- Leakage of urine.
- Urination on coughing, sneezing, laughing, or lifting, or when physically active.
- Urgent need to urinate when the bladder is not full.

Also called stress or urge incontinence, the inability to control bladder function commonly occurs with aging. Although it becomes quite common in women over sixty-five, as many as one in six women between forty and sixty-five and one in ten under forty have a problem with bladder control. Stress incontinence, the most common type, denotes a leakage of urine after coughing, sneezing, laughing, or lifting a heavy object puts pressure on the bladder. Urge incontinence occurs when the feeling that one needs to urinate is so strong that making it to the bathroom in time is impossible. (An infection in the bladder can also create an urgent need to urinate even though little urine is passed (see Urinary Tract Infections, p. 191). Regardless of what causes a bladder control problem, it can be so embarrassing that many women who have it never tell their doctors—which is unfortunate, because almost everyone can be helped.

Bladder control problems are most often the result of weak pelvic muscles that fail to properly support the bladder and urethra (the short tube through which urine flows from the bladder to a tiny opening, the meatus, above the vagina). A weak urethral sphincter, a muscle that surrounds the urethra, may also be at fault. To urinate, this muscle, along with other muscles of the lower pelvis, must relax. If they relax unintentionally, a few drops of urine may leak out or, in more extreme cases, the bladder may empty completely.

A weak urethral sphincter and/or inadequate pelvic muscle support becomes especially common in women after menopause, when estrogen levels diminish. There appears to be a genetic component to the problem, too, since it tends to occur among female relatives. Childbirth, particularly a long and difficult delivery, can stretch pelvic muscles, which may continue to sag over the years unless strengthened. Chronic constipation can also stretch the pelvic muscles. Another cause of incontinence is pressure on the urethral sphincter and bladder from abdominal fat or from a developing fetus during pregnancy. Chronic coughing, such as a smoker's cough, can also strain the urethra's ability to hold back the flow of urine.

Less often, bladder control problems, such as bed-wetting, are associated with neurological conditions such as stroke, multiple sclerosis, or Parkinson's disease. Incontinence may also be a symptom of infection.

Diagnostic Steps

For the physician to assess the extent of the problem, it helps to keep a diary in which you record the timing of urinary frequency, amount excreted, what you were doing when it occurred, what liquids you consumed, and any medications you may have taken. A bladder infection can be ruled out by testing the urine for bacteria. If blood is found in the urine, other diagnostic tests such as X rays of the kidney may follow. A cystoscopy (direct examination of the inside of the bladder and urethra through a tiny tube equipped with a magnifying lens) may be done. More complex tests of the bladder that evaluate its storage capacity and ability to empty completely may also be required.

The physician will do a pelvic exam to evaluate the strength of the muscles supporting the bladder and check that the bladder or the urethra or both are not sagging into the vaginal space.

Conventional Treatments

Estrogen replacement therapy (ERT) or direct application to the urethra of estrogen cream, such as estriol vaginal cream, once or twice a week may help. Detrol (tolterodine tartrate) is sometimes prescribed to control

◉ WORKOUT FOR PELVIC MUSCLES

Six weeks of Kegel exercises will usually strengthen the muscles of the pelvic floor, although for some women improvement may not be significant for six months. Typically, Kegel movements involve squeezing for ten seconds the muscles that would normally hold back a stream of urine. (Do not do this while actually urinating, however.) A common prescription is to perform the exercises four times a day, contracting the muscles ten times and holding each contraction for ten seconds. Women with weak muscles may begin by squeezing the muscles for only two seconds, but gradually as the muscles regain their tone, work up to ten seconds each. Since some women have trouble knowing if they are contracting the pelvic muscles (and not those of the lower abdomen), some physicians, such as Christiane Northrup, suggest putting two fingers into the vagina and spreading them apart slightly. As the vaginal muscles are squeezed, the woman should feel the muscles press on her fingers. Biofeedback tools are also available that display the exact amount of force of the muscle contraction.

Another approach is based on an ancient Chinese muscle-strengthening method that involves inserting a weighted cone and holding it in place for one to five minutes, twice a day. The cones are available in different weights, so you can increase the weight as the muscles get stronger. Of course, muscle strengthening will not relieve incontinence if it is due to infection, diuretics, or drinking caffeinated beverages.

- Consider discontinuing diuretic medications and those that acidify the urine and/or irritate the bladder, such as vitamin C or vitamin preparations that include aspartate.
- Adopt a healthy lifestyle. For example, quit smoking.
- Avoid diuretic drinks (coffee, colas, and tea), alcohol, and acidic and spicy foods that contribute to bladder irritation.
- Drink more water to dilute the urine, so that it is less irritating to the bladder.
- Avoid straining when exercising, particularly when weight training. Avoid high-impact aerobics.
- Practice bladder training—that is, go to the bathroom at regular intervals whether or not you have an urge to urinate. Then gradually increase the interval time.

urinary frequency and urge incontinence (side effects, such as dry mouth, are minimal, but be alert to the possibility of blurred vision).

A plastic or rubber pessary, inserted into the vagina, can help women whose uterus or bladder has fallen and/or whose incontinence seems to occur only during certain activities such as when exercising. A pessary looks like an oversized diaphragm. Other mechanical devices can be placed directly over the urethra.

Surgery to correct anatomical problems and reposition the bladder may be recommended.

Nutraceuticals for Incontinence

No tonics or herbs improve bladder control problems, but foods such as soy (which is high in phytoestrogens), and herbs such as wild yam and dong quai may help by toning the bladder internally to diminish excessive urination. The mechanical problem causing incontinence is best treated with appropriate exercises.

■ BOTANICAL MEDICINES

Wild yam (*Dioscorea villosa*)

How it works. The root of this vine contains an alkaloid that relaxes the muscles of the abdomen. It also contains anti-inflammatory saponins.

Recommended dosages. Wild yam is available over the counter in capsules. A tea can also be made by combining 1 to 2 teaspoons of powdered bark in a cup of boiling water and allowing it to steep for eight hours. After straining, it can be made more palatable by mixing with honey or another herbal tea.

Possible problems. None have been reported.

Dong quai (*Angelica sinensis*)

How it works. The root contains coumarin, cadinene, carotene, carvacrol, sesquiterpenes, and vitamins A, B_{12}, and E, which increase the effects of ovarian hormones.

Recommended dosages. In powder form, 500 mg a day is recommended for menopausal symptoms, which may include bladder control problems. Simmer 2 teaspoons of grated root for twenty minutes in 1½ pints of water to make a decoction.

Possible problems. Do not take during pregnancy or if you have blood-clotting problems or heavy menstrual periods. Never take dong quai if you have any tumor growth of the reproductive organs.

BREAST DISORDERS (BENIGN)

Most breast lumps are benign. Noncancerous breast lumps are grouped together under such umbrella terms as fibrocystic breast syndrome (FBS) or cysticmastitis. FBS is the most common noncancerous breast condition among women, afflicting about 20 percent of all adult women at some time in their lives. Although the breasts are uncomfortable, FBS is not serious. Fibrocystic breasts do not increase your risk of breast cancer. However, they may mask malignant tumors or make them difficult to diagnose.

Although some doctors call this condition fibrocystic breast *disease,* that's a misnomer. These lumps are not diseases. Most are simply an exaggeration of changes that normally occur in the breast over the course of the monthly menstrual cycle. Just as the uterus prepares for pregnancy every month by building a thicker lining, so do the breasts change in anticipation of the need for milk production. In the first half of the menstrual cycle, the milk-secreting glands swell and their cells, and surrounding fibrous tissue, increase in number. In the days leading up to menstruation, extra breast fluid normally is reabsorbed by the body and excess fibrous tissue recedes. If such resolution is not complete, extra fluid is trapped in small sacs called cysts, which is one of the causes of lumpy breasts. However, when incomplete reabsorption is repeated every month, the sacs may fill with fibrous tissue and are called benign tumors.

The growth of fibrous tissue most frequently appears during a woman's late thirties or forties and disappears with menopause. However, because FBS is often linked to shifts in female hormones, it is also seen in teenagers who have not yet established regular menstrual cycles; women who have children late in life; women who are on estrogen treatment; women who have gained weight; and those who are under stress. The condition tends to improve during pregnancy and breast-feeding, as well as after menopause. It is not clear whether the fibrocystic condition is related to a specific excess of estrogen, or simply to an imbalance in a woman's estrogen-progesterone ratio.

Diagnostic Steps

Any new lump in your breasts should be reported to your doctor. A basic evaluation includes a manual breast examination and may proceed to a mammogram and possibly an ultrasound evaluation. Depending on the findings, the doctor then may recommend a needle biopsy, in which

◎ SYMPTOMS

- Symptoms often ebb and flow, most commonly worsening in the week or two before menstruation.
- Tenderness and swelling.
- Breast discomfort, ranging from mild achiness to marked pain.
- Breast lumps, ranging from a few to a generalized lumpiness that pervades the breasts, making them feel "pebbly" or somewhat like bean bags.

◎ WARNING SIGNS

Although most breast lumps are harmless, always take a new one seriously, especially if:

- The lump grows larger and does not seem to change with your menstrual cycle.
- You have a discharge from your nipple or if the nipple remains tender throughout your menstrual cycle.
- Your breast begins to change shape or looks puckered or dimpled.
- The skin on your breasts is irritated or you develop a rash.
- You have severe pain in the breast that does not change during the month.

▪ Do not expect any one method to banish breast lumps overnight. Start by keeping a daily diary of your symptoms for several months. Make notes of which lifestyle, dietary, and supplement changes you have made in an effort to discern which have an impact on your symptoms.

▪ Reduce your intake of methylxanthines; these chemicals include caffeine, theophylline, and theobromine. They are found in coffee, tea (black and green), chocolate, soft drinks, and various over-the-counter drugs, including pills for alertness, and some analgesics and cold remedies. They appear to promote over-production of compounds in breasts linked to cyst fluid and fibrous tissue. Studies have shown that women who avoid these chemicals often find that their lumps disappear in one to six months.

▪ If you are overweight, try to reduce. A decreased fat intake, as well as less fat in your body, may help lower your overall estrogen levels. Studies have shown that estrogen levels decrease in women with fibrocystic breast syndrome when they are put on a low-fat diet; in turn, pain and lumpiness decrease after three months to six months. The symptoms seem most strongly related to foods containing saturated fat, such as meat and dairy products.

▪ Cut back on your salt intake. Salt promotes fluid retention, which contributes to monthly breast swelling and tenderness.

▪ Increase your fiber intake. Some studies have linked FBS to constipation and a diet low in fiber. Regular bowel movements (more than three times a week) may increase the amount of estrogen being excreted.

▪ Exercise regularly. In one study, women who ran forty-five miles per month reported less breast tenderness. These benefits may derive from a change in hormone levels due to increased activity.

a hollow needle is inserted into the lump. If fluid is easily removed, the lump is probably a harmless cyst. If no fluid can be withdrawn and the lump is solid, other diagnostic techniques are in order, including laboratory analysis of tissue removed from the lump.

If FBS is diagnosed, your doctor will likely advise that you examine your breasts at more frequent intervals to become familiar with your own pattern of lumps and related symptoms. Then you will only need to consult your doctor for regular checkups or when you identify a lump that is not consistent with your pattern.

Conventional Treatments

Because it is not a disease, FBS generally does not require medical treatment. However, sometimes medication is prescribed to alleviate severe symptoms. Analgesics alleviate pain. In all likelihood, your doctor will recommend a simple over-the-counter product such as acetaminophen or aspirin, or an NSAID such as ibuprofen. If your FBS occurs in conjunction with premenstrual syndrome (see p. 597), more potent NSAIDs may be prescribed.

Diuretics can help prevent fluid retention. Hormones may be prescribed to alter the hormonal balance; danazol and tamoxifen are most commonly used. However, because both can have long-term adverse effects, they are only used in cases with severe symptoms and should be limited to three to six months.

Nutraceuticals for Benign Breast Disorders

▪ VITAMINS AND MINERALS

Vitamin E

How it works. The mechanism underlying vitamin E's benefits for FBS are not clear. They may result from the vitamin's anti-inflammatory effects, or from some sort of balancing influence on hormones.

Recommended dosages. Supplemental vitamin E, at levels of 400 to 800 IU per day, taken with food, has been found effective in the treatment of breast tenderness.

Possible problems. If you take blood-thinning medication, do not supplement with vitamin E without consulting your physician.

Vitamin B-complex

How they work. The B-complex vitamins regulate estrogen activity by promoting healthy liver function; the liver is the primary site for estrogen clearance. In addition, B_6 also has a natural diuretic effect, helping to reduce swelling.

Recommended dosages. A standard daily multivitamin usually provides an adequate supplement of B vitamins. Some women find better benefits with B_6 doses of 200 to 500 mg per day, taken in divided doses.

Possible problems. Pregnant or breast-feeding women should not take more than 100 mg of vitamin B_6. Huge doses of B_6—1 to 5 g daily for months—can damage nerves.

Iodine

How it works. Iodine plays a pivotal role in thyroid function, and animal studies have shown that iodine deficiencies may cause changes very similar to those seen in women with FBS. Further, some women with FBS have been shown to have low thyroid function; thyroid supplementation has yielded an improvement in symptoms. It is theorized that iodine deficiency makes breast cells more sensitive to estrogen.

Recommended dosages. Studies have used 70 to 80 mcg of molecular (caseinate or liquid) iodine per kilogram of body weight. Other forms of iodine may require a total dosage of 500 mcg per day.

Possible problems. High doses (several milligrams per day) of iodine can interfere with normal thyroid function. Studies of even moderate supplementation with iodines yielded side effects in a small number of patients; these included altered thyroid function, watery nose, weakness, excessive salivation, and acne. Do not take iodine for FBS without consulting your health care practitioner.

■ BOTANICAL MEDICINES

Evening primrose (*Oenothera biennis*)

How it works. The gamma-linolenic acid (GLA), an essential fatty acid, in evening primrose oil helps in iodine absorption. It also serves as a building block for the body to use in making anti-inflammatory prostaglandins. GLA is also available in borage oil and flaxseed oil. Native American women traditionally have chewed the seeds of this plant for medicinal purposes.

Recommended dosages. Check the label for the amount of GLA in each capsule of evening primrose oil; find ones that have about 50 mg of GLA each. You'll need at least three and possibly six to ten capsules daily to achieve results.

Possible problems. You may have to take evening primrose oil daily for two to three months before you see a benefit.

Chaste berry (*Vitex agnus-castus*)

How it works. This fruit helps balance hormones and can help with menstrual-related breast lumps.

Recommended dosages. Studies suggest 175 to 225 mg extract of chaste berry daily.

Possible problems. Avoid chaste berry if you have menstrual-related depression, are pregnant or may become pregnant.

ENDOMETRIOSIS

When the tissue that normally lines the inside of the uterus, the endometrium, attaches itself to the fallopian tubes, the ovaries, or any other place outside the uterine cavity, it causes a chronic and usually progressive condition known as endometriosis. Delayed childbearing appears to be a contributing factor, and it is most prevalent among women in their thirties and forties. Both of these facts have led some people to call it the "career woman's disease." Endometriosis tends to run in families.

In severe cases endometriosis can cause scarring within the pelvis or abdomen and form tough fibrous tissue called adhesions between the internal organs. Endometrial tissue outside the uterus responds to a woman's hormonal cycles in the same ways that endometrial tissue lining the uterus does. Women who do have symptoms—and many don't—have pelvic or back pain during their periods. Occasionally there will be discomfort during sexual intercourse. The most significant problem associated with endometriosis is infertility, which can occur if fallopian tubes are blocked and/or distorted by scarring. In either case, the egg is prevented from entering the uterus or sperm cannot reach the egg.

Diagnostic Steps

Nodes or tender areas behind the woman's cervix may be noticed by a physician performing a pelvic examination. The only way to make a definitive diagnosis is to examine the pelvic cavity directly through a telescopelike instrument called a laparoscope. It is sometimes possible to remove endometrial tissue through the laparoscope. In advanced cases, endometrial tissue can form large cysts, and it's not unusual for fibroids to be present as well.

◉ SYMPTOMS

- Pelvic pain.
- Abdominal or back pain.
- Pain in the rectum.
- Painful intercourse.
- Abnormal menstrual cycles.
- Bleeding between periods.
- Inability to become pregnant.

◉ STRATEGIES FOR RELIEF

- Endometrial tissue grows when stimulated by estrogen, so dietary measures that affect hormone levels may be useful. Aim for a high-fiber diet based on fruits, leafy green and cruciferous vegetables, and soy products. Soy products contain phytoestrogens; these natural plant estrogens seem to balance the effects of your own estrogen. In addition, reduce saturated fats, refined carbohydrates, and dairy products.
- Excessive amounts of certain eicosanoids—hormonelike chemicals that include prostaglandins—can make symptoms worse, so eliminate meat and dairy foods; avoid hydrogenated oils (such as margarine); and include omega-3 fatty acids, found principally in cold-water fish such as mackerel, salmon, and swordfish, and in flaxseed.
- Acupuncture and heat (a hot bath or heating pad) help to control pain.
- Regular exercise can tame pain and discomfort and may prevent progression of the illness.

Conventional Treatments

Many women with mild endometriosis are advised to take a wait-and-see approach, unless the woman is older and wants to have children or is experiencing pain.

Endometriosis can be forced into remission with drugs such as oral contraceptives, the testosteronelike drug danazol (Danocrine), and GnRh (gonadotropin-releasing hormones) agonists (Synarel and Lupron), which inhibit the release of estrogen. Progesterone cream (¼ to ½ teaspoon of 2 percent progesterone cream twice a day from day ten to day twenty-eight of the menstrual cycle) may decrease the effects of estrogen on the endometrial tissue. Greater concentrations of progesterone are available by prescription. Surgery to remove the endometrial tissue in the pelvic cavity may be considered if cysts are forming, if symptoms are not relieved by other treatments, or if the woman has tried and failed to become pregnant. The endometrial tissue can be destroyed through cauterization or with a laser. In severe cases a hysterectomy may be necessary.

Nutraceuticals for Endometriosis

■ VITAMINS AND MINERALS

Vitamin B-complex

How it work. Each B vitamin has a different role that makes it useful for treating the symptoms of gynecologic problems. Vitamin B_6, for instance, is critical in the formation of hemoglobin and is useful in treating the anemia that may follow excessive bleeding. Riboflavin, or vitamin B_2, is involved in hormone production. Together, the B vitamins maintain the health of the liver, which helps regulate estrogen.

Recommended dosages. Recommended Dietary Allowances for each B vitamin vary, but the standard multivitamin or B-complex supplement contains an adequate amount of each in the proper balance.

Possible problems. Since B vitamins are water-soluble, excessive amounts are excreted and toxicity is rare. However, nerve damage, particularly numbness of the hands and feet, has been reported in those who take large doses of vitamin B_6, and insomnia and anxiety may also occur.

Vitamin E

How it works. Supplements may reduce the production of certain prostaglandins, hormonelike substances that promote inflammation.

Recommended dosages. Taking 100 to 800 IU of natural vitamin E (d-alpha tocopherol) daily is considered safe, although some experts recommend beginning with 200 IU daily and gradually increasing the dose to 400 to 1,000 IU a day. Take it with food.

Possible problems. Most excess vitamin E is excreted, but even so, too much can cause symptoms such as nausea, headache, muscle weakness, and skin problems. Supplements are not suggested for people taking anticoagulants, aspirin, or other blood thinners or who have hypertension, because the combination can result in bleeding problems. It should not to be taken with iron, since it interferes with absorption of that mineral.

Iron

How it works. To offset the blood loss that may accompany fibroids and to prevent anemia, supplements of this mineral are often necessary to maintain production of hemoglobin, the oxygen-carrying protein in blood, and myoglobin, the protein that stores oxygen in muscle.

Recommended dosages. The Recommended Dietary Allowance for premenopausal women is 12 mg a day, but in pregnancy the RDA jumps to 30 mg.

Possible problems. Too much iron suppresses the immune system and promotes the production of free radicals. Therapeutic doses for the treatment of anemia should be prescribed by a physician, since too much iron can cause problems such as stomachache, diarrhea, and constipation. Iron supplements should not be taken at the same time as vitamin E. Vitamin C, on the other hand, enhances iron absorption.

Magnesium

How it works. This is one of the most important minerals in the body and is present in large amounts in the liver, which helps regulate estrogen. It is also essential for the transmission of nerve impulses, muscle contraction, and bone metabolism.

Recommended dosages. The Recommended Dietary Allowance for women is 280 mg, but several situations—a calorie-restricting diet, a high-fiber diet, alcohol, stress, and strenuous exercise—can lead to a deficiency, so supplements are often recommended even in healthy women.

Possible problems. If more magnesium is taken than the kidneys can process, or if kidney function is impaired, toxicity can occur. Low blood pressure, slurred speech, and nausea are signs of an overdose.

■ BOTANICAL MEDICINES

Flaxseed oil (*Linum usitatissimum*)

How it works. Flaxseed oil contains two essential fatty acids that reduce symptoms associated with menstrual problems and endometriosis.

Recommended dosages. There is no general consensus, but some experts suggest 500 mg, up to four times a day, or pulverizing 1 to 2 tablespoons of fresh flaxseed to a fine consistency and sprinkling it into soup, cereal, or a smoothie. To prevent intestinal problems from the added fiber, be sure to drink eight to ten glasses of water during the course of the day.

Possible problems. Flaxseed oil should be refrigerated to prevent rancidity and should not to be used in cooking. (See Flax, p. 455.)

Wild yam (*Dioscorea villosa*)

How it works. The root of this vine contains an alkaloid that relaxes the muscles of the abdomen. It also contains anti-inflammatory saponins. Wild yam is also believed to have progesteronelike activity, which would be helpful in countering the effects of estrogen, and may provide some mild pain relief.

Recommended dosages. Wild yam is available over the counter in capsules. A tea can also be made by combining 1 to 2 teaspoons of powdered bark in a cup of boiling water and allowing it to steep for eight hours. After straining, it can be made more palatable by mixing with honey or another herbal tea.

Possible problems. None have been reported.

Chaste berry (*Vitex agnus-castus*)

How it works. Glycosides and flavonoids are probably responsible for chaste berry's stimulating effects on the pituitary gland, which, in turn, signals the production of progesterone. Studies have shown that chaste berry helps to normalize the balance of female hormones, particularly when too much estrogen is circulating, which makes it helpful for endometriosis.

Recommended dosages. A tea may be made using 1 teaspoon of ripe berries and a cup of boiling water; allow it to steep for ten to fifteen minutes. This tea or 1 ml of tincture may be taken three times a day. Imbalances typically require treatment lasting anywhere from ten days to six months or longer.

Possible problems. Rare side effects include gastrointestinal disturbances and itching. It should not be taken if you are or may become pregnant; it is also contraindicated if you suffer from depression.

Black cohosh (*Cimicifugua racemosa*)

How it works. The dried root and rhizome contain glycosides, isoflavones, isoferulic acid, and tannins. This powerful combination promotes menstruation, relaxes uterine muscle spasms, and relieves muscle-related pain. Some research indicates that black cohosh has an estrogenlike action, so its benefits may also be related to a hormonal effect.

Recommended dosages. Bring ½ to 1 teaspoon of fresh dried root and a cup of water to a boil and allow it to simmer for ten or fifteen minutes. This decoction or 2 ml of a tincture can be taken three times a day.

Possible problems. Occasional gastrointestinal upset has been reported. It should not be taken during pregnancy. Overdose may cause dizziness, excessive sweating, and seizures. Don't take it along with replacement hormones without first discussing it with your doctor. There is a lack of information on the toxic effects of this powerful root.

INFERTILITY

Infertility is defined as an inability to become pregnant after at least one year of regular sexual activity. Many experts consider the inability to sustain a pregnancy after conception to be a form of infertility as well.

About 40 percent of the time, the man is the infertile partner. Often he will be evaluated first, to determine whether a low sperm count or some anatomical problem that interferes with the flow of sperm is the source of the problem. (See Nutraceuticals Just for Men and Athletes, p. 609.)

As a woman ages, her ability to conceive becomes increasingly more limited. She's less fertile in her late twenties than in her early twenties, and her chances of conceiving gradually diminish with each decade. At age forty, 25 percent of women cannot conceive. Infertility may stem from one or more abnormalities that can be successfully treated, however. Moreover, the development of new reproductive technologies, including in vitro fertilization, make it possible for many more women to conceive well into their forties or even fifties.

Mechanical or structural abnormalities linked to infertility in women include endometriosis or fibroid tumors, which are quite common causes of infertility. If endometriosis or a sexually transmitted disease has created scar tissue on the fallopian tubes, surgery may be helpful to clear the opening within the tubes and/or remove adhesions. Ovulation difficulties, occurring among 10 to 15 percent of women, are another significant source of infertility. They may stem from a functional problem within the ovary or an imbalance in hormones that might stem from a variety of conditions, from thyroid disease to stress. Cycles of weight gain and weight loss may contribute, as can eating disorders, regular intense exercise, and even smoking.

Diagnostic Steps

Urine and blood tests are useful in evaluating hormone levels at different times during the menstrual cycle to determine if infertility is linked to a failure to ovulate. Too much of one hormone or not enough of another can interfere with ovulation. A sampling of endometrial tissue from within the woman's uterus can also reveal if ovulation is normal and help establish if the lining is adequately developed to nourish a fertilized egg. A test of secretions from the cervix shortly after intercourse can determine if a woman's mucus is destroying her partner's sperm. When a woman has symptoms or a history of disorders that could affect the anatomy of her reproductive tract, certain X rays can help pinpoint the defect. For example, a hysterosalpingogram is an X ray of the pelvic organs done while a special contrast material is injected into the uterus and fallopian tubes. A physician may do a laparoscopy (see Endometriosis p. 574) to directly examine the pelvic organs.

Since diagnosing the cause of infertility can be very time-consuming, costly, and stressful for couples, psychological counseling is often recommended.

Conventional Treatments

Treatment depends on the cause of the infertility. Surgery, for example, may help clear the tubes of endometrial tissue that blocks them. In some cases, microsurgical techniques permit reconstruction of blocked tubes.

If a woman is ovulating, her cycle will be monitored, and she and her partner will be advised on the best times to have intercourse. If ovulation is not occurring or is infrequent, drugs to induce it are prescribed. The most commonly used drug, clomiphene citrate, stimulates follicle-stimulating hormone (FSH) and causes ovulation. If it's going to be effective, the woman will usually conceive within six menstrual cycles. Clomiphene citrate does, however, have unpleasant side effects, including hot flashes, bloating, and abdominal pain, and may cause temporary ovarian cysts. Other fertility drugs include human menopausal gonadotropin (hMG) and gonadotropin-releasing hormone (GnRh).

Nutraceuticals for Infertility

■ VITAMINS AND MINERALS

Vitamin E

How it works. Vitamin E may alter the production of certain prostaglandins, hormonelike substances that promote inflammation.

Recommended dosage. Taking 100 to 800 IU daily is considered quite safe, athough some experts recommend beginning with 200 IU daily and gradually increasing the dose to 400 to 1,000 IU of the natural (d-alpha form) a day. Take it with food.

Possible problems. Most excess vitamin E is excreted, but even so, too much can cause symptoms such as nausea, headache, muscle weakness, and skin problems. Supplements are not suggested for people taking anticoagulants, aspirin, or other blood thinners or who have hypertension, because the combination can result in bleeding problems. It should not to be taken at the same time as iron, since it interferes with absorption of that mineral.

Selenium

How it works. Since deficiencies have been associated with fertility problems, assuring an adequate intake of this trace mineral may be useful.

Recommended dosage. The Recommended Dietary Allowance is 55 mcg for nonpregnant women. Supplements of no more than 200 mcg have been recommended.

Possible problems. Large doses may be toxic, causing nerve damage, nausea, weight loss, lethargy, and hair loss.

■ BOTANICAL MEDICINES

Various herbs can be used in an attempt to stimulate the glands responsible for producing hormones.

Chaste berry (*Vitex agnus-castus*)

How it works. Studies have shown that chaste berry helps to normalize the balance of female hormones.

Recommended dosages. A tea may be made using 1 teaspoon of ripe berries and a cup of boiling water and allowed to steep for ten to fifteen minutes. This tea or 1 ml of tincture may be taken three times a day. Imbalances require treatment lasting from ten days to six months or longer.

Possible problems. Rare side effects include gastrointestinal disturbances and itching; it should not be taken if you are or may become pregnant, or if you suffer from depression.

MENOPAUSE

Menopause is the time when, due to a decline in production of the hormone estrogen, the monthly release of eggs by a woman's ovaries ends, menstruation ceases, and she is no longer able to conceive children. Technically, menopause occurs when a woman no longer menstruates, but the biological mechanisms leading to menopause can begin years before, and symptoms can continue for several years afterward.

In some women, menopause may occur suddenly. But in most, periods become erratic over a period of months or years before stopping completely. During this time, termed perimenopause, you may miss one or two periods and then return to what seems like a normal pattern of menstruation. Some women also may experience very heavy or prolonged vaginal bleeding during perimenopause. The years after complete cessation of menstruation are called postmenopause.

Women usually reach menopause in their late forties or early fifties. Some women, however, may enter the menopause in their late thirties. Others continue to menstruate into their late fifties. If a woman's ovaries have been removed by surgery, her body is suddenly unable to supply hormones. She will enter menopause immediately unless her doctor prescribes hormones to replace those which her ovaries have been supplying.

Menopause is *not* a disease—it is a natural event in a woman's reproductive life. But after a woman enters menopause, she becomes at increased risk for a number of diseases, notably heart disease and osteoporosis, against which estrogen offers great protection during her reproductive years. But whether replacement hormones offer protection from heart disease, as has been believed for years, and whether the benefits outweigh the risks (principally of breast and uterine cancer), remains highly controversial and awaits definitive studies.

Diagnostic Steps

Irregular menstruation is usually the diagnostic key. But sometimes estrogen levels start to decline without causing such changes. Your doctor may do a blood test for follicle-stimulating hormone (FSH), which rises as the ovaries start shutting down.

Conventional Treatments

Menopause itself is natural and does not have to be treated. However, some of the side effects of menopause can be alleviated, including those that are directly related to estrogen loss, such as hot flashes and dry vaginal tissue.

Estrogen replacement therapy (ERT) or hormone replacement therapy (HRT) is the most common treatment and can considerably alleviate menopausal symptoms for women who suffer severely. It can also reduce the likelihood of osteoporosis and possibly heart attack for women at risk for those disorders, although other measures are also available. Estrogen replacement may be taken by pill or skin patch, both of which have systemic effects on the whole body, or by a cream applied to the vagina. Estrogen does, however, increase the risk for breast cancer.

Unless a woman has had a hysterectomy, ERT alone may trigger uterine cancer. Thus many women have been taking estrogen-progesterone therapy (HRT). New studies have been suggesting that this combination increases the risk of breast cancer in these women. Larger studies are expected to provide more definitive information

◉ SYMPTOMS

Some women notice few changes other than cessation of the menstrual cycle and menstrual flow. Others experience many physical and emotional changes in the several years before and after menopause. Some of these symptoms may result directly from the lack of estrogen, such as:

- Thinning of the mucous membranes lining the vagina, leading to vaginal dryness and discomfort during sexual intercourse.
- Thinning of the walls of the urethra, through which urine exits the body, leading to a higher risk of urinary tract infections.
- Hot flashes, which are feelings of heat that start at the forehead and spread down the body, sometimes causing skin reddening or sweating, which can be profuse.
- Night sweats, similar to hot flashes but interrupting sleep.
- Weight gain, especially around the waist and abdomen.
- Decrease in short-term memory.

Although the following symptoms are frequently associated with menopause or perimenopause, their cause remains unclear:

- Headache.
- Nausea.
- Joint pain.
- Mood swings and depression.
- Insomnia.
- Changes in sexual interest or functioning.

Declining estrogen and other hormones may be at fault, but other causes are possible. The symptoms may derive from decreased levels of serotonin, a body chemical that affects sleep and self-esteem. Or night sweats themselves, causing sleep deprivation, may account for irritability, headache, and depression. Some symptoms may also reflect a woman's emotional discomfort with this difficult time in life.

As a woman's body adjusts to its new hormone levels, some symptoms—such as hot flashes—go away. Others, like vaginal thinning and dryness, continue.

▪ Hot flashes and other menopausal symptoms are relatively uncommon in cultures that are all or largely vegetarian, especially those that rely on a soy-based diet, as in Japan. Beyond soy, of particular value may be alfalfa, anise, apple, barley, carrots, cherries, clover, fennel, garlic, green beans, hops, licorice, oats, peas, pomegranates, potatoes, rice, rye, sage, sesame seeds, wheat, and yeast.

▪ Make sure your bedroom is very cool. Sleep on bed linens made of natural cotton, rather than synthetic fibers, to absorb the moisture of night sweats.

▪ Acupuncture and relaxation techniques may reduce hot flashes.

▪ To ease vaginal dryness, try twice-weekly use of the moisturizer Replans. For immediate lubrication prior to intercourse, try Astroglide or K-Y Jelly. Do not use an oil-based lubricant, such as Vaseline, because it can interfere with the natural cleansing system of the vagina. Some women prefer natural aloe vera gel, which has a texture similar to that of vaginal fluids.

within the next few years. Women need to discuss their individual needs and risks with their doctors.

Other hormones that may be prescribed include testosterone or danazol, which are androgenic or "male" hormones (which women's bodies also produce); these may help fuel sexual interest and response.

Another drug that may help ease hot flashes is clonidine, an antihypertensive drug.

Nutraceuticals for Menopause

Women have been using various herbal remedies to ease the discomforts of menopause since recorded time. Some have recently received scientific validation. In particular, plants containing phytoestrogens—notably soy products—have been shown to contain weak estrogenlike compounds.

▪ VITAMINS AND MINERALS

Vitamin E

How it works. Vitamin E stabilizes blood vessels so that they do not dilate as widely in response to hormonal change. This can help reduce the intensity of hot flashes.

Recommended dosages. Some women reduce their hot flashes by taking supplements of 400 to 1,200 IU of vitamin E a day. Take it with food.

Possible problems. If you take blood-thinning medication, do not supplement with vitamin E without consulting your physician.

Boron

How it works. Boron is a trace mineral present in leafy vegetables, apples, grapes, nuts, and grains. USDA research has shown that as little as 3 mg of boron can double blood levels of circulating estrogen.

Recommended dosages. The average American eats between 1 and 2 mg of boron daily; 3 mg supplement is recommended.

Possible problems. No problems have been seen at this dose, but do not exceed it or take it long-term. (See table, Other Important Minerals, p. 262.)

▪ NUTRITIONAL SUPPLEMENTS

Dhea

How it works. Dehydroepiandrosterone (DHEA) is one of the master hormones of the body that is broken down into estrogens and androgens. Studies have shown benefit in reducing hot flashes as well as bone loss.

Recommended dosages. There is no standard dosage, but at least 50 mg is usually necessary for benefits. If 100 mg does not provide some relief from hot flashes after a week of use, you may be using a brand that is not biologically active in the body; try another.

Possible problems. Because of the androgen content, some women develop acne and an increase in facial hair. Reducing the dosage temporarily may alleviate the problem. Do not use at higher dosages. Do not combine with hormone replacements without first discussing it with your doctor.

Soy products

How they work. Considerable research has shown that high soy intake reduces menopausal symptoms.

Recommended dosages. One cup of cooked soybeans provides about 300 mg of isoflavones, the most important class of phytoestrogens. Comparable amounts are found in one-third cup of soy protein or eight ounces of tofu. This amount is equivalent to the level of estrogen provided in one tablet of Premarin, the most commonly prescribed synthetic estrogen used in ERT.

Possible problems. Some people have some gastrointestinal upset until their bodies adjust to a higher soy intake.

■ BOTANICAL MEDICINES

Black cohosh (*Cimicifuga racemosa*)

How it works. This herb has been shown to have estrogenic activity and has long been used for a variety of "female complaints," including menopause. It can reduce hot flashes and ease vaginal dryness.

Recommended dosages. Some practitioners recommend 40 mg daily, in a capsule or tincture.

Possible problems. Occasional gastrointestinal upset has been reported. It should not be taken during pregnancy. Overdose may cause dizziness, excessive sweating, and seizures. Don't take it along with replacement hormones without first discussing it with your doctor.

Chaste berry (*Vitex agnus-castus*)

How it works. This herb helps regulate hormones involved in the menstrual cycle.

Recommended dosages. A daily dose of 30 to 40 mg of the drug in capsules or tinctures has been used.

Possible problems. This drug should never be taken by a woman who is or attempting to become pregnant. It also should not be taken if you suffer from depression.

Dong quai (*Angelica polymorpha*)

How it works. Also known as Chinese angelica, this herb has been known throughout history as a women's tonic, particularly for relief of hot flashes and vaginal dryness.

Recommended dosages. Standard doses range from 3 to 15 g.

Possible problems. It has a mild laxative effect, so don't take it if you have diarrhea. It also increases sensitivity to sunlight. Like chaste berry, it should never be taken if you are or may become pregnant.

Ginseng (*Panax quinquefolius*)

How it works. This herb is recommended for its phytoestrogenic qualities.

Recommended dosages. It is commonly taken in doses of 1 to 9 g daily.

Possible problems. There have been some reports of abnormal bleeding in postmenopausal women who take ginseng.

Red clover (*Trifolium pratense*)

How it works. This herb is high in isoflavones, an important class of phytoestrogens. It is the primary ingredient in Promensil, a dietary supplement often recommended for menopausal women.

Recommended dosages. Each Promensil tablet contains 40 mg of red clover isoflavones. In a recent study at Tufts University, a single Promensil tablet daily reduced hot flashes from 8.1 to 3.6 daily and reduced intensity by 56 percent.

Possible problems. No side effects have been observed. In particular, red clover does not increase the thickness of the endometrial lining, which is a complication commonly associated with ERT.

Sage (*Salvia officinalis*)

How it works. Sage suppresses perspiration and contains phytoestrogens.

Recommended dosages. Steep 1 teaspoon of dried sage in boiling water for ten minutes. Some women find this tea helps them to sleep more comfortably.

Possible problems. Avoid sage oil, which is extremely toxic, and do not drink the tea regularly over the long term.

MENSTRUAL PROBLEMS

Menstruation ordinarily occurs about every twenty-eight days. Only a few tablespoons of blood are lost, and no significant discomfort should be associated with it. However, many women do not fit that norm.

The most common menstrual problems are cramps (dysmenorrhea), heavy bleeding (menorrhagia), and an absence of menstruation (amenorrhea). Each is treated quite differently.

Cramps just before and during the first day or so of menstruation are very common. They usually begin to occur during adolescence and tend to abate with age, especially after pregnancy. In most cases, cramps are caused by contractions of the uterus and an interference with the flow of oxygenated blood to that muscular organ. Contributing factors may include lack of exercise, excessive prostaglandin production, anxiety, a narrow cervix, or a malpositioned uterus. Less commonly, dysmenorrhea results from some underlying disorder, such as endometriosis, uterine fibroids, or pelvic inflammatory disease.

Primary amenorrhea is defined as the failure of menstruation to begin by the time a young woman is sixteen. Secondary amenorrhea is the cessation of menstruation for three months or more in a woman who has previously menstruated normally. During a woman's reproductive years, an absence of menstruation is normal only during pregnancy and breast-feeding. Amenorrhea usually indicates some type of hormonal abnormality, such as a pituitary, hypothalamic, adrenal, thyroid, or ovarian disorder. However, the most common simple cause of secondary amenorrhea is severe weight loss and inordinate exercise or overtraining. Women need a certain amount of fat on their bodies to provide the estrogen needed for normal reproductive function. Thus, it is not uncommon for women who exercise or diet excessively (especially those who are anorexic) to experience this problem.

Abnormal uterine bleeding may result in periods that are longer, heavier, or more frequent than normal—but what that means varies from one woman to the next. Concern should be raised when you vary significantly from your own personal pattern. Although heavy bleeding may be caused by an underlying disorder, usually hormonal or related to fibroids, most heavy bleeding is simply a functional problem with no known cause.

Diagnostic Steps

The diagnostic evaluation may include a pelvic examination, blood and urine tests, and imaging studies, such as ultrasonography and special X-ray techniques.

◉ SYMPTOMS

Cramps
- Low abdominal pain ranging from a dull, constant ache to spasmodic cramps.
- Pain that may spread to the lower back or legs.
- Headache, nausea, constipation, diarrhea, frequent urination, or PMS may accompany cramps.

Absence of Menstruation
- Failure to menstruate for three or more months in a woman of reproductive age.

Heavy Bleeding
- Excessive bleeding, due to longer, heavier, or more frequent menstrual periods.

◉ STRATEGIES FOR RELIEF

- Regular exercise increases circulation and helps carry off excess body fluids in the form of perspiration. Exercise also stimulates the brain to release endorphins and increases your production of serotonin, which will help you relax and sleep.
- Hot baths or heating pads often help ease menstrual cramps.
- Adequate rest and sleep may help reduce cramps.
- Raspberry leaf tea often helps ease cramps.
- Be alert to fat sources in your diet. Excessive animal fat can produce an inflammatory environment that may increase cramps. It may be useful to take add flaxseeds (sprinkle them into cereal or baked goods) or flaxseed oil (add it to your salad dressing).
- Some women report a reduction in menstrual problems after a regimen of acupuncture treatments.
- An absence of menstruation in a woman who has been exercising or dieting excessively is a signal that she needs to modify her habits to restore some fat to her body, by decreasing exercise or eating more.

Conventional Treatments

In general, medical treatment of these problems focuses on easing symptoms. Aspirin and other non-steroidal antiinflammatory drugs (NSAIDs), such as ibuprofen, help not only because they ease the pain of cramps but because they help slow down the production of hormone-like prostaglandins. These drugs may be more effective if they are taken several days before cramps are expected to begin.

Prescription of hormones is common. Most commonly, women with severe cramps are given oral contraceptives—low-dose estrogen-progesterone combinations that suppress ovulation. They should not be used if you want to become pregnant.

Cases of heavy bleeding may be helped by dilation and curettage, a surgical procedure to scrape out the lining of the uterus. Sometimes simple dilation of a narrow cervical opening, an office procedure, may relieve cramps.

Nutraceuticals for Menstrual Problems

■ VITAMINS AND MINERALS

Vitamin E

How it works. Vitamin E is a natural anticoagulant that thins the blood. It is sometimes recommended as a treatment for menstrual cramps. It can have a potent anti-inflammatory effect in the higher dose range.

Recommended dosages. Take at least 200 IU daily, or up to 800 IU daily in divided doses. Take it with meals because vitamin E needs some fat for full absorption.

Possible problems. Rarely, it may cause some gastrointestinal upset. Lowering the dose usually solves the problem. However, if you take blood-thinning medication, do not supplement with E without consulting your physician.

Calcium

How it works. Calcium helps prevent water retention, mood swings, and cramps.

Recommended dosages. Take at least 1000 mg of calcium daily, in food or as a supplement.

Possible problems. Calcium in any form is absorbed best by the body when it is taken several times a day in amounts of 500 mg or less, but taking it all at once is better than not taking it at all. Calcium supplements may reduce the absorption of the antibiotic tetracycline. Because calcium also interferes with iron absorption, the two should not be taken at the same time, unless the iron is taken with vitamin C or calcium citrate. Calcium can be constipating, but adding magnesium counteracts this problem.

Magnesium

How it works. Magnesium relaxes muscles and eases cramps. It works together with calcium.

Recommended dosages. Take half as much magnesium as you do calcium. So, if you're taking 1000 mg of calcium, take 500 mg of magnesium daily, in divided doses.

Possible problems. Taking too much magnesium often leads to diarrhea. Reducing the dose usually eliminates the problem. If you have heart or kidney problems, check with your doctor before taking magnesium supplements.

Iron

How it works. If you are bleeding more than 60 ml of fluid during menstruation, you are at risk for iron deficiency anemia.

Recommended dosages. A daily dose of 100 mg of elemental iron is often recommended for women with heavy menstrual flow.

Possible problems. No problems are associated with this dose in menstruating women.

■ BOTANICAL MEDICINES

Black cohosh (*Cimicifuga racemosa*)

How it works. This herb has been shown to have estrogenic activity and suppresses luteinizing hormones. It has long been used for a variety of "female complaints," including painful menstrual cramps and menopausal symptoms.

Recommended dosages. Doses of 40 mg daily are prescribed for premenstrual complaints.

Possible problems. Some gastrointestinal discomfort may occur. Little is known about the long-term toxic effects of this powerful herb. It should not be taken during pregnancy. Overdose may cause dizziness, excessive sweating, slow pulse and seizures. Don't take it along with replacement hormones without first discussing it with your doctor.

Dong quai (*Angelica polymorpha* or *Angelica sinensis*)

How it works. Also known as Chinese angelica, this herb has served as a women's tonic since antiquity, particularly for the relief of painful menstruation.

Recommended dosages. Standard doses are from 3 to 15 grams. Some practitioners recommend 40 mg daily, in a capsule or tincture.

Possible problems. It has a mild laxative effect, so don't take it if you have diarrhea. It also increases sensitivity to sunlight and can cause a rash. It should never be taken by pregnant women or nursing mothers.

Uva ursi (*Arctostaphylos uva ursi*)

How it works. The leaves of this herb, also known as bearberry, may help reduce cramps and heavy menstrual bleeding by gently constricting blood vessels in the lining of the uterus.

Recommended dosages. The standard dose is one full dropper of tincture in a little water or 1 or 2 capsules three to four times a day.

Possible problems. Rarely, some people experience queasiness and vomiting if the preparation was made with a high tannin content. A change of source should resolve the problem. However, uva ursi should not be taken in women who are pregnant or nursing.

Shepherd's purse (*Capsella bursa-pastoris*)

How it works. This herb has a long history of use in the management of female bleeding, especially during obstetrical hemorrhage. Some studies have shown it to be useful in treating heavy menstrual bleeding.

Recommended dosages. It can be taken in any one of several forms three times a day, such as 4 to 6 ml of a tincture or 250 to 500 mg of a powdered solid extract, or 1.50 grams of dried leaves used to make an infusion.

Possible problems. No side effects have been reported with these dosages.

PREGNANCY

After years of treating pregnancy as a "condition," finally attitudes have shifted. When a woman is pregnant, her body is passing through an utterly normal phase, with characteristic—and healthy—hormonal surges and nutritional demands. Labor and delivery, too, are once again regarded as natural events, not an emergency that calls for medical intervention—unless of course, problems arise that require special treatment. Nevertheless, there is an increase in nutritional needs during pregnancy, and the hormonal changes and the sheer physical impact of supporting a developing baby produce discomfort and stress. To ease that strain, relieve symptoms that interfere with day-to-day life, and treat conditions that may threaten the pregnancy, modern medicine—conventional and complementary—and age-old remedies have much to offer.

Healthy Eating During Pregnancy

Ideally, a woman should begin paying attention to certain nutrients, like folic acid, before she becomes pregnant, since a healthy diet in-

⊙ HERBS AND DRUGS TO AVOID

Since alcohol, smoking, prescribed and recreational drugs, and some nutraceuticals can harm the egg, sperm, or the developing fetus, especially in the critical early days of gestation, a woman and her partner should take exceptional care if they are thinking of having a baby. The most damaging effects of alcohol take place in the first weeks of pregnancy. Be aware that cocaine diminishes blood supply to the uterus and can cause neurologic damage and retard the baby's growth.

It's wise to cut back on foods that have drug-like effects. Caffeine, for example, is a diuretic and contains potentially dangerous alkaloids; recommended limits on coffee range from one to three cups a day. Artificial sweeteners haven't proved to be dangerous, but enough questions have been raised to prompt caution in their use. Women who are heavy drinkers of diet soda, for example, should consider switching to a beverage that provides

cluding a variety of foods not only enhances fertility but provides the nourishment a developing embryo needs during the critical early days after conception. A woman who is thinking about having a baby should try to achieve her ideal weight long before she conceives. (At least 2,200 calories a day are needed to support the growth of the developing fetus, so pregnancy is *not* the time for dieting.) Being overweight is a problem, because it increases the risk of complications during pregnancy, such as high blood pressure and gestational diabetes (see below), and delivery.

Being underweight isn't healthy either. Women who are more than 15 percent under normal weight are at risk of complications during pregnancy and childbirth, and they are especially at risk for having small, unhealthy babies. It's important for them to gain weight by eating nutritionally balanced meals *before* becoming pregnant if at all possible. Physicians typically recommend an average weight gain of 24 to 30 pounds during pregnancy—more if a woman is underweight to begin with.

During the first few weeks of pregnancy, an adequate supply of essential nutrients is critical, since this is when all the cells form that will develop into the baby's organs. Later on, some specific nutritional needs will change. For example, calcium is especially important during the second trimester when bone and blood development escalates. In the last trimester, the baby will have a huge growth spurt, nearly doubling in size, so more protein is required.

To be safe, review your typical diet with your obstetrician and be certain you're not getting too much of any of the "good" nutrients or creating a nutritional imbalance. Vegetarians—particularly those who do not eat eggs or dairy—would be smart to work with a nutritionist to insure they are eating the right mix of whole foods. *And no one should take any neutraceutical without first discussing the pros and cons with her health care practitioner.*

Iron

Most nutritionists recommend eating a lot of iron-containing foods, such as liver (from organically produced beef), spinach, alfalfa, watercress, cabbage, parsley, currants and raisins, blackberries, and eggs to fuel the rapidly expanding blood volume needed to supply the fetus. Certain herbs—sorrel, dandelion, and nettles, for example—are good sources of iron as well. Fresh fruits that contain vitamin C will enhance iron absorption. Still, by the end of pregnancy about 20 percent of women are anemic because of iron deficiency. Because it is so difficult to get enough iron in the diet, prenatal supplements are usually recommended.

Folate (folacin or folic acid)

Needs for this nutrient double during pregnancy, but it is especially important in the weeks immediately before and after conception in order to prevent spinal and brain defects. To get the necessary 400 mcg a day of folate, pregnant women need to eat leafy green vegetables (spinach,

◉ **HERBS AND DRUGS TO AVOID** (cont.)
some nutrients and no phenylalanine, which research has shown can reach the fetus.

Discuss with your physician the necessity of taking any drugs that are currently prescribed. The following drugs and herbs are known to cause harm:

- Retin A (isotrenoin), Accutane, and high doses of vitamin A can cause birth defects. Accutane, a derivative of vitamin A used to treat acne, can cause serious birth defects.
- Certain anticonvulsants.
- Iodine-containing drugs.
- High doses of aspirin.
- Certain high blood pressure medications known as angiotensin-converting enzyme (ACE) inhibitors.
- Certain antibiotics, such as tetracycline, streptomycin, gentamicin, and kanamycin.
- Lithium.
- Strong bitter herbs, such as feverfew, tansy, goldenseal, mugwort, and barberry.
- Herbs that contain alkaloids, including goldenseal, bloodroot, broom, mandrake, and barberry.
- Any herb oil.
- Laxative herbs, including senna and cascara.
- Peruvian bark, poke, cotton root, and male fern.

If you are pregnant or nursing, be diligent in checking with your doctor before taking *any* nutritional supplement or botanical medicine.

◉ **WHO IS AT RISK FOR GESTATIONAL DIABETES**
- Women over 35.
- Women who have had an episode of diabetes in the past, especially during pregnancy.
- Women with a family history of diabetes or high blood sugar.
- Women who are overweight.
- Women who have had a baby weighing more than nine or ten pounds.
- Women who have high blood pressure.

turnip greens, endive, broccoli), fruits, and that iron-rich favorite, liver. To guarantee an adequate folate supply, obstetricians recommend supplements of both folate and iron, but too much of either can be a problem too, leading to zinc deficiency.

B-complex vitamins

Except for vitamin B_{12}, the other B vitamins—thiamine, riboflavin, niacin, and B_6—are plentiful in a diet that includes a mix of vegetables, dairy products, and whole grains. Foods of animal origin are rich sources of all the B's. Getting enough vitamin B_{12} may be particularly problematic for vegetarians; this B vitamin is essential for the baby's developing blood supply and nervous system. Prenatal vitamin formulations provide a healthy and balanced dose of the B complex. Some physicians suggest adding 100 to 300 mg of vitamin B_6 to relieve morning sickness.

Vitamin A

At least 800 RE (3,666 IU) from foods such as vegetables and dairy products is recommended, because this nutrient is essential for growth and development of skin and eyes and the tissue that lines the respiratory, intestinal, and urinary tracts. High doses are dangerous and should be avoided.

Vitamin C

This is another example of some is good, more is dangerous. Eight ounces of orange juice delivers the 60 mg required for the nonpregnant woman, so it's easy to drink a bit more or eat more broccoli, red or green pepper, or strawberries for the additional 10 mg required in pregnancy. Most prenatal vitamins contain some vitamin C. Megadoses, however, can actually create scurvy—a vitamin C deficiency disease—in the newborn, because once outside the mother's body, the large doses of C are abruptly cut off.

Minerals

The demand for bone-building minerals such as calcium and phosphorus soar during pregnancy. Most women get enough phosphorus in the foods they eat, but calcium is a bit harder to get, especially if a woman doesn't like or has difficulty digesting milk and dairy products. Dark green, leafy vegetables are good sources, but absorption can be problematic. Supplements of calcium—and vitamin D, which is needed for absorption—may be advised.

Side Effects and Complications of Pregnancy

Most of the unpleasant side effects of pregnancy are more irritating than they are dangerous, and there are some steps you can take for relief. When side effects are severe or long-lasting, medical intervention may be necessary.

■ MORNING SICKNESS

Although the well-known nausea of pregnancy usually does occur in the morning, and magically disappears after the first trimester, it can last all day or ebb and flow for nine months. The surge in hormone levels is responsible, because, among other things, it causes the stomach to empty more quickly. Therefore, the first remedy is to eat small frequent meals, and always have something in the stomach. Here are some suggestions:

- Have a snack that includes protein and carbohydrate before bed and a carbohydrate snack, such as crackers, before getting up.
- Definitely avoid high-fat foods and possibly ease up on spicy foods.
- Carry fruit with you so you're never caught without a snack.
- Carbonated drinks—ginger ale or cola—sometimes settle an upset stomach.
- Hot or very cold drinks help.
- Herbal teas (see below) may relieve nausea and vomiting.

Medical intervention—taking drugs to control the nausea—is a last resort and is used only if there is a concern that the developing baby isn't being well nourished. In cases of severe vomiting, intravenous feeding may be necessary to prevent dehydration.

Neutraceuticals for Morning Sickness

■ BOTANICAL MEDICINES

Peppermint (*mentha piperita*)

How it works. Menthol in peppermint relaxes the muscles of the digestive system.

Recommended dosage. Commercial peppermint teas are available, or you can steep one to two heaping teaspoons of dried peppermint in a cup of boiling water for ten minutes to make a tea. A dilute tea is best during pregnancy.

Possible problems. Do not take it if you have a history of miscarriage or are subject to heartburn.

Ginger (*Zingiber officinale*)

How it works. This is a traditional remedy for morning sickness because it stimulates the flow of saliva and soothes the intestinal tract.

Recommended dosage. Commercial teas are available, or steep 1 or 2 teaspoons of grated fresh ginger in a cup of hot water and then strain it.

Possible problems. Although the FDA includes ginger on the "Generally Recognized As Safe" list, studies of the safety of ginger during pregnancy are unclear. Since some research indicates it may affect the level of sex hormones in the baby's brain, large medicinal doses should be avoided. A one-inch square of ginger candy contains about 500 mg of ginger, so be careful that nibbling on candied ginger doesn't become a habit.

Raspberry leaf (*Rubus idaeus*)

How it works. Raspberry has been recommended for a tonic throughout history to strengthen the uterus and pelvic muscles and prevent spasms that can threaten the pregnancy. After delivery, the same relaxing and toning attributes may help speed recovery.

Recommended dosage. A tea made with 2 teaspoons of dried herb and allowed to steep for 10 to 15 minutes can be taken as needed. Two to 4 ml of tincture can be taken three times a day.

Possible problems. None have been reported.

Meadowsweet (*Filipendula ulmaria*)

How it works. This herb soothes the mucous membranes lining the digestive tract and reduces stomach acidity.

Recommended Dosage. A tea made with 1 to 2 teaspoons of dried herb and allowed to steep for 10 to 15 minutes can be taken as needed.

Possible problems. Generally considered safe.

Rosemary (*Rosemarinus officinalis*)

How it works. The leaves and twigs calm the digestive tract, particularly when an upset stomach is related to tension and anxiety.

Recommended dosage. A tea made with 1 to 2 teaspoons of dried herb and allowed to steep for 10 to 15 minutes or ½ ml of a tincture can be taken three times a day.

Possible problems. Generally considered safe, but avoid rosemary oil.

Heartburn

The hormones that relax the smooth muscles of the body also affect the circular muscle (circular esophageal sphincter) just above the stomach. Because this muscle may not contract as strongly as before pregnancy, stomach contents can flow up into the esophagus, causing an uncomfortable burning. The following strategies help prevent heartburn from occurring and offer relief when it happens:

- Eat small but frequent meals.
- Avoid spicy and high-fat foods.
- Avoid alcohol, coffee, and chocolate.
- Try milk as a soothing antacid, but avoid commercial antacids, except under a doctor's direction.
- Don't lie down after eating.
- Avoid peppermint tea.
- If citrus or tomato juices cause heartburn (and they don't in everyone), avoid them.
- Eat slowly.

CONSTIPATION

As the baby grows larger, the expanding uterus presses on the abdominal organs and can make it difficult to have a bowel movement, especially if constipation was a problem before pregnancy. Physicians recommend eating more fruits and vegetables—especially fresh fruits and lightly steamed vegetables—and whole grains, and drinking a lot of water. If necessary, natural fiber laxatives, Glucomannan (see Gestational Diabetes, below), or fruits such as prunes and figs that contain the natural laxative isatin should relieve the discomfort. Do *not* take commercial laxatives or the herbs senna or cascara.

If a hemorrhoid (an engorged vein in the rectum) results from the strain of trying to have a bowel movement, warm baths and compresses soaked in witch hazel and then applied to the anal area may help.

VARICOSE VEINS

The expanding uterus also puts pressure on the veins of the legs, and about one in five women will develop varicose veins when the valves in the blood vessels fail to stop the back flow of blood. Support hose, taking frequent breaks to walk (if you spend much of your time sitting), sitting with your feet up (if you spend much of your time standing), helps prevent blood from pooling in the legs. When traveling by car, stop every hour to take a short walk. In an airplane or train, move about frequently.

GESTATIONAL DIABETES (MATERNAL HYPERGLYCEMIA)

Among the most serious complications of pregnancy, gestational diabetes occurs when not enough insulin is being produced to handle the blood-sugar swings that are common in pregnancy. As blood sugar increases, the symptoms of diabetes occur. These include profuse sweating, nervousness, inability to concentrate, headache, abdominal pain, numbness of the hands or mouth, blurred vision, and rapid heartbeat. Because symptoms may be slight and go unnoticed, health care practitioners are careful to monitor blood-sugar levels throughout pregnancy.

With or without noticeable symptoms in the mother, the health of the fetus is still at risk in women with gestational diabetes, and the condition needs to be treated. Often following a special prescribed diet that involves cutting back on sweets and spreading calories more evenly throughout the day is sufficient to manage the blood sugar; more rarely, insulin injections are necessary.

The dangers of untreated hyperglycemia include the risk of prematurity, high birth weight, and birth defects. Usually, the mother's insulin difficulties resolve after delivery of the baby.

Neutraceuticals for Gestational Diabetes

■ NUTRITIONAL SUPPLEMENTS

Glucomannan (*Konjac mannan*)

How it works. This polysaccharide passes through the intestinal tract undigested, but it does expand in the presence of water. Therefore, it's considered to be a dietary fiber and is often used in Japan and Indonesia, where it is cultivated, to treat constipation. Studies have shown that it reduces cholesterol and delays glucose absorption from the intestine, so it may be useful in regulating blood sugar.

Recommended dosage. Follow package instructions.

Possible problems. Do not take Glucomannan without first discussing it with your doctor.

■ HIGH BLOOD PRESSURE

Close medical supervision is essential if blood pressure begins to climb. Excessive swelling of the hands and feet and severe headache must be reported immediately. Medication to control blood pressure and diuretics to reduce swelling may be prescribed. Hospitalization and complete bed rest may be ordered, and in the most severe cases, labor may be induced or a cesarean section performed. After delivery, the condition typically resolves itself.

Postpartum

After the baby is born, many of the side effects of pregnancy quickly disappear. However, the first six weeks after delivery are a stressful time, and the body needs some care—mainly rest, which can be extremely difficult to achieve—and time to heal. The uterus will have mild contractions that cause some cramping or after-pains for the first few days. Gradually over the next few weeks, the uterus will become smaller and more firm. Bleeding will subside and there may be some vaginal discharge. Many experts suggest massaging the abdomen gently to encourage this process called, involution. Kegel exercises (*see* Bladder Control Problems) will help restore pelvic muscle tone.

Unless you are breastfeeding, nutritional needs return to normal, but there are some things you can do to hasten recovery.

Nutraceuticals that Speed Recovery

■ BOTANICAL MEDICINES

Raspberry leaf (*Rubus idaeus*)

How it works. Long used in pregnancy to strengthen the uterus and pelvic muscles, raspberry leaves contain polypeptides, flavonoids, and tannins, which act as an astringent and tonic. After delivery, these relaxing and toning attributes may help speed recovery.

Recommended dosage. A tea made with 2 teaspoons of dried herb and allowed to steep for 10 to 15 minutes can be taken as needed. Two to 4 ml of tincture can be taken three times a day.

Possible problems. Generally considered safe.

Black cohosh (*Cimicifuga racemosa*)

How it works. The dried root and rhizome contain glycosides, isoflavones, isofeulic acid, and tannins. This powerful combination relaxes uterine muscle spasms and may be helpful for painful uterine contractions after delivery.

Recommended dosages. Bring ½ to 1 teaspoon of fresh dried root and a cup of water to a boil and allow it to simmer for 10 or 15 minutes. This decoction or 2 ml of a tincture can be taken three times a day.

Possible problems. Occasional gastrointestinal upset has been reported. It should not be taken during pregnancy. Overdose may cause dizziness, excessive sweating, and seizures. Don't take it along with replacement hormones without first discussing it with your doctor.

Wild Yam (*Dioscorea villosa*)

How it works. The root of this vine contains an alkaloid that relaxes the muscles of the abdomen and relieves painful contractions after delivery. It also contains anti-inflammatory saponins.

Recommendation dosages. Wild yam is available over the counter in capsules. A tea can also be made by combining 1 to 2 teaspoons of powdered bark in a cup of boiling water and allowing it to steep for two hours. After straining, it can be made more palatable by mixing with honey or another herbal tea.

Possible problems. None have been reported.

How it works. This relaxing, sedative herb is useful in relaxing the uterus and easing uterine congestion and inflammation.

Recommended dosage. Bring to a boil 2 teaspoons of dried bark in 1 cup of water and simmer for 10 minutes. This decoction or 5 to 10 ml of the tincture can be taken three times a day.

Possible problems. None have been reported.

■ POSTPARTUM DEPRESSION

About 10 to 15 percent of women experience serious depression that seems to extend beyond the "baby blues" that are extremely common after the birth of a child. The symptoms are similar to those that affect nonpregnant women: they feel tired, helpless, and discouraged. Now, too, they may feel overwhelmed by the new demands of motherhood. Mood swings sometimes coincide with the decrease in estrogen and progesterone following the baby's birth, so they are often treated the same as premenstrual syndrome (see below).

The physical demands on the new mother—especially sleep deprivation—and the emotional stresses of isolation, particularly if she is not accustomed to being at home all day; frustration that she isn't recovering quickly enough, and the loss of control that the new, demanding infant creates may contribute to a full-blown depression. If the depression becomes severe or lasts more than a few weeks, some physicians prescribe antidepressants. It may help to seek a consultation with a mental health professional, especially if the doctor doesn't take the woman's concerns seriously. Lingering depression is not normal and a woman doesn't have to live with it. And it's not good for the baby. See "Depression" for a complete list of nutraceuticals (95). Women who are breast-feeding, should discuss with her doctor any nutraceuticals she wishes to take.

Lactation

Nutritional needs continue to remain high, because you are still eating for two. To insure adequate mounts of protein and calcium, four glasses of whole or low-fat milk are recommended. As much as three quarts a day is needed to supply the necessary fluid. As in pregnancy, this is not a time to diet; you'll need an extra 500 calories every day just to fuel milk production. Continue to steer clear of caffeine, alcohol, and drugs. Depending on your diet, a physician may suggest a multivitamin supplement.

Nutraceuticals for nursing mothers

■ BOTANICAL MEDICINES

Fennel (*Foeniculum vulgare*)

How it works. A wide variety of constituents in fennel seeds, including flavonoids and coumarin, make it an excellent remedy for a variety of ailments from gas pains to inflamed eyelids, but it also increases the flow of milk.

Recommended dosage. Make a tea of 1 to 2 teaspoons of slightly crushed seeds and 1 cup of boiling water. The tea or 1 to 2 ml of tincture can be taken three times a day.

Possible problems. Allergic reactions are possible, but rare.

Sage (*Salvia officinalis*)

How it works. Sage is helpful to reduce the flow of milk after you have weaned your baby.

Recommended dosage. A tea can be made by steeping 2 to 3 teaspoons of leaves in 1 cup of boiling water for 10 minutes. A teaspoon of tincture can be taken three times a day with water.

Possible problems. Avoid sage while nursing or during pregnancy. It may be toxic in high doses or when taken over the long term. Never use sage oil.

PREMENSTRUAL SYNDROME

Premenstrual syndrome, also known as PMS, is the general term used to describe the various discomforts experienced by more than half of all women during the week to ten days before their menstrual periods. The National Women's Health Resource Center reports that as many as 95 percent of women have some premenstrual discomfort, although it is severe for only about 35 percent.

Historically, women were told that their problems were psychological. However, recent medical research has demonstrated that real problems with physical causes trouble many women. The symptoms seem to be related to fluctuations in estrogen and progesterone. Women who suffer from PMS often have high levels of estrogen in relation to progesterone in their blood during the latter half of their menstrual cycle. Estrogen causes the body to retain water. Water buildup in various parts of the body can lead to pelvic congestion, as well as small amounts of brain tissue swelling and subsequent mood

SYMPTOMS

The specific symptoms, and their severity, may vary from woman to woman and from month to month. They may range from mild to seriously disabling, and last from a few hours to more than ten days.

Psychological symptoms

- Mood changes, such as irritability, anxiety, nervousness, lack of control, agitation, and anger.
- Insomnia.
- Difficulty concentrating.
- Lethargy and fatigue.
- Food cravings, especially for sweets.

Physical symptoms

- Weight gain.
- Bloating sensations.
- Swollen and tender breasts.
- Pelvic heaviness and cramps.
- Backaches and other dull muscle aches.
- Headaches.
- Dizziness.
- Heart palpitations.
- Constipation.
- Nausea and vomiting.
- Acne.
- Aggravation of other chronic health problems, such as asthma, epilepsy, depression, allergies, and eye problems.

changes. This hormonal imbalance could account for other symptoms of PMS as well. Further, some women seem to metabolize progesterone differently, producing less of a chemical (a neurosteroid or neurotransmitter) needed for healthy brain function. For example, some studies have shown that women with PMS have low levels of two substances produced in the brain: beta-endorphins, which are natural painkillers, and serotonin, an antidepressant chemical. Finally, women seem to have higher levels of prostaglandins during severe PMS. These are hormonelike substances that mediate inflammation in the body.

Diagnostic Steps

PMS is diagnosed based on a personal history, noting recurrence of the same types of symptoms in the days leading up to monthly menstruation. However, if the symptoms are severe and do not respond to standard self-care and therapies, a doctor may recommend a complete examination to rule out other possible problems that may be contributing to PMS symptoms.

Conventional Treatments

Medical treatment generally focuses on easing symptoms.

- Aspirin and other nonsteroidal anti-inflammatory drugs (NSAIDs), such as ibuprofen, ease pain and slow down the production of prostaglandins. If over-the-counter medication does not significantly relieve your symptoms, a physician can prescribe more potent NSAIDs.
- Diuretics can relieve fluid retention. Hydrocholorothiazide may be prescribed starting just before symptoms are expected.
- Hormonal manipulation may be useful for some women. This may involve taking oral contraceptives or progesterone alone.
- Tranquilizers such as a benzodiazepine may be prescribed for irritability and nervousness.
- Antidepressants, particularly of the class known as selective serotonin reuptake inhibitors (SSRIs), can markedly improve mood. Fluoxetine (Prozac) and sertraline (Zoloft) are the most commonly prescribed but must be taken for at least a month before their impact will be felt.
- Counseling and support groups may be helpful in learning to cope more effectively and to reduce stress during the latter part of the menstrual cycle.

Nutraceuticals for PMS

Women have experimented with a variety of techniques to ease PMS for years. Some have now been proven valid by scientific study.

■ VITAMINS AND MINERALS

Vitamin B$_6$

How it works. This vitamin helps reduce sugar cravings, irritability, and bloating.

Recommended dosages. Naturopaths recommend 500 mg daily in time-release form, starting ten days before the expected onset of your period.

Possible problems. Vitamin B$_6$ in this dosage is not associated with any problems.

Calcium

How it works. Calcium helps prevent water retention, mood swings, and cramps.

Recommended dosages. Take at least 1,000 mg of calcium daily, in either food or supplements.

Possible problems. Some experts think that excessive calcium may exacerbate kidney and bladder stones, although recent studies tend to discount this.

■ BOTANICAL MEDICINES

Black cohosh (*Cimicifuga racemosa*)

How it works. This herb seems to function as an estrogen substitute and a suppressor of luteinizing hormone. It helps reduce the psychological symptoms of PMS as well as painful menstrual cramps.

Recommended dosages. Doses of 40 mg daily are prescribed for premenstrual complaints.

Possible problems. Some gastrointestinal discomfort may occur. Avoid overdose, which can cause vomiting, headache, dizziness, limb pains, and lowered blood pressure.

Chaste berry (*Vitex agnus-castus*)

How it works. This fruit helps balance sex hormones, increasing the production of luteinizing hormone and inhibiting the release of follicle-stimulating hormone. The balance results in a changed estrogen-progesterone ratio.

Recommended dosage. In one study, 175 mg daily of chaste berry extract was shown to ease PMS.

Possible problems. If you have marked depression with PMS, avoid chaste berry; it also should not be taken if you are or may become pregnant. Possible side effects include upset stomach and itchiness.

◉ STRATEGIES FOR RELIEF

Many premenstrual problems can be cured by these lifestyle changes:

- Reduce your intake of salt during the second half of your menstrual cycle to ease fluid retention and subsequent bloating.
- Increase your intake of water, which in itself acts as a diuretic.
- Have small, high-protein snacks every few hours and cut back on high-carbohydrate and high-sugar foods, which can worsen irritability and moodiness.
- Cut back on coffee, tea, and colas, which contain a type of caffeine that can worsen the hormonal imbalance. All are also stimulants, which can add to nervousness.
- Avoid alcohol. Although it provides an initial lift, it is actually a depressant drug.
- Get regular exercise, which increases circulation and helps carry off excess body fluids in the form of perspiration. Exercise also stimulates the brain to release endorphins and increases your production of serotonin, which will help you relax and sleep.
- Take hot baths or use heating pads, which often help, especially if muscle stiffness or tension are symptoms.

How it works. The gamma-linolenic acid (GLA) in evening primrose oil provides a less inflammatory building block for the body to use in making prostaglandins. GLA is also available in borage oil and flaxseed oil. Native American women have chewed the seeds of evening primrose plants for centuries to alleviate various "female" disorders. Evening primrose oil is also approved for PMS treatment in Great Britain.

Recommended dosages. Check the label for the amount of GLA in each capsule of evening primrose oil; find ones that have about 50 mg of GLA each. You need at least three and possibly six to ten capsules daily to achieve results.

Possible problems. You may have to take evening primrose oil daily through two or three menstrual cycles before you see a benefit.

UTERINE FIBROIDS

Also called uterine myoma, a fibroid is a benign tumor that grows within the muscular wall of the uterus or extends from it into the cavity of the uterus. An estimated 20 to 50 percent of women have fibroids. They are much more common in African-American women. Since they tend to occur among female relatives, there probably is a genetic influence. About half of women with fibroids experience no symptoms. However, large tumors may put pressure on surrounding organs and cause pain and heavy bleeding. A fibroid may also contribute to infertility. This benign tumor only rarely become malignant.

A fibroid can grow so large that it no longer has an adequate blood supply, and it will begin to self-destruct. Sometimes it disappears entirely, particularly when the degeneration follows the hormonal changes of pregnancy or menopause. However, since this process can cause uterine contractions, it may threaten a pregnancy or cause premature birth.

Diagnostic Steps

A woman who experiences any of the above symptoms should see a physician, but if she is symptom-free, she may not know she has a fibroid until it is felt by the physician during a routine pelvic exam. When a physician feels or suspects a fibroid, pelvic ultrasonography will reveal the tumor's size and location.

◉ SYMPTOMS

- Heavy menstrual bleeding.
- Anemia and fatigue as a result of the uterine bleeding.
- Pressure or sense of fullness in the rectum, bladder, or abdomen.
- Frequent urination.
- Inability to become pregnant.
- Painful intercourse.

◉ STRATEGIES FOR RELIEF

- Fibroids grow when stimulated by estrogen, so dietary measures that affect hormone levels may be useful. To diminish menstrual bleeding and shrink fibroids, aim for a high-fiber diet based on fruits, leafy green and cruciferous vegetables, and soy products. Soy products contain phytoestrogens; these natural plant estrogens seem to balance the effects of your own estrogen. In addition, reduce saturated fats, refined carbohydrates, and dairy products. A large Italian study recently showed that fibroids are more common among women who eat a lot of red meat and ham, and less common in those whose diet is rich in green leafy vegetables and fruit.
- Try raspberry leaf tea, which many women claim helps reduce the fibroid-related heavy bleeding.
- Avoid high-dose oral contraceptives.

Conventional Treatments

Unless a fibroid is causing symptoms or growing rapidly, many doctors advise a wait-and-see approach and perform a pelvic examination every six months. Opinions differ on whether a fibroid should be removed in women who want to become pregnant. Surgery to remove the fibroid only, a myomectomy, will spare the uterus, and is an option for women who want to have children.

Surgery to remove the uterus, a hysterectomy, is sometimes recommended. It is a last resort for those in their childbearing years. Fibroids are the major cause of most hysterectomies in the United States.

Drugs such as Lupron and Synarel mimic menopause and can cause a fibroid to shrink. If the fibroid doesn't disappear completely, it may become small enough to make myomectomy an option.

Nutraceuticals for Fibroids

■ VITAMINS AND MINERALS

B-complex vitamins

How it works. Each B vitamin has a different role that makes it useful for treating the symptoms of gynecologic problems. Vitamin B_6, for instance, is critical in the formation of hemoglobin and is useful in treating the anemia that may follow excessive bleeding. Riboflavin, or vitamin B_2, is involved in hormone production. Together, the B vitamins maintain the health of the liver, which helps regulate estrogen.

Recommended dosages. Recommended Dietary Allowances for each B vitamin vary, but the standard multivitamin or B-complex supplement contains an adequate amount of each in the proper balance.

Possible problems. Since B vitamins are water soluble, excessive amounts are excreted and toxicity is rare. However, nerve damage, particularly numbness of the hands and feet, has been reported in those who take large doses of vitamin B_6, and insomnia and anxiety may occur.

Iron

How it works. To offset the blood loss that may accompany fibroids and prevent anemia, supplements of this trace mineral are often necessary to maintain production of hemoglobin, the oxygen-carrying protein in blood, and myoglobin, the protein that stores oxygen in muscle.

Recommended dosages. The Recommended Dietary Allowance for premenopausal women is 15 mg a day, but in pregnancy the RDA jumps to 30 mg.

Possible problems. Too much iron suppresses the immune system and promotes the production of free radicals. Therapeutic doses for the treatment of anemia should be prescribed by a physician, since too much iron can cause problems such as stomachache, diarrhea, and constipation. Iron supplements should not be taken with vitamin E. Vitamin C, on the other hand, enhances iron absorption.

Magnesium

How it works. This is one of the most important minerals in the body and is present in large amounts in the liver, which helps regulate estrogen. It is also essential for the transmission of nerve impulses and muscle contraction.

Recommended dosage. The Recommended Dietary Allowance for women is 280 mg, but several factors—a calorie-restricting diet, a high-fiber diet, alcohol, stress, and strenuous exercise—can lead to a deficiency, and so supplements are often recommended even in healthy women.

Possible problems. Toxicity may develop if more magnesium is taken than the kidneys can process, or if kidney function is impaired. Low blood pressure, slurred speech, and nausea are signs of an overdose.

■ NUTRITIONAL SUPPLEMENTS

Methionine

How it works. This essential amino acid contains sulfur and is involved in the synthesis of many of the body's chemicals. It is also involved in breaking down fats. Since women who eat a high-fat diet tend to have an increase in circulating estrogens, some experts recommend it to help eliminate excess estrogen.

Recommended dosages. Some experts suggest 500 to 1000 mg daily for a limited period of time.

Possible problems. Single amino acids, such as methionine, should be taken with caution and always under a physician's guidance, since they can have serious effects on the nervous system.

Choline

How it works. This component of lecithin is most well known for its involvement in the synthesis of the neurotransmitter acetylcholine, but it also helps mobilize fat, particularly if the liver is sluggish. Choline is synthesized in the body from methionine.

Recommended dosages. One expert suggests 500 to 1000 mg daily for women suffering from fibroids, along with methionine and inositol. A balanced diet that includes a variety of foods supplies about 500 to 900 mg of choline a day. The best way to supplement choline is to take lecithin, because it's easy for the body to absorb. The best dietary source of choline is eggs.

Possible problems. Since too much choline can cause nausea, vomiting, and depression, it should be taken under a doctor's supervision.

Inositol

How it works. Like methionine and choline, inosotol helps remove fats from the liver, and thereby may diminish excess estrogen levels.

Recommended dosages. Taking 500 mg to 1000 mg a day along with methionine and choline may lower estrogen levels. There is no recommended daily allowance.

Possible problems. None have been noted.

L-Arginine

How it works. This amino acid, which is involved in numerous body processes, is especially helpful in the repair of damaged tissue; it is an essential component of collagen. Because it stimulates the thymus gland, where the immune system's T-cells are produced, it's believed to boost immune function and slow the growth of tumors.

Recommended dosages. For fibroids, some experts recommend 500 mg daily taken on an empty stomach. However, it's been reported that as little as 30 mg a day enhances immunity. Some also recommend taking 500 mg of lysine daily to balance arginine.

Possible problems. High doses can cause nausea and diarrhea, and long-term use should be avoided. Pregnant women and nursing mothers should not take this supplement. Since using arginine supplements is considered experimental, it should be taken only under a doctor's supervision. Finally, since arginine can promote the proliferation of certain viruses, it should not be taken by anyone with herpes.

■ BOTANICAL MEDICINES

Plants with astringent properties may help reduce menstrual bleeding, and those that counter muscle spasms can relieve cramping and pain. Herbs that stimulate the production of progesterone help control estrogen levels.

Chaste berry (*Vitex agnus-castus*)

How it works. Studies have shown that chaste berry helps to normalize the balance of estrogen and progesterone, particularly when too much estrogen is circulating, which suggests a role in treating fibroids.

Recommended dosages. Make a tea with 1 teaspoon of ripe berries in 1 cup of boiling water and allow it to steep for 10 to 15 minutes. This tea or a 1 ml tincture may be taken three times a day. Imbalances typically require at least 10 days of treatment but may take 6 months or longer.

Possible problems. Rare side effects include gastrointestinal disturbances, itching, and headaches.

VAGINITIS

◎ **SYMPTOMS**
- Vaginal or vulvar itching, burning, redness or swelling
- Pain or stinging during intercourse.

Monilia (yeast infection)
- Vaginal discharge that is thick and white and may look like cottage cheese.

Trichomoniasis
- Thin, foamy vaginal discharge that is pale green or gray and has a foul odor.

Gardnerella
- A white or yellow vaginal discharge, which may have an unpleasant odor.

◎ **STRATEGIES FOR RELIEF**
The best approach to vaginal infections is to try to prevent them. These self-care strategies often ease simple irritation within a week:

- Wash the genital area regularly and keep dry. Avoid irrigating soaps, douches, perfumes, sprays, and strong detergents.
- Don't use other people's bathing suits, towels, or washcloths.
- Wear clean cotton underwear that fits properly. Avoid panties that are too tight in the crotch, and nylon underwear and panty hose, which retain moisture. Vaginal infections are three times more common in women who wear nylon underwear or tights rather than cotton underwear.
- Avoid getting fecal material in the vaginal area. After bowel movements, wipe yourself by cleaning from front to back.
- Make sure your sexual partner is "clean."
- If you have recurrent vaginal yeast infections and use oral contraceptives, consider switching to another form of birth control. Yeast overgrowth is more common in those using the pill.
- If extra lubrication is needed during intercourse, use a sterile, water-soluble jelly specifically designed for the purpose, such as K-Y jelly. Do not use Vaseline or cold cream.
- For minor itching, apply an over-the-counter hydrocortisone cream.
- If self-care does not produce improvement within a week, or if you have a fever or pain in the abdomen, see a physician promptly.

Vaginitis literally means inflammation of the vagina. It is the problem most frequently reported by women to their gynecologists. Most women have one or more episodes of vaginitis during their lifetimes. For some, episodes are easily treated. For others, vaginitis is a recurrent problem.

The vagina normally takes excellent care of itself, with healthy self-protective and self-cleansing mechanisms. Part of that system includes vaginal moisture and mucus that are secreted from the vagina. A normal discharge is transparent or slightly milky. However, when the vagina becomes infected, bacteria or other infectious organisms can grow out of control and change the nature of these secretions.

Sometimes vaginitis is due to simple irritation. Other times it results from invading organisms, including those that cause sexually transmitted diseases, such as gonorrhea, syphilis, and chlamydia.

More commonly, vaginal infection is simply an overgrowth of organisms that normally live in the vagina. (These organisms also affect men.) Such infections can be triggered by events that overwhelm the vagina's normal self-cleansing system. These may include: lowered resistance; excessive douching; pregnancy; use of birth control pills or antibiotics; diabetes; or cuts, abrasions or other irritations inside the vagina.

The three most common types of vaginitis are monilia, trichomoniasis, and gardnerella.

- Monilia is a yeast or fungus-like organism, also called *Candida albicans*, which normally grows in harmless quantities in the vagina. When the normal cleansing system of the vagina goes out of balance, the yeast-like organisms grow profusely. (See Candidiasis box.)
- Trichomoniasis is caused by trichomonas, is a single-celled organism, often causing no symptoms. It is usually spread through intercourse.
- Gardnerella (also called bacterial vaginitis or non-specific vaginitis) is the term physicians use for other garden-variety vaginal infections.

Rarely, vaginitis is an early sign of cancer in the reproductive system.

Diagnostic Steps

Your gynecologist can often diagnose the specific type of infection by the texture, color, and odor of the vaginal discharge. In other cases, a sample of the discharge must be taken for laboratory examination. Although many over-the-counter treatments are available for yeast infections, you need to know what type of vaginitis is causing your symptoms, which is not always possible on your own.

Conventional Treatments

Yeast grows best in a very mildly acidic environment. Fortunately, the vagina normally has a very high acidity level. While the use of an alkaline douche can help prevent the development of monilia, it is less effective once monilia proliferates. Then, topical treatment with an antifungal treatment inserted in the vagina is needed. Such medication can quickly cure monilia. Topical antifungal drugs you can buy without a prescription include clotrimazole, miconazole, and butoconazole. Read the package label carefully to discern how many days it should be used. Oral or intravenous antifungal drugs require a prescription. They include the same drugs used topically as well as other antifungals, such as fluconazole and amphotericin.

Trichomonas grows best in an alkaline environment, so acidic douches may control it if begun early, as soon as symptoms arise. Once it has fully developed, oral medication prescribed by a physician will be needed. A single dose of metronidzaole may be all that is required. However, once the parasite has entered a woman's system, trichomoniasis symptoms will recur in about one-third of all patients. These statistics improve if the sexual partner is treated.

Treatment of gardnerella and other non-specific vaginitis depends on the type of infection, although prescribed creams or suppositories usually alleviate symptoms.

Nutraceuticals for Vaginitis

■ NUTRITIONAL SUPPLEMENTS

Acidophilus (*Lactobacillus acidophilus*)

How it works. The active cultures in *lactobacillus acidophilus* help restore the normal vaginal flora. While many women are aware of its benefits for yeast infections, it also can help the vagina do battle more effectively against other bacterial invaders. Further, lactobacillus acidophilus produces lactic acid and natural antibiotic substances.

Recommended dosages. Lactobacillus can be taken orally and/or as a douche. An oral supplement should provide one to two billion live organisms. Three cups of yogurt containing the live bacteria are also effective. As a douche, use an acidophilus-containing solution twice daily. Use enough of an acidophilus supplement (or an active-culture yogurt, if you don't mind the mess) to provide one billion organisms.

◎ **CANDIDIASIS**

Candida albicans is a species of fungus that normally lives in the body, most commonly in the gastrointestinal tract and the vagina, without causing any problems. Bacteria and immune system mechanisms normally keep its growth in check. When this balance is upset, candida can overgrow and cause a yeast infection. In the vagina, it's called monilia. In the mouth, it's called thrush. When the fungus affects multiple areas of the body and is persistent, it is called chronic candidiasis or yeast syndrome and can be quite serious and may need to be treated intravenously. In the worst cases, candidiasis may be progressive and ultimately fatal. Women are eight times more likely to experience chronic candidiasis than men.

Although yeast overgrowth may arise spontaneously, it is particularly linked to the use of certain medications, especially antibiotics, corticosteroids such as prednisone, oral contraceptives, or anti-ulcer drugs such as cimetidine and ranitidine. Underlying health conditions that may predispose someone to candida overgrowth include pregnancy, diabetes, and allergies. Impaired immunity (such as from AIDS or treatments for various cancers) and decreased digestive secretions are also predisposing factors. Although yeast infections are popularly attributed to a diet high in carbohydrates and refined foods, that theory is highly controversial and lacking in scientific evidence.

When yeast infections occur systematically or in addition to the vagina, symptoms may include:

◎ **GASTROINTESTINAL YEAST INFECTIONS**
- A thick, white coating on the tongue and other mouth surfaces called thrush.
- Bloating, gas, or cramps.
- Diarrhea.
- Rectal itching.

CHRONIC CANDIDIASIS

Symptoms will depend on which organ systems are affected. In addition:

- Chronic fatigue, malaise, and loss of energy.
- Fever.
- Depression.
- Low immune function and frequent infections.
- Chemical sensitivities and allergies.
- Menstrual problems.

STRATEGIES FOR CANDIDIASIS RELIEF

- According to some experts, a well-balanced diet low in fats, sugars, simple carbohydrates, and refined foods is important for preventing candida overgrowth. Especially important, they say, is avoidance of a high-sugar diet. To follow this advice, anyone who is prone to yeast infections of any kind should limit their intake of refined sugar, fruits, fruit juices, refined carbohydrates, and alcohol. Focus on a diet of fresh fruits and vegetables, whole grains and legumes.
- Restriction or elimination of milk may help treat gastrointestinal or chronic candidiasis.
- Those with chronic candidiasis should avoid mold- and yeast-containing foods. These include alcoholic beverages, cheeses, dried fruits, and peanuts.
- If you can avoid troubling allergens and have allergies treated, chronic recurring yeast infections may be subdued.
- For chronic candidiasis, some health care providers recommend detoxification programs that include: supplements of lipotropic agents to promote the flow of fat and bile to and from the liver; promotion of elimination with daily supplements of psyllium seed, kelp, agar, pectin and/or plant gums; and probiotics to bolster intestinal flora.

Dissolve it in 10 ml of water. Insert it into the vagina with a bulb syringe, and retain it for a few minutes before expelling.

Possible problems. None are known.

Boric Acid

How it works. Boric acid capsules inserted in the vagina have been used to treat yeast vaginitis with great success. In one study of 100 women with chronic yeast vaginitis who were not successfully treated with any over-the-counter or prescription antifungal medicines, 98 percent successfully treated their infections with boric acid capsules inserted into the vagina twice per day for 2 to 4 weeks.

Recommended dosages. Studies have used a 600 mg boric acid vaginal suppository twice daily for 2 weeks.

Possible problems. Boric acid capsules should not be used in the vagina during pregnancy.

Iodine

How it works. A topical douche of providone iodine has been shown effective against multiple causes of vaginitis, including trichomonas, candida, chlamydia, and nonspecific vaginitis.

Recommended dosages. Providone iodine (Betadine) should be diluted to one part iodine in 100 parts water. Use it twice daily for 14 days.

Possible problems. Avoid excessive use. If iodine is absorbed into the body, it can affect thyroid function.

BOTANICAL MEDICINES

Garlic (*Allium sativum*)

How it works. Ingesting garlic may inhibit the growth of yeast organisms and increase resistance to vaginal, gastrointestinal, and systemic yeast infections. Garlic has antibacterial, antiviral, and antifungal/antiyeast activity.

Recommended dosages: Those with no aversion to the odor can chew one whole clove of raw garlic daily. Others can choose odor-controlled, enteric-coated tablets standardized for allicin content. Take 900 mg per day (providing 5,000 mcg of allicin), preferably divided into two equal doses. Or a tincture of 2 to 4 ml may be taken 3 times daily. For health maintenance and prevention of recurrent infections, one-half of the therapeutic doses is sufficient.

Possible problems: Some people are sensitive to garlic and may experience heartburn and flatulence. Because of its anticlotting properties, those taking anticoagulant drugs should check with their doctor before taking garlic. Those scheduled for surgery should stop taking garlic supplements two weeks before surgery and inform their surgeon if they were taking those supplements. There are no known contraindications to garlic use during pregnancy and breastfeeding.

Tea tree oil (*Melaleuca alternifolia*)

How it works. Topical use of diluted tea tree oil may be useful for vaginal yeast infections. It can be used as a diluted douche or as part of a coconut oil–based suppository (with 2 percent tea tree oil).

Recommended dosages. Concentrations of tea tree oil as strong as 40 percent may be used with caution as a vaginal douche. In suppository form, insert twice a day for a maximum of 5 days.

Possible problems. Tea tree oil should not be applied to broken skin or to areas affected by rashes. The oil can cause a burning sensation if it gets into eyes, nose, mouth, or other tender areas. Some women have allergic reactions, including rashes and itching, when applying tea tree oil. For this reason, only a small amount should be applied when first using it. The oil should never be taken by mouth.

Echinacea (*E. angustifolia*)

How it works: Echinacea is a useful immune system support for women with recurrent yeast infections. One study showed a 43 percent drop in recurrence rate in yeast infections with women using echinacea.

Recommended dosages: For immune support on an ongoing basis, take the dose recommended on the package.

Possible problems. Some experts warn that echinacea loses its effectiveness when taken continuously. Instead, take it for only 2 weeks and then resume after 2-week break. Women with autoimmune diseases such as lupus, rheumatoid arthritis, or multiple sclerosis should not take echinacea.

Nutraceuticals for Systemic Candida Infections

Berberine-containing botanicals

How it works. Berberine is an alkaloid that has been extensively studied for its activity against bacteria, protozoa, and fungi, especially candida. It has demonstrated particular success in treating the diarrhea caused by yeast overgrowth in the gastrointestinal system. Plants that contain berberine include goldenseal, goldthread, barberry, yellowroot, and Oregon grape.

Recommended doses: The easiest approach may be to purchase goldenseal tincture and, based on package directions, add it to juice 3 times a day. For other berberine sources: 2 to 4 grams of dried root can be used to make a tea; 250 to 500 mg of an 8 to 12 percent alkaloid content dry powder may be taken or ½ to 1 teaspoon of a 1:1 fluid extract.

Potential problems: Berberine should not be used during pregnancy. High doses can interfere with the metabolism of B vitamins.

Caprylic Acid

How it works. This is a naturally occurring fatty acid that has an antifungal action useful in treating gastrointestinal and systemic infections. However, because it is easily absorbed by the intestines, timed-release or enteric coated pills must be taken to allow for gradual release throughout the intestinal tract.

Recommended dosage: The standard dose is 1,000 to 2,000 mg. Take it with meals.

Possible problems. None have been reported.

Volatile Oils

How it works. Volatile oils from oregano, thyme, peppermint, and rosemary are all effective antifungal agents, based on laboratory, not human studies. One study showed oregano oil to be over 100 times more potent than caprylic acid against candida.

Recommended dosage: Enteric-coated preparations should be taken twice daily between meals at a dose of 0.2 to 0.4 ml.

Possible problems: Volatile oils can cause severe heartburn when quickly absorbed, making enteric-coating essential to prevent problems and assure delivery to the intestines.

CHAPTER 4

Nutraceuticals Just for Men and Athletes

Many people mistakenly assume that women are the only users of nutritional supplements, botanical medicines, and other nutraceuticals. In reality, however, nutraceuticals are equally beneficial for men and women. Just like women, men catch colds and other infectious diseases, and both sexes suffer from many of the same conditions—everything from allergies and arthritis to ulcers and weight problems. It's not surprising that a growing number of men are also turning to nutraceuticals not only to treat diseases but also to achieve and maintain overall health.

Some of the diseases commonly considered to be "male problems" also strike both sexes. Perhaps the best example is heart attack, which is the number-one killer of both men and women, although men are usually stricken at an earlier age than women. In combating heart disease, nutraceuticals and other lifestyle factors can literally mean the difference between life and death for both sexes. A recent Harvard study found that more than 80 percent of heart attacks could be prevented simply by adopting five lifestyle changes (see box, p. 622). In addition, study after study demonstrates the value of various vitamins, minerals, and other nutritional supplements in preventing cardiovascular disease, many cancers, and other specific disorders that affect both men and women and are discussed in chapter 2. This chapter deals with conditions that are exclusively male.

The Testosterone/Estrogen Factor

Sex hormones are chemicals responsible for reproduction and establishing as well as maintaining gender-specific characteristics. For men, it's testosterone that prompts the penis and testicles to develop before birth and to enlarge during puberty. Testosterone—which is produced mostly in the testicles—also spurs the growth of a beard and body hair, deepening of the male voice, and increased muscle development during puberty. It is responsible for acne and male-pattern balding, and is often cited as the reason why men tend to be more aggressive than women.

Men also produce small amounts of estrogen, the female sex hormone, just as women make small amounts of testosterone. The effects of too much of the opposite sex's hormone are well known. Men with abnormally high estrogen levels develop many female sex characteristics—their breasts enlarge, their voices become higher-pitched, their beards scanty, and in time, they lose muscle mass, their testicles shrink, fertility diminishes, and they may be unable to achieve an erection. Obviously, no man is going to wittingly take estrogen without a very good reason, such as the treatment of advanced prostate cancer. But what about the unwitting intake of estrogen? In recent years, there has been increasing concern about the prevalence of environmental estrogens, which are the by-products of the plastics industry; they are also released into the environment in pesticides and industrial pollutants and make their way into the food chain. Some experts cite environmental estrogens as a possible cause of the marked increase in undescended testicles among male babies as well as the rise in male infertility and prostate and testicular cancers.

Avoiding exposure to environmental estrogens is almost impossible because they are so prevalent in our foods and everyday products. But there is a possible answer: phytoestrogens, the hormonelike plant chemicals that appear to protect women against the ill effects of estrogen. There is mounting evidence that men who consume large amounts of soy products and foods high in phytoestrogens may achieve similar protective effects against environmental estrogens. Here's how phytoestrogens may help. Cells throughout the body have estrogen receptors that take up the hormone from the bloodstream. Phytoestrogens are almost chemically identical to natural and environmental estrogens, but they have a much weaker effect. Estrogen receptors recognize phytoestrogens as the real thing and allow them to occupy their receptor sites, thus blocking the action of the more potent estrogens that are potentially harmful to men. So while it may seem contradictory, in reality, an increased intake of soy and other foods high in isoflavones and other phytoestrogens may be even more important for men than for women (see also Phytoestrogens, p. 336, and Soy Products, p. 349).

Muscle-Building Nutraceuticals

Although both men and women participate in sports and bodybuilding, there are important differences. While men and women have the same number of muscles and bones, those in the male body tend to be bigger and stronger, thanks largely to male hormones.

Exercise is the key to building and maintaining strong muscles and bones. It is a well-documented fact that prolonged inactivity, such as being bedridden while recovering from a serious accident, leads to a loss of both muscle tissue and bone mass. But muscle tissue is also broken down during strenuous exercise, and to repair and rebuild the damaged muscle tissue, the body uses various amino acids, the building blocks of protein. The typical high-protein American diet provides all of the amino acids needed to maintain healthy muscles. But many weight lifters, bodybuilders, and endurance athletes turn to supplements in search of an added edge. Pharmaceutical products such as anabolic steroids increase muscle mass, but at a tremendous cost in terms of side effects, including bone loss, fertility problems, and an increased risk of heart disease. Nutraceuticals such as androstenedione and DHEA (see p. 291) are intended to boost the body's production of testosterone and anabolic steroids. There are also questions about their efficacy and long-term safety.

Carnitine, a substance that the body can make from the amino acids methionine and lysine, is another popular supplement among athletes. It enables the muscles to burn fatty acids for energy, thereby increasing endurance. Some studies suggest that it also speeds the muscles' postexercise recovery (see Carnitine, p. 279, for a more detailed discussion).

Creatine, a combination of amino acids stored in muscle tissue, is still another supplement claimed to help build muscles and enhance athletic performance. Research shows that creatine helps muscle tissue retain more water, but whether it actually increases muscle mass and strength is debatable (see Creatine, p. 289).

Perhaps the safest athletic supplements are those made from various amino acids, which give the body the building blocks needed for muscle repair. Soy protein, which is high in arginine and glutamine, is one of the most popular of the amino acid supplements; it is also high in isoflavones—the phytoestrogens discussed earlier (see Soy Products, p. 349). A recent controlled study involving athletes at Ohio State University compared the effectiveness of soy protein and whey protein in promoting muscle recovery following exercise. The athletes who consumed 20 g of soy protein a day had significantly lower levels of creatine kinase and myeloperoxidase—enzymes that are released when muscle tissue is broken down—than the whey protein group. The study director concluded that the soy protein protected the muscles and allowed the athletes to work out sooner without risking injury.

There are many other combinations of amino acids. Some emphasize the branched-chain amino acids (BCAAs), such as isoleucine, leucine, and valine; these are said to inhibit muscle breakdown and increase protein synthesis. BCAAs are often combined with arginine or glutamine, two of the important amino acids in soy protein that are thought to hasten muscle recovery following exercise.

For Men Only

The disorders discussed in the following pages are very common among men, and are often treated with a combination of medical and alternative therapies.

BENIGN PROSTATE ENLARGEMENT

Most organs get smaller with age, but for many men, the prostate—the organ that manufactures seminal fluid—actually grows larger. In men who are in their twenties, the prostate gland is about the size of a walnut and weighs about 20 grams, or less than an ounce. It is situated just below the male bladder and in front of the rectum, and the gland surrounds the urethra—the tube that carries urine from the bladder to the penis. An enlarged prostate presses against the urethra, impeding normal urine flow and causing bladder irritation.

At about age forty to fifty, the prostate gland slowly begins to change and enlarge—the medical term for this phenomenon is *benign prostatic hyperplasia,* or BPH. The initial changes are microscopic, and do not ordinarily produce symptoms. With increasing age, however, symptoms occur, and more than half of all men in their sixties suffer from some degree of BPH.

The cause of BPH is unclear, but it may be due in part to hormonal changes within the prostate itself. One theory holds that high levels of dihydrotestosterone (DHT)—a male sex hormone—in the prostate gland fosters the growth of problematic cells, which may trigger a malignant change.

Diagnostic Steps

A doctor begins the diagnostic process by taking a medical history, paying particular attention to any urinary symptoms, and conducting a thorough physical examination. Blood will be drawn for a PSA analysis. Depending upon the results, you may be referred to a urologist, a specialist in urinary-tract disorders.

Tests vary, but in addition to a digital rectal exam and PSA, they may include:

- Rectal ultrasound, in which a tube equipped with an ultrasound transducer is inserted into the rectum to examine the prostate by using high-frequency sound waves.

◉ THE SPECTER OF PROSTATE CANCER

Although most prostatic enlargement is harmless, no man can be complacent about the health of his prostate. Prostate cancer is the most common malignancy among American men, and the second leading cause of cancer death in males over age fifty-five. The incidence of prostate cancer has been rising steadily over the last few decades; according to the American Cancer Society, the lifetime risk of developing it is one in seven among African Americans and one in eight among Caucasians. It is most common after age sixty-five, but it is also diagnosed among many men in their forties and fifties. Fortunately the majority of men have a slowly growing form of prostate cancer that tends to remain confined to the gland and does not metastasize.

Early diagnosis and treatment offers the best chance for surviving prostate cancer. The American Cancer Society recommends that all men age fifty and older undergo annual screening for prostate cancer. Earlier screening may be advisable for men with a higher than average risk of prostate cancer, such as those with a family history of the disease and African Americans. Screening involves a digital prostate examination, in which a doctor inserts a lubricated gloved finger into the rectum to feel the prostate gland for any suspicious lumps and hardness. The second screening

- A urine flow study, which measures whether the bladder can be fully emptied during voiding.
- An intravenous pyelogram, a dye-enhanced X-ray study of the urinary tract to determine if there are any blockages.
- Cystoscopy, in which a lighted viewing tube equipped with magnifying devices and a tiny camera is inserted into the urethra and bladder.

Conventional Treatments

According to the National Institutes of Health, as many as a third of all mild cases of BPH resolve themselves without any need for treatment. Even so, BPH increases the risk of urinary tract infections, so frequent physician examinations are advisable.

There are a number of drugs for mild to moderate BPH. Some of these are drugs that are also used to treat high blood pressure; these include prazosin (Minipress), doxazosin (Cardura), and terazosin (Hytrin), which relieve the symptoms of BPH in about 70 percent of men. They work by relaxing the muscles located near the prostate, lessening the annoyance of prostate enlargement.

Finasteride (Proscar) is the only approved prescription medication for prostate reduction in the United States. It can cause several unpleasant side effects, however, including a waning sex drive, erectile dysfunction, and ejaculation problems. (On the plus side, the drug is also prescribed, under the name of Propecia, to treat male-pattern balding.)

More advanced cases of BPH may require one of several procedures. Transurethral microwave procedures (TMP) use microwaves to heat and destroy extraneous prostate tissue. The procedure can be performed in about an hour in a doctor's office. Another procedure, called transurethral needle ablation, also uses heat to destroy excess prostate tissue. Laser surgery, which uses powerful light beams to vaporize tissue, is also used to treat BPH.

Surgical reduction of the gland is another option. The most common procedure is transurethral resection of the prostate, or TURP. A viewing instrument is inserted through the penis and the innermost core of the gland is removed while leaving the outer shell intact.

Nutraceuticals for Prostate Enlargement

■ VITAMINS AND MINERALS

Vitamin E

How it works. Vitamin E is a powerful antioxidant that also helps control cholesterol levels, both factors that may contribute to prostate health. Population studies indicate that it may also protect against pros-

---

◙ THE SPECIFIC OF PROSTATE CANCER (cont.)

examination is a blood test to measure levels of prostate-specific antigen (PSA). An elevated level (above 4 ng/ml) suggests possible prostate cancer, and warrants further investigation. with ultrasound testing and perhaps a biopsy.

Chances of survival are excellent if the cancer is detected and treated while it is still confined to the prostate gland. Just how it should be treated, however, is an area of continuing medical debate and should be tailored to the man's age, type of cancer cell present, and other individual factors.

◙ SYMPTOMS

An enlarged prostate can block the urethra, making urination difficult. Signs and symptoms include:

- A frequent urge to urinate, especially during the night.
- Difficulty starting and maintaining a steady stream of urine.
- Dribbling of urine after urination.
- Inability to fully empty the bladder.

◙ STRATEGIES FOR RELIEF

- Early treatment is the best way to relieve BPH symptoms. It may be difficult for men to speak with their doctor about prostate problems. But doing so can pave the way to finding relief.
- Saw palmetto and other herbal preparations can provide relief, but be sure to let your doctor know if you are using these products.
- Avoid taking nonprescription decongestant cold and allergy remedies; these can cause severe urinary retention in men who have an enlarged prostate.
- Drink ample water, juice, and other fluids, but restrict intake of alcohol and caffeinated beverages, which can increase urinary urgency and worsen prostate symptoms.

tate cancer. For example, a study of thirty-thousand Finnish men found that those who took daily vitamin E supplements had a third less prostate cancer than men who did not take the vitamin.

Recommended dosages. The typical dosage is 400 IU of natural (d-alpha) vitamin E, although some experts recommend taking 800 to 1000 IU—dosages that are within the safe range.

Possible problems. High doses of vitamin E can cause bleeding problems, especially among people who are taking aspirin, Coumadin, ginkgo biloba extract, and other blood thinners. Otherwise, daily doses up to 1,500 IU are considered safe.

Selenium

How it works. Selenium is a mineral and an essential component of an antioxidant enzyme. It is thought to work with vitamin E to provide extra protection against oxidative damage to cells. It is also thought to slow prostate growth and help prevent prostate cancer.

Recommended dosages. The RDA for selenium is 70 mcg for males, but a large study of 1,400 patients found 200 mcg to be safe and enough to lower the risk of prostate cancer.

Possible problems. High doses of selenium (800 to 900 mcg a day) are toxic, and can cause nerve damage, nausea, fatigue, and a garlicky breath odor.

Zinc

How it works. Zinc is important for proper immune system function; it also is instrumental in making sex and thyroid hormones. A recent study found that zinc may help shrink an enlarged prostate, but how it works is unknown.

Recommended dosages. The RDA for zinc calls for 15 mg a day for men; supplements of up to 30 mg a day are safe. Pumpkin seeds are rich in zinc and an alternative to supplements.

Possible problems. Prolonged high doses of zinc actually reduce immunity. It also interferes with copper absorption, so the diet should be supplemented with 2 mg a day of this mineral.

■ BOTANICAL MEDICINES

Saw palmetto (*Serenoa repens*)

How it works. The fruit of the saw palmetto tree, a shrublike palm native to the southeastern United States, contains fat-soluble therapeutic compounds called sterols (e.g., beta-sitosterol, campesterol, and stigmasterol). This group of sterols is thought to reduce levels of dihydrotestosterone (DHT) in the prostate, the hormone some experts say fuels prostate tissue overgrowth. But saw palmetto extract has a number of other possible mechanisms of action that may be beneficial in treating BPH, including blocking the activity of estrogen receptors in the prostate. A number of European studies have documented improved urinary flow among men with mild to moderate BPH. At least two controlled studies compared saw palmetto extract with finasteride, and found that the two were about equally effective in relieving BPH symptoms.

Recommended dosages. The European studies used 320 mg of saw palmetto extract a day, usually divided into two doses of 160 mg each.

Potential problems. There have been some reports of stomach upset, but they are uncommon. There is some concern amongst health professionals that saw palmetto may trigger inaccurate PSA test results, so always let your doctor know if you have been taking it.

Nettle root (*Urtica dioica*)

How it works. This herb dates to medieval times when it was used as a diuretic and a therapy for joint problems. Today, it is also used to treat BPH. Nettle root extract contains compounds that inhibit the action of sex hormones, which are thought to stimulate the growth of prostate tissue.

Recommended dosages. The usual dosage is 120 mg of standardized nettle root extract twice a day. It may be taken alone, or in combination with saw palmetto or pygeum.

Potential problems. With the exception of rare allergic reactions and intestinal disturbances in some people, nettle root has no known serious side effects.

Pygeum (*Pygeum africanum*)

How it works. Africans have long used a tea made from the African prune (pygeum) to treat urinary disorders. Pygeum now has a growing following among European and American practitioners of botanical medicine. Pygeum bark extract is thought to counter BPH in three ways: it contains beta-sitosterol, which appears to interfere with prostaglandin synthesis; its pentacyclic triterpenes appear to help shrink prostate tissue; and its ferulic esters reduce levels of prolactin (a hormone) and block accumulation of cholesterol in the prostate.

Recommended dosages. The usual dosages are 100 to 200 mg a day.

Potential problems. No major side effects have been reported.

In addition, a number of ordinary foods may have a beneficial effect on the prostate, and mounting evidence shows that some may help prevent prostate cancer.

Soy products

How they work. Soy products, such as tofu, soy nuts, soy milk, and tempeh, contain isoflavones that may help prevent prostate enlargement. These plant chemicals mimic the action of estrogen, and may help detoxify DHT, which fosters prostate tissue production. Genistein and diadzein are the isoflavones in soy considered to provide the most health benefits for men.

Recommended dosages. There are no official recommendations for soy products to promote prostate health, but population studies indicate that four or five servings of soy foods weekly may reduce the risk of many diseases, especially if they are served as substitutes for animal foods, including cow's milk, meat, and poultry. Alternatively, some naturopaths and others recommend taking 25 to 50 g of powdered soy protein—a rich source of isoflavones—a day. It can be added to food or mixed with skim milk or juice to make a nutritious breakfast drink.

Possible problems. Probably none, but if you eat too many soy products without cutting back on other high-protein fare, you may be consuming excess calories, causing weight gain. Some people develop soy sensitivity from excessive soy intake.

Lycopene

How it works. Lycopene is a carotenoid, which are antioxidant plant pigments that give many fruits and vegetables their bright colors. Tomatoes are the major dietary source of lycopene; other sources include watermelon and red grapefruit. Lycopene tends to concentrate in the prostate, but how it promotes prostate health and reduces the risk of prostate cancer is unknown.

Recommended dosages. There is no recommended dosage, but Harvard researchers following the health histories of more than forty-seven thousand men for six years found the lowest incidence of prostate cancer among men who consumed ten servings a week of tomatoes, especially in cooked forms (tomato pasta sauce, pizza, tomato juice), had the lowest incidence of prostate cancer. (See Beta-Carotene-Carotenoids, p. 270.)

Possible problems. Some people are allergic to tomatoes, but the vast majority can eat them without experiencing any problems.

SEXUAL DYSFUNCTION

Only recently have large numbers of men, including some prominent public figures, talked openly about erectile dysfunction (ED or impotence) and other problems related to sexual function. The overnight success of Viagra—the first pharmaceutical product to effectively treat ED—indicates that the problem is indeed widespread.

All men now and then experience some type of ED. For many—especially younger men—it's a temporary problem caused by stress, fatigue, illness, or some other transient circumstance. After age fifty, however, repeated episodes of ED are more likely to have an organic cause; the most common are the use of certain drugs, especially alcohol,

◉ **SYMPTOMS**
- Inability to achieve an erection or to engage in sexual intercourse.
- Inability to maintain an erection long enough to achieve satisfactory sexual intercourse.
- Premature ejaculation.

recreational substances, and some prescription drugs (see box, Drugs and Substances That Can Cause Sexual Dysfunction, opposite); heart disease and circulatory problems; diabetes; nerve disorders such as multiple sclerosis; spinal cord injuries; and some hormonal disorders.

Diagnostic Steps

A doctor will do a complete physical examination and order blood and urine tests to rule out an organic cause of the problem. Tests, such as overnight observation in a sleep laboratory, may be done to determine whether normal erections occur during sleep. If a psychological cause is suspected, the patient may be referred to undergo testing for depression or other mental disorders known to cause ED.

Conventional Treatments

Treatment varies according to the cause. If ED is due to an organic disorder, treating it will often resolve the problem. If psychological problems are involved, counseling and sex therapy or couples therapy may help.

The introduction of Viagra, a drug that increases blood flow to the penis, has revolutionized the drug treatment of ED, especially for men with diabetes and other disorders that interfere with circulation. However, this drug should not be taken with nitroglycerin, an antianginal medication that many heart patients take before intercourse to prevent chest pains and other symptoms.

Nutraceuticals for Sexual Dysfunction

▪ VITAMINS AND MINERALS

Vitamin C

How it works. Vitamin C is an important antioxidant; it also helps maintain the elasticity of blood vessels, allowing blood to flow freely through them—an important aspect of achieving and maintaining an erection.

Recommended dosages. Experts usually recommend taking 200 to 500 mg a day.

Possible problems. High doses of 1,000 mg or more a day appear to have the opposite effect of an antioxidant. They also may cause diarrhea and provoke kidney stones in susceptible people and can interact with some anticlotting drugs.

◎ STRATEGIES FOR RELIEF
- Strive to maintain good overall health.
- Do not smoke or use recreational drugs and abstain from alcohol or use it only in moderation.
- Talk to your doctor about any prescription medications you are taking. If the ED is related to a medication side effect, switching to another drug may solve the problem.
- If you are under a lot of stress, try to bring it under control. Learn to set priorities and tackle tasks one at a time. Try not to worry about what doesn't get done on a particular day; instead, put it on a future list.
- Work to maintain a caring and friendly relationship with your partner. Set aside time for pleasurable activities including sex.

◎ DRUGS AND SUBSTANCES THAT CAN CAUSE SEXUAL DYSFUNCTION

Addictive, abused, or recreational substances
- Alcohol.
- Nicotine and other tobacco substances.
- Recreational drugs, including heroin, marijuana, cocaine, and amphetamines.

Pharmaceutical products
- Allergy and cold medications containing antihistamines.
- Beta-blockers (e.g., Inderal), sympathetic blockers (e.g., Aldomet and Catapres), and many other drugs used to treat high blood pressure and angina.
- Sedatives and muscle relaxants such as diazepam (Valium).
- Antispasmodic drugs used to treat nausea, irritable bowel syndrome, and Parkinson's disease.
- Some antibiotics.
- Histamine blockers (e.g., Tagamet) used to treat ulcers.
- Antiseizure medications used to treat epilepsy.

Vitamin E

How it works. Vitamin E is an antioxidant vitamin that is important in maintaining sexual health and fertility; it also improves blood flow by acting as a blood thinner.

Recommended dosage. The typical dosage calls for 400 to 800 IU of natural (d-alpha) vitamin E a day.

Possible problems. High doses of vitamin E should be used with caution, if at all, by people who are taking blood-thinning medications such as Coumadin or who are also taking ginkgo biloba or other nutraceuticals that interfere with clotting.

Vitamin B-complex

How they work. The B vitamins are important in maintaining proper nerve function—an essential aspect of sexual function. Some are important in hormone synthesis; others help maintain a healthy heart, fight depression, and counter stress.

Recommended dosages. The B-complex vitamins should be taken in balance because a high dose of one may interfere with the metabolism of others. A multivitamin that provides the RDA of all the B vitamins is adequate for most people; those with heart disease or other specific health problems may need a high-dose supplement, such as B-complex 50 or 100.

Possible problems. Very high doses of some B vitamins, especially B_6, can cause nerve damage.

Selenium and zinc

How they work. These minerals are important in the production of sperm. Zinc deficiency has been associated with testicular atrophy (shrinking) and infertility. Large amounts of zinc are lost during ejaculation, increasing the risk of deficiency.

Recommended dosages. Only a small amount of zinc is needed; supplements of 25 to 30 mg a day are more than adequate. The RDA for selenium is 70 mcg a day; supplements up to 200 mcg a day are considered safe and may also lower the risk of prostate cancer.

Possible problems. Very high doses (more than 100 mg a day) taken for more than a week or so can reduce immunity. Zinc also interferes with copper absorption; take 2 mg of copper a day if zinc is used for more than a few weeks.

■ NUTRITIONAL SUPPLEMENTS

Essential fatty acids

How they work. Fish oils and flaxseed oil are high in omega-3 fatty acids. These substances help prevent heart disease—a possible cause of

ED—by reducing inflammation and helping prevent the clogging of arteries with fatty plaque.

Recommended dosages. There is no dosage for ED per se; two or three servings of fatty, cold-water fish (tuna, salmon, sardines, etc.) a week has been shown to reduce the risk of heart disease and associated problems. If eating this much fish is not feasible, a 1,000-mg fish oil capsule taken with each meal is an alternative. The usual flaxseed oil dosage calls for 1 to 2 teaspoons of oil once or twice a day.

Possible problems. Essential fatty acids in the recommended dosages are generally safe, with a few exceptions. High doses (more than 2,000 mg a day) of fish oil supplements may raise blood sugar in people with diabetes. It can also increase the risk of bleeding problems among people who are taking blood thinners or who have uncontrolled high blood pressure.

■ BOTANICAL MEDICINES

Ginkgo (G. biloba)

How it works. Ginkgo increases blood flow, and thus may be helpful in treating ED related to circulatory problems.

Recommended dosages. Herbalists generally recommend taking 80 mg of an extract standardized to contain 24 percent flavone glycosides three times a day.

Possible problems. Some people experience an upset stomach and headache when taking ginkgo biloba. It may also cause bleeding problems in people who are taking other blood-thinning medications, such as Coumadin.

Ginseng (Panax ginseng. P. quinquefolius, and other species)

How it works. Animal studies indicate that ginseng boosts testosterone levels; the herb is widely reputed to increase libido in humans, but this claim is unproved. However, it has a long history of use by Asian healers as a general tonic and to treat sexual and fertility problems.

Recommended dosages. The typical dosage calls for 100 to 300 mg twice a day; the product should be standardized to contain 7 percent or more ginsenosides. Some practitioners recommend rotating the different types of ginseng; for example, taking Siberian ginseng for two weeks, switching to American ginseng for two weeks, and then switching to Asian ginseng. (It should be noted, however, that some physicians are wary of this approach, and advise using either the Asian or American ginseng.)

Possible problems. High doses may cause nervousness, sleep problems, and an upset stomach.

Yohimbe (*Pausinystalia yohimbe*)

How it works. Yohimbe comes from the bark of a tree in West Africa, where it has a long history of use as an aphrodisiac. It contains an alkaloid (yohimbine) that increases peripheral blood flow, which may promote an erection; it may also stimulate nerves in the genital area as well as the central nervous system. Despite its reputation of being a powerful sexual stimulant, however, this has not been verified in scientific studies.

Recommended dosages. Yohimbine is available as a prescription drug, and should be taken only under the supervision of a doctor experienced in its use.

Possible problems. Yohimbine can cause many side effects, including anxiety, tremors, insomnia, a rise in blood pressure, palpitations, nausea and vomiting, and hallucinations. Taken in high doses, it can cause a severe drop in blood pressure, weakness, and paralysis. Some states have banned the nonprescription sale of yohimbine, and the FDA has ruled it unsafe as an over-the-counter product.

CHAPTER 5

Antiaging Nutraceuticals

It is often said that the aging process begins at birth and continues throughout life. This may be something of an exaggeration, and while no one disputes the fact that all living creatures and plants inevitably grow old and die, it is increasingly clear that we can slow the process and minimize the effects of aging. Researchers have long observed that, in human beings, each individual ages in a unique manner and biological age often has little to do with one's years. We all know people who seem much older than they really are and others who look and act decades younger than their actual age. Of course, genetics and general health are key factors, but so too is lifestyle. This chapter focuses on the role of diet and specifically nutraceuticals in countering the toll of time.

Starting with the Cells

To better understand aging, we need to consider the cell, the body's most basic unit. Each cell contains a complete genetic blueprint of its host and is programmed to carry out a specific function within the organism. Our bodies are made up of trillions of cells, which are organized into tissues that make up the individual organs, such as the brain and the heart. Some organs are in a constant state of renewal, as dead cells are replaced by new ones; the skin is a prime example of this process. Other organs, such as the liver, possess remarkable regenerative capabilities. Still others, such as the heart, are programmed to grow to a certain point and then rely upon a cell-repair system to continue functioning for however long the person lives. With time, however, the process of cell destruction outpaces cell production and repair, and certain organs begin to slowly wear out. In addition, the genetic material of some cells may change, or mutate, resulting in renegade cells that are no longer programmed to function normally; they can cause cancer and other degenerative diseases.

With advancing age, the body's immune system also begins to wear down, paving the way for an increasing vulnerability to infections and a dwindling ability to seek out and destroy mutant cells that may evolve into cancer. This is one area in which lifestyle factors, especially diet and nutraceuticals, play critical roles.

How Do We Age? No One Really Knows

Since long before Ponce de Leon landed on these shores in search of the Fountain of Youth, humans have sought answers to how and why we age. The search continues today in scores of laboratories around the world, where researchers are busy unraveling the genetic code, finding cures for many of the world's killer diseases, and accomplishing other feats that can extend life. Indeed, there is mounting speculation that one day we will live for 150, 200, or more years, enjoying youthful looks and health all the while. Toward this end, we have formed dozens of theories as to how and why we age; so far, however, none fully explain the process. These theories include:

The genetic control theory holds that DNA—a cell's reproductive blue-print—is the key to how an individual ages. In other words, how we age is determined at the moment of conception. While heredity is certainly an important factor, there is ample evidence that many circumstances and interventions can alter our genetic predestination, so it seems likely that aging involves more than simple genetics.

The neuroendocrine theory holds that hormones are the key, based on the fact that hormones regulate virtually every bodily process and function. Hormone production peaks during adolescence and young adulthood, and then declines steadily with advancing years. Proponents of this theory contend that the declining hormone levels result in a drop in cellular repair and replacement, hence the degenerative changes that characterize aging.

The wear-and-tear theory is based on the premise that a living organism is similar to, for example, a lightbulb or an automobile in that after a certain amount of use, the organism simply wears out. Under this theory, overuse or abuse of an organ hastens the process and increases the risk of disease, just as a lack of preventive maintenance results in the risk of a car's breaking down. Certain aspects of this theory certainly hold true; it is well known, for example, that alcohol abuse eventually overwhelms the liver's ability to detoxify the substance and it wears out. But then there are those few individuals who smoke, are heavy drinkers, never have a checkup, and still defy the odds by living into their nineties or beyond.

The rate-of-living theory, which is similar to the wear-and-tear concept, holds that each living organism starts life with a specific energy allowance. According to this theory, aging and death simply reflect a depletion of one's lifetime energy allowance. One would assume, then, that living life in the fast lane—always on the go with poor eating habits, lots of stress, and inadequate sleep, for example—would lead to early burnout and aging, while those moving at a more moderate pace would live longer. Trouble is, there are too many examples to the contrary in each category, so it's likely that other factors are involved.

The immune system theory holds that a decline in immune-system function causes the changes related to aging. There is no question that immunity declines with aging, but an overactive immune system can also shorten life by attacking healthy tissue and causing serious autoimmune diseases such as lupus.

The free radical theory holds that these unstable substances damage cells as they travel through the body and are responsible for many of the degenerative changes associated with aging. Free radicals are the by-products of normal metabolism; they are also produced by exposure to sunlight, smog and other environmental pollutants, cigarette smoke, harmful chemicals, and other toxins. They are unstable because they are missing an electron, which prompts them to travel through the body in search of one that they can "steal" from another molecule. This can damage the formerly normal cell's DNA, resulting in a mutant cell that may evolve into a cancerous one unless it is deactivated or destroyed by the body's immune system, which recognizes these abnormal cells as "foreign invaders." Free radicals are also destroyed by enzymes such as glutathione peroxidase, which the body makes from bits of protein (amino acids) and by antioxidants (see below).

The Role of Nutraceuticals

Even though we do not fully understand the aging process, there is ample evidence that there are many things we can do to slow and minimize the effects of aging, and some of the most effective involve nutraceuticals. Here's a brief overview of some of the most important.

Antioxidants

These substances, which are found in many foods and nutraceuticals, counter the action of free radicals by attaching to them and providing their missing electron. Some of the most important and abundant antioxidants are vitamins C and E, beta-carotene (the precursor of vitamin A), selenium, and the bioflavonoids, as well as specific nutraceuticals such as coenzyme Q_{10}. There is no single magic antioxidant that protects all parts of the body; instead, the individual substances are distinguished, at least in part, by the area of the body in which they are the most effective. This is why it is so important to consume a variety of foods and supplements that have many different antioxidants. For example, vitamin E, which is dissolved in and carried through the body on fat molecules (lipids or lipoproteins), protects the fats found in cell membranes. Vitamin C, a water-soluble antioxidant, protects the watery contents inside the cells, including DNA. Still another antioxidant nutraceutical, coenzyme Q_{10}, is concentrated in heart cells.

Although the various antioxidants have specific functions, they also work together to protect against the oxidative damage caused by free radicals. The relationship between vitamins C and E is a case in point. Vitamin C helps recycle vitamin E to increase its usefulness in protecting fats from turning rancid because of exposure to oxygen (oxidation).

Antioxidants are by no means limited to a few vitamins and minerals—there are hundreds of other very beneficial antioxidants in foods. The carotenoids—pigments that give orange and red fruits and vegetables and deep green vegetables their bright colors—are very important antioxidants. So far, some six-hundred carotenoids have been identified; some of the most beneficial are alpha- and beta-carotene, beta-cryptoxanthin, lutein, lycopene, and zeaxanthin.

There are more than eight-hundred bioflavonoids, which are also referred to as flavonoids. They are also parts of brightly colored fruits and vegetables, as well as nuts, wine, and tea.

Phytoestrogens

Phytoestrogens are plant chemicals that are chemically similar to estrogen, the major female sex hormone. So far, about three hundred phytoestrogens have been identified in foods; among the most important are the isoflavones and lignans. Phytoestrogens mimic many of the effects of estrogen, which is especially beneficial for older women, whose estrogen production drops dramatically during menopause. (Men, too, need small amounts of estrogen, just as women need small amounts of testosterone, the major male sex hormone.) Among myriad functions, estrogen helps protect bones against mineral loss; it may reduce the risk of heart disease, Alzheimer's, and other age-related degenerative diseases.

In addition to mimicking some of the effects of natural estrogen, phytoestrogens appear to protect against some of the harmful effects of the hormone. For example, estrogen is known to spur the growth of certain cancers, especially some types of breast tumors. By occupying estrogen receptor sites in the breasts and other organs, phytoestrogens may reduce cancer risk by minimizing the tumor-stimulating effects of the body's estrogen. In effect, they function as estrogen blockers, similar to Tamoxifen, an antiestrogen drug that has been shown to reduce the risk of breast cancer.

Tofu and other soy foods are the richest sources of isoflavones, the most potent of the phytoestrogens. But many other foods also provide phytoestrogens. For example, whole grains, fruits, and vegetables contain lignans, while flaxseed, sesame seeds, and sunflower seeds contain the compounds that are converted to lignans. Legumes contain coumestans and isoflavones, while coumestrol is a phytoestrogen prevalent in soy, alfalfa, and clover sprouts.

The precise amount of any given phytoestrogen that is needed to prevent specific age-related diseases is unknown. Some studies indicate

◉ THE TOP 10 ANTIOXIDANT FRUITS AND VEGETABLES

All brightly colored fruits and vegetables are good sources of antioxidants, but some are much more potent than others. Here are the top ten, ranked in order of their antioxidant potency as determined by USDA scientists. But don't feel you should limit your choices to these foods—it's important to consume a variety of fruits and vegetables for their other vitamins and minerals, as well as dietary fiber.

1. Blueberries
2. Blackberries
3. Garlic
4. Kale
5. Strawberries
6. Spinach
7. Brussels sprouts
8. Plums
9. Alfalfa sprouts
10. Broccoli florets

Antioxidants at a Glance

ANTIOXIDANT	GOOD FOOD SOURCES	ROLE IN THE BODY	SUGGESTED DAILY DOSE TO COUNTER AGING
Vitamin C	Citrus fruits and vegetables	Helps form white blood cells that fight disease.	200 to 500 mg
Vitamin E	Nuts, vegetable oils, egg yolks, wheat germ; nutritional supplements	Prevents LDL oxidation; boosts immunity; protects eyes from cataracts; thwarts certain cancers, possibly by neutralizing free radicals or blocking formation of cancer-causing compounds; protects lipids from oxidation; slows progression of Alzheimer's; may protect against strokes.	400 to 800 IU (only supplements provide these therapeutic amounts)
Beta-carotene	Bright yellow, orange, or green fruits and vegetables, especially sweet potatoes, cantaloupe, broccoli, and others	Protects heart and many other organs against free-radical damage; may reduce risk of cancer.	Eat at least 5 servings of brightly colored fruits and vegetables a day; recommended supplement dosage is 15 mg or 25,000 IU, preferably as part of mixed carotenoids (see below).
Carotenoids	Bright yellow, orange, or green fruits and vegetables (e.g., pumpkin, kale, spinach, carrots, tomatoes, apricots) and nutritional supplements	May prevent certain cancers, heart disease, protect vision.	Eat at least 5 servings of fruits and vegetables a day; take mixed carotenoid (including beta-carotene) supplements in dosages up to 15 mg or 25,000 IU.
Bioflavonoids	Various fruits and vegetables, especially apricots, blackberries, black currants, broccoli, citrus fruits, among others; also tea, red wine, and nuts.	May prevent heart disease and cancer.	Eat at least 5 servings of fruits and vegetables a day.
Coenzyme Q_{10}	Nuts, oils, and many other foods; also produced in the human body and all living organisms	Works with vitamin E to protect heart cells; also important in energy metabolism of all cells.	100 to 120 mg
Selenium	Brazil nuts, halibut, shrimp, wheat germ	Vital component of glutathione peroxidase, an antioxidant enzyme that battles free radicals; works with vitamin E; may reduce cancer risk, boost immunity, and help prevent cataracts.	100 to 200 mcg

that one or two servings of soy foods a day can reduce the risk of heart disease; in addition to protective phytoestrogens, the protein in soy foods may also reduce the risk of heart disease and help control blood sugar levels. Much higher amounts may be needed to prevent hot flashes and other menopausal symptoms; for this, some experts recommend taking soy isoflavone supplements of 50 to 150 mg a day.

DHEA

DHEA (dehydroepiandrosterone) is one of several hormones produced by the adrenal glands, small organs that sit atop the kidneys. DHEA is sometimes called a "mother hormone" because the body needs it to make estrogen, testosterone, and other important hormones. At about age thirty, DHEA production begins to slack off, and it continues to decline with advancing age. In recent years, DHEA supplements have been promoted as an antiaging hormone, but doctors advise against taking it except to treat a specific disorder, and then only under careful medical supervision. Flooding the body with excessive DHEA can result in serious hormonal imbalances and an increased risk of cancers linked to high levels of estrogen and testosterone. In general, deficiencies of these hormones should be treated with specific hormone replacement therapy, rather than with DHEA. If supplements are taken, the daily dosage should not exceed 25 mg. Otherwise, DHEA may raise testosterone levels high enough to spur growth of prostate cancer, while an increased risk of some types of breast cancer is linked to high levels of estrogen.

DHEA may have other antiaging effects. For example, the body needs it to help build muscle tissue. But more study is needed to determine what role, if any, DHEA plays as an antiaging hormonal supplement. In the meantime, many natural hormonal products claim to provide a safe form of DHEA. But here the promises appear to outweigh any actual benefit. For example, some wild yam products claim to contain substances that the body can convert to DHEA. However, this conversion appears to take place only in the laboratory, not the human body.

Growth Hormone

Human growth hormone (hGH) is produced by the pituitary gland and, as its name implies, is instrumental in growth, development, and maintenance of muscle tissue and organs. Its production drops with increasing age, and in recent years, the loss of muscle mass and other effects of aging have been attributed to a lack of hGH. In fact, in the media it has been promoted as an antidote to aging, and it has been proved to help children who are deficient in the hormone grow normally. Preliminary studies involving older adults show that it may help increase muscle mass and strength and reduce the tendency to increase fatty tissue. But more study is needed to establish its safety; experts note that hGH may spur the growth of tumors and also increase the risk of diabetes, high blood pressure, and other adverse effects.

Melatonin

This is a hormone produced by the pineal gland, a tiny organ situated in the forebrain. Melatonin is instrumental in controlling the sleep-wake cycle and may play a role in other biorhythms as well. Many older people develop sleep problems, and the quality of sleep tends to decline with age. Melatonin, which is available as a dietary supplement, has been shown to help many people sleep better; it is also a popular remedy to overcome jet lag among travelers crossing several time zones. In recent years, melatonin has also been promoted as an antiaging supplement—a benefit that is supported only by animals studies. In one study, mice given melatonin lived an average of 25 percent longer than those in a control group. But it is not known whether humans achieve similar benefits.

As a sleep aid, the effects of melatonin vary greatly from one person to another. Some studies have shown that taking 1 to 3 mg of melatonin at bedtime shortens the time needed to fall asleep and reduces the number of wakenings during the night. Unlike prescription sleep medications, melatonin is not addictive, and it generally does not cause a morning hangover. However, some people do experience mental confusion, drowsiness, and headache, and it may raise blood pressure in susceptible people.

Aging-Related Changes That May Be Slowed by Nutraceuticals

As stressed earlier, nutraceuticals are not that elusive fountain of youth, but they can make a big difference in how you look and feel. Following is an overview of the body's major organ systems, and nutraceuticals that help keep them fit and functioning properly. Understanding how time affects your body helps you make the most informed choices about the nutraceuticals that can slow down the aging process.

Immune System

Our bodies are equipped with a sophisticated defense system that protects against a host of potential dangers, including bacteria, viruses, fungi, parasites, and mutant cells that could give rise to cancer. When confronted with a perceived danger, the immune system responds by producing antibodies and several types of white blood cells that seek out and destroy it.

Antibody production falls as we age, and the immune system is less efficient in fighting off infection and destroying mutant cells. Consequently, the elderly are more susceptible to infection, cancer, and other diseases. Or the immune system may go awry, attacking healthy body tissue as if it were a foreign invader and resulting in an autoimmune disease such as lupus or rheumatoid arthritis.

Maintaining a strong immune system requires a healthful balanced diet that provides ample immune-enhancing nutrients, including vitamins, minerals, and antioxidants. Nutraceutical supplements, including echinacea, ginseng, aloe gel extracts, and other botanical medicines, often speed recovery from a cold, flu, or other common viral infections. Of course lifestyle factors—managing stress, getting enough sleep, and regular exercise—also bolster immunity. For more on immunity, see Allergies, p. 25; Chronic Fatigue Syndrome, p. 75; Common Cold and Flu, p. 84; and Lupus, p. 157.

The Brain and Nervous System

Any older person who regularly misplaces keys or has trouble remembering names begins to worry about memory problems and a loss of mental function. It may be comforting to know that these are problems shared by most people, regardless of age, and are not necessarily a sign of degenerative brain disorder such as Alzheimer's disease. We just tend to worry more about them as we get older.

As with most organs, the brain shrinks a bit with increasing age. Much of this is due to water loss; as with most body tissue, the brain contains a large amount of fluids, and the body tends to shrivel as it dries out. But there is also a time-related loss of neurons, the nerve cells that are instrumental in processing information and the ability to think clearly. Still, neuroscientists assure us that the typical brain has billions more neurons than we actually need, and recent studies have found that, contrary to what was once thought, new neurons are formed as we grow older. In the large majority of people, the cerebral cortex—the part of the brain responsible for long-term memory, language, learning, and thought processes—remains remarkably intact well into advanced age, and many people in their nineties remain mentally alert.

Still, there is no question that aging affects the brain. Blood flow to the brain begins to decline as early as the mid to late thirties. This effect is particularly pronounced in people with atherosclerosis (hardening of the arteries), high blood pressure, and heart disease. Studies show that elevated blood pressure in midlife is the primary reason for the decline in nerve tissue and reduced brain volume of people in their seventies. Along with cigarette smoking, excessive alcohol consumption, and poorly controlled diabetes, chronically high blood pressure speeds up the normal changes seen in the aging brain.

Vitamin E has been shown to help maintain blood flow to the brain, and some studies suggest that it is also important in preserving memory function. Ginkgo biloba also increases blood flow to the brain and may help improve memory, although the evidence for this is largely anecdotal.

Deficiencies of some of the B vitamins also hasten the effects of aging on brain tissue. With advancing age, the body absorbs less of vitamins B_6 and B_{12}, as well as folacin (folic acid), members of the B-complex family that are especially important in preserving nerve and brain function. Supplements of these important vitamins have been found to help ward off age-related depression, confusion, and memory loss.

For more detailed information, see Vitamin B$_6$, p. 230; Vitamin B$_{12}$, p. 232; Folacin, p. 217; Vitamin E, p. 216; Ginkgo, p. 463; Alzheimer's Disease and Memory Loss, p. 29; and Depression, p. 93.

Heart and Circulatory System

A number of age-related changes affect the way blood flows through the body. The heart is a muscle that is designed to last a lifetime, but with increasing age, it may beat less forcefully than in a young person. In addition, the chest wall loses some of its elasticity, which reduces the amount of oxygen inhaled during breathing. The arteries also lose some elasticity; more pressure therefore is needed to force blood through them, resulting in high blood pressure, or hypertension.

Compounding these changes is a very common disease process—atherosclerosis—in which fatty deposits (plaque) build up along the artery walls, narrowing the channel and further reducing blood flow. Reduced circulation is one reason why older people often complain of feeling cold, even when those around them are comfortably warm. Depending upon the area of blockage, circulation to the brain, legs and feet, kidneys, and the heart muscle itself may be seriously impaired. In addition, the narrowed arteries are vulnerable to the formation of blood clots, which can result in a heart attack, stroke, or pulmonary embolism (a blood clot in the lungs).

While all this sounds inevitable and depressing, the good news is that many nutraceuticals can prevent or slow the process. Vitamin C helps maintain healthy blood vessels and recent studies suggest it may help lower blood pressure. In addition, it and other antioxidants protect against plaque formation. Vitamin E promotes circulation and reduces the likelihood of abnormal clotting; omega-3 fatty acids, red rice yeast, benecol, and many nutraceutical supplements help control blood cholesterol levels—a major risk factor in developing atherosclerosis. Dietary fiber—especially the soluble type found in oat and rice bran, pectin, and many fruits and green tea also thwart plaque formation.

For more specific information, see Cholesterol Disorders and Atherosclerosis, p. 68; Circulatory Problems, p. 80; Heart Disease, p. 118; High Blood Pressure, p. 122; Leg Cramps and Restless Legs, p. 149; and Varicose Veins, p. 194.

Musculoskeletal System

Bones and muscles give the body its shape, provide a protective cage for internal organs, and enable us to move with ease. They are also responsible for many of the aches and pains that accompany aging.

The hard exterior of bones give the false impression that nothing much is happening inside. In reality, bone is very active tissue that

At any age, you can benefit from regular exercise. You don't need to become a gym fanatic—walking twenty to thirty minutes every day and engaging in some type of weight-training or strength-building exercise at least three times a week will improve endurance, strengthen muscles, build bone mass, reduce flab, and bring an enhanced sense of well-being psychologically and physiologically through endorphin release. All you need to do is get started and stick with it. Of course, you should consult a doctor if you have been sedentary, are over age forty-five, or have any risk factors for (or a history of) heart disease, stroke, or diabetes. Once you get a medical go-ahead, here are tips to help ensure success.

- Pick an activity you really enjoy. Maybe it's walking a dog, playing tennis, dancing, jogging—it really doesn't matter what you do so long as it's vigorous enough to make your heart beat faster and pump a little harder and exercise all your large muscles. If you enjoy the activity, you're more likely to stick with it.
- Vary your routines. Doing the same thing day after day can be boring and may also increase the risk of injury. So try walking one day, swimming or cycling the next, and so forth.
- Consider exercising with a partner or group; this can increase motivation and enjoyment.
- Combine strength training with your aerobic exercise. You can work out with free weights, resistance machines, elastic bands, or surgical tubing. Weight training preserves and builds muscles and bone tissue at any age; it also improves balance and agility. It can also lessen joint and back pain.
- To get started, consider consulting a pro—this may be a physical therapist or exercise physiologist if you have arthritis or another limiting medical problem. Most gyms employ personal trainers who can show you the proper way to use various exercise machines and help design a regimen to meet your specific goals.

contains a rich network of nerves and vessels. Bone undergoes constant remodeling, characterized by a cycle of destruction and renewal of bone cells. In addition, calcium and other minerals constantly move in and out of bone tissue. Again, time takes its toll, and eventually, you lose more bone minerals and mass than you build. This can lead to osteoporosis, a very common disease characterized by thin, brittle bones that fracture easily, and a loss in height as the spinal column compresses.

A certain amount of bone loss is to be expected with age, but numerous studies show that nutraceuticals and lifestyle can hold the loss to manageable proportions. Older women are especially vulnerable to osteoporosis because the decline in estrogen during menopause hastens the loss of bone minerals. Hormone replacement therapy helps, but for some women, this increases the risk of cancer, blood clots, and other adverse side effects. For them and women who do not want to take estrogen replacement, phytoestrogens may be the answer to maintaining strong bones. While men are not as vulnerable as women to osteoporosis, they do account for 25 percent all cases and can also benefit from these nutrients.

Osteoarthritis and other joint problems also grow increasingly common with advancing age. Again, there are numerous nutraceuticals, such as glucosamine, chondroitin, and SAM-e, that can slow the process and relieve pain and other symptoms. For more on protecting bones and joints, see Arthritis, p. 40; Gout, p. 115; and Osteoporosis, p. 175.

Beginning around age twenty-five, you lose muscle tissue. The process is so slow that you probably won't notice the missing muscle mass until middle age or later. Protein is needed to make muscle tissue, but that doesn't mean that a high-protein diet translates into bigger biceps. Maintaining muscle mass means getting at least 53 grams of protein daily if you're a woman, and about 10 grams more if you're male. Of course, working out counts, because it builds new tissue and maintains what you already have. There are also nutraceuticals that may help. One that has received considerable media attention is creatine, a substance that the body makes from protein. It helps improve endurance by delaying the buildup of lactic acid, a by-product of the accelerated energy metabolism during vigorous exercise. It has not been proved that creatine supplements will actually increase endurance or muscle mass, and there is some question about their safety; for a more detailed discussion, see Creatine, p. 289.

Gastrointestinal System

People over age fifty are especially vulnerable to atrophic gastritis, an age-related condition that results in reduced production of stomach acid. In turn, this can cause inadequate absorption of vitamin B_{12}, a nutrient that is especially important in nerve function and the production of healthy red blood cells. Inadequate vitamin B_{12} can lead to pernicious anemia and higher blood levels of homocysteine, a protein that increases the risk of heart disease and stroke.

Other intestinal changes are more obvious than atrophic gastritis. Constipation is a common complaint among older people; chronic constipation increases the risk of other intestinal disorders, including diverticulosis, the formation of small pouches (diverticula) along the outer colon wall. About half of all Americans age sixty to eighty have diverticulosis, and the incidence becomes even more prevalent among people over eighty.

Older people, especially those over age sixty, also have a very high incidence of gallstones, which form when bile stored in the gallbladder hardens into rock-hard material. Liver problems also become more common after age sixty or so, which can be a problem for people who take a lot of medications. An aging liver is not as efficient in metabolizing medications and other chemical compounds. Consequently, older people often need lower dosages to achieve the same effects as would be expected in a younger person. They are also more vulnerable to adverse side effects.

For information on specific conditions, see Constipation, p. 89; Diarrhea, p. 105; Diverticular Disease, p. 109; Gallstones, p. 112; Heartburn, p. 123; Liver Diseases, p. 153; and Ulcers, p. 188.

Reproductive Systems

Age-related changes in the reproductive systems are more obvious in women than men, but for both sexes, these changes can cause big problems. In men, the prostate—a small, walnut-sized gland that encircles part of the urethra (the tube that carries urine from the bladder to the penis)—enlarges with advancing age. This can cause urinary frequency and other problems; it also increases the risk of prostate cancer, the most common malignancy in men.

Women, of course, go through menopause, which ends the reproductive years. Starting in a woman's mid- to late thirties or early forties, her ovaries start making less estrogen, which reduces fertility and can lead to irregular menstrual periods. But, as noted, estrogen does much more than control fertility; the hormone is also instrumental in maintaining bones, skin, and vaginal tissue; it is also thought to play a role in memory, promoting a healthy balance of HDL and LDL cholesterol, and promoting elasticity of blood vessels.

In the past, it was generally assumed that age brought an inevitable decline in sexuality. We now know that this is not the case, that sex is an important and pleasurable aspect of life for both men and women. While no food or supplement is a magical aphrodisiac, maintaining good nutrition and overall health are certainly important aspects of a healthy sex life.

For more information on coping with reproductive system changes, see Menopause, p. 580; Menstrual Problems, p. 585; Benign Prostate Enlargement, p. 612; Sexual Dysfunction, p. 616; Urinary Tract Infection, p. 191; and Vaginitis, p. 604.

Sensory Organs

Vision

Everyone's eyesight changes with increasing age. At about age forty, most people notice that it is more difficult to read the fine print in newspapers or telephone directories, especially in dim light. Other changes in vision include inadequate tear production, resulting in dry eyes, or making too many tears. The risk of cataracts—the clouding of the clear lens that admits light into the eye—starts in the late sixties or early seventies, and perhaps earlier among people with diabetes. Carotenoid supplements have been shown to prevent or slow the progression of cataracts. Glaucoma, a disorder characterized by a buildup of pressure inside the eyeball, is also more common among older people. It is usually asymptomatic in its early stages, and by the time symptoms develop, the disease may already have caused irreversible vision loss. This can be prevented by having an annual eye examination after age forty-five or so.

Age-related macular degeneration (AMD) damages the central part of the retina, the paper-thin tissue that lines the back of the eyeball, destroying sharp, central vision. People over the age of sixty run the greatest risk for AMD; the risk can be reduced by several nutraceuticals, including vitamin C and other antioxidants, especially lutein and zeaxanthin, carotenoids that are concentrated in the eye. It can also be reduced by stopping smoking.

Diabetic retinopathy destroys vision by damaging the tiny vessels that feed the eyes with oxygen-rich blood. A chronically elevated blood glucose level is the culprit. People with diabetes should have a complete eye exam at least once a year, and perhaps more often if the disease is not under good control. For more information on specific eye disorders, see Cataracts, p. 64; Diabetes, p. 101; and Macular Degeneration, p. 160.

Hearing

Hearing, like many of the other senses, becomes less acute with advancing age. It becomes more difficult to hear high-pitched voices and soft sounds, and many people eventually need a hearing aid. Some of this hearing loss is natural, related to a decline in the microscopic hair cells (cilla) that pick up sound waves. A reduced blood flow and nerve damage are possible contributing factors. Injury and exposure to loud noise also diminish hearing. The B vitamins that support nerve function help maintain hearing; recent studies indicate that high blood cholesterol also contributes to the problem. For more information, see Cholesterol Disorders and Atherosclerosis, p. 68.

Taste and Smell

These two senses are closely related; without a healthy sense of smell, the ability to taste foods declines. Many older people complain of a lack of appetite because "nothing tastes good." This is more often due to an impaired sense of smell than to a disorder involving the tongue taste buds. In fact, the taste buds detect just four flavors: sweet, bitter, salty, and sour. The ability to tell an onion from an apple, for example, rests with the sense of smell and a closely associated memory center in the brain. The sense of smell begins to wane at about age sixty or so; to compensate, try using stronger flavorings, such as cinnamon or garlic, that also have distinctive odors. Many botanical medicines also help perk up a flagging appetite, especially herbal remedies such as burdock, cinnamon, dill, mint, and gentian and other herbs that are rich in bitter compounds.

Touch and Skin

We all get a bit wrinkled as we get older. Gravity and a loss of skin moisture are the major reasons. The two main layers of skin, the outer epidermis and the underlying dermis, become dryer and thinner as the years go by. Exposure to sun and wind accelerates the process. In addition, collagen, a gluelike protein that holds together cells, diminishes. As a result, thinner, less elastic skin becomes more fragile; it bruises and tears more easily and takes longer to heal.

The skin also loses its ability to synthesize vitamin D, the nutrient that works with calcium to bolster bone density. This increases the risk of osteomalacia, a danger that can be minimized by taking vitamin D supplements. For more on specific skin problems, see Dermatitis/ Eczema, p. 98, and Psoriasis, p. 178.

Resources and Guidelines on Buying and Using Nutraceuticals

Christopher M. Foley, M.D., and Allen M. Kratz, Pharm.D., Co-Editors, *JANA, Journal of the American Nutraceutical Association*

There's no doubt that nutraceuticals are more than just another passing health fad. Some 60 million Americans are now using nutraceutical products on a regular basis. According to government estimates, they spent more than $12 billion on various nutraceuticals last year, and this figure is expected to go up at least 10 percent this year. More than eight hundred companies now make or distribute nutraceutical products in the United States, and their ranks are growing continually. Their products are available not only in health food stores but also pharmacies, supermarkets and corner groceries, on scores of on-line sites, by mail order, and from door-to-door salespersons.

With so many choices, it's understandable that one of the most frequent questions we hear from consumers is: "How do I pick a product I can trust?" Unfortunately, there is no easy or definitive answer. From our own experiences and practices we know that there are many nutraceutical products that are safe and effective. But there are also problems. For example, many factors—everything from the weather and quality of soil to the time of harvest and processing methods—affect the potency of the raw materials used to make botanical medicines.

Manufacturing standards and quality control varies greatly from company to company, and there have been numerous reports of disquieting results from independent analyses of popular nutraceuticals. Many products have been found to contain exactly what the label says, while others—perhaps even the same brand but from a different manufacturing lot—provided little or none of the active ingredient(s), while others contained more than the stated amount. There have also been reports of mislabeled, misidentified, and contaminated products, sometimes with adverse results. And since nutraceuticals are marketed as nutritional supplements rather than medications, most do not have package inserts that list possible side effects, adverse reactions, interactions, and other precautions required for pharmaceutical products. Obviously, this is one area in which consumers should gather as much information as possible before buying. The bulk of this book has dealt with the many uses of nutraceuticals; following are some general guidelines for selecting reliable products.

How to Read a Label

By law, nutraceutical manufacturers cannot make health claims for their products, but they can list effects—proven or otherwise—that the product may have on bodily "structure or function." Thus, a term like antidepressant cannot be used for a nutritional supplement, but a vague description such as *mood balancer* will pass muster. Take care not to read too much into these descriptive phrases; instead, rely on references such as this book to learn more about the properties and actions of the various nutraceuticals.

Some of the other words that appear on nutraceutical labels have no standard definitions, and are included more for selling or promotional purposes than to inform. Common examples include *all-natural, highly concentrated, naturally pure, scientifically or clinically proven, time tested*, and *longevity formula*. Such terms may be favored by advertising copywriters but provide little real benefit in judging the reliability of a product. Here are terms that do have standard definitions and may be useful in selecting a product:

Bulk herbs: Fresh or dried herbs, roots, or other medicinal parts of the plant.

Extract: Concentrated powder, tincture, or other form of an herb; typically made by soaking the herb in a solvent and then evaporating the solution.

High potency: Under FDA regulations, this term can be used only on products that contain 100 percent or more of the Daily Value. If a product contains more than one active ingredient, two-thirds must contain more than 100 percent of the Daily Value, and a percentage must be listed for the others.

Standardized: Botanical product that is produced to provide a constant amount of the key, or active, ingredient.

Wildcrafted: Botanicals are gathered in the wild rather than cultivated.

The Label Itself

The Food and Drug Administration mandates that all active ingredients be listed on a product's label. In addition, since 1999, the FDA has required that products sold as nutritional supplements must have a Supplement Facts panel, similar to the Nutrition Facts panel on processed foods. This panel lists the following information:

- Serving size (e.g., 1 tablet)
- Amount per serving (e.g., St. John's wort herb with flowers, 300 mg; 0.3% hypericin=0.9 mg)
- % of daily value (Percentage of the recommended daily intake, usually the Recommended Dietary Allowance (RDA) or Reference Daily Intake (RDI), if one has been established; otherwise, a statement such as "Daily Value not established.")

Also look for:
- Directions for use
- Listing of other ingredients, both active and those used as binders, fillers, dyes, and flavoring agents
- Statement of potency and purity
- Manufacturer's code or lot number, which should be referred to if problems develop
- Expiration date
- Storage instructions
- Information on how to reach manufacturer or distributor, including name, address, toll-free number, and perhaps web site or e-mail address.

Other information that may be important to individuals:
- Kosher or vegetarian
- Animal testing

Forms of Nutraceuticals

Nutraceuticals can be taken in many ways; following are the most common forms:

- *Bulk herbs*, which can be bought from various outlets, grown at home, or gathered in the wild. These are used to make various herbal remedies. It should be noted that using bulk herbs for therapeutic purposes requires a certain amount of knowledge and skill. Many plants look alike, and it's easy to confuse a poisonous plant with one that is beneficial. So when gathering wild herbs, proper identification is critical. Also, remember that the method of drying and preparation of bulk herbs greatly affects their potency.

- Pills and tablets can provide precise amounts of various nutraceuticals, including vitamins, minerals, herbal extracts, and combinations of ingredients. They are easy to take and store, and last longer than dried or bulk herbs. Some people find large pills difficult to swallow; they may also contain inert ingredients (excipients) that are there to bind (hold) the ingredients together and hasten their dissolving in the stomach. These ingredients must be considered if a person has an allergic or other adverse reaction.

- Capsules are used to "package" powdered ingredients in a dissolvable capsule, which many people find easier to swallow than a hard pill. Capsules also provide a form for convenient storage and consistent dosages of a powdered product.

- Softgels or gelcaps, which are used to "package" liquid ingredients, such as fat-soluble vitamins. As with capsules of powdered ingredients, softgels provide consistent dosages; they are also easy to swallow and more palatable than taking the liquid ingredient alone.

- Sublingual tablets are small pills that are placed under the tongue (or perhaps in the cheek pocket) where they dissolve and are more rapidly absorbed into the blood than pills that are swallowed.

- Chewable pills or tablets may be preferable for people who have difficulty swallowing whole pills, and for children. They may also be absorbed more rapidly because they are ground into small pieces.

- Time-release capsules or tablets are filled with tiny coated pellets that are designed to dissolve at different speeds to provide a constant flow of the ingredient into the bloodstream and also to avoid adverse effects that may occur if a larger dose enters the blood circulation at the same time. High-potency vitamins and iron are often packaged as time-release formulas.

- Powdered nutraceuticals, such as soy protein and other products taken in relatively large amounts, can be dissolved in juice or milk or added to food. They are ideal for people who have difficulty swallowing pills.

- Infusions, teas, and decoctions are a favored form of taking many herbal products, including those high in mucilage (e.g., slippery elm or licorice root) to soothe a sore throat or intestinal inflammation. Infusions and teas are made by pouring water over a dried or fresh herb, letting it sit (steep) for a few minutes, straining, and drinking as you would any tea. A decoction is made by simmering the plant—often a root or woody parts—for at least thirty minutes, sometimes longer. This produces a stronger brew than an infusion or tea, and it is often diluted before drinking.

- Liquid extracts are often used for children or people who are unable to swallow pills or capsules. The concentrated liquid can also be added to hot water to make an instant tea.

- Tinctures are concentrated liquid that are made by soaking a botanical product in ethyl alcohol or glycerin and water.
- Syrups are made by boiling a botanical product in a sugar solution.
- Compresses are made by dipping a cloth in a tea or decoction and applying it to the skin; they are used to treat superficial inflamation and achiness.
- Poultices are a soft mass of leaves or ground herbs spread on a piece of cheesecloth or muslin, and applied to an inflamed or aching part of the body for an hour or longer. Often, the poultice is changed when the cloth cools. Common examples include comfrey poultices to treat a spider bite or bruises, or calendula to treat minor skin wounds.
- Salves, ointments, gels, and creams are made by mixing a powdered herbal extract with a fat or oil to make a thick paste. Other ingredients, such as aromatic oils, may be added.
- Essential (aromatic) oils are concentrated oils that are derived by distilling or cold extraction. Many essential oils are highly toxic if used full-strength; instead, they are diluted with a neutral oil or water and applied to the skin, inhaled as aromatherapy. A few may be diluted and used internally, but caution is needed to make sure that the oil is safe to ingest.
- Lozenges are sucked and dissolved slowly in the mouth; they are used mostly to treat sore throats, coughs, or mouth sores. Zinc lozenges may be used to shorten the duration of a cold or other upper respiratory infection.

Picking a Product

This is more difficult in the United States than in countries like Germany where, by law, manufacturers of botanical medicines must guarantee that their products meet specific standards. In the United States, the U.S. Pharmacopeia, a nonprofit group, has set standards for some of the most-used herbal products (e.g., St. John's wort, saw palmetto, feverfew, among others). Manufacturers who meet the Pharmacopeia's standards can label their products with a NF, for National Formulary, or USP, for United States Pharmacopeia. They can also advertise that they meet the organization's standards. Unfortunately, Pharmacopeia standards have been set for only a handful of products.

Laboratory Analysis

Various independent laboratories offer chemical analysis of medications, including nutraceuticals. This is expensive and provides information only on the specific product and dosage form that is analyzed. Chemical analysis has found wide variations not only among different brand names but also among different batches or lots of the same brand name. Even so, repeated spot testing can help identify those brand names that generally contain the ingredients and amounts stated on the product labels. This service is being offered by ConsumerLab.com, a private company located in White Plains, New York. This company has contracted with independent laboratories across the country to evaluate nutraceutical products. The results are posted on the organization's web site (www.ConsumerLab.com). As of this writing, several hundred brand names have been analyzed, and those that provide labeled amounts are posted on the web site. In addition, products that have passed the ConsumerLab.com criteria can use the CL seal on their labels and in advertising.

The Role of Clinical Studies

The Food and Drug Administration is empowered to regulate nutraceuticals in much the same manner that it can regulate other food products: manufacturers cannot make unproven health claims and the FDA or other government agencies can remove from the market any product that is found to be harmful. But nutraceutical manufacturers are not required to do controlled clinical trials—scientific studies in which the effectiveness and safety of a product is measured against a dummy pill (placebo) or a proven competitive product. Because most nutraceuticals are natural substances that cannot be patented, there is little incentive for manufacturers to spend many millions of dollars on clinical studies. Even so, a growing number of manufacturers are sponsoring controlled clinical studies, not only to demonstrate that their products are safe and effective, but perhaps to give them a competitive edge in a burgeoning market.

Although an increasing number of companies are subjecting their nutraceutical products to clinical testing, there is no uniform database that a consumer can use to compare results. The American Nutraceutical Association is in the process of creating such a database, and results will be posted periodically on the ANA web site (www.ANA-JANA.org). In the meantime, the ANA has compiled the following list of brand-name products that have passed clinical evaluation, with the results either published in a peer-reviewed scientific journal or reported at a recognized scientific gathering.

It should be stressed that omission from the list does not necessarily mean that a product has not been tested clinically; the ANA is still in the process of reviewing hundreds of clinical studies and the list will be updated in future printings of this book as well as posted on the ANA web site. Additionally, inclusion in the following list does not imply endorsement by the ANA.

Brand Name Products

The following are grouped according to medical indication. Each brand name is followed by the manufacturer's name in parenthesis; in some cases, the major active ingredients are also listed.

Allergies

Eclectic Institute Stinging Nettles (Eclectic Institute Inc.)

Cancer Support

Propax (shown to counter chemotherapy side effects; Nutritional Therapeutics Inc.)

SelGuard (In vitro studies shows enhanced chemotherapeutic effect when taken with Taxol and Doxorubicin; contains selenium; VIVA Life Science)

Cardiovascular Health/Circulation

CoEnzyme Q10 (VITALINE Formulas)

HeartBar (L-arginine, Cooke Pharan Inc.)

HeartCare (hawthorn extract; Nature's Way)

Kwai (also shown to lower cholesterol; garlic; Lichtwer Pharma U.S., Inc.)

L-Carnitine USP (also improves muscle function; VITALINE Formulas)

SynX Bar (Shaman Pharmaceuticals)

Rusperin C (butcher's broom extract, hesperidin methyl chalcone plus vitamin C; Technical Sourcing International)

Q-Gel (coenzyme Q10; Tishcon Corp.)

Cervical dysplasia (CIN)

Ilndol-3-Carbinol (Designed Nutritional Products, Inc/Theranaturals, Inc.)

Cholesterol Lowering

Benecol Spread (plant stanol esters; McNeil Consumer Heathcare Inc.)

Cholestin (red rice yeast; Pharmanex)

DailyGuard (helps maintain high levels of HDL cholesterol; VIVA Life Science)

Gugulipid (Sabinsa Corp.)

Glucomannan (also for weight loss; (Hankintatukku Natural Health Products Co.)

LipoGuard (concentrated fish oils {omega-3 fatty acids}, garlic, and other nutrients; VIVA Life Science)

Colds/Sore Throats

Echinacea Plus (Traditional Medicinals)

Esberitox (Enzymatic Therapy)

SamBucol (black elderberry; Nature's Way/Razei Bar Industries of Israel)

Throat Coat Tea (slippery elm; Traditional Medicials)

Constipation

Metamucil (psyllium; Procter & Gamble Inc.)

Milk of Magnesia-Cascara (*Cascara sagrula*; Pharmaceutical Associates; Roxane)

Depression (mild)

Kira (St. John's wort; Lichtwer Pharma U.S., Inc.)

Perika (St. John's wort; Nature's Way)

Quanterra Emotional Balance (St. John's wort; Warner Lambert Inc.)

Diabetes

Chromax (chromium picolonate; Nutrition 21; AMBI Nutrition Company)

Diarrhea

Normal Stool Formula (Shaman)

Digestive Disorders

Iberogast (shown to help prevent GI side effects of certain medications; Enzymatic Therapy)

Cynara-SL (artichoke extract; Lichtwere Pharma U.S., Inc.)

Hypertension

Cardia Salt (potassium and magnesium salt; Nutrition 21)

Immune Support

ACKYROL (Scandinavian Natural Health & Beauty Products, Inc.)

EchinaGuard (echinacea; Nature's Way)

Echinacea Herb (Pharmative)

Grifon-Pro (beta-1,3/1,6 glucan from maitake mushroom fraction D extract; Maitake Products Inc.)

JuicePlus (carotenoids; NSA)

Manapol (aloe extract; Caraloe Inc, subsidiary of Carrington Laboratories)

Moducare Sterinol (beta-sitosterol and beta-sitosterol glucoside; Essential Sterolin Products)

New Life Colostrum (Symbiotics)

Norwegian Beta 1,3/1,6 Glucan (beta glucan; Immunocorp)

Pleuran (beta glucan; Vita Health Labs)

VIVA Shield (antioxidant formula; VIVA Life Science)

Intestinal Inflammation plus Immune Support

Manapol Powder (aloe extract; Caraloe Inc, subsidiary of Carrington Laboratories)

Irritable Bowel Syndrome

Calm Colon (based on formula of 20 Chinese Herbs; Samra Health & Beauty)

Insomnia

Circadian (melatonin; Neurim Pharmaceutical Labs)
Sedonium (valerian; Lichtwer Pharma U.S., Inc.)
QLife Melatonin (Batory AM Inc.)

Liver Disorders

Thisilyn (silymarin/milk-thistle extract; Nature's Way)

Memory/Cognitive Function

Ginkai (ginkgo biloba; Lichtwer Pharma U.S., Inc.)
Ginkgo 5 (Pharmline)
Ginkgold and Gkingo (Nature's Way)
Vinpocetine (periwinkle extract; Intelectol (covex))
Quanterra Mental Sharpness (Warner-Lambert)

Menopausal symptoms

Promensil (red clover extract; Novogen)
Remifemin (black cohosh; Enzymatic Therapy)

Migraine headaches

Migrafew (feverfew extract; Nature's Way)
Migra-Lieve (combination of feverfew, magnesium and riboflavin; Natural Science Corp. of America)

Osteoarthritis

Cosamin DS (Nutramax Laboratories, Inc.)

Glucosamine Sulfate (Phytopharmacia)

SAM-e (S-adenosylmethionine 1,4-butanedisulfonate; Nature Made or General Nutrition Corp.)

Prostate Disorders (Benign)

Masculex (saw palmetto; Enzymatic Therapy)

Permixon (saw palmetto; P.F. Medicaments)

Prostactive (saw palmetto; Nature's Way)

ProstaMed and Saw Palmetto Complex (Enzymatic Therapy)

Rheumatoid arthritis

PhytodolorN (also shown to relieve pain of osteoarthritis; Enzymatic Therapy)

SeaRX/Glycomarine (also shown to improve symptoms of osteoarthritis; extract from New Zealand green lipped mussel; Marine Nutraceutical Corp.)

Weight loss

Natrol's Glucomannan (Natrol Inc.)

Miscellaneous Products

The following are supplements or botanical products have been used in clinical studies and have multiple uses:

Black Cohosh

Reminemin (Schaper & Brummer)

Chaste Tree Berry

Vitex (Nature's Way)

Evening Primrose Oil

Efamol's Pure Evening Primrose Oil (standardized to 9 percent GLA; Efamol)

Fish Oils

ProOmega (Nordic Naturals)

Horse Chestnut

Venestat (Pharmaton Natural Health Products)

Kava

Nature's Way Kava (Nature's Way)

L-Carnitine

Carnitor (L-carnitine; requires MD prescription; Sigma Tau Pharmaceuticals)

Selenium

SelenoExcell (high selenium yeast, Cypress Systems)

Vitamin C

Ester-C (Inter-Cal Corp.)

Selected Bibliography

Reference Works

Blumenthal, M.J., W.T. Busse, A. Goldberg, J. Gruenwald, et al, eds. *The Complete German Commission E Monographs: Therapeutic Guide to Herbal Medicines*. Austin: American Botanical Council/Boston: Integrative Medicine Communications, 1998.

Castleman, M. *The Healing Herbs: The Ultimate Guide to the Curative Power of Nature's Medicines*. New York: Bantam Books, 1995.

Chevallier, A. *The Encyclopedia of Medicinal Plants: A Practical Reference Guide to More Than 550 Key Medicinal Plants and Their Uses*. New York: Dorling Kindersley Publications, 1996.

Crawford, A.M. *The Herbal Menopause Book*. Freedom, CA: The Crossing Press, 1996.

Duke, J.A. *CRC Handbook of Medicinal Herbs*. Boca Raton, FL: CRC Press, 1985.

Duke, J.A. *The Green Pharmacy*. Emmaus, PA.: Rodale Press, 1997.

Food and Nutrition Board Commission on Life Sciences, National Research Council. *Recommended Dietary Allowances, 10th Edition*. Washington, D.C.: National Academy Press, 1989.

Green, J. *The Male Herbal: Health Care for Men and Boys*. Freedom, CA: The Crossing Press, 1991.

Herbert, V., G.J. Subak-Sharpe. *Total Nutrition: The Only Guide You'll Ever Need*. New York: St. Martin's Press, 1995.

Hsu, H.Y., W.G. Preacher. *Chinese Herb Medicine and Therapy, Revised Edition*. Los Angeles: Oriental Healing Arts Institute of USA, 1994.

Lee, W., H. Lee, J.A. Friedrich. *Medicinal Benefits of Mushrooms*. New Canaan, CT: Keats Publishing, 1997.

Lininger, S., J. Wright, S. Austin, D. Brown, A. Gaby eds. *The Natural Pharmacy*. Rocklin, CA: Prima Publishing, 1998.

Mindell, E. *Earl Mindell's Herb Bible*. New York: Simon & Schuster, 1992.

Mowrey, D.B. *The Scientific Validation of Herbal Medicine*. New Canaan, CT: Keats Publishing Inc., 1986.

Murray, M.T. *The Healing Power of Herbs: The Enlightened Person's Guide to the Wonders of Medicinal Plants*. Revised and expanded Second Edition. Rocklin, CA: Prima Publishing, 1995.

Murray, M.T., J.E. Pizzorno. *Encyclopedia of Natural Medicine*. Rocklin, CA: Prima Publishing, 1991.

Ody, P. *The Complete Medicinal Herbal*. New York: Dorling Kindersley Publications, 1993.

PDR for Herbal Medicines, First Edition. Montvale, NJ: Medical Economics Company, 1998.

Schulz, V., R. Hansel, V.E. Tyler. *Rational Phytotherapy: A Physicians' Guide to Herbal Medicine*. Heidelberg: Springer-Verlag, 1998.

Peirce, A. *The American Pharmaceutical Association Practical Guide to Natural Medicines*. New York: William Morrow & Co., 1999.

Shandler. N. *Estrogen: The Natural Way*. New York: Villard, 1998.

Tyler, V.E. *Herbs of Choice: The Therapeutic Use of Phytomedicinals*. Binghamton, NY: Pharmaceutical Products Press/The Haworth Press, 1994.

Tyler, V.E. *The Honest Herbal*. Binghamton, NY: Pharmaceutical Products Press/The Haworth Press, 1993.

Weil, A. *Natural Health, Natural Medicine: A Comprehensive Manual for Wellness and Self-Care*. Boston: Houghton Mifflin Company, 1990.

Weiner, M. *Herbs and Immunity*. San Rafael, CA: Quantam Books, 1990.

Selected Monographs and Articles

Adler, A.J., B.J. Holub. "Effect of garlic and fish oil supplementation on serum lipid and lipoprotein concentrations in hypercholesterolemic men." *American Journal of Clinical Nutrition* 1997; 65:445–50.

Ames, B.N., M.K., Shigenaga, T.M. Hagen. "Oxidants, antioxidants, and the degenerative diseases of aging." *Proceedings of the National Academy of Sciences (USA)* 1993; 90:7915–22.

Anderson, J.W. "Meta-analysis of the effects of soy protein intake on serum lipids." *New England Journal of Medicine* 1995; 333:276–82.

Anonymous. "Herbal Rx: The Promises and Pitfalls." *Consumer Reports*, March 1999: 44–8.

Bassett, I.B., et al. "A comparative study of tea tree oil vs. benzoyl peroxide in the treatment of acne." *Medical Journal of Australia* 1990; 153:455–58.

Bergner, P. "Goldenseal and the common cold." *Medical Herbalism: A Journal for the Clinical Practitioner.* Winter 1996–97.

Bone, K. "Kava: A safe herbal treatment for anxiety." *British Journal of Psychotherapy* 1994; 3:145–53. 2j

Brinker, F. "Inhibition of endocrine function by botanical agents." *Journal of Naturopathic Medicine* 1990; 1:10–18.

Brown, D., A. Gaby, R. Reichert. "Migraine," *Condition-Specific Monograph Series,* Natural Product Research Consultants, 1997.

Collins, A., A. Cerin, G. Coleman et al. "Essential fatty acids in the treatment of premenstrual syndrome." *Obstetrics and Gynecology* 1993; 81:93–98.

Diehm, C. et al. "Comparison of leg compression stocking and oral horse chestnut seed extract therapy in patients with chronic venous insufficiency." *Lancet* 1996; 347, 292–4.

Dorant E., P.A. vander Brandt. "Garlic and its significance for the prevention of cancer in humans: A critical review." *British Journal of Cancer* 1993; 67"474–29.

Elmer, G.W., C.M. Surawicz, L.V. McFarland. "Biotherapeutic agents." *JANA* 1996; 275(11)870–76.

Frankos, V.H., D. J. Brusick, E. M. Johnson, et al. "Safety of Sanguinaria (bloodroot)

extract as used in commercial toothpaste and oral rinse products." *Journal of the Canadian Dental Association* 1990; 56 (supplement 7): 41–47.

Garfinkel, D., M. Laudon, D. Nof et al. "Improvement of sleep quality in elderly people by controlled-release melatonin." *Lancet* 1995; 346:541–44.

Glore, S.R., D. Van Treeck, A. W. Knehans et al. "Soluble fiber and serum lipids: A literature review." *Journal of the American Dietetic Association* 1994; 94:425–36.

Hilton, E., H.D. Isenberg et al. "Ingestion of yogurt containing Lactobacillus acidophilus as prophylaxis for candidal vaginitis." *Annals of Internal Medicine* 1992; 116:353–7.

Hobbs, C. "Overcoming Chronic Fatigue: Traditional Remedies for a Modern Disease," *Veggie Life*, Vol. 5, January 1997.

Hobbs, C. "St. John's Wort (Hypericum Perforatum L.): A Review." *Herbal Gram*, The American Botanical Council, 1996.

Horrobin, D.F., M. Manku, M. Brush et al. "Abnormalities in plasma essential fatty acid levels in women with PMS and nonmalignant breast disease." *Journal of Nutritional Medicine* 1991; 2:2591–64.

Hungerford, D., R. Navarro, T. Hammad. "Use of Nutraceuticals in the Management of Osteoarthritis." *JANA* Spring 2000, 23–27.

Jacques, P. F., L. T. Chylack. "Epidemiologic evidence of a role for the antioxidant vitamins and carotenoids in cataract prevention." *American Journal of Clinical Nutrition* 1991; 53:352S–55S.

Jantti, J., E. Seppala, H. Vapaatalo et al. "Evening primrose oil and olive oil in treatment of rheumatoid arthritis." *Clinical Rheumatology* 1989; 8:238–44.

Kleen, H. J. Payan, J. Allawi, et al. "Treatment of diabetic neuropathy with gamma-linolenic acid." *Diabetes Care* 1993; 16:2–15.

Kleijnen, J., et al. "Garlic, onions, and cardiovascular risk factors: A review of the evidence from human experiments with emphasis on commercially available preparations." *British Journal of Clinical Pharmacology* 1989; 28:535–44.

Kubena, K.S., D.N. McMurray. "Nutrition and the immune system: A review of nutrient-nutrient interactions. *Journal of the American Dietetic Association* 1996: 96(11): 1156–64.

Lynn, B. "Capsaicin: Actions on nociceptive C-fibers and therapeutic potential." *Pain* 1990; 41:61–69.

Mossad, S.B., M.L., Macknin, S. V. Medendorp et al. "Zinc gluconate lozenges for treating the common cold." *Annals of Internal Medicine* 1996; 125:81–88.

Potter, S.M., J. A. Baum, H. Teng et al. "Soy protein and isoflavones: Their effects on blood lipids and bone density in postmenopausal women." *American Journal of Clinical Nutrition* 1998; 68:1375S–79S.

Russel, R.M. "A minimum of 13,500 deaths annually from coronary artery disease could be prevented by increasing folate intake to reduce homocysteine levels." *JANA* 1996; 275:1828–29.

Sauvaire, Y., G. Ribes, J. C. Baccou, et al. "Implication of steroid saponins and sapogenins in the hypocholesterolemic effect of fenugreek." *Lipids* 1991; 26:191–97.

Schelosky, L., et al. "Kava and dopamine antagonism." *Journal of Neurology, Neurosurgery and Psychiatry* 1995; 58(5): 639–40.

Seydel, R. "Herbal Healing for the Seasons of Womanhood." *Co-op Connection Newsletter*, May 2000.

Sobota, A.E. "Inhibition of bacterial adherence by cranberry juice: Potential use for the treatment of urinary tract infections." *Journal of Urology* 1984; 131:1013–16.

Stampfer, M.J., C.H. Hennekens, J.E. Manson, et al. "Vitamin E consumption and the risk of coronary disease in women." *New England Journal of Medicine* 1993; 328:1450–56.

Stansbury, J. "Botanical Therapies for Fibrocystic Breast Disease." *Medical Herbalism: A Journal for the Herbal Practitioner* (available at: http:/www.medherb.com).

Steiner, M., A.H. Khan, D. Holbert, R. I. Lin. "A double-blind crossover study in moderately hypercholesterolemic men that compared the effect of aged garlic extract and placebo administration on blood lipids." *American Journal of Clinical Nutrition* 1996; 64(6): 866–70.

Subhan, Z, I. Hindmarch. "The psychopharmacological effects of Ginkgo biloba extract in normal healthy volunteers." *International Journal of Clinical Pharmacology Research* 1984; 4:89–93.

Warshafsky, S., et al. "Effect of garlic on total serum cholesteorl." *Annals of Internal Medicine* 1993; 119:599–605.

Weil, A. "A New Look at Botanical Medicine." *Whole Earth Review* 64, Fall 1989.

Weil, A. "Boost immunity with mushrooms." *Natural Health*, May–June, 1993.

Winslow, L.C., D. J. Kroll. "Herbs as medicines." *Archives of Internal Medicine* 1998; 158 (9): 2192–99.

Wise, J.A., R.O. Voy. "Nutritional Supplements for Sports: Aids to Exercise Performance and Recovery, *JANA* Spring 2000, 28–33.

Index